LIPPINCOTT

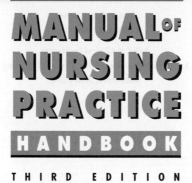

MANUAL OF NURSING PRACTICE HANDBOOK

THIRD EDITION

SANDRA M. NETTINA, MSN, APRN,BC, ANP

Nurse Practitioner
Columbia, Maryland

Adjunct Clinical Instructor
Johns Hopkins University School of Nursing
Baltimore, Maryland

LIPPINCOTT

MANUAL OF NURSING PRACTICE

HANDBOOK

THIRD EDITION

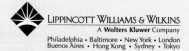

LIPPINCOTT WILLIAMS & WILKINS
A Wolters Kluwer Company

Philadelphia • Baltimore • New York • London
Buenos Aires • Hong Kong • Sydney • Tokyo

STAFF

Executive Publisher
Judith A. Schilling McCann, RN, MSN

Acquisitions Editor
Patricia Casey

Editorial Director
H. Nancy Holmes

Clinical Director
Joan M. Robinson, RN, MSN

Senior Art Director
Arlene Putterman

Editorial Project Manager
Jennifer Lynn Kowalak

Editor
Naina B. Chohan

Copy Editors
Kimberly Bilotta (supervisor),
Tom DeZego, Heather Ditch,
Dona Perkins, Pamela Wingrod

Designers
Lesley Weissman-Cook
(book design),
Lynn Foulk (project manager),
Joseph John Clark

Digital Composition Services
Diane Paluba (manager),
Joyce Rossi Biletz, Donna S. Morris

Manufacturing
Patricia K. Dorshaw (director),
Beth J. Welsh

Editorial Assistants
Megan L. Aldinger, Karen J. Kirk,
Katherine Rothwell, Linda K. Ruhf

Design Assistant
Georg W. Purvis, IV

Indexer
Barbara Hodgson

LMNPHB3011105—050411

**Library of Congress
Cataloging-in-Publication Data**

Nettina, Sandra M.
    Lippincott manual of nursing practice handbook / Sandra M. Nettina. — 3rd ed.
        p. ; cm.
    Rev. ed. of: Lippincott's pocket manual of nursing practice. 2nd ed. c2003.
    Based on: The Lippincott manual of nursing practice. 8th ed. c2006.
    Includes index.
    ISBN-13: 978-1-58255-631-4
    ISBN-10: 1-58255-631-8 (alk. paper)
    1. Nursing—Handbooks, manuals, etc. I. Lippincott Williams & Wilkins. II. Lippincott's pocket manual of nursing practice. III. Lippincott manual of nursing practice. IV. Title. V. Title: Manual of nursing practice handbook.
    [DNLM: 1. Nursing Care—Handbooks. 2. Nursing Assessment—Handbooks. WY 49 N474L 2006]
    RT51.N377 2006
    610.73—dc22   2005022887

CONTENTS

PART ONE

DISEASES AND DISORDERS 1

REVIEWERS

Margaret C. Dirienzo, RN, BSN, CEN
Director Critical Care Services
North Austin (Tex.) Medical Center

Marge Lantz, MS, CCRN, CNRN
Assistant Director Intensive Care/Neuro Intensive
  Care and Neurostepdown Units
Hinsdale (Ill.) Hospital

Laurie Moore, RN, CCRN
Intensive Care Clinical Educator
North Austin (Tex.) Medical Center

Kirk Sinclair, RN, BSN, CEN
Critical Care Educator-Emergency Department
North Austin (Tex.) Medical Center

Keiko L. Torgersen, RNC, BSN, MS
Commander
60th Medical Operations Squadron,
Travis, AFB CA

Susan J. Waltz, RN, MSN
ASN Program Chair, Associate Professor of Nursing
Ivy Tech State College
Columbus, Ind.

Debra Woodard, BSN, MA
Psychiatric Nurse and Health Care Consultant
Sykesville, Md.

Rita K. Young, RN, MSN, CDE
Visiting Instructor
University of Akron (Ohio) College of Nursing

PREFACE

Lippincott Manual of Nursing Practice Handbook, Third Edition, is the perfect resource for your health care information collection. This compact book contains concise yet thorough summaries of both medical and nursing practice information. Like its companion, The *Lippincott Manual of Nursing Practice,* Eighth Edition, the handbook contains comprehensive assessment, treatment, and nursing intervention information for virtually all areas of nursing practice. This is the only handbook covering medical-surgical, pediatric, psychiatric, and maternity conditions.

Like the last edition, conditions and disorders are organized in an alphabetical format for medical-surgical, pediatric, and psychiatric conditions. This allows direct and quick access to information about a particular condition and, in this edition, new alphabetical tabs on the pages speed your search. Maternity conditions are covered in a separate section organized in terms of prenatal care, labor and delivery, postpartum and newborn care, and specific complications of the childbearing experience. Conditions can also be accessed through the Table of Contents as well as the index. The index not only contains major conditions, but also contains important procedures, treatments, medications, signs and symptoms, and referral sources.

Another way to access information is through extensive cross-referencing from one condition to another throughout the book.

The format within each condition contains a description of the condition, assessment, diagnostic evaluation, collaborative management (therapeutic interventions, pharmacologic interventions, surgical interventions), nursing diagnoses, and nursing interventions (monitoring, supportive care, education, and health maintenance). Surgeries are described by their own format, containing a description of the procedure, potential complications, nursing diagnoses, preoperative care, postoperative care, and education and health maintenance. Key points in the text are highlighted by boxed logos identified as Emergency Alert, Drug Alert (new!), Gerontologic Alert, Pediatric Alert, Community Care Considerations, and Alternative Intervention.

Several new features have been added to this edition. Conditions added to the third edition include Severe Acute Respiratory Syndrome (SARS) and Other Emerging Infections, and Anaphylactic Syndrome of Pregnancy. New tables have been added and existing tables have been rewritten and redesigned for readability. A variety of procedures have been added, highlighting steps in nursing care. Each condition has been extensively updated, particularly for treatment information.

I hope you will enjoy *Lippincott Manual of Nursing Practice Handbook*, Third Edition, find it easy to use, and find that it will enhance your nursing practice. As a student or a practicing nurse in any setting, you'll have the information you need at your fingertips.

Sandra M. Nettina, MSN, APRN,BC, ANP

Diseases and Disorders

ABDOMINAL SURGERY

See *Gastrointestinal or Abdominal Surgery.*

ACQUIRED IMMUNODEFICIENCY SYNDROME

See *HIV Disease and AIDS.*

ADD

See *Attention Deficit Disorder and Learning Disabilities.*

ADDISON'S DISEASE

See *Adrenocortical Insufficiency.*

ADRENOCORTICAL INSUFFICIENCY

Adrenocortical insufficiency occurs when the adrenal cortex secretes inadequate amounts of adrenocortical hormones, primarily glucocorticoids and mineralocorticoids. The disorder occurs in two forms in adults and children. Primary adrenocortical insufficiency (Addison's disease) results from destruction and subsequent hypofunction of the adrenal cortex, usually caused by an autoimmune process. Presentation may be insidious or acute. Secondary adrenocortical insufficiency occurs because of adrenocorticotropic hormone (ACTH) deficiency from pituitary disease, or from suppression of the hypothalamic-pituitary axis by corticosteroids administered to treat nonendocrine disorders, which causes the adrenal cortex to atrophy.

Inadequate aldosterone produces disturbances of sodium, potassium, and water metabolism. Cortisol deficiency produces abnormal fat, protein, and carbohydrate metabolism. Absence of cortisol during a period of stress can precipitate addisonian (acute adrenal) crisis, an exaggerated state of adrenal cortical insufficiency, which is fatal if not immediately treated.

Assessment

1. Anorexia, nausea, vomiting, diarrhea, constipation, abdominal pain; craving salty foods
2. Muscular weakness, fatigue, weight loss
3. Hyperpigmentation ("bronzing") of skin caused by melanocyte-stimulating hormone secretion from the pituitary
4. Mental changes, such as depression, irritability, anxiety, and apprehension; behavioral problems in children
5. Hypotension, low basal metabolic rate, increased insulin sensitivity
6. Hyponatremia and hyperkalemia

PEDIATRIC ALERT Neonates with the condition are gravely ill after birth, with tachycardia, tachypnea, fever, cyanosis, cold and clammy skin, and hypotension.

Diagnostic Evaluation

1. Chemistry panel: decreased glucose, decreased sodium, increased potassium.
2. Complete blood count: increased lymphocytes.
3. Low fasting plasma cortisol level; low aldosterone level.
4. 24-hour urine studies show decreased levels of 17-ketosteroids, 17-hydroxycorticoids, and 17-ketogenic steroids.
5. ACTH stimulation test may show no increase in plasma cortisol and urinary 17-ketosteroids.
6. Possibly increased adrenal antibody titers in children.

Collaborative Management

Therapeutic Interventions

1. High-sodium, low-potassium diet and fluids to restore normal fluid and electrolyte balance.
2. Cardiovascular support may be indicated, with cardiac and hemodynamic monitoring, oxygen therapy.
3. Recognition and treatment of underlying cause of addisonian crisis (for example, treatment of infection).

Pharmacologic Interventions

1. Hydrocortisone or prednisone to treat glucocorticoid deficiency

GERONTOLOGIC ALERT Elderly patients and those with chronic obstructive pulmonary disease and heart failure may require preparations with low mineralocorticoid activity (such as methylprednisolone) to prevent fluid retention.

2. Fludrocortisone to treat mineralocorticoid deficiency

DRUG ALERT Mineral corticoid overtreatment may be manifested by hypertension, edema from sodium and water retention, and weakness caused by potassium loss.

3. If addisonian crisis or circulatory collapse is imminent, provide immediate treatment:
    a. I.V. sodium chloride solution
    b. I.V. hydrocortisone
    c. Injection of circulatory stimulants such as atropine, calcium chloride, and epinephrine

Nursing Diagnoses
1, 23, 24, 78, 136

Nursing Interventions
Monitoring
1. Monitor vital signs frequently; a decrease in blood pressure and increase in temperature may suggest an impending addisonian crisis.
2. Monitor serum sodium and potassium levels.
3. Monitor intake and output, daily weight, and edema during corticosteroid therapy.

Supportive Care
1. Encourage high-calorie, high-protein diet rich in sodium and fluid content, if tolerated.
2. Administer or teach self-administration of prescribed glucocorticoids and mineralocorticoids, documenting the response.
3. Administer I.V. infusions of sodium, water, and glucose as indicated.
4. Assess comfort and emotional status of the patient. Minimize stressful situations to avoid risk of adrenal crisis.

5. Protect the patient from infection by using good handwashing technique and avoiding contact with staff and visitors who may be carriers.
6. Assist the patient with activities of daily living if weak and fatigued.
7. Provide periods of rest and activity to avoid overexertion.
8. Maintain constant room temperature and avoid drafts, dampness, or extremes in temperature to prevent addisonian crisis.
9. Report early signs of addisonian crisis (sudden decrease in blood pressure, nausea and vomiting, high temperature).

Education and Health Maintenance

1. Instruct about the need for lifelong therapy and follow-up.
   a. Emphasize the importance of not missing a dose and of taking more hormones when under stress. Dose may be doubled for minor illness or tripled for an illness keeping patient home from school or work. An injection of hydrocortisone may be needed for trauma, surgery, severe fatigue, and other highly stressful situations.
   b. Suggest that the patient carry an identification card indicating medication being taken and health care provider's telephone number.
2. Teach I.M. injection technique as indicated.
3. Advise the patient that excessive long-term use of corticosteroids may cause such adverse effects as fluid overload, osteoporosis, pathologic fractures, hyperglycemia, masking of signs of infection, poor tissue regeneration and growth, peptic ulcer, and psychosis.

PEDIATRIC ALERT In children, weight gain and poor growth may occur with long-term corticosteroid therapy.

4. Identify factors that may precipitate addisonian crisis (infection, extremes of temperature, trauma) and that additional corticosteroids may be necessary.

AIDS

See *HIV Disease and AIDS*.

ALDOSTERONISM, PRIMARY

Primary aldosteronism refers to excessive secretion of aldosterone by the adrenal cortex, which is usually caused by a cortical adenoma (tumor) or bilateral adrenal hyperplasia. Hyperaldosteronism, in turn, causes excessive sodium and water retention and excessive potassium excretion by the kidneys and GI tract. A secondary form of the disease occurs in conjunction with heart failure, renal dysfunction, or cirrhosis of the liver. One to 2 percent of cases of hypertension are caused by primary aldosteronism, which can be treated by adrenalectomy.

Seventy percent of patients with aldosterone-secreting adenomas are women, and the incidence of primary aldosteronism is four times higher among blacks than among the general population. Complications include the long-term effects of untreated hypertension — stroke, renal failure, and heart failure.

Assessment
1. Excessive thirst (polydipsia) caused by hypernatremia
2. Muscle weakness caused by hypokalemia
3. Possible paresthesias, tetany, and polyuria caused by alkalosis
4. Hypertension

Diagnostic Evaluation
1. Suspect primary aldosteronism in all hypertensive patients with spontaneous hypokalemia; also suspect it if hypokalemia develops concurrently with start of diuretics and remains after diuretics are discontinued.
2. Salt-loading screening test — ingestion of at least 200 mEq per day (approximately 12 g salt) for 4 days will depress serum potassium to less than 3.5 mEq/L in a patient with aldosteronism. No effect is seen if aldosteronism is absent.
3. CT scanning to determine and localize cortical adenoma.

Collaborative Management
Pharmacologic Interventions

1. Spironolactone, a potassium-sparing diuretic to treat both hypertension and potassium depletion; used as long-term therapy for bilateral adrenal hyperplasia, or short-term therapy until adrenalectomy is successful for cortical adenoma.
   a. Therapy is needed 4 to 6 weeks before the full effect on blood pressure is seen.
   b. Adverse effects include reduced testosterone in men or boys (decreased libido, impotence, gynecomastia) and GI discomfort. Amiloride may be given instead in sexually active men or in cases of GI intolerance.
   c. Restrict sodium: Avoid saline infusions, give low-sodium diet.
   d. Give potassium supplement if indicated by severity of hypokalemia.
2. Antihypertensive agent such as thiazide diuretic may be needed.
3. Management of underlying cause of secondary aldosteronism (heart, kidney, or liver disease).

Surgical Interventions

1. Unilateral adrenalectomy may be done to remove adrenal tumor.

Nursing Diagnoses
24, 42, 78, 136

Nursing Interventions
Also see *Gastrointestinal or Abdominal Surgery*, page 381.

Monitoring

1. Monitor fluid intake and output and daily to weekly weights.
2. Monitor serum potassium and observe for electrocardiogram changes (sagging ST segment and low T wave) caused by hypokalemia.
3. Monitor blood pressure.

4. Monitor for complications of adrenalectomy (hemorrhage, adrenal crisis).
5. After adrenalectomy, monitor serum sodium, potassium, and glucose; report abnormalities.
   a. Sodium and potassium may normalize, or potassium may become elevated (because of transient adrenal insufficiency after surgery).
   b. Electrolyte imbalances may persist for 4 to 18 months after surgery.
   c. Hypertension may persist for 3 to 6 months after surgery.
   d. Temporary corticosteroid treatment causes glucose level to increase and worsens control in diabetics; may require additional treatment.

Supportive Care

1. Provide low-sodium diet and potassium supplements as ordered and teach patient to carry out these measures.
2. Administer or teach self-administration of antihypertensives as ordered.
3. Assess for dependent edema; encourage activity, frequent repositioning, and elevation of feet periodically to reduce edema.
4. Prepare the adrenal surgery patient by reinforcing explanation of procedure given by health care provider; describe nursing care.
5. Advise about the need for frequent blood pressure checks and glucocorticoid infusions before and after surgery to cover period of stress (surgery), because one adrenal gland is removed and it will take time for the remaining gland to compensate.
6. Perform usual postoperative care for abdominal surgery, including frequent check of vital signs, assessing for hemorrhage, turning, coughing and deep breathing, early ambulation, slow progression of diet when bowel sounds return, and control of pain with scheduled opioid administration or patient-controlled analgesia.
7. Administer hydrocortisone I.V. as ordered.
8. Maintain nonstressful environment, promote rest, and provide meticulous care to protect the patient against in-

fection and other complications that could cause adrenal crisis.

Education and Health Maintenance

1. Instruct the patient regarding the nature of illness, the necessary treatment, and the need for continued medical care.
2. Instruct the patient on the importance of following prescribed medical treatments.
   a. The patient must remain on spironolactone for life. Advise on reporting significant adverse effects and if drug interferes with sexual performance and quality of life.
   b. Advise the patient that glucocorticoid administration may be temporary (after subtotal or unilateral adrenalectomy) or long term (for bilateral adrenalectomy); dose may need to be increased during times of illness or stress.
3. Teach the patient and family members how to take blood pressure readings, if indicated.

ALS

See *Amyotrophic Lateral Sclerosis*.

ALZHEIMER'S DISEASE

Alzheimer's disease is a degenerative disorder of the cerebral cortex characterized by dementia with progressive impairment of memory, cognitive function, language, and self-care ability. Although there is no known cause, genetics and female gender are thought to be risk factors. Several chromosomes have been identified in early- and late-onset Alzheimer's disease. Viruses, environmental toxins, silent brain infarcts, and previous head injury may also play a role. Profound structural changes in brain tissue (amyloid deposition, granulovascular degeneration, and neurofibrillary tangles) along with neurotransmitter impairment are known to occur. Complications include infection, injury, and malnutrition.

A

Assessment

1. Early signs are difficulty with planning meals, managing finances, using the telephone, or driving without getting lost. Personality changes such as irritability, suspiciousness, neglect of appearance, and disorientation to time and space may also occur.
2. The middle stage may bring repetitive actions, nocturnal restlessness, apraxia (inability to perform purposeful activity), aphasia, and agraphia (inability to write).
3. Further disease progression brings frontal lobe dysfunction with loss of spontaneity and social inhibitions, delusions and hallucinations, aggression, and wandering.
4. Advanced Alzheimer's disease results in urinary and fecal incontinence, emaciation, increased irritability, and, possibly, unresponsiveness and coma.

Diagnostic Evaluation

1. Laboratory testing such as blood chemistry, thyroid function tests, and urinalysis to rule out metabolic disorders
2. Imaging studies such as MRI and CT scan of the brain to rule out treatable forms of dementia
3. Neuropsychological evaluation to establish clinical criteria for diagnosis
4. Assay for cerebrospinal fluid (protein and beta amyloid and genetic testing are available but not ready for widespread use)

Collaborative Management
Therapeutic Interventions

1. Environmental control to provide structure and routine that the patient can cope with; goal is to maximize function and improve quality of life

Pharmacologic Interventions

1. Anxiolytics and antipsychotics control behavioral disturbances; antidepressants treat depressive symptoms.
2. Cholinesterase inhibitors such as donepezil and galantamine improve cognitive functioning and quality of life for some patients.

    a. May cause elevation of liver enzymes; monitor liver function tests frequently.

    b. Possible drug interactions in this class include theophylline, cimetidine, anticholinergics, and nonsteroidal anti-inflammatory drugs (NSAIDs).

3. Research with estrogen, NSAIDs, and botanical agents has not proved consistent effectiveness. Memantine is currently under study.

ALTERNATIVE INTERVENTION

Ginkgo biloba is an herbal preparation that has shown some promise in memory impairment or dementia in several studies; however, its benefits are unproven and it interacts with antiplatelet agents such as aspirin and warfarin. Vitamin E has not proven to be of benefit in Alzheimer's disease.

Nursing Diagnoses
8, 10, 34, 35, 36, 45, 136, 162

Nursing Interventions
Monitoring

1. Watch for signs and symptoms of respiratory and urinary tract infections. Sudden worsening of cognitive status may be the only symptom of infection.

2. Monitor fluid and food intake to check for malnutrition or imbalances caused by inattention to mealtime and hunger or lack of ability to prepare meals. Monitor intake and output, and weigh patient weekly.

3. Inspect the skin for evidence of injury attributable to lack of insight, hallucinations, and confusion.

4. Monitor neurologic function, including emotional and mental states and motor capabilities, for changes indicating further deterioration.

5. Monitor response to antipsychotic medications.

Supportive Care

1. Simplify the patient's environment.

    a. Reduce noise levels.

   b. Provide a structured routine to reduce the number of choices available to the patient. Use pictures to identify daily activities.
   c. Maintain consistency in interactions, and introduce new people slowly.
2. Protect the patient from accidents.
   a. Try to avoid using restraints, but keep the patient under observation as needed.
   b. Provide adequate lighting to help the patient interpret environment.
   c. Remove unneeded furniture and other obstacles from the room to reduce risk of falling.
   d. Make sure patient's shoes or slippers are easy to put on and to remove.
3. Provide the patient with an identification tag or medical alert bracelet.

COMMUNITY CARE CONSIDERATIONS

Remind family members of possible dangers around the house as patient becomes less responsible for behavior. Encourage them to reduce the temperature of hot water heater, to remove dials from the stove and other electrical appliances, to remove matches and lighters, and to store away tools and other potentially dangerous items.

4. If possible, help the patient maintain a level of social interaction.
   a. Instruct the family that their presence is helpful even though actual interaction with the patient may be limited.
   b. Encourage the family to interact at a level appropriate to the patient. Ask them to bring in objects from home that are meaningful to the patient.
5. Ensure adequate rest, alternating with periods of exercise to expend energy.
6. Maintain usual sleep habits and bedtime rituals, including changing into pajamas, consuming a bedtime snack

or warm decaffeinated beverage, listening to music, or engaging in prayer.

7. Provide familiar foods that are high in calories and fiber in small, frequent meals. Include finger foods and adequate fluids.

8. Make sure that dentures fit well and that dental care is maintained.

9. Provide support to the caregivers, encouraging them to take care of their own health needs and to use community resources to prevent caregiver burnout.

Education and Health Maintenance

1. Advise caregiver to encourage activities that provide physical exercise and repetitive movement but take little thought, such as dancing, painting, doing laundry, or vacuuming.

COMMUNITY CARE CONSIDERATIONS

Agitation and wandering can be managed at home by using soft background music or white noise, having the patient wear a wander alarm, and providing repetitive stimulation such as music or rocking.

2. Teach about the need to eliminate stimulants (such as caffeine) from the diet.

3. Discuss the need to organize finances and make advance directive decisions and guardianship arrangements (while the patient is still able) to allow patient to participate in the process.

4. For additional information, refer to agencies such as Alzheimer's Association, *www.alz.org*.

AMNESIC DISORDER

See *Delirium, Dementia, and Amnesic Disorder.*

AMPUTATION

Amputation is the total or partial surgical removal of an extremity or digit. It is done in cases of inadequate tissue perfusion not responsive to other treatments, such as with diabetes mellitus or other peripheral vascular diseases; severe trauma; malignant tumor; or congenital deformity. The extent of amputation is based on the level of maximal viable tissue available for wound healing.

In a closed amputation, the stump is covered by a flap of skin sutured posteriorly; this is the most common procedure. Open (guillotine) amputation is used in emergencies, such as in severe infection and in patients who are poor surgical risks; the wound heals by granulation or secondary closure in approximately a week. Dressings may be either soft or rigid. Soft dressings permit wound inspection and are used primarily in patients who should avoid early weight-bearing (eg, those with peripheral vascular disease). Rigid dressings shape the residual limb, reduce edema, and allow early ambulation and attachment of a prosthesis.

Potential Complications

1. Infection, sepsis
2. Hematoma, necrosis
3. Unrelieved phantom pain
4. Delayed healing of residual limb

Nursing Diagnoses

3, 62, 78, 88, 123

Collaborative Interventions

Preoperative Care

1. Hemodynamic evaluation is performed through testing, such as angiography or arterial blood flow xenon-133 scan, to determine optimal amputation level.
2. Culture and sensitivity tests of draining wounds are done to assist with infection control preoperatively.
3. Evaluation of contralateral extremity is performed to determine functional postoperative potential.
4. Evaluation of cardiovascular, respiratory, renal, and other body systems is needed to determine the patient's preoperative condition, thereby reducing the risks of surgery by optimizing function of these systems.

GERONTOLOGIC ALERT Amputation of the lower extremity can be a life-threatening procedure, especially in patients older than age 60 with peripheral vascular disease. In such patients, significant morbidity accompanies above-knee amputations because of associated poor health and disease as well as the complications of sepsis and malnutrition and the physiologic insult of amputation.

5. Nutritional status is evaluated; supplemental protein may be added to enhance wound healing.
6. Exercises are taught to patients who are about to undergo a lower-limb amputation to strengthen upper-extremity muscles for use of ambulatory aids.
7. The patient is familiarized with ambulatory aids to instill self-confidence and prepare for postoperative mobility.

Postoperative Care

1. Monitor for signs of excessive blood loss: hypotension, widening pulse pressure, tachycardia, diaphoresis, restlessness, decreased alertness.
2. Watch for excessive wound drainage.
   a. Keep tourniquet ready to apply to residual limb if excessive bleeding occurs.
   b. Reinforce dressing as required, using aseptic technique.
   c. Maintain accurate record of bloody drainage on dressing and in drainage system.
3. Monitor intake and output for fluid balance.
4. Elevate residual limb to promote venous return.
5. Maintain pressure dressing; reapply if necessary, using sterile dressing secured with elastic bandage.
6. Notify surgeon if rigid cast dressing comes off.
7. Control surgical pain with opioids as prescribed, and use other techniques such as distraction, progressive muscle relaxation, and imagery.
8. Recognize that increasing discomfort may indicate presence of hematoma, infection, or necrosis.
9. Use physical modalities (eg, wrapping, temperature changes) and transcutaneous electrical nerve stimulation, if prescribed, to relieve phantom limb pain; encourage patient activity to decrease awareness of pain.

10. Reassure patient that phantom limb pain will diminish over time.

A

11. Support patient through psychological acceptance of body image change. Expect anger, denial, withdrawal, and depression. Obtain psychological referral and use such resources as a social worker, the clergy, family, and friends to help strengthen patient's coping skills.

12. Encourage participation in rehabilitation planning and self-care.

13. Teach the patient to avoid long periods in bed in one position, to prevent dependent edema, flexion deformity, and skin pressure areas.

    a. Lower-extremity amputations — hip flexion contracture (avoid placing residual limb on pillow; encourage prone position twice a day) and abduction deformity (use trochanter roll; avoid pillow between legs)

    b. Upper-extremity amputations — postural abnormalities (encourage good posture)

14. Encourage active range-of-motion exercises and muscle-strengthening exercises when prescribed, to minimize atrophy, increase muscle strength, and prepare residual limb for prosthesis.

15. Promote reestablishment of balance (amputation alters distribution of body weight).

    a. Transfer the patient to a chair within 48 hours of surgery.

    b. Instruct and guard lower-limb amputee during balance exercises.

    c. Support plan developed by physical therapist.

GERONTOLOGIC ALERT Diabetes mellitus, heart disease, infection, stroke, chronic obstructive pulmonary disease, peripheral vascular disease, and increasing age are factors that may limit rehabilitation.

Education and Health Maintenance

1. Teach the patient and family how to wrap residual limb with elastic bandage to control edema and to form a firm conical shape for prosthesis fitting.

2. Teach the patient residual limb conditioning:

    a. Push the residual limb against a soft pillow.

    b. Gradually push residual limb against harder surfaces.

    c. Massage healed residual limb to soften scar, decrease tenderness, and improve vascularity.

3. Instruct the patient to wash and dry limb thoroughly at least twice per day (removing all soap residue), to prevent skin irritation and infection. Also, teach the patient to avoid soaking residual limb because this results in edema.

4. Inspect residual limb and skin under prosthesis harness daily for pressure, irritation, and actual skin breakdown.

5. Have patient wear residual limb sock or cotton underwear to absorb perspiration and to avoid direct contact between prosthetic socket or harness and skin. Avoid wrinkles in residual limb sock to prevent potential pressure areas.

6. Wipe the socket of prosthesis with a damp cloth when prosthesis is removed for evening.

7. Have prosthesis checked periodically.

8. Teach the patient to protect the remaining extremity from injury and to secure prompt treatment of problems.

AMYOTROPHIC LATERAL SCLEROSIS

Amyotrophic lateral sclerosis (ALS), also known as *Lou Gehrig disease,* is an incapacitating disease of unknown cause that results from degeneration of upper and lower motor neurons or of the cerebral cortex, brain stem, and spinal cord. This causes progressive loss of voluntary muscle contraction and functional capacity, accompanied by other lower motor neuron signs such as atrophy or fasciculations. ALS usually affects men between ages 40 and 70. It is invariably fatal, usually within 2 to 5 years of diagnosis; death usually results from a complication such as respiratory failure, aspiration pneumonia, or cardiopulmonary arrest.

Assessment

1. Progressive weakness and wasting of muscles of arms, trunk, and legs

2. Muscle fasciculations and spasticity

TABLE A-1	Cranial Nerve Function

A

CRANIAL NERVE	FUNCTION
I Olfactory	▪ Sense of smell
II Optic	▪ Visual acuity, visual fields
III Oculomotor IV Trochlear VI Abducens	▪ Together control extraocular muscles ▪ Oculomotor, also controls pupil constriction
V Trigeminal	▪ Motor—strength of jaw, corneal reflex ▪ Sensory—light touch and pain of face
VII Facial	▪ Symmetry and strength of facial movements
VIII Acoustic	▪ Cochlear branch—hearing ▪ Vestibular branch—equilibrium
IX Glossopharyngeal X Vagus	▪ Motor-pharyngeal movement (gag reflex, movement of uvula and palate)
XI Spinal Accessory	▪ Strength of sternocleidomastoid and trapezius muscles (turning head, shrugging shoulders)
XII Hypoglossal	▪ Movement of tongue

3. Tachypnea, hypopnea, restlessness, poor sleep, and excessive fatigue caused by hypoxia from respiratory weakness
4. Cranial nerve dysfunction, particularly gag reflex and swallowing difficulty, as well as nasal and unintelligible speech (see *Table A-1*)

Diagnostic Evaluation

1. Laboratory testing, such as creatine kinase, heavy metal screen, thyroid function tests, and cerebrospinal fluid evaluation, to rule out other disorders
2. Pulmonary function testing to evaluate respiratory status
3. Barium swallow to evaluate ability to control swallowing
4. Brain imaging such as MRI and CT scanning to rule out other disorders
5. Electromyography to evaluate denervation and muscle atrophy; nerve conduction testing to evaluate nerve pathways

Collaborative Management
Therapeutic Interventions

1. Enteral nutrition through gastrostomy or jejunostomy tube when high risk for aspiration develops
2. Intubation, tracheostomy, and mechanical ventilation when indicated for respiratory failure

Pharmacologic Interventions

1. Antispasticity drugs such as baclofen and diazepam
2. Antidepressants and sleep aids as needed
3. Riluzole (first drug to be approved by the U.S. Food and Drug Administration for ALS); however, effects are limited

Nursing Diagnoses
51, 62, 75, 135, 159

Nursing Interventions
Monitoring

1. Monitor respiratory rate, depth, and tidal volume frequently. Document pattern and report any decrease below patient's baseline.
2. Monitor for drooling or regurgitation of fluids through nose, which indicates deteriorating swallowing ability.
3. Monitor for fever and tachycardia and obtain sputum, urine, and other cultures as indicated to evaluate for infection.

4. Because standard call lights cannot be activated by the severely disabled ALS patient, arrange for constant monitoring and surveillance to meet patient needs.

A

Supportive Care

1. Position the patient upright, suction the upper airway, and perform chest physical therapy as tolerated to enhance respiratory function.
2. Encourage use of an incentive spirometer to exercise respiratory muscles.
3. Establish the patient's wishes regarding life support measures; obtain a copy of advance directives for chart, if applicable.
4. Provide meticulous care to patient with artificial airway to prevent infection.
5. Encourage the patient to continue usual activities as long as possible, but alternate with rest periods to avoid fatigue.
6. Encourage physical therapy exercises to strengthen unaffected muscles and carry out range-of-motion exercises to prevent contractures.
7. Obtain assistive devices as needed to help patient maintain independence, such as special feeding devices, remote controls, and a motorized wheelchair.
8. Provide high-calorie, small, frequent feedings to patient who can still swallow.
   a. Semisolids are usually easiest to swallow.
   b. Position patient upright for meals with neck flexed to protect the airway.
   c. Instruct the patient to take a breath before swallowing, hold breath to swallow, exhale or cough after swallowing, and swallow again.
9. Examine the oral cavity before and after swallowing and provide frequent mouth care.
10. Encourage rest periods before meals to alleviate muscle fatigue.
11. Remember that the patient with ALS maintains full alertness, sensory function, and intelligence. Try to spend time with the patient and let him know that you recognize this.

Use mechanical speech aids or communication board when needed. Eye movements/blinking may be the last voluntary movement; develop a code system to serve as a communication method. Be aware that patients with locked-in syndrome remain fully aware despite their inability to respond.

Education and Health Maintenance

1. Stress the importance of maintaining physical exercise; discourage bed rest to prevent pulmonary stasis.
2. Review with the patient and family proper eating mechanics to avoid fatigue and aspiration of food.
3. Inform the patient of right to make decisions regarding advance directives, and provide palliative care referrals as required.
4. Encourage the family to seek support and respite care.
5. Remind the family that the patient with ALS maintains full alertness, sensory function, and intelligence. Encourage them to maintain interaction, socialization, and stimulation and to explore using emerging technology such as mind-activated, computer-driven communication devices.
6. Refer the family for counseling as needed and to supportive agencies such as The Amyotrophic Lateral Sclerosis Association, *www.alsa.org*.

ANAPHYLAXIS

Anaphylaxis is an immediate, life-threatening systemic reaction that occurs on exposure to a particular substance. It results from a type I hypersensitivity reaction in which release of chemical mediators from mast cells results in massive vasodilation, increased capillary permeability, bronchoconstriction, and decreased peristalsis. Anaphylaxis may be caused by immunotherapy, skin testing, medications, contrast media infusion, insect stings, certain foods, or exercise. Prompt identification of signs and symptoms and immediate intervention are essential; the more quickly a reaction occurs, the more severe it tends to be. Complications include cardiovascular collapse and respiratory failure.

EMERGENCY ALERT With immunotherapy (allergy shots), the risk of systemic reaction is always present. Skin testing can also cause systemic reactions. Make sure that epinephrine 1:1,000 (with syringe and tourniquet) is available during these procedures, and observe the patient for at least 30 minutes after administration.

Assessment

1. Immediately assess airway, breathing, and circulation if presentation is severe, and intervene with cardiopulmonary resuscitation as appropriate.
2. If presentation is less severe, assess vital signs, degree of respiratory distress, and presence of angioedema.
3. Signs and symptoms include:
   a. Urticaria (hives), angioedema, pruritus, flushing
   b. Laryngeal edema, bronchospasm, cough, wheezing, feeling of lump in throat
   c. Hypotension, tachycardia, palpitations, syncope
   d. Nausea, vomiting, diarrhea, abdominal pain, bloating

DRUG ALERT Before administering any medication, ask patient if he or she has ever had a reaction to it. Do not rely on the chart alone.

Diagnostic Evaluation

None necessary; diagnosis is made by clinical presentation.

Collaborative Management

Therapeutic and Pharmacologic Interventions

1. Immediate treatment should include application of a tourniquet above site of antigen injection (allergy injection, insect sting) or skin test site, to slow the absorption of antigen into the system.
2. Epinephrine 0.1 to 0.5 mg (0.01 mg/kg) is injected into opposite arm subcutaneously (S.C.) or I.M. May repeat every 15 to 20 minutes, if necessary, to cause vasoconstriction, decrease capillary permeability, relax airway smooth muscle, and inhibit mast cell mediator release.
3. Subsequently, an adequate airway is established and hypotension and shock are treated with fluids and vasopressors.

4. Bronchodilators are given to relax bronchial smooth muscle.
5. Antihistamines, such as diphenhydramine and, possibly, H_2-histamine blockers, such as ranitidine, may be given to block the effects of histamine.
6. Corticosteroids are given to decrease vascular permeability and diminish the migration of inflammatory cells; may be helpful in preventing late-phase responses.

Nursing Diagnoses
6, 19, 24, 75

Nursing Interventions
Monitoring
1. Continually monitor respiratory rate and depth and breath sounds for respiratory effort and effectiveness of ventilation.
2. Monitor blood pressure using continuous automatic cuff.
3. Monitor central venous pressure to ensure adequate fluid volume and to prevent fluid overload.
4. Insert indwelling catheter and monitor urine output hourly to ensure kidney perfusion.

Supportive Care
1. Establish and maintain an adequate patent airway. If epinephrine has not stabilized bronchospasm, assist with endotracheal intubation, emergency tracheostomy, or cricothyroidotomy as indicated.
2. Administer nebulized epinephrine and/or other bronchodilators, as ordered. Monitor heart rate (increased with bronchodilators).
3. Provide oxygen by nasal cannula at 2 to 5 L/minute or by alternate means, as ordered.
4. Rapidly infuse I.V. fluids to fill vasodilated circulatory system and raise blood pressure. Titrate vasopressors based on blood pressure response.
5. Remain responsive to the patient, who may remain alert but not completely coherent because of hypotension, hypoxemia, and effects of medication.

A

6. When the patient is stable and alert, give a concise explanation of anaphylaxis and the treatment that was given.
7. Keep family and significant others informed of the patient's condition and the treatment being given.

ALTERNATIVE INTERVENTION

Warn people who are allergic to ragweed, chrysanthemums, marigolds, daisies, and other members of the Asteraceae plant family that they may have a severe allergic reaction to certain herbal products, such as chamomile, milk thistle, echinacea, and feverfew. Combination supplements and remedies should be avoided if ingredients are not clearly identified.

Education and Health Maintenance

1. Instruct the patient to read labels and be familiar with the scientific name of the drug thought to cause a reaction.
2. Advise patient to discard all unused drugs. Make sure any drug kept in the medicine cabinet is clearly labeled.
3. Help the patient become familiar with drugs that may cross-react with the allergen.
4. Advise extreme care about diet if patient has known sensitivity to a food product—allergic compounds (such as caseinate or lactalbumin) are often hidden in a preparation.
5. Teach the patient at risk for anaphylaxis about the potential seriousness of these reactions.
6. Educate patients to recognize the early signs and symptoms of anaphylaxis.
7. Instruct a patient allergic to bee stings to avoid wearing brightly colored or black clothes, perfumes, and hair spray. Shoes should be worn at all times.
8. For exercise-induced anaphylaxis, patients should exercise in moderation, preferably with another person, and in a controlled setting where assistance is readily available.

9. If food is associated with exercise-induced anaphylaxis, instruct patient to wait at least 2 hours after eating before exercising.

10. Instruct the patient to wear a medical alert bracelet or tag at all times.

COMMUNITY CARE CONSIDERATIONS

Instruct the patient in self-injection of epinephrine (Epi-Pen) and to carry it at all times. Explain the importance of prompt administration at the first sign of a systemic reaction, and advise person to follow up with a visit to the health care provider or emergency facility as response warrants. Check medication periodically to make sure it has not expired.

ANEMIA, IRON DEFICIENCY AND OTHER TYPES

Iron deficiency anemia is a condition in which total body iron content is inadequate for optimal development of red blood cells (RBCs). The defective RBCs are fewer in number and have lower hemoglobin content. This reduces the blood's ability to deliver sufficient oxygen to the tissues.

Iron deficiency anemia is the most common type of anemia in all age-groups and results from one or more causes: 1) chronic blood loss; 2) iron malabsorption, as in small-bowel disease or gastroenterostomy; 3) increased iron requirement, as in pregnancy or periods of rapid growth; or 4) insufficient intake caused by inadequate diet or weight loss. The disease primarily occurs in premenopausal women, children in rapid growth spurts, and pregnant women. Without treatment, advanced disease may cause growth retardation in children, heart failure, and ischemic organ damage such as myocardial infarction or stroke.

Other major types of anemia include pernicious anemia, folic acid deficiency anemia, aplastic anemia, and thalassemia major. (See *Table A-2*.)

TABLE A-2 Other Important Anemias

TYPE AND CAUSES	FEATURES	TREATMENT
Pernicious Anemia Vitamin B_{12} deficiency from small-bowel disease, gastric resection, or genetic cause	• GI symptoms and neuropathy. Increased mean corpuscular volume (MCV), Schilling test is positive	• Monthly parenteral replacement with cyanocobalamin (B_{12})
Folic Acid Deficiency Dietary deficiency, alcoholism, jejunal malabsorption, pregnancy, and some medications	• Implicated in congenitally acquired neural tube defect • Folate level is decreased, and MCV is increased	• Oral folic acid replacement and diet • Treatment of underlying cause
Aplastic Anemia Bone marrow hypoplasia resulting in pancytopenia (insufficient numbers of red blood cells (RBCs), white blood cells, and platelets). May be idiopathic or caused by exposure to chemical toxins, radiation, viral infections, certain drugs (chloramphenicol), or may be congenital.	• In addition to anemia, causes increased risk of overwhelming infection due to neutropenia, and gross and occult bleeding due to thrombocytopenia. • Course is variable, if severe, is usually fatal.	• Removal of causative agent or toxin • Allogeneic bone marrow transplantation (BMT) in severe cases • Immunosuppressants, bone marrow stimulating factors, and care: supportive platelet and RBC transfusions, antibiotics, monitoring *(continued)*

Other Important Anemias *(continued)*

TYPE AND CAUSES	FEATURES	TREATMENT
Thalassemia Major (Cooley's anemia) A genetic microcytic, hemolytic anemia most commonly seen in people of Mediterranean descent. The heterozygous form, beta-thalassemia minor, does not cause the severe manifestations.	■ In addition to anemia, causes skeletal deformities, growth failure, heart failure, hepatosplenomegaly, and hemosiderosis (deposition of iron in skin and organs). ■ RBC indices indicate low MCV and mean corpuscular hemoglobin concentration	■ Frequent transfusions of packed RBCs for hemoglobin less than 10 ■ Iron chelation therapy with deferoxamine to decrease iron effects on body ■ Splenectomy (possible), BMT

GERONTOLOGIC ALERT The elderly person who may be consuming a soft diet because of dental problems is also at risk for iron deficiency anemia.

Assessment
1. Headache, dizziness, tinnitus, fatigue
2. Tachycardia, palpitations, chest pain
3. Dyspnea on exertion
4. Pallor of conjunctivae, nail beds, skin, lips, and oral mucosa
5. Smooth, sore tongue
6. Lesions at corners of mouth (cheilosis)
7. Spoon-shaped fingernails (koilonychia)
8. Irritability, inability to concentrate, possible pica (craving to eat unusual substances [eg, mud, ice])
9. Listlessness, poor feeding in infants and children

PEDIATRIC ALERT Children in rapid growth stages — toddlers and adolescents — as well as pregnant and lactating women are at risk for iron deficiency. Cow's milk is deficient in iron, so should not be used for infants, who do not have significant food intake.

Diagnostic Evaluation

1. Complete blood count shows decreased hemoglobin and hematocrit and elevated red cell distribution width.
2. Iron profile shows decreased serum iron and ferritin and normal or elevated total iron-binding capacity.
3. Parvovirus B19 titer is elevated in transient erythroblastopenia of childhood (parvovirus infection causing transient anemia).
4. Sigmoidoscopy, colonoscopy, upper and lower GI studies, and stool and urine (for occult blood examination) may determine source of chronic blood loss.

Collaborative Management
Pharmacologic Interventions

1. Iron therapy — oral ferrous sulfate is the therapy of choice and continues until hemoglobin level is normalized and iron stores are replaced (up to 6 months); parenteral therapy is rarely used because of risk of anaphylaxis.
   a. Dose is up to 6 mg/kg of elemental iron per day.
   b. Ferrous sulfate 325 mg contains 65 mg of elemental iron.
2. Source of blood loss is treated (treatment of ulcers, menorrhagia).

Nursing Diagnoses
1, 24, 51, 88

Nursing Interventions
Supportive Care

1. Assess diet for foods rich in iron. Arrange for a referral to a nutritionist as appropriate.
2. Use Z-track method of deep I.M. injection for parenteral iron.

> ⚡ **EMERGENCY ALERT** Anaphylactic reactions may occur after parenteral iron administration. Monitor patient closely for hypotension, angioedema, and stridor after injection. Do not administer in conjunction with oral iron.

3. Determine activities that cause fatigue; assist in developing a schedule of activity, rest periods, and sleep.
4. Encourage conditioning exercises to increase strength and endurance.
5. Assess patient for palpitations, chest pain, dizziness, and shortness of breath; minimize any activities that cause these symptoms.
6. Elevate head of bed and provide supplemental oxygen as ordered.

Education and Health Maintenance

1. Educate patient on proper nutrition and good sources of iron; select a well-balanced diet including animal proteins, iron-fortified cereals and bread, green leafy vegetables, dried fruits, legumes, and nuts.
2. Teach patient about iron supplementation:
   a. Take iron on empty stomach with full glass of water or fruit juice. (Iron is absorbed best in acidic environment.)
   b. Liquid forms may stain teeth; mix well and use straw. Dental stains can be removed by brushing teeth with sodium bicarbonate.
   c. Limit amount of milk to 16 to 24 ounces per day and do not give with iron because it impairs iron absorption.
   d. Anticipate some epigastric discomfort, change in color of stool to green or black and, in some cases, nausea, constipation, or diarrhea.

COMMUNITY CARE CONSIDERATIONS

Make sure that iron medications are kept secure and away from children as an overdose may be fatal.

3. Encourage follow-up laboratory studies and visits to health care provider, especially for children, for evaluation of growth and development.

ANEURYSM, AORTIC

An aneurysm is distention of an artery caused by structural weakening of the arterial wall. Under hemodynamic pressure, the weakened area enlarges, causing serious complications by compressing surrounding structures. Aneurysms result from degeneration of the medial wall, which occurs as a normal part of the aging process as well as with hypertension, atherosclerosis, trauma or infection, immunologic conditions, and as a complication of Marfan syndrome.

Thoracoabdominal aortic aneurysms may originate in the ascending aorta and aortic arch (frequent site of dissection) or in the lower descending thoracic aorta and upper abdominal aorta.

Abdominal aneurysms originate in the abdominal aorta, typically between the renal arteries and iliac branches. Many of these patients (mostly male) are asymptomatic.

Aneurysms may also occur in peripheral arteries (femoral, popliteal, renal, subclavian) or any major artery. Aneurysms may be saccular (distention of vessel projecting from one side), fusiform (distention of entire circumference), or dissecting (tear of the intima and separation of the medial layers causing hemorrhage or intramural hematoma). Complications include fatal hemorrhage, paraplegia caused by interruption of anterior spinal artery, abdominal ischemia, stroke, myocardial ischemia, lower extremity ischemia, renal failure, impotence, and cardiac tamponade.

Assessment

1. Thoracoabdominal aortic aneurysm
   a. Constant, boring pain or pressure in chest
   b. Intermittent neuralgic pain caused by nerve compression

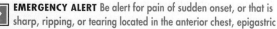

EMERGENCY ALERT Be alert for pain of sudden onset, or that is sharp, ripping, or tearing located in the anterior chest, epigastric

area, shoulders or back; this indicates acute dissection or rupture of thoracoabdominal aneurysm.

    c. Dyspnea, cough, and hoarseness because of pressure against trachea and recurrent laryngeal nerve

    d. Dysphagia because of pressure on esophagus

    e. Dilated superficial veins of chest and cyanosis caused by compression of chest vessels

    f. Ipsilateral dilation of pupils caused by pressure against cervical sympathetic chain

    g. Pulse or blood pressure variations between arms caused by interference with circulation in left subclavian artery

2. Abdominal aneurysm

    a. Persistent or intermittent abdominal pain, often localized to middle or lower left side of abdomen

> **EMERGENCY ALERT** Be alert for left lower quadrant abdominal pain and intense low back pain; this indicates rapid expansion, followed by syncope, tachycardia, and hypotension due to rupture.

    b. Pulsating mass with bruit

    c. Blood pressure elevated in arm more than in thigh

3. Predisposing factors include:

    a. Local infection, pyogenic or fungal (mycotic aneurysm)

    b. Congenital weakness of vessels

    c. Arteriosclerosis

    d. Trauma

    e. Syphilis

> **GERONTOLOGIC ALERT** Most abdominal aneurysms occur in people between ages 60 and 90. Rupture is likely if there is coexistent hypertension or if the aneurysm is larger than 6 cm.

Diagnostic Evaluation

1. Abdominal or chest X-rays may show calcification that outlines the aneurysm.
2. CT scan and ultrasonography are used to detect and monitor size of aneurysm.
3. MRI or magnetic resonance angiography further evaluate circulation.
4. Arteriography allows visualization of aneurysm and vessel.

Collaborative Management
Therapeutic Interventions
1. Reassure the patient that small aneurysms (4 cm or less) may be monitored with CT scans or ultrasound every 6 months, concurrent with aggressive blood pressure control.

Surgical Interventions
1. Surgery may be required to remove the aneurysm and restore vascular continuity with a bypass graft. Complications of surgery include arterial occlusion, graft hemorrhage, infection, ischemic colon, and impotence.
2. Endovascular grafting using a stent inserted via catheter through the femoral artery may be warranted.

Nursing Diagnoses
3, 88, 123, 135

Nursing Interventions
Monitoring
1. Monitor for signs and symptoms of spinal cord ischemia — pain, numbness, paresthesias, and weakness — caused by dissection.
2. Monitor for signs of stroke or cardiac tamponade caused by dissection.
3. Postoperatively, monitor vital signs continuously.
4. Monitor for arterial occlusion; check extremities for sensation, temperature, pulses, color, capillary refill, and petechiae.
5. Monitor for bleeding from the wound and for signs of hemorrhage — hypotension, tachycardia, pallor, and diaphoresis.
6. Monitor temperature and incision for signs of infection.
7. Measure abdominal girth or limb girth (of graft site) daily.
8. Monitor for watery, bloody diarrhea, which indicates ischemic bowel caused by reduced perfusion during surgery.
9. Monitor urinary output hourly.

Supportive Care

1. Maintain I.V. infusion to administer blood pressure medications and provide fluids postoperatively.
2. Administer antibiotics, if ordered, to prevent infection.
3. Administer pain medication, as ordered, or monitor patient-controlled analgesia.
4. Position the patient appropriately to enhance circulation.
   a. Elevate the head of the bed no more than 45 degrees for first 3 days postoperatively to prevent pressure on the repair and graft site.
   b. Warn the patient not to cross legs or sit for long periods to prevent thrombus formation.

Education and Health Maintenance

1. Teach the patient about blood pressure medications and the importance of taking them as prescribed.
2. Teach the patient to recognize and report signs and symptoms of an expanding aneurysm or rupture.
3. For postsurgical patients, discuss signs of postoperative complications (fever, inflammation of operative site, bleeding, and swelling).
4. Encourage adequate nutritional intake to enhance wound healing.
5. Teach the patient to maintain a postoperative exercise regimen.

ANEURYSM, INTRACRANIAL OR RUPTURED ARTERIOVENOUS MALFORMATION

An *intracranial aneurysm* is a saccular dilation of a cerebral artery whose walls are congenitally weakened. Constant blood flow against the weakened area causes the aneurysm to enlarge. The enlarging aneurysm may compress nearby cranial nerves or brain tissue to create symptoms, or it may rupture. The resulting hemorrhage within the subarachnoid space causes increased intracranial pressure (ICP), vasospasm, and ischemia, producing symptoms of a hemorrhagic stroke. Intracranial aneurysm may result from unknown causes or may be related to atherosclerosis, intracranial arteriovenous malformation (AVM; see below), infection, severe hypertension, or head trauma. They are most common in middle-aged adults and are classified by shape as saccular (most common), berry, or fusiform (encompassing the entire circumference of the artery).

An AVM is a tangle of abnormally formed cerebral arteries and veins that lack a normal interconnecting capillary bed. Because of backflow pressure, a fistula develops, resulting in vascular dilation and chronic hypoperfusion. Approximately 50% of patients with AVMs present with rupture and hemorrhage.

Intracranial aneurysm and AVM are graded from 0 (unruptured, asymptomatic) to IV (deep coma, decerebrate rigidity). Complications include rebleeding, cerebral vasospasm, hydrocephalus, and seizures.

Assessment

1. Sudden onset of severe headache, nausea, and photophobia but no neurologic deficits; may result from a "warning bleed" caused by leaking of aneurysm or rupture of the AVM.
2. Sudden, severe headache (commonly described as worst headache of patient's life) with meningeal signs (nuchal rigidity, photophobia, irritability); decreasing level of consciousness and focal neurologic deficits result from subarachnoid hemorrhage. The patient may present with loss of consciousness and severe deficits if bleed is massive.
3. Neurologic deficits occur specific to vascular territory (see page 903).

Diagnostic Evaluation

1. CT and MRI or magnetic resonance angiography scans may determine presence of blood in subarachnoid space and rule out other lesions.
2. Cerebral angiography may detect presence and location of cerebral aneurysm and provide information about vasospasm.
3. Lumbar puncture may detect blood in cerebrospinal fluid; observe for elevated opening pressure. If increased ICP

is suspected, lumbar puncture is contraindicated due to the danger of brain stem herniation.

4. Transcranial Doppler evaluates cerebral perfusion and monitors for changes.

Collaborative Management
Pharmacologic Interventions

1. Osmotic diuretics to control increased ICP.
2. Antifibrinolytic therapy with aminocaproic acid to inhibit clot lysis and prevent additional bleeding (infrequently used).
3. Nitroprusside or other I.V. agent to manage systemic hypertension. Monitor closely to prevent sharp decrease in blood pressure, aggravating ischemia.
4. Calcium channel blockers, specifically nimodipine, and plasma expanders, to prevent vasospasm.
5. Seizure prophylaxis with phenytoin or phenobarbital.
6. Antibiotics if aneurysm is mycotic.

Surgical Interventions

1. Craniotomy for clipping, ligation, clot evacuation, or strengthening the vessel wall by wrapping (if no other option).
2. Radiosurgery with gamma knife or LINAC scalpel for intact AVM.
3. Endovascular management through the use of coiling or balloon occlusion.
4. Ventricular shunt to control hydrocephalus.

Nursing Diagnoses
3, 6, 20, 88

Nursing Interventions
Also see page 239 for care of craniotomy patient.

Monitoring

1. Perform and document frequent neurologic assessments, including level of consciousness, pupillary changes, cra-

nial nerve function, and motor function. Focal neurologic deficits may indicate vasospasm.

2. Be alert for increasing headache, which may indicate re-bleeding (highest risk within first 6 hours).

3. Monitor for signs of increased ICP — increasing temperature, decreasing pulse, increasing blood pressure, widening pulse pressure, tachypnea, decreased level of consciousness, pupillary changes, and vomiting.

Supportive Care

1. Keep the patient free from agitation, and institute seizure precautions.

2. Institute subarachnoid precautions:
   a. Maintain absolute bed rest with head elevated 30 degrees to reduce cerebral edema.
   b. Maintain quiet, tranquil environment with low lighting and no noise or unnecessary activity to prevent photophobia, agitation, and pain.
   c. Provide physical care such as bathing and feeding.
   d. Restrict visitors to the immediate family or significant other who have been counseled to ensure tranquility.
   e. Encourage the conscious patient to avoid activities that increase blood pressure or ICP, such as Valsalva's maneuver for position changing, straining, sneezing, acute flexion or rotation of the neck, and cigarette smoking.
   f. Teach the conscious patient to exhale through the mouth during defecation to reduce strain; administer stool softeners, as ordered.
   g. Advise the patient to avoid caffeinated beverages.

3. Assess level of pain and pain relief; report any increase in headache.

4. Be alert for arrhythmias and electrocardiogram changes as well as electrolyte changes that may occur due to abnormal hormonal responses.

5. If opioid is being given with a sedative, monitor for central nervous system depression, decreased respirations, and decreased blood pressure.

6. Use reassurance and therapeutic conversation to relieve the patient's fear and anxiety.

7. Encourage distraction with soft music and other measures that will promote calm.
8. Prepare patient and family for surgery (see page 240).
9. Encourage discussion of risks and benefits with the surgeon.

Education and Health Maintenance

1. Educate the patient to the risk of rebleeding, which is highest during the first 6 months following rupture, but may remain for rest of his life.
2. Advise the patient to avoid strenuous activities to prevent sudden increased ICP—heavy lifting, straining, and so forth.
3. Encourage lifelong medical follow-up and immediate attention if severe headache develops.
4. Teach the patient and his family how to deal with permanent neurologic deficits, and make sure that they obtain rehabilitation referral.

ANOREXIA NERVOSA

See *Eating Disorders*.

ANTHRAX

Anthrax is a serious infection caused by the gram-positive, spore-forming bacteria, Bacillus anthracis. In industrialized nations, infection in humans was all but nonexistent until the threat of bioterrorism became apparent in late 2001. Infection occurs through contact with infected animals, products from infected animals, and intentionally tainted materials. Anthrax is a potential biologic weapon because spores can be distributed easily through the mail or other means. People exposed to airborne particles may develop cutaneous, inhalation, or GI anthrax, based on the route of exposure. Complications include meningitis, circulatory collapse, and death.

Assessment

1. Cutaneous anthrax: After incubation period of 1 to 12 days, a papule develops and progresses to a vesicle and,

ultimately, to a necrotic ulcer; fever, malaise, headache, and lymphadenopathy may also occur.

2. Inhalation anthrax: After an incubation period of several days to 60 days, a brief prodrome of fever, cough, fatigue, and mild chest discomfort occurs and may rapidly progress to severe respiratory distress, diaphoresis, stridor, cyanosis, and signs of meningitis (nuchal rigidity, headache, photophobia, altered mental status); may proceed to shock and death within 24 to 36 hours.

3. GI anthrax: Approximately 1 to 7 days after ingestion of tainted material or undercooked contaminated meat, nausea, anorexia, fever, severe abdominal pain, hematemesis, and bloody diarrhea may occur; the oropharyngeal form may also occur, characterized by lesions at base of tongue, dysphagia, fever, and cervical lymphadenopathy.

Diagnostic Evaluation

1. Nasal swab testing may be conducted on several people to detect contamination by anthrax in the environment, but this does not confirm infection by anthrax in an individual.

2. Testing to confirm disease in an individual includes blood, tissue, and spinal fluid cultures (before antibiotics); polymerase chain reaction testing; and chest X-ray to identify mediastinal widening in inhalation anthrax.

Collaborative Management
Pharmacologic Interventions

1. Antibiotic prophylaxis after exposure to spores is warranted, and 60-day therapy is advised. Drug recommendations include:
   a. Ciprofloxacin 500 mg bid for adults; 10 to 15 mg/kg bid for children
   b. Doxycycline 100 mg bid for those weighing 99 pounds (45 kg) and over; 2.2 mg/kg bid for children at least age 8 but weighing 99 pounds or less
   c. Amoxicillin 500 mg bid for adults; 80 mg/kg divided into three doses for children (if penicillin sensitivity of organism is confirmed)

2. Treatment of cutaneous anthrax involves 60-day treatment using the antibiotics listed above; however, signs of systemic involvement, including lesions of the head and neck and extensive edema, require I.V. treatment with multiple drugs as for inhalation anthrax.

3. Treatment of inhalation, GI, and oropharyngeal anthrax requires observation in a critical care unit with a combination of two or three I.V. antibiotics.

   a. Ciprofloxacin 400 mg q12h for adults; 10 to 15 mg/kg q12h for children OR doxycycline 100 mg q12h for adults; 2.2 mg/kg q12h for children at least age 8 and weighing 99 pounds (45 kg) or less

   b. AND one or two of the following: rifampin, vancomycin, penicillin, ampicillin, chloramphenicol, imipenem, clindamycin, clarithromycin.

   c. I.V. therapy can be switched to oral antibiotic therapy after clinical improvement is noted; total therapy is 60 days.

   d. Treatment is the same for pregnant women; potential benefits of therapy outweigh the risks.

4. I.V. corticosteroids may be given as adjunct therapy in severe cases (for all forms).

5. Symptomatic treatment includes analgesics, antiemetics, and emergency drugs for circulatory collapse.

6. Prognosis for cutaneous anthrax is good with antibiotic treatment; however, mortality rate is 25% to 60% for GI anthrax and up to 80% for inhalation anthrax, despite antibiotic treatment.

7. An anthrax vaccine has been available for veterinarians (not routinely used due to low incidence of animal disease), animal product handlers at high risk for exposure, and U.S. military personnel. It is a six-dose series requiring annual boosters. Its role in routine prophylaxis and adjunct treatment is controversial. Refined vaccines are being developed.

Nursing Diagnoses
44, 49, 57, 123

Nursing Interventions
Monitoring
1. Monitor vital signs and hemodynamic parameters closely for circulatory collapse.
2. Monitor temperature for response to antibiotic therapy.
3. Auscultate chest for crackles, indicating need for better secretion mobilization.
4. Monitor oxygen saturation and arterial blood gases periodically to determine oxygenation status and acid–base balance.
5. Monitor intake and output to determine fluid volume balance.
6. Monitor level of consciousness and for meningeal signs such as nuchal rigidity.

Supportive Care
1. Provide supplemental oxygen or mechanical ventilation, as needed.
2. Position for maximum chest expansion and reposition frequently to mobilize secretions.
3. Suction frequently and provide chest physiotherapy to clear airways, prevent atelectasis, and maximize oxygen therapy.
4. Administer I.V. fluids or encourage oral fluid intake to replace the fluid lost through hyperthermia and tachypnea.
5. For GI anthrax, maintain GI decompression, monitor emesis and liquid stool output, and medicate for abdominal pain, as needed.

Education and Health Maintenance
1. Anthrax is a reportable disease. Advise patient and family that a public health official will investigate the case for source of infection.
2. Advise the patient and family that anthrax is not transmitted person to person; one must come in contact with the spores to contract infection.
3. Long-term nature of antibiotic therapy may present adverse effects. Educate patient taking ciprofloxacin to be

on the alert for and report dizziness, agitation, impaired cognitive function, hallucinations, joint pain, muscle pain, or severe tendon pain. Interactions with other drugs include theophylline (should not be taken simultaneously because theophylline toxicity may occur) and sucralfate and antacids (interfere with absorption, so should not be taken for 1 hour before or 2 hours after ciprofloxacin).

4. Although the benefits may outweigh the risk of antibiotic therapy, educate parents that doxycycline may cause discoloration of teeth in children younger than age 8 and that it may have adverse effects on a developing fetus.

5. Advise extended follow-up for those who received prophylactic treatment for exposure as well as those recovering from any form of anthrax.

6. Further information can be obtained through the Centers for Disease Control and Prevention, *www.cdc.gov.*

ANXIETY, SOMATOFORM, AND DISSOCIATIVE DISORDERS

Anxiety is a subjective feeling of apprehension and tension that is manifested by psychophysiologic arousal and a variety of behavioral patterns. The common theme among all anxiety-related disorders is that affected people experience a level of anxiety that interferes with functioning in personal, occupational, or social spheres, as well as with psychophysiologic well-being.

According to the *Diagnostic and Statistical Manual of Mental Disorders*, 4th edition, Text Revision (*DSM-IV-TR*), *anxiety disorders* include panic disorder, posttraumatic stress disorder (PTSD), phobias, obsessive-compulsive disorder (OCD), substance-induced anxiety disorder, generalized anxiety disorder (GAD), and acute stress disorder.

Related disorders include *somatoform disorders*, including somatization disorder, undifferentiated somatoform disorder, conversion disorder, pain disorder, hypochondriasis, and body dysmorphic disorder; and *dissociative disorders*, including dissociative amnesia, dissociative fugue, dissociative identity disorder, and depersonalization disorder.

Anxiety disorders result from combinations of biochemical, genetic, psychosocial, and sociocultural factors.

Assessment

Diagnostic criteria for common anxiety disorders are as follows:

1. Panic disorder
   a. Recurrent unexpected anxiety attacks; onset is sudden, and patient experiences intense apprehension and dread
   b. Four or more of the following symptoms: Dyspnea; chest discomfort; dizziness; hot or cold flashes; tingling of hands or feet; feelings of unreality; palpitations; syncope; diaphoresis; trembling; or fear of losing control, going crazy, or dying
2. PTSD
   a. After experiencing a psychologically traumatic event outside the range of usual experience (eg, rape, combat, bombings, kidnapping), the patient continues to experience the event through recurrent and intrusive dreams and flashbacks.
   b. Emotional numbness, detachment, and estrangement may be used to defend against anxiety.
   c. May experience sleep disturbance, hypervigilance, survivor's guilt, poor concentration, and avoidance of activities that trigger memory of the event.
3. Phobias — irrational fear of an object or situation that persists, although the person may recognize it as unreasonable. Anxiety is severe if the object, situation, or activity cannot be avoided. Types include:
   a. Agoraphobia: Fear of being alone or in public places where escape might be difficult; may not leave home
   b. Social phobia: Fear of situations in which one might be seen and embarrassed or criticized (eg, eating in public, public speaking, performing)
   c. Specific phobia: Fear of a single object, activity, or situation (eg, snakes, closed spaces, flying)
4. OCD

      a. Preoccupation with persistent intrusive thoughts (obsessions), repeated performance of rituals designed to prevent some event (compulsions), or both.

      b. Anxiety occurs if obsessions or compulsions are resisted or from feeling powerless to resist the thoughts or rituals.

5. Substance-induced anxiety disorder
   a. Prominent anxiety, panic attacks, or obsessions or compulsions
   b. Symptoms develop within 1 month of substance intoxication or withdrawal.
   c. Medication use is related to disturbance.
   d. Disturbance does not occur exclusively during the course of delirium.
   e. Significant distress or impaired social and occupational functioning results.

6. GAD—persists for at least 6 months. Symptoms present from three of the four following categories:
   a. Motor tension
   b. Autonomic hyperactivity
   c. Apprehensiveness
   d. Hypervigilance

7. Acute stress disorder—person has witnessed or experienced a traumatic event; duration of 2 days to 4 weeks. Develops three or more of the following dissociative symptoms:
   a. Subjective sense of numbing
   b. Absence of emotional responsiveness
   c. Feeling dazed
   d. Derealization
   e. Depersonalization
   f. Dissociative amnesia

Diagnostic Evaluation

1. Measurement tools for anxiety:
   a. Hamilton Anxiety Scale
   b. Graphic Anxiety Scales
   c. Yale-Brown Obsessive-Compulsive Scale
   d. Acute Panic Inventory

2. Sodium lactate infusion or carbon dioxide inhalation will likely produce a panic attack in a patient with panic disorder.

3. Increased arousal may be measured through studies of autonomic functioning (eg, heart rate, electromyography, sweat gland activity) in a patient with posttraumatic stress disorder.

Collaborative Management
Therapeutic Interventions

1. Determine the level and place of care to be provided — psychiatric inpatient, outpatient, day treatment, or psychiatric home care.
2. Psychoeducational strategies:
   a. Relaxation techniques
   b. Progressive muscle relaxation
   c. Guided imagery and visualization
3. Psychotherapy
   a. Psychodynamic: Assist patients with understanding their experiences by identifying unconscious conflicts and developing effective coping behaviors.
   b. Behavioral: Focus on the patient's problematic behavior and work to modify or extinguish the behavior. Systematic desensitization is often successful.
   c. Hypnotherapy can be used as part of therapy for those suffering dissociative disorders.
   d. Cognitive: Helps patients to question faulty thought patterns and examine alternatives.
4. Biofeedback: Relaxation through biofeedback is achieved when a person learns to control physiologic mechanisms that are not ordinarily within his or her awareness. Awareness and control are accomplished by monitoring body processes, including muscle tone, heart rate, and brain waves.

Pharmacologic Interventions

1. Antianxiety drugs traditionally include benzodiazepines, which are effective; however, use is limited due to the po-

tential for dependence and additive effects with other central nervous system (CNS) depressants.

2. A nonbenzodiazepine anxiolytic, buspirone, may be used for long-term therapy; however, it often takes up to 4 weeks for it to produce therapeutic effects and is not always effective. Adverse effects include dizziness, headache, insomnia, nervousness, nausea, and dry mouth. CNS depressants should also be avoided.

3. Several antidepressants (fluoxetine, paroxetine, sertraline) have been approved for treatment of anxiety disorders; therapeutic effects may be seen in 3 to 4 weeks.

4. Propranolol may also be used control the autonomic symptoms of panic and anxiety; however, blood pressure and cardiovascular effects should be monitored.

ALTERNATIVE INTERVENTION

Ask the patient if he or she is taking any over-the-counter products, herbal remedies, or supplements. St. John's wort should not be taken with antidepressants, and kava kava should not be mixed with alcohol or other CNS depressants.

Nursing Diagnoses
6, 35, 44, 78, 84, 96, 136, 159

Nursing Interventions
Monitoring
1. Monitor for objective and subjective manifestations of anxiety.
   a. Tachycardia, tachypnea
   b. Verbalization of feelings of anxiety
   c. Signs and symptoms associated with autonomic stimulation: Perspiration, difficulty concentrating, insomnia
2. Monitor effects of medication and functional ability.

Supportive Care
1. Develop an honest, nonjudgmental relationship with the patient.

A

2. Help patient develop assertiveness and communication skills.
3. Maintain a calm, serene manner.
4. Use short, simple sentences and low tone when communicating with patient.
5. Teach relaxation techniques to diminish distress that interferes with concentration ability.
6. Help patient identify anxiety-producing situations and develop strategies to avoid them.
7. Encourage patient to discuss reasons for and feelings about social isolation.
8. Help patient identify specific situations that serve to inhibit social interaction.
9. Recommend participation in programs directed at specific conflict areas or skill deficiencies. Such programs may focus on assertiveness skills, body awareness, managing multiple role responsibilities, and stress management.
10. Identify secondary benefits, such as decreased responsibility and increased dependency, that inhibit patient's move to independence.
11. Explore alternative methods of meeting dependency needs.
12. Explore beliefs that support a helpless or dependent mode of behavior.
13. Teach and role-play assertive behaviors in specific situations.
14. Assist patient with improving skills based on performance.
15. Provide experiences in which patient can be successful.

Education and Health Maintenance
1. Teach patient and family members about anxiety.
2. Describe the medication regimen, potential adverse reactions, and dangerous interactions (particularly with other CNS depressants and alcohol).
3. Identify, describe, and practice deep-muscle relaxation techniques, relaxation breathing, imagery, and other relaxation therapies.
4. Teach family to give positive reinforcement for use of healthy behaviors.

5. Teach family not to assume responsibilities or roles normally assigned to the patient.
6. Teach family to give attention to the patient, not to the patient's symptoms.
7. Teach alternative ways to perform activities of daily living if physical disability inhibits function and performance.
8. For additional information and support, refer to agencies such as Anxiety Disorders Association of America, *www.adaa.org*.

AORTIC ANEURYSM
See *Aneurysm, Aortic*.

APPENDICITIS
Appendicitis is inflammation of the vermiform appendix caused by an obstruction attributable to infection, stricture, fecal mass, foreign body, or tumor. Appendicitis can affect either gender at any age, but is most common in males ages 10 to 30. Appendicitis is the most common disease requiring surgery. If left untreated, appendicitis may progress to abscess, perforation, subsequent peritonitis, and death.

Assessment
1. Generalized or localized abdominal pain occurs in the epigastric or periumbilical areas and in the upper right abdomen.
2. Within 2 to 12 hours, the pain localizes in the right lower quadrant and intensity increases.
3. Anorexia, fever, nausea, vomiting, and constipation may also occur.

GERONTOLOGIC ALERT Be aware of vague symptoms in elderly patients: Milder pain, low-grade fever, and leukocytosis with shift to the left (immature neutrophils) on white blood cell (WBC) differential.

4. Bowel sounds may be diminished.
5. Tenderness anywhere in the right lower quadrant
   a. Often localized over McBurney's point, just below midpoint of line between umbilicus and iliac crest on the right side

b. Guarding and rebound tenderness in right lower quadrant and referred rebound when palpating the left lower quadrant

6. Positive psoas sign
   a. Have the patient attempt to raise the right thigh against the pressure of your hand placed over the right knee.
   b. Increased abdominal pain indicates inflammation of the psoas muscle in acute appendicitis.
7. Positive obturator sign
   a. Flex the patient's right hip and knee and rotate the leg internally.
   b. Hypogastric pain indicates inflammation of the obturator muscle.

Diagnostic Evaluation

1. WBC count shows moderate leukocytosis (10,000 to 16,000/mm) with shift to the left (increased immature neutrophils) in WBC differential.
2. Urinalysis rules out urinary disorders.
3. Abdominal X-ray visualizes shadow consistent with fecalith in appendix.
4. Pelvic sonogram rules out ovarian cyst or ectopic pregnancy.

Collaborative Management
Surgical Interventions

1. Surgical removal is the only effective treatment (simple appendectomy or laparoscopic appendectomy).
2. Preoperatively, maintain patient on bed rest, NPO status, I.V. hydration, possible antibiotic prophylaxis, and analgesia, as directed.

> **EMERGENCY ALERT** When appendicitis is suspected, analgesics with antipyretic property should be avoided to prevent masking of fever; cathartics are contraindicated because they may cause rupture.

Nursing Diagnoses
3, 16, 130, 135

Nursing Interventions

Also see *Gastrointestinal or Abdominal Surgery*, page 381.

Monitoring

1. Monitor frequently for signs and symptoms of worsening condition, indicating perforation, abscess, or peritonitis (increasing severity of pain, tenderness, rigidity, distention, absent bowel sounds, fever, malaise, and tachycardia).
2. Notify health care provider immediately if pain suddenly ceases; this indicates perforation, a medical emergency.

Supportive Care

1. Assist patient to position of comfort such as semi-Fowler's with knees flexed.
2. Restrict activity that may aggravate pain, such as coughing and ambulation.
3. Apply ice bag to abdomen for comfort.
4. Avoid indiscriminate palpation of the abdomen to avoid increasing the patient's discomfort.
5. Promptly prepare patient for surgery once diagnosis is established.

Education and Health Maintenance

1. Explain signs and symptoms of postoperative complications to report — elevated temperature, nausea or vomiting, or abdominal distention; these may indicate infection.
2. Instruct patient on turning, coughing, deep breathing, use of incentive spirometer, and ambulation. Discuss purpose and continued importance of these maneuvers during the recovery period.
3. Teach incisional care and avoidance of heavy lifting or driving (until cleared by surgeon).
4. Advise avoidance of enemas or harsh laxatives; increased fluids and stool softeners may be used for postoperative constipation.

ARTERIAL OCCLUSIVE DISEASE

A

Arterial occlusive disease (also known as *peripheral vascular* or *arterial disease*) is a common complication of arteriosclerosis in which the vascular system of the legs becomes blocked. Diabetes, hypertension, and cigarette smoking are major risk factors. Chronic occlusive arterial disease occurs much more frequently than acute disease (which usually results from sudden and complete blocking of a vessel by a thrombus or embolus).

There are two main types of arterial occlusive disease: *arteriosclerosis obliterans* occurs at bifurcations of a vessel, most commonly at aortoiliac, femoropopliteal, and popliteal-tibial sites; *thromboangiitis obliterans*, or Buerger's disease, is an inflammatory process of the arterial walls that may lead to thrombosis. It frequently occurs in men ages 35 to 45 who are heavy smokers. Untreated, chronic occlusive arterial disease may progress to ulceration of feet and toes; severe occlusion causes gangrene and may necessitate partial or complete limb amputation.

Acute arterial occlusion results from an arterial embolus that causes complete arterial obstruction; such emboli tend to lodge at bifurcations and atherosclerotic narrowings.

Assessment

1. Intermittent claudication or predictable pain in extremity upon activity; may progress to pain at rest, aggravated by elevation of legs (may cause patient to get out of bed at night).
2. Numbness and tingling in the toes (indicates occlusion of the femoral, popliteal, and distal arteries).
3. Changes in color (pallor to mottling in acute arterial embolism), sensation, and temperature (coldness) from one side to the other. See *Table A-3*, page 52, for comparison with venous disease.
4. Thickened, opaque nails; shiny, atrophic, hairless skin with dry apperance reflects long-term changes.
5. Diminished or absent pulses distal to affected artery; bruits on auscultation.
6. Possible ulcers of toes and feet.

TABLE A-3	Comparison of Arterial and Venous Obstruction	
FACTOR	**ARTERIAL OBSTRUCTION**	**VENOUS OBSTRUCTION**
Onset	▪ May be sudden	▪ Gradual
Color	▪ Pale ▪ Later — mottled, cyanotic	▪ Slightly cyanotic ▪ Rubescent
Skin temperature	▪ Cold	▪ Warm
Leg size	▪ May be reduced	▪ Enlarged
Leg hair and nails	▪ Decreased hair; thick, brittle nails	▪ No change
Edema	▪ None to mild	▪ Typically calf to foot
Sensation	▪ Sensory changes	▪ Normal sensation
Arterial pulses	▪ Pulse deficit	▪ Normal
Effect of elevating leg	▪ Condition worsens	▪ Slight improvement

7. Acute onset of severe pain may signal an acute arterial embolism. Pain may be aggravated by movement of and pressure on the extremity.
8. Sharp line of color and temperature demarcation distal to the site of occlusion as a result of ischemia in acute arterial embolism.
9. Aortoiliac disease may cause mesenteric ischemic pain, weight loss, renal insufficiency, poorly controlled hypertension, impotence, as well as intermittent claudication.

Diagnostic Evaluation

1. Vascular examination, including brachial and ankle systolic pressures, before and after exercise. Ankle-brachial index (ratio) 0.9 or greater is normal; below 0.9 indicates mild, moderate, or severe occlusion.
2. Doppler ultrasound may show increased flow velocity through a stenotic vessel or no flow with total occlusion; segmental plethysmography shows decreased pressure through region of occlusion.
3. Arteriography or imaging studies (magnetic resonance angiography, spiral CT) confirm arterial occlusion.

Collaborative Management

Therapeutic Interventions

1. Conservative treatment to manage intermittent claudication includes walking program, weight reduction, smoking cessation, and control of other conditions, such as hypertension and diabetes mellitus.
2. Hyperbaric oxygen therapy (only available at specialized centers) may be implemented for nonhealing ulcers and gas gangrene.

Pharmacologic Interventions

1. Pentoxifylline may be given to improve blood flow; drug increases erythrocyte flexibility and reduces blood viscosity. Contraindicated in patients who have recently undergone surgery, experienced hemorrhage, or have a caffeine or methylxanthine intolerance.
2. Cilostazol or aspirin, which act as antiplatelet agents to inhibit thrombosis, may be used together with caution. Monitor for bleeding; cilostazol is contraindicated in heart failure.
3. Anticoagulants and thrombolytics to treat acute arterial embolism.
   a. Heparin I.V. reduces tendency of emboli to form or expand (useful in smaller arteries).
   b. Thrombolytics I.V. dissolve clot.

    c. Low molecular weight heparin or oral anticoagulation
      with Coumadin may be used to prevent a recurrence,
      following initial treatment.
4. Treatment of shock in the event of acute arterial embolism
   of large artery.

ALTERNATIVE INTERVENTION

Patients may be taking "natural" preparations to improve circulation, such as ginkgo, grapeseed, horse chestnuts, and garlic. Encourage patients to divulge all over-the-counter and prescription
medications they may be taking because there may be an interaction with prescribed anticoagulant or antiplatelet medication.

EMERGENCY ALERT Arterial embolization of a large artery (such
as the iliac) that has major systemic effects is life-threatening and
requires emergency surgery.

Surgical Interventions
1. Reconstructive arterial surgery (endarterectomy, arterial
   bypass grafting, or a combination) may be required.
2. Percutaneous transluminal angioplasty may be used alone
   or with reconstructive surgery to dilate localized noncal-
   cified segments of narrowed arteries.
3. Microvascular surgery may be required for small artery occlusive disease.
4. Embolectomy must be performed within 6 to 10 hours of
   acute arterial occlusion to prevent muscle necrosis and
   loss of extremity.
5. Amputation may be necessary with gangrene.

Nursing Diagnoses
33, 88, 108, 135

Nursing Interventions
Monitoring
1. Monitor the condition of extremities for injury, ulceration, and signs of infection.

2. In anticoagulant therapy for acute arterial embolism, monitor patient for signs of bleeding (gums, urine, stool). Also monitor coagulation studies.
3. Monitor the postoperative embolectomy patient for tachycardia, fever, pain, erythema, warmth, swelling, and drainage at the incision site, indicating infection.

Supportive Care

1. For patients with chronic arterial disease, encourage walking or range-of-motion exercises to increase blood flow and provide analgesics as indicated.
2. In acute arterial embolism, protect the extremity by keeping it at or below the body's horizontal plane. Provide and encourage a well-balanced diet to enhance wound healing.
3. Postoperatively, check the surgical wound for bleeding, swelling, erythema, and discharge.
4. To prevent arterial ulcers, provide and teach proper foot care:
   a. Encourage the patient to wear protective footwear such as rubber-soled slippers or shoes with closed, wide toe-box when out of bed.
   b. Avoid using adhesive tape on affected skin.
   c. Wash and carefully dry feet, trim toenails, and inspect feet daily.
   d. Apply lanolin or petrolatum to lower extremities to prevent drying and cracking of skin.
   e. Encourage the patient to wear clean hose daily; woolen socks for winter, cotton socks for summer.

Education and Health Maintenance

1. Teach patient the importance of maintaining/improving circulation:
   a. Walking
   b. Not sitting or standing in one position for long periods; not crossing legs when sitting or lying
   c. Not using tight-fitting, elastic-topped socks

BOX A-1	Selected Substances that Interact with Coumadin

SUBSTANCES THAT DECREASE COUMADIN EFFECT*
- Barbiturates
- Antacids
- Hormonal contraceptives and estrogens
- Corticosteroids
- Quinidine
- Tamoxifen
- Rifampin
- Vitamin K–rich foods
- Grapefruit juice

SUBSTANCES THAT INCREASE COUMADIN EFFECT*
- Aspirin
- Heparin
- Nonsteroidal anti-inflammatory drugs
- Cimetidine
- Penicillins (high dose), macrolides, cephalosporins
- Fluconazole
- Ticlopidine
- Thyroxine
- Sulfa compounds
- Alcohol
- Ginkgo biloba, ginseng, garlic

*Consult a pharmacist or medication reference for a complete list.

2. Teach patient methods to promote vasodilation by keeping extremity warm, not smoking, and stopping use of other vasoconstricting substances such as caffeine.
3. Reinforce dietary teaching to promote healing (vitamin C, protein, balanced diet).
4. Tell patient to have a podiatrist cut corns and calluses; do not use corn pads or strong medications.
5. Teach the patient to recognize and report early signs of skin irritation (redness, swelling, blistering, itching) and bruises, cuts, and other skin lesions that do not heal quickly.

6. Teach patient not to add any other medications (without consulting the health care provider) because there are many interactions with Coumadin. (See *Box A-1.*)

ARTERIOVENOUS MALFORMATION, RUPTURED

See *Aneurysm, Intracranial*.

ARTHRITIS

See *Osteoarthritis, Rheumatoid Arthritis, and Rheumatoid Arthritis, Juvenile*.

ARTHROPLASTY AND TOTAL JOINT REPLACEMENT

Arthroplasty is reconstructive surgery to restore joint motion and function and to relieve pain. It generally involves replacement of bony joint structure by a prosthesis. In total joint replacement, both articulating surfaces are replaced with metal or plastic components. The most common types of joint replacement are total hip replacement, usually with a metal femoral component topped by a spherical ball fitted into a plastic acetabular socket; and total knee replacement, an implant procedure in which tibial, femoral, and patellar joint surfaces are replaced.

Indications for total joint replacement include unremitting pain and irreversible joint damage, as in primary degenerative arthritis (osteoarthritis) and rheumatoid arthritis; selected fractures (eg, femoral neck fracture); failure of previous reconstructive surgery; congenital hip disease; pathologic fractures from metastatic cancer; and joint instability.

Potential Complications
1. Deep infection, sepsis, thromboembolism
2. Increased pain or decreased function associated with loosening of prosthetic components
3. Implant wear
4. Dislocation or fracture of components
5. Avascular necrosis or dead bone caused by loss of blood supply

6. Heterotrophic ossification (formation of bone in periprosthetic space)

Nursing Diagnoses
3, 8, 24, 62, 128, 136

Collaborative Interventions
Also see *Orthopedic surgery*, page 680.

Preoperative Care
1. Assess the patient for bladder, dental, or skin infections that may be a source for prosthesis infections.
2. Provide preoperative patient teaching.
   a. Educate the patient concerning postoperative regimen (eg, extended exercise program).
   b. Teach isometric exercises (muscle setting) of quadriceps and gluteal muscles; teach active ankle motion.
   c. Teach bed-to-wheelchair transfer without going beyond the hip flexion limits (usually 90 degrees).
   d. Practice nonweight- and partial weight-bearing ambulation with ambulatory aid (walker, crutches) to facilitate postoperative ambulation.
   e. Demonstrate abduction splint, knee immobilizer, or continuous passive motion if equipment will be used postoperatively.
3. Use antiembolism stockings to minimize the risk of thrombophlebitis.
4. Give meticulous skin preparation with antimicrobial solution to minimize potential infection.
5. Administer antibiotics, as prescribed, to ensure therapeutic blood levels during and immediately after surgery to prevent osteomyelitis.
6. Thoroughly assess cardiovascular, respiratory, renal, hepatic, hydration, and nutritional status, and institute measures to maximize general health condition.

Postoperative Care
1. Employ appropriate positioning to prevent dislocation of prosthesis.

2. After hip arthroplasty, position the patient supine in bed. Keep the affected extremity in slight abduction using an abduction splint or pillow or Buck's extension traction to prevent dislocation of the prosthesis.

⚡ **EMERGENCY ALERT** The patient must not adduct or flex operated hip because this may produce dislocation. Signs of joint dislocation include shortened extremity, increasing discomfort, and inability to move joints.

   a. With the aid of a coworker, turn the patient on unoperated side while supporting operated hip securely in an abducted position; support the entire leg on pillows.

   b. Use overhead trapeze to assist with position changes.

   c. Do not elevate the bed more than 45 degrees; placing the patient in an upright sitting position puts a strain on the hip joint and may cause dislocation.

   d. Use a fracture bedpan when needed. Instruct the patient to flex the unoperated hip and knee and pull up on the overhead trapeze to lift buttocks onto pan. Instruct the patient not to bear down on the operated hip in flexion when getting off the pan.

3. After knee arthroplasty, the knee will be immobilized in extension with a firm compression dressing and an adjustable soft extension splint or long-leg plaster cast.

   a. Elevate the leg on pillows to control swelling.

   b. Alternatively, initiate continuous passive motion to facilitate joint healing and restore range of motion.

4. While the patient is in bed, prevent thromboembolism by continuous use of antiembolism stockings and use of a sequential compression device (SCD); discontinue SCD when patient is ambulatory.

5. Promote early mobility. When the patient is ready to ambulate, teach to advance the walker and then advance the operated extremity to the walker to permit weight bearing as prescribed.

   a. Use an abduction splint or pillows while assisting the hip replacement patient to get out of bed.

   b. Keep the hip at maximum extension.

   c. Instruct the patient to pivot on unoperated extremity.

   d. Assess the patient for orthostatic hypotension.

    e. With increased joint stability, help the patient use crutches or cane, as prescribed.

    f. Encourage practicing physical therapy exercises to strengthen muscles and prevent contractures.

6. Assist the knee replacement patient with transfer out of bed into wheelchair with extension splint in place.

    a. Ensure that no weight bearing is permitted until prescribed by the orthopedic surgeon.

    b. Apply continuous passive motion equipment or carry out passive range-of-motion exercises as prescribed.

Education and Health Maintenance

1. Advise wearing elastic stockings until full activities are resumed.

2. Warn against excessive hip adduction, flexion, and rotation for 6 weeks after hip arthroplasty:

    a. Avoid sitting in low chair/toilet seat.

    b. Keep knees apart; do not cross legs.

    c. Limit sitting to 30 minutes at a time to minimize hip flexion and risk of prosthetic dislocation and to prevent hip stiffness and flexion contracture.

3. Encourage quadriceps setting and range-of-motion exercises as directed.

    a. Have a daily program of stretching, exercise, and rest throughout lifetime.

    b. Do not participate in activities that place undue or sudden stress on joint (eg, jogging, jumping, lifting heavy loads, becoming obese, excessive bending and twisting).

    c. Use a cane when taking long walks.

4. Teach patient to use self-help and energy-saving devices:

    a. Handrails by toilet

    b. Raised toilet seat if there is some residual hip flexion problem

    c. Bar-type stool for shower and kitchen work

5. Tell the patient to lie prone twice daily for 30 minutes.

6. Encourage follow-up evaluation.

7. Teach proper use of supportive equipment (crutches, canes, raised toilet seat) as prescribed.

8. Advise patient to notify dentist and other doctors of need to take prophylactic antibiotic if undergoing any procedure (tooth extraction, manipulation of genitourinary tract) known to cause bacteremia.
9. Advise of need to avoid MRI studies because of implanted metal component.
10. Advise patient that metal components may set off metal-detector alarms in airports, and so forth.

ASTHMA

Asthma is a chronic inflammatory disease of the airways, associated with recurrent, reversible airway obstruction with intermittent episodes of wheezing and dyspnea. Bronchial hypersensitivity is caused by various stimuli, which innervate the vagus nerve and beta-adrenergic receptor cells of the airways, leading to bronchial smooth muscle constriction, hypersecretion of mucus, and mucosal edema. Immunoglobulin (Ig) E-mediated antigen-antibody reaction (type I, immediate hypersensitivity) also occurs in susceptible individuals causing degranulation of mast cells and release of powerful mediators of bronchoconstriction and inflammation. Asthma occurs in all ages but is the most common chronic disease of childhood, with 5% to 10% of school-age children having symptoms of asthma. Asthma may develop in infants, but it usually develops after the third birthday. It is more common in blacks from urban settings.

Asthma is classified by severity as mild intermittent, mild persistent, moderate, and severe. There are six main types: *extrinsic asthma,* caused by inhaled allergens (eg, dust mites, cockroaches, mold, pollens, feathers, and animal dander); *intrinsic asthma,* caused by infection (often viral) and environmental stimuli (such as air pollution), with no inciting allergen; *mixed asthma,* in which type I reactivity appears to be combined with intrinsic factors; *aspirin-induced asthma,* caused by ingestion of aspirin and related compounds; *exercise-induced asthma,* in which respiratory symptoms occur within 5 to 20 minutes of exercise; and *occupational asthma,* caused by industrial fumes, dust, and gases.

BOX A-2 Status Asthmaticus

Status asthmaticus is a severe form of acute asthma in which airway obstruction resists conventional drug therapy and lasts longer than 24 hours. Unless treated promptly, status asthmaticus progresses to respiratory failure. Status asthmaticus is characterized by:

- Tachypnea, labored respirations, with increased effort on expiration
- Decreased ability to speak in sentences or long phrases
- Suprasternal retractions, use of accessory muscles
- Diminished breath sounds
- Fatigue, headache, irritability, dizziness, impaired mental functioning caused by hypoxia
- Muscle twitching, somnolence, diaphoresis caused by carbon dioxide retention
- Tachycardia, elevated blood pressure
- Heart failure and death from suffocation

MANAGEMENT AND NURSING INTERVENTIONS

- Continuously or frequently monitor respiratory rate, oxygen saturation, arterial blood gas (ABG) levels, blood pressure, and electrocardiogram.

  ⚡ EMERGENCY ALERT In status asthmaticus, the return to a normal or increasing partial pressure of carbon dioxide does not necessarily mean that the patient is improving. It may indicate a fatigue state that develops just before the patient slips into respiratory failure. Correlate ABG levels with respiratory effort and level of consciousness.

- Administer repeated aerosol treatments with albuterol or levalbuterol and ipratropium noting effectiveness of each treatment and monitoring for tolerance of adverse effects (nervousness, tremor, tachycardia).
- Give prescribed I.V. corticosteroids to treat inflammation of airways. Because these act slowly, their beneficial effects may not be apparent for several hours.
- Give fluids to treat dehydration and loosen secretions.
- Provide continuous humidified oxygen by way of nasal cannula as prescribed. Use oxygen cautiously in patients with chronic obstructive pulmonary disease because hypoxemia stimulates their respiratory drive.
- Initiate mechanical ventilation for severe acidosis, hypoxemia, or respiratory fatigue.
- Perform chest physiotherapy (chest wall percussion and vibration), administer expectorant and mucolytic drugs as

Status Asthmaticus *(continued)*

prescribed, and suction as needed to prevent obstruction by secretions. Bronchoscopy may be needed.
- Administer antibiotics for underlying infection.
- Alleviate the patient's anxiety and fear by acting calmly and reassuring the patient during an attack. Stay with the patient until the attack subsides.

Severe, acute asthma that fails to respond to bronchodilators is called *status asthmaticus* and is a medical emergency (see *Box A-2*). Other complications include pneumonia, atelectasis, dehydration, arrhythmias, cor pulmonale, respiratory failure, and death.

Assessment

1. Feeling of chest tightness
2. Episodes of coughing
3. Wheezing, dyspnea
4. Anxiety, apprehension
5. Nasal flaring, use of accessory muscles

EMERGENCY ALERT On auscultation, do not be misled by lack of wheezing when the patient complains of severe shortness of breath. Airflow may be so restricted that wheezing ceases.

Diagnostic Evaluation

1. Increased levels of IgE in extrinsic asthma.
2. Pulmonary function testing shows obstruction: more than 12% increase over baseline in the first second of forced expiratory volume (FEV_1) following inhalation of a bronchodilator; more than 20% variability between a.m. and p.m. measurements.
3. Bronchial methacholine challenge test (inhalation of a cholinergic agent in serial concentrations delivered by nebulizer) demonstrates airway hyperreactivity; positive response is indicated by a 20% decrease in FEV_1 from baseline.
4. Skin tests identify causative allergens.

5. Sputum and nasal cytology may detect eosinophilia.
6. Chest X-ray rules out other lung diseases.

Collaborative Management

Therapeutic Interventions

1. Environmental control: Minimize contact with offending allergens, regardless of other treatment.
2. Foods that contain tartrazine (yellow dye #5) may cause asthma in aspirin-sensitive patients and should be avoided.
3. Regular aerobic exercise. Use of an inhaled beta-agonist or cromolyn taken 15 to 20 minutes before exercise will decrease exercise-induced bronchospasm.
4. Prompt recognition and treatment of respiratory infections and exacerbation of asthma symptoms.
5. During acute attacks:
   a. Supplemental oxygen is given to maintain oxygen saturation above 95%.
   b. Cardiorespiratory monitoring and possible placement of arterial line for frequent blood gas measurements.
   c. Respiratory support may be necessary with mechanical ventilation.
   d. Dehydration and thickened secretions caused by fever and increased insensible loss (through expired air) may require I.V. fluids.

ALTERNATIVE INTERVENTION

Acupuncture, herbal preparations, yoga, and chiropractic treatment have been suggested for acute and chronic asthma control; however, none is a substitute for usual medical treatment. In fact, glucosamine and chondroitin have been suspected of causing asthma exacerbations in some patients.

Pharmacologic Interventions

Drug therapy should be maximized to allow the patient to be fully active; the management plan should be individualized to prevent and treat exacerbations.

1. Quick-relief medications

a. Short-acting inhaled beta-agonist bronchodilators such as albuterol, pirbuterol, and levalbuterol; short-acting oral preparations such as albuterol syrup

b. Inhaled anticholinergic agent, ipratropium

c. Short course of systemic corticosteroid

2. Long-term controller medications

a. Inhaled corticosteroids such as beclomethasone, triamcinolone, budesonide, fluticasone

b. Long-acting inhaled beta-agonists, such as salmeterol and formoterol

c. Combination inhalation treatment with fluticasone and salmeterol

d. Leukotriene modifiers, such as montelukast and zafirlukast

e. Inhaled mast cell stabilizers, such as cromolyn sodium and nedocromil with IgE-mediated asthma

f. Long-acting albuterol extended-release tablets

g. Oral corticosteroids at maintenance dose

h. Oral methylxanthines such as theophylline

i. IgE blocker, omalizumab, may reduce exacerbations.

3. Immunotherapy-desensitization of immune system to known allergens that cause type I hypersensitivity

EMERGENCY ALERT Beta-adrenergic blockers, such as propranolol, should not be given to patients with asthma because of the potential to cause bronchoconstriction. They also should not be given to patients receiving immunotherapy because they would make it difficult to reverse a systemic reaction, should one occur.

Nursing Diagnoses
6, 24, 75, 108

Nursing Interventions
Monitoring

1. Monitor vital signs, skin color, and degree of restlessness, which may indicate hypoxia.

2. Monitor airway functioning through peak flow measurements to assess effectiveness of treatment.

a. Place the indicator at base of the numbered scale.

b. Have the patient stand or sit upright and take a deep breath.

c. Have the patient place the meter in the mouth and close lips around it, with tongue under mouthpiece.

d. Ask the patient to blow out as hard and fast as possible; coughing or spitting will result in falsely elevated measurement.

e. Note the measurement that the indicator is pointing to on the number scale.

f. Repeat twice more and record the highest measurement.

3. Monitor oxygen saturation through finger oximetry and correlate to arterial blood gas measurement as indicated.

4. Monitor outpatient's peak flow record, which may indicate change is needed in treatment plan.

5. Monitor patient's understanding of treatment plan, appropriate use of medications, and correct technique for inhaler and spacer at regular intervals to ensure optimum therapy.

EMERGENCY ALERT Be aware of the following demographic and history factors that increase risk of asthma-related death: Adolescence, black ethnicity, at least two hospitalizations or three emergency department visits in the past year, use of two canisters per month of short-acting bronchodilator, current or recent use of oral corticosteroids, poor perception of severity, poor access to health care, history of depression, sensitivity to mold, and illicit drug use.

Supportive Care

1. Provide nebulization and oxygen therapy as prescribed.

2. Encourage fluid intake to liquefy secretions.
   a. Avoid iced fluids, which may cause bronchospasm.
   b. Avoid carbonated beverages, which may contribute to acidosis.

3. Instruct patient on positioning to facilitate breathing, for example, sitting upright (leaning forward on a table).

4. Employ chest physical therapy and postural drainage to mobilize secretions as needed.

5. Encourage patient to use pursed-lip breathing to decrease the work of breathing.

A

BOX A-3   How to Use an Inhaler

- Make sure that the medication canister is attached to the plastic inhaler and shake well, or load the medication disc according to manufacturer's instructions (for some dry powder inhaler [DPI] systems).
- Attach a spacer if recommended with your metered dose inhaler (MDI). A spacer is preferred, especially for children and anyone having difficulty with technique.
- Breathe out through your mouth while standing or sitting.
- If not using a spacer, the open-mouth method is preferred with an MDI:
  - Hold the inhaler up to 2 inches (5 cm) away from your mouth.
  - While starting to inhale through your open mouth, press down firmly on the top of the canister with your index finger.
  - Continue to inhale for 3 to 5 seconds to obtain a full breath, then try to hold your breath for 5 to 10 seconds.
- If using the closed-mouth method (recommended for DPI systems):
  - Place the mouthpiece of the inhaler in your mouth and close your lips tightly around it.
  - While starting to inhale, press down firmly on the canister with your index finger.
  - Continue to inhale for 3 to 5 seconds to obtain a full breath, then hold your breath for 5 to 10 seconds.
  - Remove the inhaler from your mouth before you exhale.
- Wait at least 30 seconds before you take your next inhalation if more than one is prescribed.

Education and Health Maintenance

1. Provide information on the nature of asthma and methods of treatment, including proper use of inhaler devices; warn against overuse of inhalers and nebulizers. (See *Box A-3*.)

COMMUNITY CARE CONSIDERATIONS

Review techniques for using the metered-dose inhaler and spacer at every follow-up visit.

2. Demonstrate the use of peak flow meter and recording of peak flow measurements. Review action plan (as prescribed by health care provider) for exacerbations. Make sure that the patient understands that long-acting bronchodilating inhalers (such as salmeterol) are not effective for asthma exacerbations.

3. Help patient to identify what triggers asthma, warning signs of an impending attack, and strategies for preventing an attack. Inform the patient of the link between attacks and emotional stress.

4. Warn the patient about using a central nervous system depressant after an asthma attack because these medications slow respirations and make breathing more difficult.

5. Teach deep-breathing exercises to prevent atelectasis. Suggest breathing exercises for children at home, such as blowing a cotton ball across a tabletop or blowing large soap bubbles.

6. Discuss methods of environmental control.
   a. Avoid persons with respiratory infections.
   b. Avoid substances and situations known to precipitate bronchospasm, such as irritants, gases, fumes, and smoke.
   c. Wear a scarf across nose and mouth if cold weather precipitates bronchospasm.
   d. Stay inside when air pollution is high.

■ **PEDIATRIC ALERT** Assist the family with obtaining a written asthma management plan from the health care provider; this will ensure quick access to medication at school.

7. Promote optimal health practices, including nutrition, rest, and exercise.
   a. Encourage regular exercise to improve cardiorespiratory and musculoskeletal conditioning.
   b. Drink liberal amounts of fluids to keep secretions thin.
   c. Try to avoid upsetting situations.
   d. Use relaxation techniques, biofeedback management.
   e. Use community resources for smoking-cessation classes, stress management, exercises for relaxation, and so forth.

8. Help families to maintain sense of normalcy in everyday activities despite chronic disease. Physical activity should

be encouraged when asthma is controlled; children may benefit from participating in sports.

9. For additional information and support, refer patient to American Academy of Allergy, Asthma, and Immunology, *www.aaaai.org*.

ATOPIC DERMATITIS

See *Dermatitis, Atopic*.

ATTENTION DEFICIT DISORDER AND LEARNING DISABILITIES

Attention deficit disorder (ADD) and attention deficit hyperactivity disorder (ADHD) are characterized by a cluster of symptoms, such as developmentally inappropriate short attention span, impulsivity, and distractibility — hyperactivity is not always present. Learning disabilities are defined as individual achievement that is significantly below what is expected for age, schooling, and level of intelligence. It is a problem with how the brain processes information that it receives, not a problem with the reception of information. Learning disabilities and ADD often occur together.

The exact causes of ADD and learning disabilities are not known; however, chromosomal abnormalities, inborn errors of metabolism, various prenatal and postnatal factors, neurotransmitter disturbances in the brain, and affinity with other handicapping conditions (eg, spina bifida, cerebral palsy, and seizure disorders) are being investigated. There is no evidence linking ADD or learning disabilities with a history of brain damage.

ALTERNATIVE INTERVENTION

Diet has not been proven to be a causative factor in ADD, ADHD, or learning disabilities. Also, diet therapies have shown no effect on the treatment of any of these disorders.

Assessment

Estimates of the incidence of ADD among children range from 2% to 9%; learning disability is reportedly present in approximately 13% of children at the end of second grade. Boys are diagnosed twice as frequently as girls, and girls are less likely to exhibit disruptive behaviors. These disorders may also be diagnosed in college-age and adulthood, characterized as an inability to focus.

1. ADD — According to the American Psychiatric Association, a child must have at least 8 of the 14 symptoms listed below and meet the following criteria: Symptoms for more than 6 months, symptoms are maladaptive, behavior is inappropriate for child's developmental level, ADD symptom onset before age 7, symptoms apparent in at least two settings, and another disorder cannot explain symptoms.

   a. Fidgeting with hands or feet or squirming in seat
   b. Difficulty remaining seated when required to do so
   c. Easily distracted by extraneous stimuli
   d. Difficulty awaiting his turn
   e. Blurts out answers to questions before they have been completed
   f. Difficulty following instructions from others
   g. Difficulty sustaining attention in tasks or at play
   h. Shifts from one uncompleted activity to another
   i. Difficulty playing quietly
   j. Talks excessively
   k. Interrupts or intrudes on others
   l. Does not seem to listen to what is being said to him or her
   m. Often loses things necessary for tasks or activities at school or at home
   n. Often engages in physically dangerous activities without considering possible consequences

2. Learning disabilities — School achievement is significantly below that expected for age, schooling, and level of intelligence
   a. No diminished mental capacity.
   b. Intelligence is usually normal or above normal.
   c. Difficulty learning basic education skills (reading, math).
   d. Skills in certain areas fall below performance in other areas.

Diagnostic Evaluation

1. Complete medical review, family history, and physical examination, including vision and hearing assessment and neurologic evaluation are performed to rule out other disorders.
2. Psychological testing is done to determine the exact nature of cognitive and perceptual dysfunctions.
3. Behavioral and social assessment.
4. Assessment of academic performance.
5. School evaluation, school psychologist, IQ testing, teacher input. Historically, preschool and kindergarten screening tools have not been accurate in predicting learning disabilities; newer tests of language and memory appear to be better predictors.
6. Occupational and physical therapy, speech and language evaluations as necessary to determine therapeutic plan.
7. MRI and other testing determine underlying neurologic abnormalities if indicated.

Collaborative Management
Therapeutic Interventions

1. Multidisciplinary approach, including behavioral and environmental approaches
2. For children with learning disabilities, special teaching strategies:
   a. For visual perceptual deficit: Present material verbally; use hands-on experience; tape-record teaching sessions.
   b. For auditory perceptual deficit: Provide materials in written form; use pictures; provide tactile learning.
   c. For integrative deficit: Use multisensory approaches; print directions while you verbalize them; use calendars and lists to organize tasks and activities.
   d. For motor/expressive deficits: Break down skills and projects into their multiple component parts; verbally describe the component parts; provide extra time to perform; allow child to type work rather than using cursive writing.

 e. For highly distractible child: Provide a structured environment; have child sit in front of class; place child away from doors or windows; decrease clutter on desk.

Pharmacologic Interventions

1. Central nervous system (CNS) stimulants are effective in 70% to 75% of ADD children (usually reserved for children older than age 7). Commonly used drugs are methylphenidate, dextroamphetamine, pemoline, clonidine, and atomoxetine.
2. Adverse effects of CNS stimulants:
 a. Insomnia may result from increased dosage or if administered too late in the day.
 b. Anorexia weight loss, hair loss, and temporary growth retardation. Height will catch up after medication is discontinued.
 c. Increased pulse and respiratory rates, nervousness, nausea, and stomach ache.
 d. Liver dysfunction with pemoline; periodic liver function tests are required.
 e. Altered effects of many antiseizure drugs and tricyclic antidepressants.
3. Does not cause euphoric effect or addiction in children.

Nursing Diagnoses
24, 53, 78, 90, 129, 133

Nursing Interventions
Supportive Care and Education

1. Educate family and school on drug regimen.
 a. Teach parents to administer medications before breakfast and lunch (sustained-release forms do not require a lunchtime dose).
 b. Work with school system to ensure lunch dose is administered.
 c. Recommend "drug holidays" during vacations and weekends to monitor effectiveness and the need for change; this is especially recommended at the start of each academic school year.

d. Advise parents that the child is usually started on a small dose, which is gradually increased until the desired response is achieved.

e. Evaluate the child's response to medication by direct observation and consultation with others, such as parents and teachers.

2. Promote family function.

a. Educate parents on nature of diagnosis.

b. Emphasize need for consistency in routines, rules, acceptable behavior, and so forth.

c. Identify situations in which the child may have difficulties.

d. Encourage parents to accept their child, celebrating strengths.

e. Teach parent to apply behavioral techniques of discipline.

f. Discuss long-term damage to self-esteem if child receives constant negative feedback.

3. Refer to resource groups such as Learning Disability Association of America, *www.ldanatl.org*, Children and Adults with Attention Deficit Disorders (CHADD), *www.chadd.org*.

B

BACK PAIN, LOW

Low back pain is characterized by uncomfortable or acute pain in the lumbosacral area related to severe spasm of the paraspinal muscles, often with radiating pain. Low back pain may result from joint disease, muscular strain, or ligamentous sprains; disk infection, degeneration, or herniation; weakness and deconditioning; arthritis; bone diseases; metastatic carcinoma; spinal cord tumors; congenital or systemic disorders; or vertebral infections. It may also result from referred pain from other areas. Complications include spinal instability, sensory and motor deficits, and chronic pain.

Assessment

1. Pain localized to low back or radiating to buttocks or one or both legs
2. Paresthesia, numbness, weakness of lower extremities
3. Reflex loss
4. Bowel or bladder dysfunction (with cauda equina compression)

Diagnostic Evaluation

1. X-rays of lumbar spine are usually negative.
2. CT scan of spine detects arthritic changes, degenerative disk disease, tumor, and other abnormalities.
3. Myelography confirms and localizes disk herniation.
4. MRI detects pathology: disc herniation, soft tissue injury, and so forth.
5. Electromyography of lower extremities detects nerve changes related to back pathology.
6. Diskogram detects herniated disk.

Collaborative Management

For management of herniated disk, see page 461.
For management of spinal cord tumors, see page 898.

Therapeutic Interventions

1. Bed rest in a supine to semi-Fowler's position with hips and knees flexed (bed rest limited to phase of acute pain and spasm). Relieves painful muscle strain and ligament sprain, heals soft tissue injury, removes stress from lumbar sacral area and sciatic nerves, and opens the posterior part of the intervertebral spaces.

   a. Acute spasm and pain should subside in 3 to 7 days if there is no nerve involvement or other serious underlying disease.

   b. Isometric exercises should be done hourly while in bed.

2. Heat or ice may be applied to relax muscle spasm and relieve discomfort. Follow heat by massage.

3. Lumbosacral support may be used to provide abdominal compression and to decrease load on lumbar intervertebral disks.

4. Transcutaneous electrical nerve stimulation may be helpful in relieving pain.

5. Physical therapy may be needed for acute stage and rehabilitation.

6. Psychiatric intervention may be needed for the patient with chronic depression, anxiety, and low back syndrome.

7. Focus on getting the patient back to functional state after long disability and prevention of recurrence through maintaining an ideal body weight, exercising, and protecting back from injury.

Pharmacologic Interventions

1. Nonsteroidal anti-inflammatory drugs (NSAIDs) are used for analgesic and anti-inflammatory properties. Oral corticosteroids may also be used.

2. Painful trigger points may be injected with hydrocortisone or lidocaine for pain relief.

3. Oral and parenteral opioid pain medication may be used in acute severe pain syndromes.

4. Muscle relaxants, including diazepam and cyclobenzaprine, are used to relieve spasm.

5. Psychotropic medication may be used for chronic pain and treatment of depression and anxiety, which exacerbate pain.

Nursing Diagnoses
3, 13, 107, 141, 144, 148

Nursing Interventions
Monitoring
1. Monitor pain level and compliance with activity restrictions.
2. Monitor for neurologic deficits indicating spinal nerve involvement, including reflex, sensory, and strength changes.

Supportive Care
1. Advise bed rest on firm mattress or with bed boards beneath mattress for support. Bed rest may reduce the need for pain medications. Patient may get up to go to the bathroom and to eat meals.
2. Keep pillow between flexed knees while patient is in side-lying position to minimize strain on back muscles.
3. Apply heat or ice as prescribed.
4. Administer or teach self-administration of pain medications and muscle relaxants as prescribed.
   a. Give NSAIDs with meals to prevent GI upset and bleeding.
   b. Muscle relaxants may cause drowsiness.
5. Encourage range-of-motion exercises of all uninvolved muscle groups.
6. Suggest gradual increase of activities and alternation of activities with rest in semi-Fowler's position.
7. Avoid prolonged periods of sitting.
8. Encourage the patient to discuss problems that may be contributing to his low back pain.
9. Encourage the patient to do prescribed back exercises to keep postural muscles strong, help recondition the back and abdominal musculature, and allow an outlet for emotional tension. (See *Figure B-1*.)

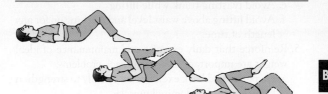

FIGURE B-1 Back exercises to strengthen abdominal and postural muscles, to stretch contracted back muscles, and to maintain flexibility.

Education and Health Maintenance

1. Instruct the patient to avoid recurrences as follows:
   a. Avoid prolonged sitting (intradiskal pressure in lumbar spine is higher during sitting), standing, and driving.
   b. Change positions and rest at frequent intervals.
   c. Avoid assuming tense, cramped positions.
   d. Sit in a straight-back, fairly high-seated chair. Sit with the knees higher than the hips. Use a footstool.
   e. Flatten the hollow of the back by sitting with the buttocks "tucked under." Pelvic tilt (small of back is pressed against a flat surface) decreases lordosis.
   f. Avoid knee and hip extension. When driving a car, have the seat pushed forward as necessary for comfort. Place a cushion in the small of the back for support.
2. Tell the patient to rest one foot on a small stool to relieve lumbar lordosis when sitting or standing for an extended period of time.
3. Tell the patient to avoid fatigue, which contributes to spasm of back muscles.
4. Teach the patient how to pick up objects or loads correctly:
   a. Maintain a straight spine.
   b. Flex knees and hips while stooping.
   c. Keep load close to body.
   d. Lift with the legs.

    e. Avoid twisting trunk while lifting.

    f. Avoid lifting above waist level and reaching up for any length of time.

5. Reinforce that daily exercise and maintenance of ideal weight are important to prevent back problems.

    a. Do prescribed back exercises twice daily to strengthen back, leg, and abdominal muscles.

    b. Walking outdoors (progressively increasing distance and pace) is recommended.

BACTERIAL ENDOCARDITIS

See *Endocarditis, Infective.*

BARTHOLIN CYST OR ABSCESS

Bartholin cyst or abscess, also called bartholinitis, results from obstruction and infection of the greater vestibular (Bartholin's) glands, which lie on both sides of the vagina at the base of the labia minora and serve to lubricate the vagina. (See *Figure B-2.*) Most cases are sterile, but some may result from cellulitis caused by mixed vaginal flora (abscesses). The abscess or cyst may spontaneously rupture or enlarge and become painful. Infection is often caused by sexually transmitted disease (STD).

Assessment

1. May be asymptomatic

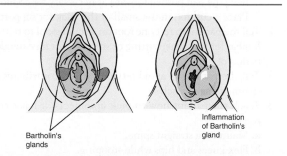

Inflammation
of Bartholin's
gland

Bartholin's
glands

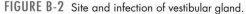

FIGURE B-2 Site and infection of vestibular gland.

2. Warmth, erythema, pain, swelling in labia minora
3. If abscess is present—pain, edema, cellulitis

Diagnostic Evaluation
1. Culture of drainage or aspirated fluid identifies infectious organisms.
2. Biopsy (indicated for women over age 40) rules out cancer.

B

Collaborative Management
Therapeutic and Pharmacologic Interventions
1. Provide warm soaks or sitz baths.
2. If cellulitis or STD is present, administer antibiotics.

Surgical Interventions
1. Abscess or cyst may require incision and drainage. Although this provides immediate relief, problem may recur.
2. Marsupialization, for recurrent abscesses:
   a. Contents are opened and drained; Ward catheter is then inserted to keep cavity open.
   b. Healing occurs from within the area of the abscess.

Nursing Diagnoses
3, 67, 135

Nursing Interventions
Supportive Care
1. Administer pain medications as indicated.
2. Instruct the patient to apply warm soaks or take sitz bath three to four times a day for 15 to 20 minutes to promote comfort and drainage.
3. Encourage the patient to remain in bed as much as possible, because pain is exacerbated by activity.
4. Prepare the patient for incision and drainage if indicated.
5. For marsupialization: Apply ice packs intermittently for 24 hours to reduce edema and provide comfort; thereafter, warm sitz baths or a perineal heat pack or lamp can be used.

6. If caused by STD:
   a. Tell the patient to instruct her partner to be tested and treated for STD.
   b. Advise the patient to abstain from intercourse until cyst or abscess has completely resolved and she has completed her antibiotic regimen.

Education and Health Maintenance
1. Review principles of perineal hygiene with the patient.
2. Discuss STD and methods of prevention.
3. Encourage patient to follow up for recurrent abscess to rule out malignancy. Surgical treatment is often necessary for recurrence.

BIPOLAR DISORDERS

Bipolar disorders are characterized by depressive episodes and one or more elated mood episodes. Although its exact cause is unknown, genetic, biochemical, and psychological factors are thought to play a role. In its most intense presentation, bipolar disorder produces altered thought processes that can produce bizarre delusions. Bipolar disorder can lead to physical exhaustion, if left untreated.

Assessment
Characteristics according to the American Psychiatric Association's *Diagnostic and Statistical Manual of Mental Disorders*, 4th edition, Text Revision (*DSM-IV-TR*):
1. Bipolar I disorder:
   a. Presence of only one manic episode.
   b. No past major depressive episodes.
   c. Manic episode is not accounted for by schizoaffective disorder.
   d. Manic episode is not superimposed on schizophrenia, schizophreniform disorder, delusional disorder, or psychotic disorder.
   e. May be further specified as mixed symptoms, psychotic, in remission, with catatonic features, or postpartum onset.
2. Bipolar II disorder:

a. Presence/history of one or more major depressive episodes.
b. Presence/history of at least one hypomanic episode.
c. No manic or mixed episodes have occurred.
d. The symptoms cause clinically significant distress or impaired social or occupational functioning.
e. May be further specified as hypomanic or depressed.

3. Cyclothymic disorder:
a. Over a period of 2 years, there are numerous periods with hypomanic symptoms and numerous periods with depressive symptoms that do not meet criteria for a major depressive episode.
b. During the 2-year period, the patient has not been without these symptoms for more than 2 months at a time.
c. During the 2-year period, no major depressive episode, manic episode, or mixed episode has occurred.
d. Symptoms are not caused by physiologic aspects.
e. Symptoms cause clinically significant distress or impairment in all aspects of functioning.

Diagnostic Evaluation

1. Complete psychologic examination and rating scale assessment tools:
a. Mania Rating Scale
b. Young Manic State
2. Laboratory testing to rule out other disorders.

Collaborative Management
Therapeutic Interventions

1. Psychotherapy includes individual therapy and family therapy.
2. Psychiatric home care nursing may be required to facilitate compliance with medications and therapeutic interventions.
3. Community-based support group participation may be recommended.

Pharmacologic Interventions

1. For acute mania: usually treated in the hospital to ensure a safe environment to initiate and stabilize medication.
   a. Lithium carbonate, aripiprazole, carbamazepine, and valproate may be used as mood stabilizers.
   b. Adjunctive treatment includes neuroleptic agents, such as risperidone for psychotic thinking, and benzodiazepines such as clonazepam for agitation.

DRUG ALERT Lithium toxicity is often related to decreased serum sodium level and inadequate hydration. Patients should have a liberal sodium intake and consume 2 or 3 qt (2 or 3 L) of water daily. Lithium level should be monitored frequently.

2. Maintenance therapy is instituted once stabilized, to control depression and mania. Use of a selective serotonin reuptake inhibitor antidepressant is cautioned because it may stimulate mania.

Nursing Diagnoses

34, 35, 136, 152

Nursing Interventions

Monitoring

1. Monitor mood for range of affect.
2. Monitor behavior for hyperactivity, increased appetite, indiscriminate sexual activity, poor concentration, little or no sleep, spending large sums of money, and other inappropriate acts.
3. Monitor thought processes for flight of ideas, sexually explicit speech, delusions, hallucinations, and clang associations (sound of word [rather than meanings] directs subsequent associations).
4. Monitor vital signs, weight, and urine output for patient in acute mania.
5. Monitor serum thyroid function tests, white blood cell count, lithium levels, and electrolytes for patient on lithium.
6. Monitor liver function tests, platelet count, and serum drug levels for patient on valproate.
7. Monitor for suicidal ideation or planning.

Supportive Care

1. Assess patient's degree of distorted thinking; redirect the patient if it becomes difficult to follow patient's thought processes.
2. Use brief explanations; remain consistent in approach and expectations.
3. Frequently reality-orient the patient; speak in a clear, simple manner.
4. Provide the patient with a relaxing area with decreased environmental stimulation.
5. Assist the patient with a gradual and progressive integration into the social environment while observing for behavioral changes that indicate readiness for participation in additional activities.
6. To facilitate adequate sleep, establish a distraction-free environment at bedtime. Help the patient find ways to avoid caffeine and nicotine.
7. Administer prescribed medications as ordered and monitor the patient's response.
8. Maintain accurate documentation of food and fluid intake.
9. Offer small, frequent meals of high-calorie food. Include finger foods, which are easy to eat.
10. Serve the patient meals in a low-stimulus environment.
11. Observe and assess interaction patterns within the family and discuss their influence on the patient and his family functioning.

Education and Health Maintenance

1. Reinforce instructions to patient and family about bipolar illness; teach about symptoms of relapse.
2. Instruct patient and family members about psychopharmacologic treatment, including its purpose, effects, adverse effects, and management. Encourage follow-up for blood work and monitoring by psychiatrist.
3. Advise patient and family members about community-based support groups or health care agencies that are relevant to their care such as National Alliance for Mental Health, *www.nami.org*.

BLADDER CANCER

See *Cancer, Bladder*.

BONE CANCER

See *Cancer, Bone*.

BRAIN TUMORS IN ADULTS

A brain tumor is a localized intracranial neoplasm. Tumors may originate in any tissue in the central nervous system or may metastasize from tumors elsewhere in the body. There are many types of benign or malignant brain tumors, and all produce effects of a space-occupying lesion (cerebral edema, increased intracranial pressure [ICP]). Malignancy may be related not to cell type or invasiveness but, rather, to location and inoperability.

Tumor types include astrocytoma (arising from connective tissue of the brain, highly invasive); glioblastoma (grade 3 and 4 astrocytomas); oligodendroglioma (arising from frontal and temporal lobes of the cerebrum); colloid cyst (develops with lateral or third ventricles); meningioma (arising from linings of the brain); acoustic neuroma (develops in or on eighth cranial nerve); metastatic lesions (usually multiple and unresectable); developmental tumors (pituitary, pineal, and other tumors); hemangioma (from blood vessels of the brain); and congenital tumors. Complications include increased ICP and brain herniation and neurologic deficits from the expanding tumor or treatment.

Assessment

1. Signs and symptoms of tumor caused by increased ICP, including morning headaches, vomiting, papilledema, altered mental status, and malaise.
2. Cranial nerve, motor, sensory, behavioral, affect, and cognitive dysfunction are possible.
3. Focal neurologic deficits related to region of tumor:
   a. Parietal area — motor or sensory alterations, speech and memory disturbances, visuospatial deficits

    b. Frontal lobe — personality changes, contralateral motor weakness, Broca's aphasia

    c. Temporal area — memory disturbances, auditory hallucinations, Wernicke's aphasia, complex partial seizures, visual field deficits

    d. Occipital area — visual agnosia and visual field deficits

    e. Cerebellar area — coordination, gait and balance disturbances

    f. Brain stem — dysphagia, incontinence, cardiovascular instability, cranial nerve dysfunction

    g. Hypothalamus — loss of temperature control, diabetes insipidus

    h. Pituitary/sella turcica — visual field deficits, amenorrhea, galactorrhea, impotence, cushingoid symptoms

4. Seizures

Diagnostic Evaluation

1. CT scan or MRI visualize tumor, associated edema, and shift of structures caused by mass effect.
2. EEG detects locus of irritability.
3. Lumbar puncture may be done for cytology; however, if increased ICP is suspected, caution should be used due to danger of brain stem herniation.
4. Angiogram detects vascular tumors.
5. Cerebral blood flow studies determine progression of tumor.
6. MRI spectroscopy differentiates tumor from infectious lesion; functional MRI determines the eloquence of brain tissue affected by the tumor (affects treatment).

Collaborative Management
Therapeutic and Pharmacologic Interventions

1. Effectiveness of treatment depends on tumor type and location, capsulation, or infiltrative status. Tumors in vital areas such as the brain stem or those that are nonencapsulated and infiltrating may not be surgically accessible, and treatment may produce severe neurologic deficits (blindness, paralysis, mental impairment).

2. Whole-brain radiation may begin after scalp incision heals (may cause brain edema and delayed necrosis), or brachytherapy (radioisotopes implanted directly into tumor to allow for high doses) may be performed.

3. Single or combination chemotherapy may be used. Autologous bone marrow transplantation may be performed, in which bone marrow is aspirated before chemotherapy and reinfused afterward to treat bone marrow depression.

Surgical Interventions

1. Procedures include removal or debulking by craniotomy, laser resection, or ultrasonic aspiration.
   a. Awake craniotomy allows for intraoperative brain mapping.
   b. Image-guided surgery uses computer images for removal and debulking.

2. Preoperative endovascular treatment allows embolization of the vascular supply to the tumor.

3. Anticonvulsants and corticosteroids are used as supportive therapy.

Nursing Diagnoses
3, 6, 51, 67, 135, 136

Nursing Interventions
Monitoring

1. Monitor the patient's response to therapy. Be alert for change in level of consciousness (LOC), neurologic deficits, increased ICP, and abnormal respirations.

2. Report immediately any signs of increased ICP (decreased LOC, elevated temperature, widening pulse pressure, bradycardia, irregular respirations, pupillary changes, headache, vomiting) or worsening condition.

3. Monitor for seizure activity and have medications available for management of status epilepticus.

4. Monitor fluid and electrolyte balance to prevent dehydration.

Supportive Care

1. Provide analgesics and comfort measures according to patient's level of pain, as ordered.
   a. Maintain a quiet environment to increase the patient's pain tolerance.
   b. Provide scheduled rest periods to help the patient recuperate from stress of pain.
   c. Darken the room or provide sunglasses if the patient is photophobic.
2. Instruct the patient to lie with the operative side up.
3. Maintain the head of the bed at 15 to 30 degrees to reduce cerebral venous congestion; if the patient is dysphagic or unconscious, position the head to the side to prevent aspiration.
4. Position dysphagic patient upright, and instruct him in sequenced swallowing to facilitate feeding.
   a. Keep oxygen and suction equipment at bedside in case of aspiration.
   b. Alter diet as tolerated if the patient has pain when chewing.
5. If the patient has visual field deficits, place materials in visual field; teach the patient to scan to the "other side" and place weak extremities in safe position when moving in bed or chair.
6. Pad the side rails of the bed and have tongue blade available to prevent injury if seizures occur.
7. Explain possible adverse effects of chemotherapy and provide supportive care for anorexia, fatigue, nausea and vomiting, mucositis, anemia, neutropenia, thrombocytopenia, and alopecia.
8. Explain possible adverse effects of radiation therapy and provide supportive care for skin irritation, fatigue, nausea and vomiting, diarrhea, esophagitis, mucositis, xerostomia, dry cough, and cystitis.
9. Provide support and appropriate preoperative and postoperative care for the patient undergoing craniotomy (see page 239.)
10. Help the patient verbalize fears about growth of the tumor, surgery, loss of hair, neurologic deficits, inability to

work and care for family, and, possibly, death. Provide information, support, and referral to counseling as needed.

Education and Health Maintenance

1. Explain the adverse effects of treatment, such as nausea, vomiting, alopecia, and bone marrow depression.
2. Encourage close follow-up after diagnosis and treatment.
3. Explain the importance of continuing corticosteroids and how to manage adverse effects, such as weight gain and hyperglycemia.
4. Encourage the use of community resources for physical and psychological support, such as transportation to medical appointments, financial assistance, and respite care.
5. Refer the patient and family to American Brain Tumor Association, *www.abta.org*; American Cancer Society, *www.cancer.org*.

BRAIN TUMORS IN CHILDREN

Brain tumors in children, as in adults, are localized intracranial neoplasms that produce effects of a space-occupying lesion. They are the second most common cancers in children. There are four main types of brain tumors in children.

Cerebellar astrocytoma is a slow-growing, often cystic type of tumor of the cerebellum.

Medulloblastoma (the most common type of brain tumor in children) is a highly malignant, rapidly growing tumor, usually found in the cerebellum. As the tumor grows, it seeds along cerebrospinal fluid (CSF) pathways.

Brain stem glioma interferes early on with the function of cranial nerve nuclei, pyramidal tracts, and cerebellar pathways. This type accounts for approximately 15% of brain tumors in children.

Ependymoma is a tumor derived from the ependyma (the lining of the central canal of the spinal cord) and cerebral ventricles. It commonly arises on the floor of the fourth ventricle, obstructing CSF flow. These tumors may invade the cardiorespiratory center, cerebellum, and spinal cord.

Prognosis is improved with early diagnosis and adequate therapy. The 5-year survival rate is increasing, especially in children with low-grade astrocytomas or ependymomas. Without treatment, however, brain stem herniation and hydrocephalus may occur.

Assessment

1. Cerebellar astrocytoma — insidious onset and slow course
   a. Increased intracranial pressure (ICP) (see Box B-1)
   b. Cerebellar signs — ataxia, dysmetria (inability to control the range of muscular movement), and nystagmus
   c. Seizures
   d. Precocious puberty
2. Medulloblastoma
   a. Similar to manifestations of cerebellar astrocytoma, but condition develops more rapidly.
   b. The child may present with unsteady gait, anorexia, vomiting, and early-morning headache, and later de-

---

BOX B-1 | **Signs and Symptoms of Increased ICP in Infants and Children**

- Vomiting
- Restlessness and irritability
- High-pitched, shrill cry (infants)
- Rapid increase in head circumference (infants)
- Tense, bulging fontanelle (infants)
- Changes in vital signs:
  - Increased systolic blood pressure
  - Decreased pulse
  - Decreased and irregular respirations
  - Increased temperature
- Pupillary changes
- Papilledema
- Possible seizures
- Lethargy, stupor, coma
- Older children may also experience:
  - Headache, especially on awakening
  - Lethargy, fatigue, apathy
  - Personality changes
  - Separation of cranial sutures (may be seen in children up to age 10)
  - Visual changes such as double vision

velop ataxia, nystagmus, papilledema, head tilt cranial nerve palsies, drowsiness, and increased head circumference.
  c. Obstructive hydrocephalus may result.
3. Brain stem glioma
  a. Cranial nerve palsies, such as strabismus, fasciculations of the tongue, and swallowing difficulties
  b. Hemiparesis, cerebellar ataxia
  c. Signs of ICP (advanced disease)
4. Ependymoma
  a. Signs of ICP that are nonspecific and nonlocalizing

Diagnostic Evaluation

1. Several or all of the following procedures may be used to localize and determine tumor extent:
  a. CT scan
  b. MRI
  c. Myelogram
  d. Positron emission tomography
  e. Lumbar puncture
  f. Angiography

Collaborative Management
Surgical Interventions

1. Surgery is performed to determine the type of the tumor and the extent of invasiveness and to excise as much of the lesion as possible.
2. A ventriculoperitoneal shunt is often necessary for children who develop hydrocephalus.
3. Corticosteroids may be used as adjunct therapy to reduce cerebral swelling.

Therapeutic and Pharmacologic Interventions

1. Radiation therapy is usually initiated as soon as the diagnosis is established and the surgical wound is healed.
2. Chemotherapy is used in children younger than age 4 with medulloblastoma (to avoid early radiation) and in children with ependymomas.

Nursing Diagnoses

3, 30, 44, 51, 62, 135, 136

Nursing Interventions

Monitoring

1. Monitor vital signs, level of consciousness, and pupillary reaction frequently.
2. Observe for signs of brain stem herniation (a neurosurgical emergency).
   a. Attacks of opisthotonos (see *Figure B-3*)
   b. Tilting of the head; neck stiffness
   c. Poorly reactive pupils
   d. Increased blood pressure; widened pulse pressure
   e. Change in respiratory rate and nature of respirations
   f. Irregularity of pulse or lowered pulse rate
   g. Alterations of body temperature

⚡ **EMERGENCY ALERT** Signs of brain stem herniation, especially opisthotonos, are ominous. The health care provider should be called immediately, and the child should be prepared for ventricular tap to relieve pressure. Resuscitation equipment should be on hand.

3. Monitor temperature closely after surgery.
   a. A marked rise in temperature may be attributable to trauma, disturbance of the heat-regulating center, or to intracranial edema.

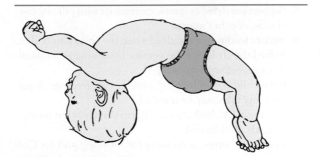

FIGURE B-3 Opisthotonos, a sign of brain stem herniation.

    b. If hyperthermia occurs, administer antipyretics and sponge baths as ordered. Temperature should not be reduced too rapidly.

4. Observe for signs of shock, increased ICP, and altered level of consciousness.

Supportive Care

1. Prepare the parents for the postoperative appearance of their child; advise that the child might be comatose immediately after surgery.
2. Prepare the child for surgery; explain procedures at the appropriate developmental level.
3. Prepare the child for postoperative expectations (ie, child may feel sleepy or have a headache and will need to remain supine).
4. Administer opioids as ordered in the immediate postoperative period; assess the child's level of consciousness before administration.
5. Position the child according to surgeon's request, usually on unaffected side with head level. Raising the foot of the bed may increase ICP and bleeding.
6. Change the child's position frequently and provide meticulous skin care to prevent hypostatic pneumonia and pressure sores.
7. Move the child carefully and slowly, being certain to move the head in line with the body.
8. Support paralyzed or spastic extremities with pillows, towel rolls, or other means.
9. Initiate feeding for the child when the child is fully alert. Refeed the child after he vomits. (Vomiting is not usually associated with nausea.)
10. If the child is unable to eat, provide tube feedings. A gastrostomy tube may be inserted.
11. Maintain I.V. hydration or hyperalimentation and intralipids, if indicated.
12. Check the surgical dressing for bleeding and for CSF drainage.
13. Assess the child for edema of the head, face, and neck.

14. Carefully regulate fluid administration to prevent increased cerebral edema.
15. Have equipment readily available for cardiopulmonary resuscitation, respiratory assistance, oxygen inhalation, blood transfusion, ventricular tap, and other potential emergency situations.
16. If the child is receiving chemotherapy or radiation, instruct the parents to report a fever of over 101° F (38.4° C) or nausea and vomiting unrelated to chemotherapy.
17. Encourage the child to express feelings regarding the changes in body image (ie, hair loss).
18. Reassure the child that he will be able to wear a wig or a hat after recovery; hair will grow back following surgery, but does not grow back at radiation site.
19. Help the parents to see the child's increasing capabilities and encourage them to foster independence.

Education and Health Maintenance

1. Provide parents with written information regarding the child's needs—medications, activity, care of the incision, and follow-up appointments.
2. Teach the parents about radiation or chemotherapy treatments and their adverse effects. Corticosteroids may cause cushingoid changes (moonface, weight gain, edema) if used for extended period.
3. If a child has a ventriculoperitoneal shunt, teach parents to recognize and report fever, nausea, vomiting, irritability, or a bulging anterior fontanelle.
4. Initiate a referral to a community health nurse to reinforce teaching and to maintain therapeutic support for the family.
5. For additional resources, refer family to agencies such as American Brain Tumor Association, *www.abta.org*; Candlelighters, *www.candlelighters.org*.

BREAST CANCER

See *Cancer, Breast.*

BRONCHIECTASIS

Bronchiectasis is a chronic dilatation of the bronchi and bronchioles caused by inflammation and destruction of bronchiolar walls. Sputum accumulates and obstructs the bronchioles; poor airway clearance results in severe coughing, which permanently dilates the bronchi. This disorder usually involves the lower lung lobes and may progress to atelectasis, fibrosis, and respiratory insufficiency. Bronchiectasis is commonly caused by pulmonary infections; bronchial obstruction; aspiration of foreign bodies, vomitus, or material from the upper respiratory tract; and immunologic disorders.

Complications include progressive suppuration, major pulmonary hemorrhage, emphysema, and chronic respiratory insufficiency.

Assessment

1. Persistent cough, with copious amounts of purulent sputum; intermittent hemoptysis; breathlessness.
2. Diffuse rhonchi and coarse crackles heard over involved lobes during inspiration.
3. Recurrent fever and pulmonary infections.
4. Finger clubbing commonly occurs late in the disorder.

Diagnostic Evaluation

1. Chest radiographs detect areas of atelectasis with widespread dilatation of bronchi.
2. Sputum specimens for smears and cultures identify causative organisms.
3. High-resolution CT scan confirms diagnosis.

Collaborative Management

Therapeutic Interventions

1. Smoking-cessation program to reduce infections
2. Chest physiotherapy and postural drainage to mobilize bronchial secretions

Pharmacologic Interventions

1. Antimicrobials to treat exacerbations of infection.

2. Bronchodilators are effective for selected patients with increased airway hyperreactivity.
3. Influenza immunization yearly and pneumococcal pneumonia vaccine to protect the patient against potential pulmonary pathogens.

Surgical Interventions
1. Segmental resection of the lung is performed when conservative management fails.

Nursing Diagnoses
49, 73, 75, 107

Nursing Interventions
Also see *Thoracic Surgeries*, page 914.

Monitoring
1. Monitor respiratory effort, sputum production, temperature, and breath sounds for change in condition.

Supportive Care
1. Encourage regular coughing and deep-breathing exercises. Use secretion clearance techniques such as with a positive expiratory pressure valve, flutter valve, Acapella valve (along with percussion vibration), and postural drainage as the patient tolerates.
2. Encourage increased fluid intake, and use a vaporizer to reduce viscosity of sputum and facilitate expectoration.
3. Be alert to exacerbations characterized by change in sputum production.

Education and Health Maintenance
1. Instruct the patient to avoid noxious fumes, dusts, smoke, and other pulmonary irritants.
2. Teach the patient to watch for and report changes in sputum quantity or character.
3. Encourage regular dental care because copious sputum production may affect dentition.

4. Instruct the patient and family to implement drainage exercises and chest physical therapy. Encourage the patient to use postural drainage before rising in the morning, to remove nocturnal sputum accumulation.
5. Advise engaging in physical activity throughout day to help mobilize secretions and increase endurance.
6. Emphasize the importance of influenza and pneumonia immunizations and prompt treatment of all respiratory infections.

BRONCHITIS, ACUTE

Acute bronchitis is an infection of the lower respiratory tract that generally follows an upper respiratory tract infection. As a result of this viral (most common) or bacterial infection, the airways become inflamed and irritated, and mucus production increases.

Assessment
1. Fever, tachypnea, mild dyspnea, pleuritic chest pain (possible).
2. Cough with clear to purulent sputum production.
3. Diffuse rhonchi and crackles (contrast with localized crackles usually heard with pneumonia).

Diagnostic Evaluation
1. Chest X-ray may rule out pneumonia. In bronchitis, films show no evidence of lung infiltrates or consolidation.

Collaborative Management
Therapeutic Interventions
1. Chest physiotherapy to mobilize secretions, if indicated
2. Hydration to liquefy secretions

Pharmacologic Interventions
1. Inhaled bronchodilators to reduce bronchospasm and promote sputum expectoration
2. A course of oral antibiotics such as a macrolide may be instituted, but is controversial.
3. Symptom management for fever and cough

Nursing Diagnoses
49, 73

Nursing Interventions
Supportive Care
1. Encourage mobilization of secretions through ambulation, coughing, and deep breathing.
2. Ensure adequate fluid intake to liquefy secretions and prevent dehydration caused by fever and tachypnea.
3. Encourage rest, avoidance of bronchial irritants, and a good diet to facilitate recovery.

Education and Health Maintenance
1. Instruct the patient to complete the full course of prescribed antibiotics and explain the effect of meals on drug absorption.
2. Caution the patient on using over-the-counter cough suppressants, antihistamines, and decongestants, which may cause drying and retention of secretions. However, cough preparations containing the mucolytic guaifenesin may be appropriate.
3. Advise the patient that a dry cough may persist after bronchitis because of irritation of airways. Suggest avoiding dry environments and using a humidifier at bedside. Encourage smoking cessation.
4. Teach the patient to recognize and immediately report early signs and symptoms of acute bronchitis.

BRONCHOGENIC CANCER
See *Cancer, Lung*.

BULIMIA NERVOSA
See *Eating Disorders*.

BURNS
Burns are a form of traumatic injury caused by thermal, electrical, chemical, or radioactive agents. Most burn-related accidents occur at home; others occur at work. Flame injury is

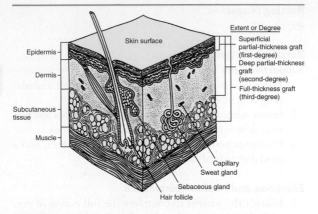

FIGURE B-4 Cross section of skin depicting blood supply, depth of burn, and relative thickness of skin grafts. (Courtesy of Ethicon)

the leading cause of accidental burns for adults, and scalding is the leading cause of accidental burns for children.

Burns may be partial or full thickness (see *Figure B-4*). *Partial-thickness* burn injuries involve the epidermis and upper portions of the dermis. The wound can spontaneously reepithelialize from the remaining dermal appendages. In *full-thickness* injuries, all layers of the skin and sometimes underlying tissues are destroyed. Grafting usually is required to close the wound.

Inhalation injury (from smoke particles, toxic gases such as carbon monoxide, sulfur dioxide, nitrous oxide, and fumes from burning plastics) causes 50% to 60% of fire deaths. Infection and pulmonary complications also significantly increase morbidity and mortality.

Systemic changes occur in major burns (more than 25% total body surface area [TBSA]), creating a life-threatening situation. These changes include fluid shift away from intravascular compartment in first 24 to 36 hours; loss of protein-rich fluid through burn tissue; possible shock and renal failure; electrolyte shifts; and catabolic shock.

Assessment

1. Assess airway, breathing, and circulation as indicated and intervene as necessary.
2. Assess burn severity.
   a. Depth: first-, second-, third-degree (see *Table B-1*, page 100)
   b. Extent: percentage of TBSA. Use Rule of Nines chart (see *Figure B-5*, page 101) or Lund and Browder chart for children.

 EMERGENCY ALERT Burns affecting hands, feet, face, and perineum require specialized care. Circumferential burns also require special attention and may require escharotomy.

3. Assess for signs of smoke inhalation: upper body burns; erythema or blistering of lips, buccal mucosa, or pharynx; singed nares hair; soot in oropharynx; dark gray or black sputum; hoarseness; crackles on auscultation.

 EMERGENCY ALERT Increasing hoarseness, stuttering, or drooling indicates the need for intubation.

4. Evaluate all patients in closed-space fires for symptoms of carbon monoxide poisoning: headache, visual changes, confusion, irritability, decreased judgment, nausea, ataxia, collapse.

Diagnostic Evaluation

1. Arterial blood gas (ABG) levels, carboxyhemoglobin levels, and spirometry may be measured to assess for inhalation injury.
2. Bronchoscopy visualizes vocal cord damage.
3. Chest X-ray determines baseline information.
4. Complete blood count, blood urea nitrogen, and creatinine, electrolytes, and other laboratory tests are performed at baseline and monitored periodically.

Collaborative Management
Therapeutic Interventions

1. Immediate I.V. fluid resuscitation is indicated for:
   a. Adults with burns over more than 15% to 20% of TBSA
   b. Children with burns involving more than 10% of TBSA

TABLE B-1	Assessment of Burn Injuries

DEGREE AND ASSESSMENT	TREATMENT CONSIDERATIONS
First-Degree Burn ■ Pink to red; slight edema, subsides quickly ■ Pain may last up to 48 h, relieved by cooling	■ Epidermis peels in about 5 days ■ Itching and pink skin persist for about 1 week ■ No scarring occurs ■ Heals spontaneously in 10 days to 2 weeks in absence of infection

Second-Degree Burn
■ Superficial
  – Pink or red; vesicles form — weeping, edematous
  – Superficial skin layers destroyed; leaves moist, painful wound
■ Deep dermal
  – Mottled white and red; edematous reddened areas blanch on pressure
  – May be yellowish, soft and elastic; may or may not be sensitive to touch; sensitive to cold air
	■ Takes several weeks to heal
	■ Scarring may occur
	■ Pain control is important

Third-Degree Burn ■ Destruction of epidermis, dermis, fat, muscle, and bone ■ Reddened areas do not blanch with pressure ■ Wound not painful; inelastic; coloration varies from waxy white to brown (leathery devitalized tissue — eschar)	■ Eschar must be removed by debridement. Granulation tissue forms to nearest epithelium from wound margins or support graft ■ Grafting is required for areas larger than 1 to 2 inches (3 to 5 cm) ■ Expect scarring and loss of skin function

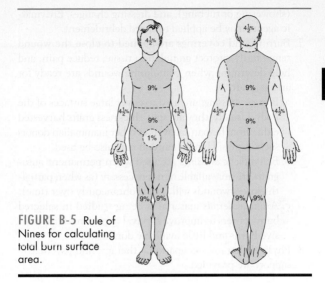

FIGURE B-5 Rule of Nines for calculating total burn surface area.

   c. Patients with electrical injury, the elderly, or anyone with cardiac or pulmonary disease and compromised response to burn injury

2. Generally, a crystalloid (lactated Ringer's) solution is used initially. Colloid is used during the second day (5% albumin or plasma).

3. The Parkland formula is most commonly used to determine fluid requirements in the first 48 hours. The Brooks & Evans formulas may also be used.

4. Initially, the patient is kept NPO until bowel sounds return (1 to 2 days). However, small amounts (5 to 10 mL/hour) of isotonic enteral tube feedings are often started within 24 hours to help maintain a functioning GI tract.

5. When caloric requirements cannot be met by enteral feedings, total parenteral nutrition is initiated.

6. Treatment of the burn wound includes daily or twice-daily wound cleaning with debridement, hydrotherapy

(showering or tubbing), and dressing changes. Enzymatic agents may be applied to speed debridement.

7. Burn wound coverings are applied to close the wound temporarily, protect granulation tissue, reduce pain, and help determine when granulating wounds are ready for an autograft.

   a. *Biologic dressings* are used to cover large surfaces of the body. Usually, they are split-thickness grafts harvested either from human cadavers or other mammalian donors such as pigs. Human amnion may also be used.

   b. *Biosynthetic dressings* are used when permanent autografts are unavailable or not necessary (as when partial-thickness wounds will heal spontaneously over time).

   c. *Artificial dermis* material is being studied in selected burn centers to improve survival of patients with massive burns and little available donor skin.

8. Physical therapy, occupational therapy, and psychiatric support are provided.

Pharmacologic Interventions

1. Opioids to control pain.
2. Topical antimicrobials are applied directly to the burn area or incorporated in single-layer dressings that do not stick to the wound but permit drainage.
3. I.V. antibiotics may be given prophylactically to prevent gram-positive infection. Wounds, urine, and sputum are cultured, and specific antibiotics are given as indicated.
4. Diuretics may be necessary to prevent fluid overload during period of fluid shifting and I.V. fluid resuscitation.
5. Tetanus prophylaxis if indicated.
6. Potassium, vitamins, and mineral replacements.
7. Histamine-2 blockers and antacids to prevent stress ulcers.

Surgical Interventions

1. Early excision of nonviable skin and grafting reduce wound infection and speed recovery; however, this incurs significant blood loss and increases metabolic demands.

a. Tangential excision (excision of thin layers of damaged skin until live tissue is evidenced by capillary bleeding) is done for deep partial-thickness burns.

b. Fascial (primary) excision (skin, lymphatics, and subcutaneous tissue removed down to fascia) is done for full-thickness burns.

2. Skin grafting is usually required or preferred for full-thickness burns greater than 2 cm in diameter or for deep partial-thickness burns.

3. Grafts of the patient's own skin (autografts) are applied after gradual eschar removal and development of a base of granulating tissue or in the presence of viable tissue after excision. Sheet grafts or meshed grafts, which provide wider expansion from donor sites, may be used.

4. Three to 4 days after grafting, blood flow is established, and, after 7 to 10 days, vascular continuity and wound closure are established.

5. Cultured epithelial autografts may be used for patients with large burns and little available donor skin.

Nursing Diagnoses
3, 8, 15, 19, 30, 36, 49, 51, 57, 63, 87, 108, 130, 135

Nursing Interventions
Monitoring

1. Check vital signs every 15 minutes until stabilized, then as indicated by condition.

2. Monitor respiratory rate, depth, rhythm, and cough; observe for signs of respiratory distress.

3. Monitor tidal volume in the patient with chest burns; report decreasing volume to health care provider.

4. Monitor central venous pressure and pulmonary artery pressure as indicated to help guide fluid resuscitation.

GERONTOLOGIC ALERT Elderly patients and those with impaired renal function, cardiovascular disease, and pulmonary disease are more likely to develop fluid overload from fluid replacement therapy. Proceed with caution.

5. Monitor peripheral pulses and neurovascular status with burns of extremities. Use Doppler as necessary. Escharotomy may be necessary if circulation is impaired.
6. Monitor hydration status, intake and output, daily weight, and urine specific gravity.
7. Monitor serum levels of potassium and other electrolytes.
8. Monitor temperature, white blood cell count, and differential.
9. Monitor ABG levels and oxygen saturation (in inhalation injury).
10. Monitor wounds for signs of infection.
11. Monitor the patient's response to pain control.

Supportive Care

1. Provide humidified 100% oxygen until blood level of carbon monoxide is known. (*Caution:* Adjust oxygen flow rate for the patient with chronic obstructive pulmonary disease as prescribed.)
2. In mild inhalation injury, provide humidification of inspired air and encourage coughing and deep breathing.
3. In moderate to severe inhalation injury, initiate frequent suctioning, administer bronchodilators, and monitor closely.
4. Be prepared to intubate patient and provide mechanical ventilation, continuous positive airway pressure, or positive end-expiratory pressure, if requested.
5. Place the patient in semi-Fowler's position to permit maximal chest excursions if there are no contraindications, such as hypotension or spinal cord injury.
6. Ensure that chest dressings are not constricting.
7. Elevate extremities to prevent edema.
8. Cleanse wounds and change dressings twice daily. Use an antimicrobial solution and saline solution or mild soap and water. Dry gently. This may be done in the hydrotherapy tank, bathtub, shower, or at the bedside.
9. Perform débridement of dead tissue at this time. May use gauze, scissors, or pickups or forceps as appropriate. Try to limit time to 20 to 30 minutes, depending on the patient's tolerance. Additional analgesia may be necessary.

10. Apply topical antimicrobial agents as directed. Cream or ointment is applied ⅛ to ¼ inch (3 to 6 cm) thick unless otherwise indicated.

 PEDIATRIC ALERT To prevent eye irritation (if the child rubs eyes with antibiotic ointment on hands), use ophthalmic ointment on open burns of the head.

11. Dress wounds as appropriate, using burn pads, gauze rolls, or any combination. Dressings may be held in place as necessary with gauze rolls or netting.

12. Describe hydrotherapy to the patient who is experiencing it for the first time, coordinate timing of pain medication, and assure the patient that you will stay.

    a. If the patient has an indwelling catheter, drain and plug it, or maintain a closed system to avoid contamination.

    b. Use aseptic technique in preparing the patient for hydrotherapy, during hydrotherapy, and in re-dressing wounds after therapy.

    c. After cleansing of the wounds, débride wounds, shave adjacent areas at health care provider's direction, shampoo hair, and gently wash normal skin.

    d. Limit hydrotherapy to as brief a time as possible to minimize loss of body heat and subsequent chilling.

13. For grafted areas, use extreme caution in removing dressings; observe for and report serous or sanguineous blebs or purulent drainage. Re-dress grafted areas according to your facility's protocol.

PEDIATRIC ALERT Prevent children from rubbing or scratching burns or graft sites by applying protective mitts to hands.

14. Observe all wounds daily, and document wound status on the patient's record.

15. Use radiant warmers, warming blankets, or adjust the room temperature to keep the patient warm because thermoregulatory ability is impaired.

16. Use meticulous handwashing and barrier garments (isolation gown or plastic apron) for all care requiring contact with the patient or the patient's bed; cover hair and wear mask when wounds are exposed or when performing a sterile procedure.

17. Ensure consultation with physical and occupational therapists who will help the patient with exercise at least once or twice daily, and order splints to prevent contractures.
18. Consult with dietitian for calculation of nutritional needs based on age, weight, height, and burn size.
19. Explore coping mechanisms and facilitate psychological counseling as indicated.
20. Arrange for the patient to see face (if burned) with appropriate supportive personnel before being transferred to a room with a mirror.
21. Encourage participation in a burn survivors' group, such as the Phoenix Society. Use and emphasize the concept of being a burn survivor, rather than a "burn victim," which enhances the sick role.

Education and Health Maintenance

1. Demonstrate and explain wound care procedures to be continued after discharge:
   a. Wash hands.
   b. Cleanse small open wounds with mild soap in tub or shower.
   c. Rinse well with tap water.
   d. Pat dry with clean towel.
   e. Apply prescribed topical agent or dressing.
2. Teach the patient to recognize and report local signs of wound infection.
3. Instruct the patient in measures to lubricate and enhance comfort of healing skin:
   a. After cleansing, use moisturizers, such as cocoa butter or other nonperfumed lotions, at least twice per day.
   b. Wear clean, white underwear and clothing free from irritating dyes.
   c. Apply antipruritics as prescribed.
   d. Stay in a cool environment if itching occurs.
   e. Protect skin from further trauma. Use a sunscreen with sun protection factor of 24 or higher.

   f. Discuss summer precautions to include a hat with a full wide brim if there were facial or neck burns. Also limit exposure to sun because the affected areas will sunburn more easily and tan more deeply.

4. Advise the patient that, if wearing a pressure vest with or without sleeves or tights, the U.S. Occupational Safety & Health Administration standards for work in a hot environment as well as the need for oral fluid replacement should be used.

5. Advise the patient to develop a schedule for his exercise regimen as prescribed by physical therapist.

6. Instruct the patient in use and care of splints and pressure garments.

7. Review with the patient and family common emotional responses during convalescence (depression, withdrawal, grieving, dreaming, anxiety, guilt, excessive sensitivity, emotional lability, insomnia, fear of future) and discuss usual temporary nature of these and effective coping mechanisms. Make sure that the patient has a phone number or referral to the counselor for follow-up appointments if desired.

8. For additional information and support, refer to American Burn Association, *www.ameriburn.org*; Phoenix Society for Burn Survivors, *www.phoenix-society.org*.

C

CANCER, BLADDER

Cancer of the bladder is the second most common urologic malignancy. Approximately 90% of all bladder cancers are transitional cell tumors that arise from the epithelial lining of the urinary tract. The remaining 10% are adenocarcinoma, squamous cell carcinoma, or sarcoma. Most are superficial and easily resected, but metastasis may occur to the bladder wall and pelvis, para-aortic or supraclavicular nodes, and the liver, lungs, and bone.

Although the specific cause is unknown, bladder cancers have been linked to cigarette smoking (two to three times higher risk), to prolonged exposure to aromatic amines (industrial dyes), to the drug cyclophosphamide, to pelvic radiation therapy, and to chronic bladder irritation (as in long-term indwelling catheterization). Bladder cancer occurs three times more commonly in men, with peak incidence between ages 60 and 80.

Assessment

1. Painless hematuria, either gross or microscopic, is the most characteristic sign.
2. Dysuria, frequency, urgency.
3. Pelvic or back pain may indicate distant metastases; leg edema may result from invasion of pelvic lymph nodes.

Diagnostic Evaluation

1. Cystoscopy visualizes the number, location, and appearance of tumors, and may be used to obtain biopsy specimens.
2. Urine and bladder washing for cytology to detect cancer cells.
3. Urine flow cytometry uses fluorescence microscopy to scan for abnormal cells.

4. Intravenous urogram may show a filling defect indicative of bladder cancer; also helps determine status of upper urinary tract.
5. Additional tests evaluate metastatic disease, such as chest X-ray, CT scan, or MRI bone scan.

Collaborative Management
Therapeutic and Pharmacologic Interventions
1. Intravesical (within the bladder) chemotherapy allows a high concentration of drug to come in contact with the tumor and urothelium with minimal systemic toxicity.
2. Instillation of immunotherapeutic agent, bacille Calmette-Guérin (BCG), to stimulate immune response to prevent recurrence of transitional cell tumors.
   a. Adverse reaction is a systemic BCG reaction—fever greater than 100° F (38° C) for more than 24 hours.
   b. Treated with antituberculosis agents.
   c. Weekly instillations may be performed for 6 to 8 weeks.
3. Systemic chemotherapy to treat metastatic bladder cancer; combination therapy.
4. Radiation therapy may be internal or external.

Surgical Interventions
1. Transurethral resection and fulguration may be used for superficial tumors, usually with intravesical chemotherapy to prevent tumor recurrence. (Some tumors may be treated with lasers, but this does not allow biopsies.)
2. Partial cystectomy may be used when tumors are located only in the dome of the bladder, away from the ureteral orifices.
3. Radical cystectomy (bladder removal) with urinary diversion may be used for invasive or poorly differentiated tumors.
   a. Requires urinary diversion.
   b. *In a male*, includes removal of bladder, prostate and seminal vesicles, proximal vas deferens, and part of proximal urethra.

    c. *In a female,* includes anterior exenteration with removal
    of bladder, urethra, uterus, fallopian tubes, ovaries, and
    segment of anterior wall of the vagina.
    d. Cystectomy may be combined with chemotherapy and
    radiation.

Nursing Diagnoses
3, 6, 69, 135

Nursing Interventions
Also see *Kidney Surgery and Urinary Diversion,* page 555.

Monitoring
    1. Monitor for complications of therapy:
      a. Hemorrhage, infection, bladder perforation, and tem-
      porary irritative voiding in transurethral resection
      b. Urinary tract infection, irritative voiding symptoms,
      allergic reaction, bone marrow suppression or systemic
      BCG reaction in intravesical chemotherapy
    2. After transurethral surgery, monitor intake and output,
    including irrigation solution.
    3. Monitor urine output for clearing of hematuria.

Supportive Care
    1. After transurethral surgery, maintain patency of indwelling
    urinary drainage catheter. Manual irrigation is not rec-
    ommended because of the risk of bladder perforation. Con-
    tinuous bladder irrigation may be used if necessary. Do
    not irrigate unless specifically ordered.
    2. Ensure adequate hydration, either orally or I.V.
    3. Administer an analgesic for pelvic discomfort.
    4. Administer an anticholinergic as directed to relieve blad-
    der spasms.
    5. Remove indwelling catheter as soon as possible after pro-
    cedure, to reduce risk of infection.
    6. To relieve anxiety, allow the patient to verbalize fears and
    concerns, and provide information about diagnostic stud-
    ies, surgery, and treatments. Be prepared to discuss con-

cerns about sexual dysfunction and incontinence after surgery.
7. For intravesical chemotherapy:
   a. Minimize fluids and avoid diuretics for several hours before instillation to maximize concentration of drug during treatment.
   b. Help the patient change position as directed during instillation to allow drug to contact as much of urothelial surface as possible.
   c. Tell the patient not to void for 1 to 2 hours after instillation; then have the patient increase fluid intake and void frequently.
   d. Tell the patient to wash hands and perineal area after voiding, to prevent contact dermatitis caused by medication.

Education and Health Maintenance

1. Advise the patient that irritative voiding symptoms and intermittent hematuria are possible for several weeks after transurethral resection.
2. Emphasize the importance of adhering to follow-up schedule: cystoscopy every 3 months for 1 year, then every 6 months to 1 year thereafter for the rest of the patient's life (70% of superficial tumors will recur).
3. Encourage cessation of smoking.

CANCER, BONE

Bone cancer refers to primary malignant tumors, such as chondrosarcoma and osteogenic sarcoma, which arise from areas of rapid growth of cartilage or bone structure (occur most frequently at the peak of the adolescent growth spurt); and metastatic bone tumors (seeded from another site), which may accompany cancers of the breast, the prostate, and, most commonly, the lung. Metastatic tumors most frequently occur in the vertebrae and cause pathologic fractures. Benign bone tumors include osteoid osteoma, chondroma, and osteoclastoma (benign giant cell tumor); some may become malignant. Complications of malignant tumors include fractures, hypercalcemia, and metastasis.

Assessment

1. Generally mild to constant pain, which may be worse at night or with activity. Pain will be acute with pathologic fracture.
2. Swelling and limitation of motion and joint effusion.
3. Numbness, tingling, weakness may present with nerve root compression.
4. Palpable, tender, fixed bony mass.
   a. Increase in skin temperature over mass
   b. Superficial veins dilated and prominent

Diagnostic Evaluation

1. X-ray studies and tomograms usually reveal the tumor; may show increased or decreased bone density.
2. CT scan and MRI demonstrate soft tissue involvement and location of tumors.
3. Serum alkaline phosphatase usually elevated.
4. Bone biopsy may be necessary to confirm diagnosis.
5. Bone scan detects extent of malignancy and helps follow therapy.
6. Additional tests include arteriography to further assess soft tissue involvement, and chest X-ray and lung scan to detect metastasis.

Collaborative Management

Therapeutic Interventions

1. Radiation therapy may be used to irradiate tumors, usually in combination with other therapies.
2. Prophylactic radiation to lungs may suppress metastases.
3. If pathologic fracture occurs, the fracture is managed conservatively or with open reduction and internal fixation as appropriate.

Pharmacologic Interventions

1. Chemotherapy may be administered before surgery to shrink the tumor and afterward to prevent metastases.
   a. May be used in combination with other therapies to achieve greater patient response at lower toxicity, and to minimize potential drug resistance problems.

b. May be given in varying courses separated by rest periods.

2. Immunotherapy may be used.

3. Hormone therapy may be used to treat metastatic tumors of the breast and prostate.

Surgical Interventions

1. Tumor curettage or resection with bone grafting may be used.

2. Limb-saving procedures involve resection of affected bone and surrounding normal muscle tissue, with reconstruction using metallic prostheses or allografts and skin grafts as needed.

3. Amputation is necessary in some cases.

Nursing Diagnoses

3, 21, 53, 62, 136

Nursing Interventions

Also see *Amputation*, page 14 and *Orthopedic Surgery*, page 680.

Monitoring

1. Monitor the patient's response to pain control measures.

2. Monitor for adverse effects of chemotherapy (see page 119).

3. Monitor for adverse effects of radiation therapy (see page 119).

Supportive Care

1. Prepare the patient for amputation (page 14) or other orthopedic surgery (page 680) as indicated.

2. Administer an analgesic 30 minutes before ambulation or other uncomfortable movement; use relaxation and diversion techniques.

3. Support painful extremities on pillows; support joints when repositioning the patient.

4. Assist the patient in movement with gentleness and patience.

5. Avoid jarring the patient or the bed.
6. To avoid pathologic fractures, create a hazard-free environment.
7. Create a supportive environment to help family deal with diagnosis of cancer and possible amputation.
8. Answer questions and clear up misconceptions about treatment options. Refer for counseling as indicated.

Education and Health Maintenance
1. Teach the patient about the particular treatment selected.
2. Encourage appropriate follow-up and diagnostic testing for recurrence.
3. Refer for additional information and support to American Cancer Society, *www.cancer.org*.

CANCER, BREAST

Breast cancer or carcinoma is the leading type of cancer in American women. One in eight women will develop it, and about 1,000 cases in men occur each year in the United States. It is second only to lung cancer as the highest cause of cancer deaths in American women. Most breast cancer begins in the lining of the milk ducts, sometimes in the lobule. Eventually, the cancer grows through the wall of the duct and into the fatty tissue. Breast cancer metastasizes most commonly to axillary nodes, lung, bone, liver, and the brain.

Age, staging, histologic differentiation, and treatment are important prognostic factors for survival. If the cancer is localized to the breast, the 5-year survival rate is 97%.

Women at high risk for breast cancer include those with prior breast cancer and those with a family history (especially mother, sisters), and those who are older. Other probable risk factors include nulliparity, first child after age 30, late menopause, early menarche, long-term estrogen replacement therapy, and benign breast disease. Controversial risk factors include oral contraceptive use, alcohol use, obesity, and increased dietary fat intake. Family history accounts for about 7% of breast cancer cases. Familial breast cancer is associated with the BRCA-1 and BRCA-2 susceptibility genes. Screening for these genes is offered to women with family history; prophylactic treatment may be given.

GERONTOLOGIC ALERT Age is the greatest single risk factor for the development of cancer. Cancer warning signals may be unheeded in older women.

Assessment

1. A firm lump or thickening in breast, usually painless; 50% are located in the upper outer quadrant of the breast.
2. Spontaneous nipple discharge; may be bloody, clear, or serous.
3. Asymmetry of the breasts may be noted as the woman changes positions; compare one breast with the other.
4. Nipple retraction or scaliness, especially in Paget's disease.
5. Enlargement of axillary or supraclavicular lymph nodes may indicate metastasis.

GERONTOLOGIC ALERT Normal breast changes in the elderly include drooping, flaccid breasts caused by decreased subcutaneous tissue from decreased estrogen levels. Nipple size and erection are also reduced.

6. Late signs of breast cancer include pain, ulceration, edema, and orange peel skin (peau d'orange) from impaired lymphatic drainage.

Diagnostic Evaluation

1. Mammography (most accurate method of detecting nonpalpable lesions) shows lesions and cancerous changes, such as microcalcification. Ultrasonography may be used to distinguish cysts from solid masses.
2. Biopsy or aspiration confirms diagnosis and determines the type of breast cancer.
3. Estrogen or progesterone receptor assays, proliferation/ S phase study (tumor aggressiveness), and other tests of tumor cells determine appropriate treatment and prognosis.
4. Blood testing detects metastasis; this includes liver function tests to detect liver metastasis and calcium and alkaline phosphatase levels to detect bony metastasis.

5. Chest X-rays, bone scans, or possible brain and chest CT scans detect metastasis.

Collaborative Management

Measures are based on the type and stage of breast cancer, receptor studies, and menopausal status. For women with localized breast cancer, clinical trials indicate that treatment with a breast-preserving surgery yields similar survival rates to modified radical mastectomy.

Therapeutic Interventions

1. Radiation is an adjuvant therapy to breast-preserving surgery to decrease incidence of local tumor recurrence.
   a. Radiation is directed to breast, chest wall, and remaining lymph nodes.
   b. A course usually involves five treatments per week for 6 or 7 weeks. A "booster" or second phase of treatment may be given.
   c. May include implants of radioactive material after external treatments are completed.
   d. A balloon device (MammoSite) may be temporarily implanted into the breast to deliver radiation twice per day for 5 days.
2. Also used as primary therapy to shrink a large tumor to operable size, and to alleviate pain caused by metastasis.
3. May be used after mastectomy in patients with large tumors that involve the chest wall or many positive axillary lymph nodes.
4. Treatment is individualized in pregnant women, with chemotherapy that follows the appropriate surgery in the second or third trimester, and radiation delayed until after delivery.

Pharmacologic Interventions

1. Chemotherapy is primarily used as adjuvant treatment postoperatively; usually begins 4 weeks after surgery (very stressful for a patient who just finished major surgery).
   a. Treatments are given every 3 to 4 weeks for 6 to 9 months. Because the drugs differ in their mechanisms

of action, various combinations are used to treat cancer.

b. Principal breast cancer drugs include cyclophosphamide, methotrexate, fluorouracil, doxorubicin, and paclitaxel.

c. Additional agents for advanced breast cancer include docetaxel, vinorelbine, mitoxantrone, and fluorouracil.

d. Herceptin is a monoclonal antibody directed against Her-2/neu oncogene; may be effective for patients who express this gene.

2. Indications for chemotherapy include large tumors, positive lymph nodes, premenopausal women, and poor prognostic factors.

3. Chemotherapy is also used as primary treatment in inflammatory breast cancer and as palliative treatment in metastatic disease or recurrence.

4. Anti-estrogens, such as tamoxifen, are used as adjuvant systemic therapy after surgery.

a. Given orally for at least 5 years.

b. Greatest benefit is seen in estrogen- or progesterone receptor-positive patients; it may also be used for metastases or recurrence.

5. Anastrozole and letrozole may be used as second-line therapy after tamoxifen in patients whose cancer has returned.

6. Estrogen-receptor modulators, such as raloxifene (Evista), may be used in place of estrogen for bone and heart protective benefits in patients with breast cancer.

7. Hormonal agents may be used in advanced disease to induce remissions that last for months to several years. Agents commonly used include:

a. Estrogens, such as diethylstilbestrol or ethinyl estradiol, given in high doses to suppress follicle-stimulating hormone (FSH) and luteinizing hormone; may also reduce endogenous estrogen production.

b. Progestins may decrease estrogen receptors.

c. Androgens may suppress FSH and estrogen production.

d. Aminoglutethimide suppresses estrogen production by blocking adrenal steroids; this "medical adrenalecto-

my" is especially useful for women with bone and soft tissue metastases.
    e. Corticosteroids suppress estrogen–progesterone secretion from the adrenals.

ALTERNATIVE INTERVENTION

Alternative products may be tried to control hot flashes in breast cancer patients, including clonidine, soy (phytoestrogens), black cohosh, and dong quai. Advise patients to discuss product use with their health care providers.

Surgical Interventions

1. Surgeries include lumpectomy (breast-preserving procedure), mastectomy (breast removal), and mammoplasty (reconstructive surgery).
2. Endocrine-related surgeries to reduce endogenous estrogen as a palliative measure:
    a. Oophorectomy (removal of ovaries) is used to treat recurrent or metastatic disease in estrogen receptor-positive premenopausal women. This deprives the breast tumor of its primary estrogen source and obtains remissions of 3 months to several years.
    b. Adrenalectomy (removal of adrenal glands) eliminates androgens, which convert to estrogen. Although this procedure yields remissions of 6 months to several years, it is rarely done because of need for long-term steroid replacement therapy.
3. Bone marrow transplantation may be combined with chemotherapy.
    a. Autologous method after high-dose chemotherapy may be curative because it allows for high doses of drugs.
    b. Especially indicated for stage 3 disease.

Nursing Diagnoses
6, 24, 30, 51, 78, 92

Nursing Interventions
Also see *Breast Surgery*, page 606.

Monitoring

1. Monitor for adverse effects of radiation therapy:
   a. Mild fatigue, sore throat, dry cough, nausea, anorexia; later, skin will look and feel sunburned, and, eventually, the breast becomes more firm.
   b. Complications include increased arm edema, decreased arm mobility, pneumonitis, and brachial nerve damage.
2. Monitor for adverse effects of chemotherapy: bone marrow suppression, nausea and vomiting, alopecia, weight gain or loss, fatigue, stomatitis, anxiety, and depression.
3. Monitor for adverse effects of endocrine therapy: hot flashes, irregular periods, vaginal irritation, nausea and vomiting, and headaches.

Supportive Care

1. Realize that a diagnosis of breast cancer is a devastating emotional shock to the woman. Provide psychological support to the patient throughout the diagnostic and treatment process.
2. Interpret the results of each diagnostic test in language the patient can readily understand.
3. Involve the patient in planning treatment.
4. Describe surgical procedures.
5. Prepare the patient for the effects of chemotherapy, and plan ahead for alopecia, fatigue, and so forth.
6. Administer antiemetics prophylactically, as directed, for patients receiving chemotherapy.
7. Encourage frequent light meals and fluids as tolerated.
8. Administer I.V. fluids and hyperalimentation as indicated.
9. Help patient identify and use support persons in family or community.

Education and Health Maintenance

1. Encourage the patient to continue in close postoperative follow-up. Most women are scheduled for examinations every 3 months for the first 2 years, every 6 months for the next 3 years, and once a year after 5 years.

2. Stress importance of continued yearly mammogram.

3. Suggest to the patient that psychological intervention may be necessary for anxiety, depression, or sexual problems.
4. Teach all women the recommended cancer-screening procedures:
   a. Breast self-examination: once per month, ages 20 and older
   b. Clinical examination by a physician or nurse every 3 years (ages 20 to 40) or every year (older than age 40).
   c. Mammography: Have first mammogram by age 40; have a mammogram every 1 to 2 years (ages 40 to 49); every year (ages 50 and older).
5. Refer for additional information to National Cancer Institute, *www.nci.nih.gov*; American Cancer Society, *www.cancer.org*.

CANCER, CERVICAL

Cervical cancer is a common gynecologic malignancy. Types of cervical cancer include dysplasia (atypical cells with some degree of surface maturation); carcinoma in situ (CIS), which is confined to the cervical epithelium; and invasive carcinomas (the stroma is involved, 90% are of the squamous cell type). Invasive cancer spreads by local invasion and lymphatics to the vagina and beyond.

Cervical cancer most commonly occurs in women ages 35 to 55. There is a decreasing mortality rate in the United States due to screening, but it is the most common malignancy in women in developing countries.

Major risk factors include early sexual activity, multiple sexual partners, and history of sexually transmitted diseases, especially human papillomavirus and herpes simplex virus. Cervical cancer may involve the bladder and rectum and may metastasize to the lungs, mediastinum, bones, and liver.

Assessment

1. Early disease is usually asymptomatic.
2. Initial symptoms are postcoital bleeding, irregular vaginal bleeding or spotting between periods or after menopause, and malodorous discharge.
3. As disease progresses, bleeding becomes more constant and is accompanied by pain that radiates to buttocks and legs.
4. Weight loss, anemia, and fever signal advanced disease.

Diagnostic Evaluation

1. Papanicolaou (Pap) smear for cervical cytology is usual screening test. A computerized screening program may increase the accuracy of manual laboratory Pap screening by as much as 30%.
2. If Pap test is abnormal, colposcopy and biopsy or conization may be done.
3. Additional testing includes metastatic workup (chest X-ray, I.V. urogram, cystoscopy, barium studies of colon and rectum, sigmoidoscopy).

Collaborative Management
Therapeutic and Pharmacologic Interventions

1. Intracavitary radiation for earlier localized stages — radium by way of applicator in endocervical canal.
   a. Applicator remains in place for 24 to 72 hours.
   b. Complications include cystitis, proctitis, vaginal stenosis, uterine perforation.
2. External radiation for generalized pelvis effect in later stages.
3. Laser therapy may be used to treat dysplasia.
4. Chemotherapy may be used as adjuvant to surgery or radiation treatments. Cisplatin is used as a radiosensitizer.

Surgical Interventions

1. Conization is performed for microinvasize stage if childbearing is desired.
2. Cryosurgery, laser ablation, and loop electrosurgical excision procedure may be done for dysplasia or CIS.
3. Hysterectomy, simple or radical depending on stage.
   a. Performed if childbearing no longer desired.
   b. Usually combined with radiation therapy for CIS and invasive carcinoma.
   c. May cause impaired bladder function.
4. Pelvic exenteration for very advanced disease if radiation therapy cannot be used; also for recurrent cancer.
   a. Removal of the vagina, uterus, uterine tubes, ovaries, bladder, rectum, and supporting structures.
   b. Creation of an ileal conduit and fecal stoma.
   c. Vaginal reconstruction may be done.

Nursing Diagnoses
6, 24, 30, 92

Nursing Interventions
Also see *Hysterectomy*, page 535.

Monitoring

1. During intracavitary radiation, check radioisotope applicator position every 8 hours, and monitor amount of bleeding and drainage (a small amount is normal).
2. Observe for signs and symptoms of radiation sickness — nausea, vomiting, fever, diarrhea, abdominal cramping.
3. Monitor for complications of surgery — bleeding, infection.

Supportive Care

1. Help the patient seek information on stage of cancer, treatment options.
2. Prepare the patient for hysterectomy or other surgery (see page 535).
3. Prepare the patient for radiation therapy to the uterus (see page 174).

4. Provide emotional support during treatment.

Education and Health Maintenance

1. Advise patient on expected discharge after surgical procedure and need to report excessive, foul-smelling discharge or bleeding.
2. Explain the importance of lifelong follow-up regardless of treatments to determine the response to treatment and to detect spread of cancer.
3. Refer the patient to a local cancer support group.
4. Encourage all women to receive regular cervical cancer screening.

CANCER, COLORECTAL

Colorectal cancer refers to malignancies of the colon and rectum. Colorectal tumors are nearly always adenocarcinomas, and they represent the second most common visceral cancer in the United States.

Colorectal tumors occur most frequently in the rectum and sigmoid areas. A tumor starts in the mucosal layers of the colonic wall and eventually penetrates the wall and invades surrounding structures and organs (bladder, prostate, ureters, vagina). Cancer spreads by direct invasion and through the lymph system and bloodstream (see *Box C-1*). The liver and

BOX C-1	Dukes' Staging of Colorectal Cancer

Class A — Negative nodes, tumor limited to mucosa and submucosa
Class B_1 — Negative nodes, tumor extends through mucosa but is still within bowel wall
Class B_2 — Negative nodes, tumor extends through entire bowel wall
Class C_1 — Positive nodes, tumor is limited to bowel wall
Class C_2 — Positive nodes, tumor extends through entire bowel wall
Class D — Advanced and widespread regional metastasis

lungs are the most common metastatic sites. Other complications are hemorrhage, obstruction, and anemia.

Risk factors include age (older than age 50), chronic ulcerative colitis (CUC; increasing risk after 10-year history), Crohn's disease, previous history of resected colorectal cancer, high-fat and low-fiber diet, genetic predisposition, polyposis syndromes, and immunodeficiency diseases.

Assessment

1. May be asymptomatic or symptoms vary according to the location of the tumor and the extent of involvement
2. Right-sided tumors — change in bowel habits, usually diarrhea; vague abdominal discomfort; black tarry stools; anemia; weakness; weight loss; palpable mass in right lower quadrant
3. Left-sided tumors — change in bowel habits, often increasing constipation with bouts of diarrhea caused by partial obstruction; bright red blood in stool; cramping pain; weight loss; anemia; palpable mass
4. Rectal tumors — change in bowel habits with possibly urgent need to defecate, alternating constipation and diarrhea, and narrowed caliber of stool; bright red blood in stool; feeling of incomplete evacuation; rectal fullness progressing to dull constant ache

 GERONTOLOGIC ALERT Fatigue, weight loss, and iron deficiency anemia in the elderly, even without rectal bleeding or bowel changes, should prompt investigation for colorectal cancer.

Diagnostic Evaluation

1. Fecal occult blood testing — commonly reveals evidence of carcinoma when the patient is otherwise asymptomatic.
2. Barium enema is useful in detecting smaller tumors.
3. Colonoscopy with biopsy is procedure of choice.
4. Pelvic MRI and endorectal ultrasonography provide information about penetration and lymph node involvement.
5. CT scan of liver, lung, and brain may show metastatic disease. Newer liver scans are also available.

6. Carcinoembryonic antigen — elevated in 70% of cases; used to monitor metastasis or tumor recurrence.

Collaborative Management
Therapeutic Interventions
1. Blood replacement or other treatment if severe anemia exists.
2. Radiation therapy may be used preoperatively to improve resectability of the tumor or postoperatively as adjuvant therapy to treat residual disease.

Pharmacologic Interventions
1. Chemotherapy may be used as adjuvant therapy to improve survival time.
2. May be used for residual disease, recurrence of disease, unresectable tumors, and metastatic disease.

Surgical Interventions
1. Wide segmental bowel resection of tumor, including regional lymph nodes and blood vessels.
2. Transanal excision for small, localized, accessible tumors.
3. Low anterior resection for upper rectal tumors; possible temporary diversion loop colostomy while rectal anastomosis heals; second procedure for takedown of colostomy.
4. Colonic J-pouch is a new technique that may be offered for rectal tumors. Laparoscopic procedures are controversial.
5. Abdominoperineal resection with permanent end colostomy for lower rectal tumors when adequate margins cannot be obtained or anal sphincters are involved.
6. Temporary loop colostomy to decompress bowel and divert fecal stream, followed by later bowel resection, anastomosis, and takedown of colostomy.
7. Diverting colostomy or ileostomy as palliation for obstructing, unresectable tumor.
8. Total proctocolectomy and possible ileal reservoir — anal anastomosis for patients with familial adenomatous polyposis and CUC before cancer is confirmed.

9. More extensive surgery involving removal of other organs if cancer has spread (bladder, uterus, small intestine).

Nursing Diagnoses
3, 6, 16, 27, 43, 51, 123

Nursing Interventions
Also see *Gastrointestinal or Abdominal Surgery*, page 381.

Monitoring
1. Monitor amount, consistency, frequency, occult blood, and color of stools.
2. Monitor the patient's dietary intake and weight.
3. Monitor for excess fluid and electrolyte loss through vomiting and diarrhea, and watch for dehydration.
4. Monitor the patient's response to radiation or chemotherapy, and watch for adverse reactions.

Supportive Care
1. Meet the patient's nutritional needs by serving a high-calorie, low-residue diet for several days before surgery, if condition permits.
2. Serve smaller meals spaced throughout the day to maintain adequate calorie and protein intake if patient is able to take nutrition orally.
3. Adjust diet before and after treatments such as chemotherapy or radiation. Serve clear liquids, bland diet, or NPO as directed.
4. Maintain hydration through I.V. therapy, and record urinary output. Metabolic tissue needs are increased, and more fluids are needed to eliminate waste products.
5. Instruct the patient to take prescribed antiemetic as needed, especially if receiving chemotherapy.
6. For constipation, encourage exercise and adequate fluid or fiber intake to promote bowel motility.
7. For diarrhea related to radiation or chemotherapy (not caused by obstruction), administer antidiarrheal medications and discuss foods that may slow transit time of bowel, such as bananas, rice, peanut butter, and pasta.

8. Maintain nasogastric decompression for obstruction. Measure and document amount of drainage.
9. Evaluate effectiveness of analgesic regimen. Investigate different approaches, such as relaxation techniques, repositioning, imaging, laughter, music, reading, and touch for control or relief of pain.
10. Institute an individualized activity plan after assessing the patient's activity level and tolerance, noting shortness of breath or tachycardia. Allow for frequent rest periods to regain energy.
11. To minimize fear, provide information and answer questions about disease process, treatment modalities, and complications. Offer additional educational materials, and refer to American Cancer Society for information and support.

Education and Health Maintenance
1. Teach and demonstrate colostomy management skills. Enlist the help of an enterostomal therapist.
2. Initiate a home care nursing referral to assist with wound care and management of treatment adverse effects, and to continue teaching colostomy care.

CANCER, ESOPHAGEAL

Esophageal cancer occurs in four types: squamous cell, adenocarcinoma, carcinosarcoma, and sarcoma. Its cause is unknown, but usually occurs after age 60. Predisposing factors include Barrett's esophagus (epithelial changes in esophagus), other head and neck cancers, achalasia, long-term alcohol and tobacco use, genetic predisposition (more common in nonwhite men), and chemical esophagitis, which causes esophageal strictures. Squamous cell and adenocarcinoma are the most common types.

Complications include malnutrition, aspiration pneumonitis, hemorrhage, sepsis, and tracheoesophageal fistula. Postoperatively, dumping syndrome, nutritional deficiencies, reflux esophagitis, and leakage of anastomosis may occur.

Assessment

1. Dysphagia is late, but is usual presenting sign.
   a. Mild, atypical chest pain associated with eating usually precedes dysphagia but is overlooked.
   b. Pain on swallowing (odynophagia) may occur.
2. Progressive weight loss and dietary changes.
3. Hoarseness with laryngeal involvement.
4. Later, hiccups, respiratory difficulty, foul breath, and regurgitation of food and saliva may occur.
5. Supraclavicular or cervical lymphadenopathy and hepatomegaly occur with metastatic involvement.

Diagnostic Evaluation

1. Chest X-ray may show adenopathy, mediastinal widening, metastasis, or a tracheoesophageal fistula.
2. Barium swallow shows polypoid, infiltrative, or ulcerative lesions.
3. Endoscopy is done to obtain biopsy specimen.
4. CT scan may be helpful in delineating the extent of the tumor, as well as in identifying adjacent tissue invasion and metastases.

Collaborative Management

Therapeutic and Pharmacologic Interventions

1. The goal of treatment may be cure or palliation, depending on the tumor stage and the patient's overall condition. Palliative treatment aims to reduce tumor-related complications and improve quality of life. One or more therapies can be used for palliative treatment. The wide variety of treatments reflects overall poor results from a single approach.
2. Radiation and chemotherapy appear to be more effective when used in combination.
3. Endoscopy or laser dilation provides palliative treatment of dysphagia.

Surgical Interventions

1. Lesions of the middle and lower esophagus are excised by way of thoracotomy with esophagogastrectomy or colon

interposition (section of colon is used to replace the excised portion of the esophagus).
2. Lesions of the cervical esophagus are excised by way of bilateral neck dissection and esophagogastrectomy; laryngectomy and thyroidectomy may be necessary.
3. A two-step approach may be selected, in which resection with cervical esophagostomy and feeding gastrostomy are performed initially, followed by reconstructive surgery.

Nursing Diagnoses
3, 44, 51, 78, 119, 123, 135

Nursing Interventions
Monitoring
1. Monitor nutritional status, weight, and dietary intake.
2. Monitor vital signs to note early onset of hemorrhage, infection, arrhythmias, aspiration, or anastomosis leakage.
3. Observe for drainage from incision nasogastric tube or for bleeding or purulence from chest tube.
4. Be alert for pain caused by dumping syndrome or reflux esophagitis.

EMERGENCY ALERT Signs of leaking esophageal anastomosis postoperatively are increased pain, dyspnea, tachycardia, and fever. Notify the surgeon immediately.

Supportive Care
1. Administer oxygen as directed to facilitate tissue oxygenation.
2. Prior to definitive therapy, provide high-protein nutritional supplements as indicated. Expect to provide I.V. hyperalimentation if the patient cannot take adequate calories.
3. Postoperatively, maintain nasogastric suction with care not to manipulate the tube, and administer I.V. fluids as directed. Initially the patient may require large volumes if many lymph nodes were removed.
4. Position the patient in semi-Fowler's to Fowler's position to prevent reflux of gastric secretions and reduce dyspnea.
5. Administer analgesics as directed.

6. Upon return of bowel sounds, restart feedings through gastrostomy or enteral feeding tube as directed.
7. Once nasogastric tube is removed and patency of anastomosis is confirmed, restart oral feeding slowly.
8. Encourage the patient to advance diet from liquids to high-energy, soft foods.
9. Remind the patient to remain in upright position for approximately 2 hours after eating to promote digestion and discourage reflux.
10. Provide mouth care for comfort and hygiene, and have oral suction available if excess salivation is a problem.

Education and Health Maintenance
1. When advanced to a full diet, encourage the patient to avoid overeating, take small bites, chew food well; avoid chunks of meat and stringy raw vegetables and fruit.
2. Depending on type of surgery, advise patient that frequent, small meals may be better tolerated.
3. Encourage the patient to rest postoperatively and to increase activities as tolerated.
4. Instruct the patient to recognize and report signs and symptoms of complications: nausea, vomiting, elevated temperature, cough, or difficulty in swallowing.

CANCER, GASTRIC

Gastric cancer, or malignant tumor of the stomach, is usually an adenocarcinoma. It spreads rapidly to the lungs, lymph nodes, and liver. Risk factors include chronic atrophic gastritis with intestinal metaplasia; pernicious anemia or having had gastric resections (greater than 15 years prior); and adenomatous polyps. This cancer is most common in men older than age 40 and in blacks. Complications are hemorrhage and dumping syndrome from surgery or widespread metastasis and death.

Assessment
1. Most often, the patient presents with the same symptoms as gastric ulcer. Later, evaluation shows the lesion to be malignant.

2. Gastric fullness (early satiety), dyspepsia lasting more than 4 weeks, progressive loss of appetite are initial symptoms.
3. Stool samples are positive for occult blood.
4. Vomiting may occur and may have coffee-ground appearance.
5. Later manifestations include pain in back or epigastric area (often induced by eating, relieved by antacids or vomiting); weight loss; hemorrhage; gastric obstruction.

Diagnostic Evaluation
1. Upper GI X-ray with contrast media may initially show suspicious ulceration that requires further evaluation.
2. Endoscopy with biopsy and cytology confirms malignant disease.
3. Imaging studies (bone scan, liver scan, CT scan) help determine metastasis.
4. Complete blood count (CBC) may indicate anemia from blood loss.

Collaborative Management
Surgical Interventions
1. The only successful treatment of gastric cancer is gastric *resection*, surgical removal of part of the stomach with involved lymph nodes; postoperative staging is done and further treatment may be necessary.
2. Surgical options include proximal or distal subtotal gastric resection; total gastrectomy (includes adjacent organs such as tail of pancreas, portion of liver, duodenum); or palliative surgery such as subtotal gastrectomy with gastroenterostomy to maintain continuity of the GI tract.
3. Surgery may be combined with chemotherapy to provide palliation and prolong life.

Nursing Diagnoses
3, 51, 135, 136

Nursing Interventions
Monitoring
1. Monitor nutritional intake and weigh patient regularly.

2. Monitor CBC and serum vitamin B_{12} levels to detect anemia, and monitor albumin and prealbumin levels to determine if protein supplementation is needed.
3. Monitor for postoperative complications of hemorrhage, shock, pneumonia, and pulmonary embolus.
4. Monitor for signs of dumping syndrome after gastric resection — nausea, weakness, perspiration, palpitations, dizziness, and diarrhea after eating.

Supportive Care

Also see *Gastrointestinal or Abdominal Surgery*, page 381.

1. Provide comfort measures and administer analgesics as ordered.
2. Frequently turn the patient and encourage deep breathing to prevent pulmonary complications, to protect skin, and to promote comfort.
3. Maintain nasogastric suction to remove fluids and gas in the stomach and prevent painful distention.
4. Provide oral care to prevent dryness and ulceration.
5. Keep the patient nothing by mouth as directed to promote gastric wound healing. Administer parenteral nutrition, if ordered.
6. When nasogastric drainage has decreased and bowel sounds have returned, begin oral fluids and progress slowly.
7. Avoid giving the patient high-carbohydrate foods and fluids with meals, which may trigger dumping syndrome because of excessively rapid emptying of gastric contents.
8. Administer protein and vitamin supplements to foster wound repair and tissue building.

Education and Health Maintenance

1. Instruct the patient to avoid dumping syndrome:
   a. Eat small, frequent meals rather than three large meals.
   b. Suggest a diet high in protein and fat and low in carbohydrates, and avoid meals high in sugars, milk, chocolate, and salt.
   c. Reduce fluids with meals, but take them between meals.
   d. Take anticholinergic medication before meals (if prescribed) to lessen GI activity.

  e. Relax when eating; eat slowly and regularly, and rest
   after meals.
 2. Teach the patient how to avoid phytobezoar formation
  (mass of compact vegetable matter that does not pass into
  intestine):
  a. Avoid fibrous foods such as citrus fruits, skins, and seeds
   because they tend to form phytobezoars.
  b. Chew food adequately before swallowing.
 3. Provide information on support groups for patients with
  cancer.
 4. Stress the importance of long-term vitamin B_{12} injections
  after gastrectomy to prevent surgically induced pernicious
  anemia.
 5. Encourage follow-up visits with the health care provider
  and routine blood studies and other testing to detect complications or recurrence.

CANCER, LARYNGEAL

Laryngeal cancer refers to carcinoma of the vocal cords or other portions of the larynx, which occurs more frequently in men
older than age 60. In North America, approximately two-
thirds of carcinomas of the larynx arise in the vocal cords (glottis), almost one-third arise in the supraglottic region, and approximately 3% arise in the subglottic region. Carcinoma of
the vocal cords spreads slowly because of minimal blood supply. Other laryngeal cancers spread more rapidly because of
abundant supply of blood and lymph and soon involve the
lymph nodes of the neck. However, if treated early, these cancers may be cured.

 Risk factors include a history of smoking, high alcohol intake, vocal straining, chronic laryngitis, industrial exposure,
nutritional deficiency, and family predisposition.

Assessment

 1. Supraglottic cancer
  a. Tickling sensation in throat
  b. Dryness and fullness (lump) in throat
  c. Painful swallowing (odynophagia) — associated with
   invasion of extralaryngeal musculature

    d. Coughing on swallowing

    e. Pain radiating to ear (late symptom)

  2. Glottic (vocal cord) cancer

    a. Hoarseness or voice change

    b. Aphonia (loss of voice)

    c. Dyspnea

    d. Pain (in later stages)

  3. Subglottic cancer

    a. Coughing

    b. Short periods of difficulty in breathing

    c. Hemoptysis; fetid odor — results from ulceration and disintegration of tumor

Diagnostic Evaluation

1. Indirect mirror examination of larynx or direct laryngoscopy and biopsy identifies lesion
2. CT scan and other special radiologic tests detect tumor
3. Laryngography — contrast study of larynx — defines blood vessels and lymph nodes

Collaborative Management

Therapeutic Interventions

1. Endoscopic removal of early malignancy
2. Radiation administered alone or in combination with surgery
   a. Complications of radiation: edema of larynx; soft tissue and cartilage necrosis; chondritis (inflammation of cartilage)

Surgical Interventions

1. Carbon dioxide laser to treat early-stage lesions.
2. Partial laryngectomy — removal of small lesion on true cord, along with adjacent healthy tissue.
3. Supraglottic laryngectomy — removal of hyoid bone, epiglottis, and false vocal cords; tracheostomy may be done to maintain adequate airway; radical neck dissection may be done.

4. Hemilaryngectomy — removal of one true vocal cord, false cord, one-half of thyroid cartilage, arytenoid cartilage.

5. Total laryngectomy — removal of entire larynx. A radical neck dissection also may be done because of metastasis to cervical lymph nodes.

6. Total laryngectomy with laryngoplasty — voice rehabilitation may be attempted through the Asai operation to construct a tube from the upper end of the trachea, which may be blocked by finger to produce speech.

C

Nursing Diagnoses
3, 51, 66, 70, 75, 107, 135, 136

Nursing Interventions
Also see *Neck dissection*, page 652.

Monitoring

1. Postoperatively, monitor for signs of difficult breathing, suprasternal and intercostal retractions, tachypnea, dyspnea, tachycardia, decreased alertness, which may indicate stomal stenosis, aspiration, or respiratory infection.

2. Monitor for complications of radiation, such as laryngeal edema and pain and inflammation of tracheal cartilage.

3. Monitor I.V. fluids; assess hydration, and measure intake and output.

4. Monitor for saliva collecting beneath the skin flaps or leaking through suture line or drain site — indicates salivary fistula. Management includes nasogastric tube feeding, meticulous local wound care with frequent dressing changes, and promotion of drainage.

 EMERGENCY ALERT Salivary fistula or skin necrosis usually precedes carotid artery rupture, which requires immediate operative repair.

5. Monitor nutritional status through frequent weighing and serum albumin and prealbumin levels.

Supportive Care

1. Prepare the patient before surgery for alternate means of communication until speech can be relearned.

2. Arrange for the patient to be visited by laryngectomee for hope and encouragement.

3. Provide information about alternate modes of restoring communication (eg, artificial larynx, Electrolarynx, tracheoesophageal puncture with voice prosthesis, esophageal speech [accomplished by training the patient to force air down the esophagus and release it in a controlled manner], and surgical reconstructive procedures to restore voice).

4. Postoperatively, suction secretions frequently to prevent obstruction or aspiration. Employ chest physical therapy and humidification through tracheal collar to help remove secretions. Also suction the mouth and nose.

EMERGENCY ALERT No air can reach lungs of a total laryngectomee (total neck breather) when stoma is clogged. In the event of clogging or obstruction of the stoma, attempt to relieve the obstruction and begin mouth-to-neck breathing immediately. If the chest fails to rise, the patient is a partial neck breather. Place the palm of your hand over the patient's mouth and pinch off the nostrils and continue mouth-to-neck breathing.

5. Be aware that the postoperative patient is unable to cough. Teach to bend forward until stoma is below lung level and to exhale rapidly, then wipe resultant secretions away from tracheostoma with a handkerchief.

6. Encourage breathing exercises, because most patients have been heavy smokers.

7. To provide adequate nutrition, administer enteral tube or gastrostomy feedings until sufficient healing of pharynx has occurred (10 to 12 days) and the patient can consume sufficient oral feedings to meet body needs. Avoid manipulation of the nasogastric tube during this time so it does not disrupt the suture line.

8. Encourage the patient to relearn swallowing. Have standby suction available.

   a. Place the patient in sitting position, leaning slightly forward, which allows larynx to move forward and hypopharynx to partially open. (Explain that the epiglottis normally prevents fluid and food from entering larynx during swallowing.)

b. Teach patient to inhale, swallow, cough gently while exhaling, and reswallow. This ensures enough air in the lungs to cough out any obstruction, thus preventing aspiration.

9. Encourage communication by writing and agreed-on signals until voice work can begin with speech therapist. Discourage forced whispering, which increases pharyngeal tension.

10. Perform and teach tracheostoma care and changing gauze dressing and tracheostomy ties when they become soiled. A laryngectomy or tracheostomy tube is worn until stoma heals (1 to 2 months); the patient then starts gradual process of leaving tube out 1 hour at a time.

COMMUNITY CARE CONSIDERATIONS

Teach the patient to wash hands before touching stoma and clean tracheostoma with warm water and clean washcloth. Avoid using soap, tissues, and cotton balls, which may enter airway. Apply petroleum jelly around stoma to prevent skin irritation and report any redness, swelling, bleeding, or drainage.

Education and Health Maintenance

1. Advise patient to provide humidification at home: use pans of water in the rooms, a humidifier, or a cool mist vaporizer, especially in the bedroom.

2. Advise patient to use a stoma cover made of cotton or crocheted yarn, or wear an ascot, turtleneck, or scarf over the stoma to filter air and manage secretions. Instruct the patient to use a protective shield for bathing, showering, or shampooing or cutting hair.

3. Encourage liberal intake of fluids (2 to 3 qt [2 to 3 L] daily) to help liquefy secretions.

4. Tell the patient to counteract any loss of smell and impairment of taste sensation with additional seasoning of food.

5. Advise patient to follow a high-fiber diet and use stool softeners because he or she may not be able to hold his or her breath and bear down for bowel movements.
6. Advise patient to avoid antihistamines and other medications that tend to dry mucous membranes.
7. Advise patient to report pain, difficulty in breathing or swallowing, or the appearance of pus or blood-streaked sputum.
8. Advise the patient that swimming is not recommended.
9. Encourage the patient to join a local laryngectomy support group (Lost Chord Club; New Voice Club).

CANCER, LIVER

Liver cancer occurs in three major forms. *Hepatocellular carcinoma*, a primary cancer of the liver, arises in normal tissue as a discrete tumor or in end-stage cirrhosis in a multinodular pattern. *Cholangiocarcinoma* is a primary malignant tumor of the bile ducts, which can be intrahepatic or extrahepatic. The third type of liver cancer results from metastasis from an extrahepatic site and invades the liver through the portal system, lymphatic channels, or by direct extension from an abdominal tumor.

Cirrhosis, hepatitis B virus, and hepatitis C virus have been implicated in the cause of primary liver cancer, and possibly hemochromatosis, alpha$_1$-antitrypsin deficiency, and a variety of toxins.

Major complications include malnutrition, biliary obstruction with jaundice, abscesses, sepsis, fulminant liver failure, and metastasis.

Assessment

1. Most common presenting symptom is right upper quadrant abdominal pain, usually dull or aching and may radiate to the right shoulder.
2. Right upper quadrant mass, abdominal distention, fever, malaise, weight loss, and anorexia become evident. Patients with pre-existing liver disease will have rapid deterioration.

3. Jaundice is present in few patients at diagnosis in primary liver cancer. In cholangiocarcinoma, the presenting symptom is usually obstructive jaundice.
4. If there is portal vein obstruction, ascites and esophageal varices occur.

Diagnostic Evaluation

1. Serum bilirubin, alkaline phosphatase, and serum transaminases are all increased.
2. Alpha-fetoprotein: principal tumor marker for hepatocellular carcinoma—elevated in 70% to 95% of patients with the disease.
3. Ultrasonography, CT, and MRI are used to detect cancer and assess if the tumor can be surgically removed.
4. Positron emission tomography detects metastasis or recurrent disease.
5. Percutaneous needle biopsy or biopsy through ultrasonography may be done.
6. Laparoscopy with liver biopsy may be performed.

Collaborative Management
Therapeutic Interventions

1. Therapy prior to surgery to reduce the size of the tumor may include transarterial chemoembolization, combination chemotherapy, chemotherapy with radiation, hepatic artery infusion of chemotherapy, and radioimmunotherapy.
2. Radiation therapy can help reduce pain and discomfort as palliative therapy. Liver cancer is radiosensitive, but treatment is restricted by the limited radiation tolerance of normal liver.
3. Hyperthermia has been used to treat hepatic metastasis.

Pharmacologic Interventions

1. Chemotherapy is used as an adjuvant therapy after surgical resection of liver cancer.
   a. Systemic chemotherapy is the only treatment applicable once the cancer has spread outside the liver.

    b. Regional infusion chemotherapy by implantable pump has been used to deliver a high concentration of chemotherapy directly to the liver through the hepatic artery.

2. Percutaneous alcohol injection is used as an ablative therapy for small tumors.

Surgical Interventions

1. Surgery is the best treatment but is feasible only in 25% of cases, after the extent of tumor and hepatic reserve has been considered.
2. Surgical resection may be along anatomic divisions of the liver or nonanatomic resections.
3. Repeated freezing and thawing of hepatic tumors by cryosurgery is a new modality that preserves normal liver; can be used for large tumors.
4. Radiofrequency ablation uses heat produced by electrodes through the percutaneous or laparoscopic approach to treat small tumors.
5. Liver transplantation has been performed to treat liver tumors, but results have been poor because of the high rate of recurrent primary liver malignancy. It is now recommended that the patient be treated before and after transplantation with chemotherapy and radiation therapy.
6. Percutaneous transhepatic biliary drainage (PTBD) is used to drain obstructed biliary ducts in patients with inoperable tumors or in patients considered poor surgical risks. A percutaneous catheter drains the biliary tree to relieve jaundice, decrease pruritus, and decrease anorexia.
7. Percutaneous or endoscopic placement of internal stents may also be used as palliative treatment for a patient with obstructed bile ducts with a terminal diagnosis.

Nursing Diagnoses
3, 5, 42, 51, 135

Nursing Interventions
Also see *Gastrointestinal or Abdominal Surgery*, page 381.

Monitoring
1. Assess the patient's response to pain control measures.
2. Monitor vital signs, intake and output, and daily weights to detect fluid balance.
3. Measure and record abdominal girth daily.
4. Monitor laboratory values for liver function, such as bilirubin, prothrombin time, aspartate aminotransferase, and alanine aminotransferase.
5. Note subtle changes in mental status indicating hepatic encephalopathy.
6. Monitor for signs of malnutrition, including weight loss, loss of strength, or anemia.

Supportive Care
1. Administer pain control agents as ordered, keeping in mind decreased liver metabolism. Monitor for signs of drug toxicity.
2. Provide nonpharmacologic methods of pain relief, such as massage and guided imagery.
3. Position the patient for comfort—usually in semi-Fowler's position.
4. Encourage the patient to eat small meals and supplementary liquid feedings.
5. Assess and report factors that may increase nutritional needs: Increased body temperature, pain, signs of infection, stress level. Encourage additional calories as tolerated.
6. Restrict sodium and fluid intake as prescribed.
7. If the patient has PTBD, monitor catheter exit site for bleeding or bile drainage, and assess drainage in bag for color, amount, and consistency. The drainage initially may have some blood mixed with bile but should clear within a few hours.
   a. Flush catheter if ordered.

b. Check for and report signs of peritonitis from bile leaking into abdomen: fever, chills, abdominal pain and tenderness, distention.

8. Provide psychological support to patient and family to help them cope with uncertain prognosis.

Education and Health Maintenance

1. Instruct the patient and family on preparation for surgery, reinforce and clarify proposed surgical procedure, and review postoperative instructions.

2. Instruct the patient to recognize and report signs and symptoms of complications.

3. Instruct the patient in continued surveillance for recurrence.

4. Instruct the patient and family in care of any tubes or drains.

CANCER, LUNG

Lung cancer or *bronchogenic cancer* is a malignant tumor of the lung arising within the bronchial wall or epithelium. Bronchogenic cancer is classified according to cell type: epidermoid (squamous cell—most common), adenocarcinoma, small cell (oat cell) carcinoma, and large cell (undifferentiated) carcinoma. The lung is also a common site of metastasis from cancer elsewhere in the body through venous circulation or lymphatic spread.

The primary predisposing factor in lung cancer is cigarette smoking. Lung cancer risk is also high in people occupationally exposed to asbestos, arsenic, chromium, nickel, iron, radioactive substances, isopropyl oil, coal tar products, and petroleum oil mists. Complications include superior vena cava syndrome, hypercalcemia (from bone metastasis), syndrome of inappropriate antidiuretic hormone (SIADH), pleural effusion, pneumonia, brain metastasis, and spinal cord compression.

Assessment

1. New or changing cough, dyspnea, wheezing, excessive sputum production, hemoptysis, chest pain (aching, poor-

ly localized), malaise, fever, weight loss, fatigue, or anorexia.
2. Decreased breath sounds, wheezing, and possible pleural friction rub (with pleural effusion) on examination.

Diagnostic Evaluation
1. Chest X-ray may be suspicious for mass; CT or positron emission tomography scan will better visualize tumor.
2. Sputum and pleural fluid samples for cytologic examination may show malignant cells.
3. Fiberoptic bronchoscopy determines the location and extent of the tumor and may be used to obtain a biopsy specimen.
4. Lymph node biopsy and mediastinoscopy may be ordered to establish lymphatic spread and help plan treatment.
5. Pulmonary function tests, which may be combined with a split-function perfusion scan, determines if the patient will have adequate pulmonary reserve to withstand surgical procedure.

Collaborative Management
Therapeutic Interventions
1. Oxygen through nasal cannula based on level of dyspnea
2. Enteral or total parenteral nutrition for malnourished patient who is unable or unwilling to eat
3. Removal of pleural fluid (by thoracentesis or tube thoracostomy) and instillation of sclerosing agent to obliterate pleural space and prevent fluid recurrence
4. Radiation therapy in combination with other methods

Pharmacologic Interventions
1. Expectorants and antimicrobial agents to relieve dyspnea and infection.
2. Analgesics given regularly to maintain pain at tolerable level. Titrate dosages to achieve pain control.
3. Chemotherapy using cisplatin in combination with a variety of other agents and immunotherapy treatments may be indicated.

Surgical Interventions
1. Resection of tumor, lobe, or lung

Nursing Diagnoses
3, 6, 51, 75

Nursing Interventions
Also see *Thoracotomy*, page 914.

Monitoring
1. Monitor blood work for hypercalcemia from bone metastasis, neutropenia from chemotherapy, and hyponatremia that may result from SIADH.
2. Monitor for upper body edema because of superior vena cava obstruction as a complication.
3. Monitor nutritional status through serial weights, dietary log, and albumin and prealbumin measurements.

Supportive Care
1. Elevate the head of the bed to ease the work of breathing and to prevent fluid collection in upper body (from superior vena cava syndrome).
2. Teach breathing retraining exercises to increase diaphragmatic excursion and reduce work of breathing.
3. Augment the patient's ability to cough effectively.
   a. Splint the patient's chest manually with hands.
   b. Instruct the patient to inspire fully and cough two to three times in one breath.
   c. Provide humidifier or vaporizer to provide moisture to loosen secretions.
4. Teach relaxation techniques to reduce anxiety associated with dyspnea. Allow the severely dyspneic patient to sleep in a reclining chair.
5. Encourage the patient to conserve energy by decreasing activities.
6. Ensure adequate protein intake — milk, eggs, oral nutritional supplements; and chicken, fowl, and fish if other meats are not tolerated — to promote healing and prevent edema.

   a. Advise the patient to eat small amounts of high-calorie and high-protein foods frequently, rather than three daily meals.
   b. Suggest eating the major meal in the morning if rapid satiety is a problem.
   c. Change diet consistency to soft or liquid if patient has esophagitis from radiation therapy.
7. Consider alternative pain control methods, such as biofeedback and relaxation methods, to increase the patient's sense of control.
   a. Evaluate problems of insomnia, depression, anxiety, and so forth, which may be contributing to the patient's pain.
   b. Suggest referral to pain clinic or specialist if pain does not respond to usual control methods.

Education and Health Maintenance

1. Teach the patient to use prescribed medications as needed for pain without being overly concerned about addiction.
2. Advise the patient to report any new or persistent pain; it may be attributable to some other cause such as arthritis.
3. Encourage the patient to keep busy and to continue with usual activities (work, recreational, sexual) as much as possible.
4. Suggest the patient talk to a social worker about financial assistance or other services that may be needed.
5. For additional information and support, refer to American Cancer Society, *www.cancer.org*.

CANCER, ORAL CAVITY, PHARYNGEAL, AND SINUSES

Cancers of the oral cavity may arise from the lips, buccal mucosa, gums, hard palate, floor of the mouth, salivary glands, and the anterior two-thirds of the tongue. *Cancers of the oropharynx* may arise from the tonsillar fossa, pharyngeal wall, and facial arch (soft palate, uvula, anterior portion of tonsillar pillars). These cancers are more common in men ages 50 to 70 and most are squamous cell carcinoma. Risk factors include use of tobacco (cigarette smoking, smokeless tobacco, pipe smoking), heavy alcohol intake (especially in combination with smoking), use of marijuana, and chronic sun exposure. *Nasopharyngeal carcinoma* is more common in people whose diet contains salted fish, as in China, and may be associated with the Epstein-Barr virus. The maxillary sinuses are most involved with *cancer of the paranasal sinuses*, and cancer is usually of squamous cell origin. Complications result from surgery and radiation to wide areas that contain vital structures, and the development of second primary cancers of the larynx, hypopharynx, esophagus, and lungs.

Assessment

1. Often asymptomatic in early stages; may note mucosal erythroplasia — red inflammatory or erythroplastic mucosal changes; appears smooth, granular, and minimally elevated, with or without a white component (leukoplakia), persisting longer than 10 to 14 days
2. Cancer of the lip — presence of a lesion that fails to heal
3. Cancer of the tongue — swelling, ulceration, areas of tenderness or bleeding, abnormal texture, or limited tongue movement
4. Cancer of the floor of the mouth — red, slightly elevated, mucosal lesions with ill-defined borders, leukoplakia, induration, ulceration, or wartlike growths
5. Involvement of other areas — neck mass, throat swelling, painful swallowing, dysphagia, ear pain, difficulty opening mouth, epistaxis, cranial nerve II, III, IV, VI, IX-XII palsies.
6. Advanced stages characterized by ulceration, bleeding, pain, induration, cervical lymphadenopathy, and weight loss.

Diagnostic Evaluation

1. Inspection of the oral cavity and pharynx with indirect mirror locates abnormal tissue.
2. Flexible or rigid nasopharyngoscopy.

3. Staining of oral lesions with toluidine blue distinguishes abnormal from normal tissue (lesions stain dark blue after rinsing with acetic acid; normal tissues retain their pink color).
4. Excisional biopsy of suspected mass identifies or rules out malignancy.
5. Chest X-ray, CT scan, MRI detect local invasiveness and metastasis.

Collaborative Management
Surgical and Other Interventions
1. Selection of treatment depends on size and site of lesion and involvement of surrounding tissues. Surgery, radiation, and chemotherapy may be considered.
2. Small lesions of the oral cavity and oropharynx can be excised widely or treated with radiation therapy or interstitial irradiation.
3. Large lesions of the oral cavity or oropharynx may be excised widely or treated by radical neck dissection for extensive lymphatic involvement, followed by external irradiation to decrease recurrence rate while preserving external appearance.
4. Surgical resection of nasopharyngeal cancer and base of tongue cancer may be difficult due to its location and its relationship to many important structures. Radiation is the treatment of choice in early stages; chemotherapy and radiation are used in combination in advanced cases.
5. Combination of surgery, radiation, and chemotherapy is used for sinus cancer.

Nursing Diagnoses
3, 30, 44, 51, 78, 135, 136

Nursing Interventions
Also see page 606 if radical neck dissection has been performed.

Monitoring

1. Evaluate the patient's emotional status as well as adjustment to cancer and altered appearance with therapy.
2. Monitor nutritional status through intake and output, weight, and laboratory studies.
3. Monitor for adverse effects of radiation: loss of taste, dry mouth, caries, blindness, nasopharyngeal stenosis, cerebrospinal fluid leak, and osteomyelitis.
4. Monitor for complications of surgery: infection, fistula formation, aspiration, salivary gland obstruction, hemorrhage, and voice changes.

Supportive Care

1. Provide analgesics and comfort measures.
2. Provide wound care as directed.
3. If the patient can tolerate it, provide mouth care with soft toothbrush and flossing between teeth.
   a. If patient cannot tolerate brushing and flossing, provide gentle oral lavage with nonirritant mouthwashes.
   b. Use power water spray to clean inaccessible areas.
4. Manage excessive salivation and mouth odors by insertion of a gauze wick in corner of mouth to absorb excess saliva, suctioning of secretions, and instruction to the patient on suctioning methods.
5. Manage decreased salivation, if necessary, by intake of adequate fluids; avoidance of dry, bulky, and irritating foods; and lozenges to moisten mucous membranes.
6. Encourage oral feedings and supplements high in protein and vitamin content and low in acidity and salt, or provide alternate enteral or parenteral nutrition as indicated.
7. Maintain clean and odor-free environment for meals.
8. If swallowing difficulties persist, suggest consultation with an occupational or speech therapist.
9. Assist the patient in caring for personal appearance and provide emotional support.
10. Observe for reaction to cancer such as acting out or withdrawn behavior and suggest psychological consultation, if necessary.

Education and Health Maintenance
1. Reinforce teaching about good oral hygiene.
2. Emphasize adequate nutrition and food preparation with blender, if necessary.
3. Provide detailed instructions on postoperative wound care.
4. Instruct patient to report any bleeding, infection, problems with salivation, or depression.
5. Encourage cessation of high-risk behaviors, such as smoking, alcohol consumption, use of smokeless tobacco, or pipe smoking.
6. Emphasize the need for routine follow-up examinations.

CANCER, OVARIAN

Ovarian cancer is a common gynecologic malignancy that carries a high mortality because it is not usually diagnosed until well advanced. Although its exact cause is not known, about 10% of cases are associated with family history of breast, endometrial, colon, or ovarian cancer. High-fat diet; smoking; alcohol; environmental toxins; patient history of breast, colon, or endometrial cancer; and low parity are additional risk factors. Ninety percent of ovarian tumors arise in epithelial tissue, with germ cell and stromal tissue making up the rest. Incidence peaks in women age 50 or older. Ovarian tumors spread intra-abdominally and through the lymph system.

Assessment
1. First manifestations include vague abdominal discomfort, indigestion, flatulence, anorexia, pelvic pressure, weight loss or gain, and palpable ovarian enlargement.
2. Late manifestations include abdominal pain, ascites, pleural effusion, and intestinal obstruction.

COMMUNITY CARE CONSIDERATIONS

A combination of a long history of ovarian dysfunction and persistent undiagnosed GI complaints raises the suspicion of ovarian cancer. A palpable ovary in a postmenopausal woman is abnormal and should be evaluated as soon as possible.

Diagnostic Evaluation

1. Pelvic sonography (with transvaginal probe) and CT scan may be done. Unfortunately, these are not sensitive to early detection of ovarian cancer.
2. Color Doppler imaging may be used to detect vascular changes within the ovaries.
3. Paracentesis or thoracentesis are done if ascites or pleural effusion is present.
4. Laparotomy is necessary to stage the disease and determine effectiveness of treatment.
5. CA 125 is a serum tumor marker that is not reliable for screening because its level may be elevated due to inflammation; however, an increase signifies progression of disease.

Collaborative Management

Therapeutic and Pharmacologic Interventions

1. Chemotherapy is more effective if tumor is optimally debulked; usually follows surgery because of frequency of advanced disease; may be given I.V. or intraperitoneally.
2. Immunotherapy with interferon or hormonal therapy with tamoxifen, an antiestrogen agent, may be used.

Surgical Interventions

1. Total abdominal hysterectomy with bilateral salpingo-oophorectomy and omentectomy is usual treatment because of delayed diagnosis.
2. Second-look laparotomy may be done after adjunct therapies to take multiple biopsy specimens and determine effectiveness of therapy.

Nursing Diagnoses

3, 6, 24, 30, 51, 78, 92

Nursing Interventions

Also see *Gastrointestinal or Abdominal Surgery*, page 381.

Supportive Care

1. Administer anxiolytic and analgesic medications as prescribed and provide support throughout the diagnostic process.
2. Administer or teach the patient or caregiver to administer antiemetics as needed for nausea and vomiting due to chemotherapy.
3. Encourage small, frequent, bland meals or liquid nutritional supplements as able. Assess the need for I.V. fluids if the patient is vomiting.
4. Prepare the patient for body image changes resulting from chemotherapy (eg, hair loss). Encourage the patient to prepare ahead of time with turbans, wig, hats, and so forth.
5. Stress the positive effects of the patient's treatment plan.
6. Prepare the patient for surgery as indicated; explain the extent of incision, presence of I.V. tubes, catheter, packing and drain tubes expected.
7. Postoperatively, reposition frequently and encourage early ambulation to promote comfort and prevent adverse effects.
8. Refer the patient to cancer support group.

Education and Health Maintenance

1. Explain to the patient that ovary removal will cause menopausal symptoms.
2. Tell the patient that disease progression will be monitored closely by laboratory tests and that a second-look laparoscopy may be necessary.
3. Explain that female relatives of the patient should notify their physicians; biannual pelvic examinations may be necessary.
4. Advise that, for women who have not had breast or ovarian cancer, oral contraceptives may decrease the risk of ovarian and endometrial cancer.

CANCER, PANCREATIC

Pancreatic cancer is the fourth leading cause of cancer deaths, and it is most common among people ages 60 to 80 but may occur in younger adults. Most pancreatic cancers (70%) occur in the head of the pancreas. The tumor may block bile flow as it compresses the common bile duct, causing pain and digestive enzyme dysfunction as well. Symptoms are usually vague and nonspecific, preventing early detection. Risk factors include prolonged exposure to industrial chemicals, high-fat diet, diabetes mellitus, and chronic pancreatitis. Complications include biliary, gastric, or duodenal obstruction; liver failure secondary to metastasis; and portal hypertension due to involvement of blood vessels in the area.

Assessment

1. Symptoms are usually vague and nonspecific, preventing early detection.
2. Anorexia, weight loss, weakness, nausea, and vomiting occur.
3. Gnawing or boring pain usually occurs in the upper abdomen and may radiate to the back.
   a. Pain is usually worse at night. Patients tend to lie with legs drawn up. Patient bends over while walking.
   b. Pain becomes more localized, severe, and unremitting as the disease progresses.
4. Pancreatic enzyme dysfunction causes early satiety and a feeling of bloating after eating.
5. Biliary obstruction produces jaundice, tea-colored urine, clay-colored stools (steatorrhea), and pruritus.

Diagnostic Evaluation

1. Elevated liver function tests and prolonged coagulation studies; possibly elevated levels of carcinoembryonic antigen and CA 19-9.
2. Ultrasound and CT scans detect tumors larger than 1 cm.
3. Endoscopic retrograde cholangiopancreatography is performed to visualize structures and obtain biopsy specimen; magnetic resonance cholangiopancreatography can be done without contrast material.
4. Percutaneous needle aspiration or biopsy through ultrasonography or CT scanning may be performed.
5. Endoscopic ultrasonography for preoperative staging.

Collaborative Management
Therapeutic and Pharmacologic Interventions
1. Chemotherapy may be used in combination with radiation therapy for resectable and unresectable tumors with and without surgery.
2. Radiation therapy may be used alone for palliation or as adjuvant to surgery.
   a. External beam irradiation for local control, reduction of pain, and to palliate obstruction.
   b. Intraoperative radiation therapy has been successful in some centers for palliation.
3. Chemical splanchnicectomy (injection of alcohol into the celiac axis nerves) may be performed to denervate the pancreas for pain relief; may be performed intraoperatively or percutaneously under CT guidance.
4. Combination chemotherapies, immunotherapy, and gene therapy are being investigated.

Surgical Interventions
1. Whipple procedure (pancreatoduodenectomy) for carcinoma of the head of the pancreas and periampullary area; also done for chronic pancreatitis of the head of the pancreas and trauma. Involves removal of the head of the pancreas, distal portion of the common bile duct, gallbladder, duodenum, and distal stomach, with anastomosis of the remaining pancreas, stomach, and common bile duct to the jejunum. The pyloric region of the stomach is preserved in the pylorus-sparing pancreatoduodenectomy.
2. Total pancreatectomy including a splenectomy may be performed for diffuse tumor throughout the pancreas.
3. Distal pancreatectomy, removal of the distal pancreas and spleen for tumors localized in the body and tail.
4. Palliative bypass of the bile duct (choledochojejunostomy or cholecystojejunostomy) or stomach (gastrojejunostomy) for unresectable pancreatic tumors.
5. Endoscopic or percutaneous stent may be placed to relieve biliary obstruction.

ALTERNATIVE INTERVENTION

Many patients may be using herbal or nutraceutical products for potential immune-strengthening or cancer-fighting effects. No alternative products have shown effectiveness in pancreatic cancer and they may interact with chemotherapy agents. Encourage patients to discuss use of all complementary and alternative therapies with their health care providers and pharmacists.

Nursing Diagnoses
3, 5, 44, 51, 63, 67, 92, 123

Nursing Interventions
Also see *Gastrointestinal or Abdominal Surgery*, page 381.

Monitoring
1. Monitor nutrition and hydration status through vital signs, intake and output, calorie count, skin turgor, and daily weights.
2. Monitor for changes in vital signs or increased pain, which may indicate hemorrhage or leak from anastomosis.
3. Monitor serum glucose level for hyperglycemia or hypoglycemia.
4. Monitor stools for signs of malabsorption—foul smelling, floating, greasy appearance.

Supportive Care
1. Administer opioids as ordered or monitor patient-controlled analgesia. Assess the patient's response to pain control measures and consider consultation with hospice service for pain control if tumor is nonresectable. Administer antiemetics as directed.
2. Teach relaxation techniques, such as relaxation breathing, progressive muscle relaxation, and imagery, as adjuncts for pain relief.
3. Assist with frequent turning and comfortable positioning.
4. Administer parenteral nutrition as prescribed preoperatively and postoperatively.

5. Maintain nasogastric decompression, and measure and record gastric output.

6. Progress diet slowly when oral intake is tolerated; observe for nausea, vomiting, and gastric distention.

7. Administer high-protein, high-carbohydrate diet with vitamin supplements and pancreatic enzymes as prescribed.

8. Evaluate laboratory values for hypoalbuminemia, hyponatremia, hypochloremia, and metabolic alkalosis; give replacement therapy as directed.

9. Observe skin for jaundice, breakdown, irritation, or excoriation. Administer antipruritics; provide frequent skin care without soap and rinse thoroughly; apply emollient lotions; and keep fingernails short to prevent scratching.

10. Inspect skin around drains and tubes for irritation and protect from fluid leakage.

11. Inspect surgical dressings and incision for bleeding, drainage, or signs of infection.

12. Prevent tension on suture lines of anastomoses by monitoring for abdominal distention and maintaining patency of tubes and drains.

Education and Health Maintenance

1. Instruct the patient and family on self-care measures for pancreatic insufficiency.
   a. Glucose monitoring, insulin administration, signs and symptoms of hypoglycemia and hyperglycemia
   b. Pancreatic enzyme replacement, high-protein, high-carbohydrate diet

2. Teach the patient about wound and drain care.

COMMUNITY CARE CONSIDERATIONS

Advise the patient that the skin around drainage tubes can be washed with soap and water, dried well, and then protected by generous application of petroleum jelly or zinc oxide before dressing is applied.

3. Explore options for pain management.

4. Coordinate referral for home care for I.V. therapy, post-operative management, or hospice care. Obtain assistive devices for energy conservation; teach caregivers how to help transfer patient, how to perform range-of-motion exercises, and so forth.

5. Instruct the family to report constipation and abdominal distention so that patient can be assessed for bowel obstruction.

CANCER, PROSTATE

Cancer of the prostate is the second leading cause of cancer death among American men and is the most common carcinoma in men older than age 65. Incidence of prostate cancer is higher in black men, and onset is earlier. The cause of prostate cancer is unknown; there is an increased risk for people with a family history of the disease, and the influence of dietary fat, serum testosterone, vasectomy, and industrial toxins is under investigation. Most prostate cancers are adenocarcinoma and are palpable on rectal examination because they arise from the posterior portion of the gland. Prostate cancer is usually multifocal, slow growing, and can spread by local extension, by lymphatics, or through the bloodstream. Complications include bone metastasis leading to vertebral collapse, spinal cord compression, and pathologic fractures, or spread to urinary tract or pelvic lymph nodes.

Assessment

1. First symptoms are caused by obstructed urinary flow, including hesitancy and straining on voiding, frequency, nocturia, reduced size and force of urinary stream.

2. A firm to hard nodule may be felt on rectal examination of the prostate (see *Figure C-1*).

3. Symptoms due to metastasis include:
   a. Pain in lumbosacral area radiating to hips and down legs (from bone metastases).
   b. Perineal and rectal discomfort.
   c. Anemia, weight loss, weakness, nausea, oliguria (from uremia).
   d. Hematuria (from urethral or bladder invasion, or both).

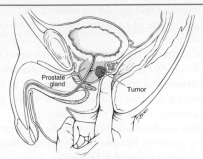

FIGURE C-1 The prostate gland can be felt through the wall of the rectum. The size of the gland, overall consistency, and the presence of any firm areas and nodules are noted.

C

    c. Lower-extremity edema — occurs when pelvic node metastases compromise venous return.

Diagnostic Evaluation

1. Needle biopsy (through anterior rectal wall or through perineum) for histologic study of biopsy tissue or aspiration for cytologic study.
2. Transrectal ultrasonography delineates tumor.
3. Prostate-specific antigen (PSA) — greater than 4 ng/mg; usually greater than 10 ng/mL. A free PSA level can help stratify the risk of elevated PSA levels.
4. Metastatic workup may include skeletal X-ray, bone scan, and CT or MRI to detect local extension, bone, and lymph node involvement.

Collaborative Management
Therapeutic Interventions

1. In many patients older than age 70, no treatment may be indicated because the cancer may be slow growing and will not be the cause of death. Instead, these patients should be followed closely with periodic serum PSA testing and examined for evidence of metastasis.
2. In advanced prostatic cancer not responsive to treatment, palliative measures include:

    a. Analgesics and opioids to relieve pain.

    b. Short course of radiation therapy for specific sites of bone pain.

    c. I.V. administration of a beta-emitter agent (strontium chloride 89) to directly irradiate metastatic sites.

    d. Transurethral resection of the prostate to remove obstructing tissue if bladder outlet obstruction occurs.

    e. Suprapubic catheter placement.

3. External beam radiation (using linear accelerator) focused on the prostate: Focuses maximum radiation on tumor while sparing uninvolved tissues.

4. Interstitial radiation (brachytherapy): Interstitial implantation of isotopes into prostate delivers radiation directly to tumor while sparing uninvolved tissue.

    a. Complications include radiation cystitis (urinary frequency, urgency, nocturia), urethral injury (stricture), radiation enteritis (diarrhea, anorexia, nausea), radiation proctitis (diarrhea, rectal bleeding), and impotence.

Pharmacologic Interventions

1. Hormone manipulation deprives tumor cells of androgens or their by-products and thereby alleviates symptoms and retards progress of disease.

2. Analogs of luteinizing hormone-releasing hormone (LHRH), such as leuprolide, reduce testosterone levels.

3. Antiandrogen drugs (flutamide and nilutamide) block androgen action directly at the target tissues (testes and adrenals) and block androgen synthesis within the prostate gland.

4. Combination therapy with LHRH analogs and flutamide blocks the action of all circulating androgen.

5. Complications of hormonal manipulation include hot flashes, nausea and vomiting, gynecomastia, and sexual dysfunction.

Surgical Interventions

1. Radical prostatectomy—removal of entire prostate gland, prostatic capsule, and seminal vesicles; may include pelvic lymphadenectomy.
   a. Complications include urinary incontinence, impotence, and rectal injury.
   b. Sexual potency may be preserved with newer surgical dissection techniques.
2. Cryosurgery freezes prostate tissue, killing tumor cells without prostatectomy.
3. Bilateral orchiectomy (removal of testes) results in reduction of the major circulating androgen, testosterone, as a palliative measure to reduce symptoms and progression.

Nursing Diagnoses
3, 6, 69, 136, 156

Nursing Interventions
Also see *Prostate Surgery*, page 759.

Supportive Care

1. Assess pain control. Make sure that the patient is not undermedicated; help the family and patient understand that addiction is not a concern.
2. Teach relaxation techniques such as imagery, music therapy, and progressive muscle relaxation as adjunct to pain control.
3. Employ safety measures to prevent pathologic fractures, such as prevention of falls if bone metastasis is present.
4. To reduce anxiety, give repeated explanations of diagnostic tests and treatment options, and help the patient gain some feeling of control over disease and decisions.
5. To help achieve optimal sexual function, give the patient the opportunity to communicate his concerns and sexual needs.
6. Inform the patient that decreased libido is expected after hormonal manipulation therapy, and that impotence may result from some surgical procedures and radiation.

7. Suggest options such as sexual counseling, learning other options of sexual expression, and consideration of penile implant.

Education and Health Maintenance

1. Emphasize the importance of follow-up for check of PSA levels and evaluation for disease progression.
2. Teach the patient to administer hormonal agents intramuscularly or subcutaneously as indicated.
3. If bone metastasis has occurred, encourage safety measures around the home to prevent pathologic fractures, such as removal of throw rugs, using handrail on stairs, and using nightlights.
4. Advise the patient to report symptoms of worsening urethral obstruction, such as increased frequency, urgency, hesitancy, and urinary retention.
5. Encourage all men to seek medical screening for prostate cancer.

COMMUNITY CARE CONSIDERATIONS

Although the PSA is not a perfect screening test, the American Cancer Society recommends an annual rectal examination and blood PSA levels for all men age 50 and older, or starting at age 40 if black or if there is family history of prostate cancer.

6. For additional information and support, refer to such agencies as US TOO International Inc., *www.ustoo.com*.

CANCER, RENAL CELL

Renal cell carcinoma is the most common malignant renal tumor, occurring twice as frequently in men as in women. Most renal cell tumors arise as adenocarcinoma in the renal parenchyma and develop with few if any symptoms. There is no known cause, although they may be associated with cigarette smoking.

Renal tumors are aggressive and metastasize rapidly to the lung, liver, bone, and brain, often before diagnosis. They most frequently occur in people ages 40 to 60.

Assessment

1. Commonly asymptomatic and may be found late on routine examination as palpable abdominal mass.
2. Intermittent, painless hematuria may occur.
3. Fatigue, anemia, anorexia, weight loss, fever may prompt the patient to get evaluation.
4. Classic triad of symptoms occurs late as hematuria, flank pain, and palpable mass in flank.

Diagnostic Evaluation

1. I.V. urography may be used as a screening procedure, but it is not sensitive to all renal tumors.
2. Renal ultrasonography may be used to differentiate renal cysts picked up on other imaging studies from renal tumors.
3. CT scan or MRI scans for patients with urographic findings suggesting tumor; useful to detect, categorize, and stage a renal mass.

Collaborative Management
Pharmacologic Interventions

1. Renal cell carcinomas are generally refractory to chemotherapeutic agents, radiation, and hormonal therapy.
2. Interleukin-2 (a lymphokine that stimulates growth of T lymphocytes) may offer some benefit in metastatic disease, but toxicity is severe.
3. Interferon is also being investigated for treating metastatic cancer.

Surgical Interventions

1. Radical nephrectomy:
   a. Removal of kidney and associated tumor, adrenal gland, surrounding perirenal fat, Gerota's fascia, and possibly regional lymph nodes to provide maximum opportunity for disease control.
   b. Performed through a vertical midline, subcostal, thoracoabdominal, or flank incision.

2. Renal artery embolization:
   a. Preoperative occlusion of renal artery followed by nephrectomy, performed if the patient has large vascular tumor.
   b. Embolizing material (Gelfoam, steel coils, blood clot) is injected through catheter into the renal artery and carried with arterial blood flow to occlude the tumor vessels.
   c. Procedure decreases tumor vascularity, minimizes blood loss, relieves pain, and devitalizes the tumor, thereby decreasing the chance for tumor cell implantation at time of surgery.
   d. Complications include arterial obstruction, bleeding, and reduced renal function.

Nursing Diagnoses
3, 6, 49, 123, 135

Nursing Interventions
Also see *Kidney Surgery and Urinary Diversion*, page 555.

Monitoring
1. Assist in evaluating cardiovascular and nutritional status prior to surgery.
2. Monitor patient comfort level and need for additional analgesia.
3. If renal artery embolization is performed, monitor for postinfarction syndrome (lasts 2 to 3 days): severe abdominal pain, nausea, vomiting, diarrhea, and fever.

Supportive Care
1. Assess the patient's understanding about diagnosis and treatment options. Answer questions and encourage more thorough discussion with health care provider as needed.
2. Encourage the patient to discuss fears and feelings; involve family and significant others in teaching.
3. To control symptoms of postinfarction syndrome:
   a. Administer analgesics as prescribed to control flank and abdominal pain.

    b. Encourage rest and assist with positioning for 2 to 3 days until syndrome subsides.

    c. Obtain temperature every 4 hours, and administer antipyretics as indicated.

    d. Restrict oral intake and provide I.V. fluids and antiemetics to control nausea.

4. Provide postoperative nephrectomy care (see page 559).

Education and Health Maintenance

1. Make sure that the patient understands where and when to go for follow-up (nephrologist; surgeon; primary care provider; oncologist and radiologist for metastatic workup and treatment).

2. Explain the importance of follow-up for evaluation of renal function, even if the patient feels well.

3. Advise the patient with one kidney to wear a medical alert bracelet and notify all health care providers because all potentially nephrotoxic medications and procedures must be avoided.

CANCER, SKIN

Skin cancer is the most common malignancy. Three major types of skin cancer are recognized. The most common type, *basal cell carcinoma*, arises from basal layers of the epidermis or hair follicles and rarely metastasizes. *Squamous cell carcinoma* arises from the epidermis; metastasis occurs more often than with basal cell carcinoma. *Malignant melanoma*, the rarest type, arises from nevocytic cells in the epidermis and metastasizes widely. Most basal and squamous cell carcinomas are located on sun-exposed areas and are directly related to ultraviolet radiation. Basal cell carcinomas are easily curable because of early diagnosis and slow progression.

    Risk factors for skin cancer include fair complexion, blue eyes, blond or red hair; working outdoors; elderly with sun-damaged skin; history of X-ray treatment of skin conditions; exposure to certain chemical agents (arsenicals, nitrates, tar and pitch, oils and paraffins); burn scars, damaged skin in areas of chronic osteomyelitis, fistulae openings; long-term immunosuppressive therapy; genetic susceptibility; and personal or family history of dysplastic nevi; congenital nevi greater than 8 inches (20 cm) in size.

Assessment

⚡ **EMERGENCY ALERT** Any skin lesion that changes in size or color, bleeds, ulcerates, or becomes infected may be skin cancer.

1. Basal cell carcinoma
   a. Lesions often begin as small nodules with a rolled, pearly, translucent border with telangiectasia, crusting, and occasionally ulceration.
   b. Appear most frequently on sun-exposed skin, frequently on face between hair line and upper lip.
   c. If neglected, may cause local destruction, hemorrhage, and infection of adjacent tissues, producing severe functional and cosmetic disabilities.
2. Squamous cell carcinoma
   a. Appears as reddish, rough, thickened, scaly lesion with bleeding and soreness, or may be asymptomatic; border may be wider, more indurated, and more inflammatory than basal cell carcinoma
   b. May be preceded by leukoplakia (premalignant lesion of mucous membrane) of the mouth or tongue, actinic keratoses, scarred or ulcerated lesions
   c. Seen most commonly on lower lip, rims of ears, head, neck, and backs of the hands
3. Malignant melanoma
   a. Melanoma in situ: earliest phase, difficult to recognize because clinical changes are minimal
   b. Superficial spreading melanoma (most common) — circular, with irregular outer portions; the margins may be flat or elevated and palpable; has combination of colors — hues of tan, brown, and black mixed with gray, bluish-black, or white; may be dull pink-rose color in a small area within the lesion; occurs anywhere on body; usually affects middle-aged people
   c. Nodular melanoma — spherical blueberry-like nodule with relatively smooth surface and relatively uniform blue-black, blue-gray, or reddish-blue color; may be polypoidal and elevated, with smooth surface of rose-gray or black color; occurs commonly on torso and ex-

tremities; invades directly into the subjacent dermis (vertical growth) and hence has a poorer prognosis

d. Lentigo melanoma—first appears as tan, flat macule; malignant degeneration is manifested by changes in color, size, and topography; slowly evolving; occurs on exposed skin surfaces of persons in the fifth or sixth decade

e. Acrolentiginous melanoma (uncommon, occurs more frequently in Blacks and Asians)—irregular pigmented macules, which develop nodules; may become invasive early; occurs commonly on palms, soles, nail beds, and rarely on mucous membranes

Diagnostic Evaluation

1. Excisional biopsy for histopathologic diagnosis and microstaging determines the thickness and level of invasion and guides treatment and prognosis.

Collaborative Management
Therapeutic Interventions

1. Radiation therapy can be done for cancer of eyelid, tip of nose, in or near vital structures (eg, facial nerve), where tissue sparing is difficult with other forms of treatment; also used for extensive malignancies where goal is palliation or when other medical conditions contraindicate other forms of therapy.

Pharmacologic Interventions

1. Systemic chemotherapy—generally used for recurrence of malignant melanoma or palliation in advanced cases; may be combined with autologous bone marrow transplantation or several agents used in combination.
2. Other regimens that may be used for basal and squamous cell carcinomas include topical fluorouracil, interferon, and retinoids.

Surgical Interventions

1. Curettage followed by electrodesiccation; usually done on tumors smaller than 1 cm of basal or squamous cell type.

2. Surgical excision for all malignant melanoma and for larger basal cell or squamous cell cancers or in areas more likely to recur (around nose, eyes, ears, lips); may be followed by simple closure, flap, or graft.

3. Lymph node biopsy; may be done for malignant melanoma recurrence with wider area of excision.

4. Microscopically controlled excision, called Mohs' surgery, may be done. Immediate microscopic examination is made of frozen or chemically fixed sections for evidence of cancer cells; layers are removed until no more cancer cells are seen.

Nursing Diagnoses
3, 6, 63, 67, 107

Nursing Interventions
Supportive Care and Education

1. Provide dressing change and wound care instructions after biopsy or surgical excision. Inspect for unusual redness, swelling, warmth, tenderness, or discharge.

2. Discuss patient's feelings about the diagnosis, treatment, and prognosis.

3. Teach the patient and all individuals to use a sunscreen with a sun protection factor of at least 15 routinely for the rest of life and avoid becoming sunburned. Teach methods of minimizing sun exposure with appropriate clothing and hats.

PEDIATRIC ALERT Adolescents may become interested in using a tanning bed or natural tanning. Teach them that sunlight as well as artificial light of a tanning bed damages the skin and that cumulative effects may cause skin cancer. They should avoid tanning, especially if their skin burns easily or tans poorly.

4. Encourage lifelong follow-up with dermatologist or primary care provider, with skin examinations every 6 months.

5. Encourage all people to have moles evaluated that are accessible to repeated friction and irritation, congenital, or suspicious in any way.

6. Demonstrate skin self-examination to all people, using mirrors and magnifying glass to examine all skin surfaces,

including scalp, genital area, buttocks, feet, and so forth, for suspicious lesions.
7. Encourage reporting any skin lesion that changes in size or color, bleeds, ulcerates, or becomes infected.

CANCER, TESTICULAR

Testicular cancer is a relatively uncommon cancer that occurs in younger men between ages 15 and 35. Most testicular cancers originate in the germ cells, and most are potentially curable. The most common germinal tumors in adults are seminoma, embryonal carcinoma, teratoma, and choriocarcinoma. The direct cause of testicular cancer is unknown; it has been linked to cryptorchidism (failure of the testes to descend into the scrotum). Complications include metastasis to the retroperitoneal lymph nodes with subsequent involvement of the mediastinal lymph nodes, lungs, and liver, resulting in death.

Assessment
1. Painless swelling or enlargement of the testis; accompanied by sensation of heaviness in scrotum
2. Pain in the testis (if patient has epididymitis or bleeding into tumor)
3. Signs and symptoms of metastatic disease: cough, lymphadenopathy, back pain, GI symptoms, lower extremity edema, and bone pain

Diagnostic Evaluation
1. Elevated serum markers of human chorionic gonadotropin and alpha-fetoprotein; tumor marker assays also used for diagnosis, detection of early recurrence, staging of tumors, and monitoring response to therapy.
2. Scrotal ultrasonography locates tumor and differentiates between solid and cystic lesions.
3. Chest X-rays locates pulmonary or mediastinal metastases.
4. CT scanning of the chest, abdomen, and pelvis evaluates retroperitoneal lymph nodes and follows progress of therapy.

Collaborative Management
Therapeutic and Pharmacologic Interventions

1. Radiation therapy to lymphatic drainage pathways is used after orchiectomy in seminomas.
   a. Achieves close to 99% cure rate.
   b. During this therapy, the uninvolved testicle is shielded, usually preserving fertility.
2. Chemotherapy with cisplatin combination therapy is used to treat nonseminomatous primary tumor and regional lymphatic metastases and in managing distant metastatic disease.

Surgical Interventions

1. Inguinal orchiectomy: removal of testis and its tunica and spermatic cord
2. Retroperitoneal lymph node dissection (RPLND): Usually performed after orchiectomy in nonseminomas for staging and therapeutic purposes
3. Complications of surgery
   a. RPLND causes infertility because of retrograde ejaculation unless modified nerve-sparing unilateral lymphadenectomy can be done to preserve ejaculation.
   b. Unilateral orchiectomy eliminates half of germinal cells, thus reducing sperm count.
   c. Libido and ability to attain an erection are preserved in both procedures.

Nursing Diagnoses
6, 30, 92, 136, 156

Nursing Interventions
Supportive Care

1. Discuss with patient the possibility of depositing sperm in sperm bank before surgery if fertility may be desired in the future.
2. Provide realistic information about impending surgery or treatment; dispel myths associated with testicular disease, and emphasize high positive cure rates.

3. Reassure the patient that orchiectomy will not diminish virility, and RPLND may cause retrograde ejaculation (into the urinary bladder) but not affect libido, erection, and sensation.
4. Advise the patient that a gel-filled testicular prosthesis can be implanted that will preserve scrotal appearance and feel.
5. Provide routine postoperative care, including early ambulation, respiratory care, and administration of pain medication.
6. After RPLND, monitor for paralytic ileus, which is common after extensive resection.
   a. Auscultate bowel sounds frequently and observe for abdominal distention.
   b. Withhold oral fluids until bowel sounds have returned.
   c. Report complaints of nausea and vomiting.
   d. Begin nasogastric decompression, if indicated.
7. For patients receiving chemotherapy, intervene for common adverse effects, including nausea and vomiting, alopecia, myalgias, abdominal cramping, and mucositis.
8. Refer the patient to a social worker or counselor as needed for problems and concerns with relationships, peers, or work life.

Education and Health Maintenance
1. Teach all young men to perform monthly testicular self-examination; after orchiectomy, the patient should examine the remaining testicle monthly.
2. Review schedule for radiation treatments or chemotherapy; teach the patient and family possible adverse effects; discuss expectations for treatment period.
3. Provide information about retrograde ejaculation after RPLND and alternatives for fertility.

CANCER, THYROID
Thyroid cancer is a malignant neoplasm of the gland that is especially likely to occur in patients who have received radiation treatments to the head and neck in early life. Incidence

increases with age; the average age at time of diagnosis is 45. Thyroid cancer occurs in several forms.

Papillary and well-differentiated adenocarcinoma is the most common type. It grows slowly and does not spread beyond the lymph nodes surrounding the thyroid. The cure rate is excellent after removal of involved tissues.

Follicular carcinoma is a rapidly growing, widely metastasizing cancer that occurs predominantly in middle-aged and elderly persons. Although X-ray treatments may temporarily retard this cancer, it has a high mortality rate.

Parafollicular or medullary thyroid carcinoma is a rare, inheritable cancer that can be completely cured if detected early enough by radioimmunoassay for calcitonin.

Undifferentiated anaplastic carcinoma is highly aggressive and lethal but, fortunately, is rare.

Assessment
1. Patient is usually asymptomatic, but hyperthyroidism may occur.
2. Palpation shows a firm, irregular, fixed, painless mass or nodule.

Diagnostic Evaluation
1. A thyroid scan with 99m-technetium pertechnetate differentiates between malignant "cold" nodules, which absorb little of the isotope, compared with nonmalignant nodules or uninvolved tissue.
2. Biopsy using fine-needle aspiration may be done.

Collaborative Management
Therapeutic and Pharmacologic Interventions
1. Thyroid hormone is administered to suppress secretion of thyroid-stimulating hormone after surgical intervention. Treatment is continued indefinitely and requires annual checkups.
2. For unresectable cancer, patient is referred for treatment with ^{131}I treatment or radiation therapy.

Surgical Interventions

1. Thyroidectomy is partial or complete, as required to remove tumor.
2. Postsurgical radiation therapy is often done to reduce chances of recurrence.
3. Follow-up includes periodic radioiodine uptake scan to detect evidence of recurrence.

Nursing Diagnoses
6, 108, 136

Nursing Interventions
Also see *Thyroidectomy,* page 927.

Monitoring

1. Monitor the patient postoperatively for hemorrhage, dyspnea due to tracheal compression caused by swelling, and difficulty speaking due to laryngeal nerve damage.

Supportive Care

1. Provide all explanations in a simple, concise manner and repeat important information as necessary to reduce anxiety, which may interfere with the patient's ability to process information.
2. Reinforce the positive aspects of treatment and high cure rate as outlined by the health care provider.
3. Support the patient through surgery, recovery, and the thyroid replacement process.

Education and Health Maintenance

1. Instruct the patient on the need for compliance with thyroid hormone replacement regimen.
2. Advise the patient about the need for follow-up to monitor replacement therapy and to check for recurrence of malignancy.
3. Supply the patient with additional information or suggest appropriate community resources dealing with cancer prevention and treatment.

CANCER, UTERINE

Uterine cancer usually occurs as adenocarcinoma of the endometrium of the fundus or body of the uterus. Its cause is unknown, but it is linked to increased estrogen stimulation, as in obesity, late menopause, nulliparity, and unopposed estrogen replacement; it is also more prevalent in those with diabetes mellitus and hypertension. Uterine cancer is the most common gynecologic cancer, and the third leading cancer in women. Most cases occur in women older than age 55. This cancer may spread to involve all pelvic structures and metastasizes to lungs, liver, bone, and brain.

Assessment

1. Irregular bleeding before menopause or postmenopausal bleeding; anemia secondary to bleeding.
2. Vaginal discharge — watery, usually malodorous.
3. Pain, fever, and bowel and bladder dysfunction are late signs.

Diagnostic Evaluation

1. Pelvic examination may reveal an enlarged uterus, and endocervical aspirate may show abnormal cells.
2. Endometrial biopsy — may be helpful, but is not sensitive.
3. Dilation and curettage — most accurate diagnostic tool.
4. Additional testing includes metastatic workup (X-ray studies and cystoscopy).

Collaborative Management
Therapeutic Interventions

1. Radiation therapy is the usual treatment, either after surgery, or instead of surgery in advanced cases. Therapy may be intracavitary or external; it is individualized according to the stage of disease and the patient's response to and tolerance of radiation.
2. Intracavitary radiation — radium by way of applicator in endocervical canal.
   a. Applicator remains in place 24 to 72 hours.

   b. Complications include hemorrhagic cystitis, proctitis, vaginal stenosis, uterine perforation.
3. External radiation—by way of linear accelerator or cobalt.
   a. External radiation over pelvis may supplement intracavitary radiation to eliminate cancer spread by way of lymphatic system.
   b. Complications include bone marrow depression, bowel obstruction, fistula.

Pharmacologic Interventions
1. Hormonal therapy (progestational agents) to alter receptor sites in endometrium for estrogen and thus decrease growth in metastatic disease.
2. Chemotherapy is given for metastatic and recurrent disease; low response rate of short duration.

Surgical Interventions
1. Hysterectomy with bilateral salpingo-oophorectomy is treatment of choice for early stage I cancer; advanced stage I and stage II require lymph node dissection as well.

Nursing Diagnoses
3, 22, 24, 43, 44, 92, 136

Nursing Interventions
Also see *Hysterectomy*, page 535.

Monitoring
1. Monitor the patient's response to pain control medications.
2. Observe for signs and symptoms of radiation sickness—nausea, vomiting, fever, diarrhea, abdominal cramping.
3. Monitor for complications of surgery—bleeding, infection.

Supportive Care
1. Administer pain medications and encourage use of relaxation techniques such as deep breathing, imagery, and distraction to help promote comfort.

2. Support the patient through the diagnostic process, and reinforce information given by the health care provider about treatment options.
3. If indicated, prepare the patient for intracavitary radiation.
   a. Advise the patient that you will be administering an enema and vaginal douche and inserting an indwelling catheter before placement of the applicator in the operating room under anesthesia. X-ray confirms placement.
   b. Encourage the patient to bring diversional materials because she will remain on bed rest during radiation treatment.
   c. Instruct the patient on radiation safety measures.
   d. Reassure the patient that radioactivity is monitored by specially trained personnel, that neither the patient nor secretions are radioactive, and that when applicators are removed, no radioactivity remains.
   e. Reinforce that help is readily available.
4. During intracavitary radiation treatment, perform the following:
   a. Maintain the patient on strict bed rest on her back with head of bed elevated 20 to 30 degrees. The patient may be log-rolled three to four times per day. Use egg-crate mattress.
   b. Have the patient bathe her upper body. Perineal care and linen changes are done only when absolutely necessary.
   c. Maintain the patient on a low-residue diet to prevent bowel movements, which could dislodge the apparatus. Encourage the patient to eat a variety of small servings.
   d. Inspect indwelling catheter frequently to ensure proper drainage. A distended bladder may cause severe radiation burns.
   e. Encourage fluids to prevent bladder infection.
   f. Check the patient frequently to minimize anxiety, but minimize time spent at bedside to reduce radiation exposure.

5. During radiation removal, perform the following:
   a. Make sure that sterile gloves, long forceps, and lead container are available.
   b. Check number of tubes removed against number applied; should be noted in chart.
   c. Practice radiation precautions in handling and returning source to radiation department.
   d. Administer a cleansing enema and douche before the patient gets out of bed.
   e. Provide assistance during ambulation because of postural hypotension from prolonged bed rest.

Education and Health Maintenance

1. Explain the importance of reporting any postmenopausal bleeding.
2. Encourage keeping follow-up visits.
3. Explain that surgery or radiation treatment does not prevent satisfying sexual activity.
4. Refer the patient to a local cancer support group.

CANCER, VULVAR

Vulvar cancer most commonly occurs as squamous cell carcinoma of the labia majora or clitoris; it may also originate as a urethral tumor. Its cause is unknown, but it has been linked to viral infections such as human papilloma virus or herpes simplex virus. It spreads primarily through the lymphatic system. Distant metastasis is rare. Vulvar cancer is most common in women older than age 60. Incidence is rising because of an increasingly elderly population, and the disease now represents approximately 4% of gynecologic cancers. If cancer is confined to the vulva, the 5-year survival rate after surgery is 90%.

Assessment

1. Lesion present for several months; may be reddened, pigmented, white, or slightly elevated or ulcerated
2. Vulvar pruritus, pain
3. Discharge or bleeding; may be foul-smelling because of secondary infection

4. Dysuria caused by invasion of urethra with bacteria
5. Lymphadenopathy, edema of vulvar tissue

Diagnostic Evaluation
1. Biopsy of lesion and lymph nodes to confirm diagnosis.
2. If lesion is small, it may be excised at time of biopsy.

Collaborative Management
Pharmacologic Interventions
1. Chemotherapy is primarily investigational. May shrink lesion so surgery can be less extensive.

Surgical Interventions
1. A precancerous lesion, vulvar intraepithelial neoplasia, is usually treated by simple vulvectomy, local excision, or laser ablation.
2. Noninvasive carcinoma in situ is treated with radical local incision, radical vulvectomy, or modified radical vulvectomy.
   a. Postoperative complications of vulvectomy include wound breakdown, lymphedema, leg cellulitis, and vaginal stenosis.
3. Invasive carcinoma is treated by radical or modified radical vulvectomy with bilateral resection of groin lymph nodes. Pelvic nodes may also be removed if involvement is suspected.
4. Advanced carcinoma is treated by pelvic exenteration, or surgery and radiation as a palliative measure. Radiation may be used preoperatively and postoperatively.

Nursing Diagnoses
3, 30, 44, 67, 135, 136, 156

Nursing Interventions
Supportive Care
1. Emphasize the positive outcomes of the prescribed treatment plan; reinforce what the surgeon has already described to her.

2. Prepare the patient for surgery and describe to her the postoperative appearance of the wound, use of drains, urinary catheter, and so forth (see *Figure C-2*).

3. Administer an enema to evacuate intestinal tract before surgery; there will be no bowel movement for 2 or 3 days after surgery.

4. After surgery, maintain drainage and compression of tissues to remove fluid that could cause edema and prevent wound healing. Empty drains as needed (at least every 8 hours).

5. Provide meticulous wound care.
   a. Keep wound clean and dry.
   b. Change sterile dressings as prescribed.
   c. Apply heat lamp if prescribed to increase circulation and healing.

6. Perform perineal care or sitz baths after each bowel movement or voiding (after catheter removed).

7. Maintain patency of urinary catheter (about 10 days) to prevent wound contamination.

8. Encourage low Fowler's position to promote comfort and reduce tension on sutures.

9. Prevent straining with defecation by providing a low-residue diet initially, stool softeners later, as ordered.

10. While patient is on bed rest, administer mini-dose heparin, if prescribed, and encourage leg exercises to prevent thrombus or embolus formation.

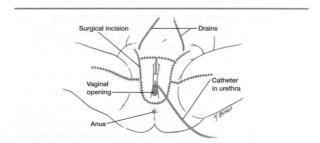

FIGURE C-2 Vulvectomy.

11. Encourage careful ambulation the day after surgery while preventing perineal tension.
12. Inform the patient of changes that may occur because of surgery—loss of sexual arousal if clitoris is removed, shortening of vagina, decreased lubrication.
    a. Tell the patient that if vagina is still intact, vaginal intercourse is still possible.
    b. Help the patient explore alternate methods of sexual intimacy and encourage her to discuss feelings with her partner.

Education and Health Maintenance
1. Encourage follow-up visits for additional therapy if required.
2. Encourage regular health checkups and screening for cancer and other age-related illness.
3. Encourage early evaluation of any suspicious lesions, bleeding, or discharge.

CARDIAC DYSRHYTHMIAS
See *Dysrhythmias*.

CARDIAC SURGERY
Cardiac surgery, or open-heart surgery, is performed for coronary artery bypass grafting (CABG), valve replacement with prosthetic or biologic valves, and repair of congenital defects. The procedure requires temporary cardiopulmonary bypass (diversion of the blood from the heart and lungs for mechanical oxygenation and recirculation) to provide a dry, bloodless field during the operation. Off-pump CABG may be done for patients with poor left ventricular function who would not tolerate the pump.

Newer and less invasive procedures include *minimally invasive direct coronary artery bypass (MIDCAB)* and *port access procedures*. MIDCAB is done through a small thoracotomy incision and is limited to single-vessel disease. A graft may be taken from the internal thoracic artery, and the heart may be slowed during anastomosis, but cardiopulmonary bypass is not needed. Postoperative length of stay is 2 to 4 days. Port access

procedures are performed through a small thoracotomy incision and a few 0.4-inches (1-cm) lateral port incisions that
allow viewing through a thoracoscope and direct access to the
heart to perform multiple vessel bypass, mitral valve surgery,
or repair of atrial septal defect. Port access procedures do require cardiopulmonary bypass, but postoperative length of stay
is cut to 1 to 3 days.

Additional procedures including transmyocardial laser
revascularization are being investigated. Also see *Box C-2*,
pages 180 and 181, for nursing care of other cardiac procedures.

Potential Complications

1. Cardiac dysrhythmias (common)
2. Cardiac tamponade
3. Myocardial infarction
4. Cardiac failure (low-output syndrome)
5. Persistent bleeding (blood clotting disturbance usually
   transient after cardiopulmonary bypass, but may be severe)
6. Hypovolemia, hypotension, renal insufficiency or failure
7. Embolization (common sites include lungs, coronary arteries, mesentery, extremities, kidneys, spleen, and brain)
8. Postpericardiotomy syndrome (unknown cause, may be
   related to anticardiac antibodies; characterized by fever,
   arthralgias, pericardial effusion, and pleural effusion)
9. Postperfusion syndrome (characterized by fever,
   splenomegaly, lymphocytosis)
10. Pulmonary complications—pneumothorax, pulmonary
    edema, phrenic nerve damage, pneumonia, atelectasis.
11. GI bleeding, ileus, cholecystitis, pancreatitis, hepatitis.
12. Neuropsychological dysfunction.
13. Wound infection, febrile complications.

Nursing Diagnoses

3, 6, 19, 57, 67, 80, 130, 135, 136, 158

BOX C-2 Other Cardiac Procedures

Interventional invasive cardiac procedures include cardiac catheterization (primarily diagnostic), percutaneous transluminal coronary angioplasty (PTCA), intracoronary atherectomy, intracoronary stenting, pacemaker insertion, and automatic implantable defibrillator (AID) insertion. These are generally outpatient or short-stay procedures done in a cardiac suite rather than operating room.

PREPROCEDURE CARE

1. Make sure that the patient has not had anything by mouth for directed length of time (usually 6 hours) prior to procedure.
2. Review results of chest X-ray, complete blood count with differential, electrocardiogram, and any other testing ordered before the procedure; make sure that physician and anesthesia care provider know results.
3. Obtain allergy history and complete list of medications (over-the-counter and prescriptions). Make sure that aspirin and other agents that affect blood clotting have been held.
4. Assess, document, and mark distal pulses for reference for postprocedure comparison with cardiac catheterization and PTCA.
5. Make sure that consent is signed and that patient knows what to expect — possible urge to cough and feeling of warmth if contrast medium is injected.

POSTPROCEDURE CARE

1. Monitor vital signs every 15 minutes for 1 hour, every 30 minutes for 1 hour, then hourly as directed. Also monitor urine output and alertness hourly.
2. Maintain bedrest with immobilization of affected extremity for 12 to 24 hours as directed.
3. Maintain cardiac monitoring and report dysrhythmias or signs of ischemia (indicating restenosis after PTCA).
4. Watch for signs of vasovagal reaction that may occur with catheter removal 4 to 6 hours after procedures — hypotension, bradycardia, and diaphoresis; place patient in Trendelenberg position.
5. Assess percutaneous incision site for oozing or hematoma formation and check extremity for color, sensation, temperature, and pulses.
6. Report chest pain.

Other Cardiac Procedures (continued)

7. Be alert for dyspnea, restlessness, cyanosis, and change in breath sounds — which may indicate hemothorax or pneumothorax — and auscultate heart every 4 hours for pericardial friction rub.
8. Record pacemaker settings and make sure that patient understands how to maintain electrical safety with pacemaker or AID (avoid magnetic resonance imaging and electric razors). Tell patient that airport security devices will alarm.
9. If a patient with an AID develops cardiac arrest, begin cardiopulmonary resuscitation. Although a slight buzz will be felt as the device fires, it is not harmful.

Collaborative Interventions

Preoperative Care

1. Review the patient's condition to detect underlying problems such as history of cardiac arrhythmias, chronic lung disease, depression, alcohol intake, and smoking that may impact postoperative recovery.
2. Obtain samples for preoperative laboratory studies, including complete blood count, electrolytes, lipids, renal and hepatic function tests, antibody screen, coagulation studies, and cultures for any underlying infection.
3. Review the patient's medication regimen for drugs that may affect surgery such as digoxin (may be stopped preoperatively to prevent toxicity associated with cardiopulmonary bypass); diuretics (may be associated with electrolyte imbalance); beta-adrenergic blockers (usually continued); psychotropic drugs (postoperative withdrawal may cause extreme agitation); reserpine (stopped in advance to allow norepinephrine repletion); anticoagulants (discontinued several days preoperatively); antiplatelet agents (may be stopped 1 to 2 weeks before surgery to prevent excess bleeding); corticosteroids (if taken within the year before surgery, may be given in supplemental doses to prevent adrenal crisis due to surgical stress); and any over-the-counter, herbal, natural, or al-

ternative product that may have deleterious effect on anesthesia or the cardiovascular syndrome.

ALTERNATIVE INTERVENTION

Many cardiac patients may be taking herbal or "natural" supplements such as hawthorn, coenzyme Q10, garlic, ginkgo, and large amounts of vitamin E or C. Although these products are generally safe, garlic and ginkgo may have antiplatelet activity and hawthorn may interact with digoxin. St. John's wort, taken for depression, may potentiate hypotension caused by anesthesia. Urge patients to discontinue supplement use well before surgery and discuss all medication use with their health care providers.

4. Improve underlying pulmonary disease and respiratory function to reduce risk of complications.
   a. Encourage the patient to stop smoking.
   b. Treat infection and pulmonary vascular congestion.

GERONTOLOGIC ALERT Elderly and debilitated patients are at greater risk for postoperative respiratory complications. Close monitoring and aggressive coughing and deep breathing are indicated.

5. Prepare the patient and family for events in the postoperative period, including chest physical therapy procedures, pain management plan, and the loose restraint of hands for several hours after surgery to avoid risk of inadvertent removal of tubes and I.V. lines.
6. Evaluate the patient's emotional state and try to reduce anxieties.
7. Prepare the patient for the procedure:
   a. Shave anterior and lateral surfaces of trunk and neck; shave entire body down to ankles (for coronary bypass).
   b. Have the patient shower or bathe with Betadine soap.
   c. Give a sedative as directed before moving patient to the operating room.

Postoperative Care

1. Monitor and support respiratory status because respiratory insufficiency is common after open-heart surgery.

a. Provide care while on mechanical ventilator (usually the first 24 hours); assist with weaning and extubation when indicated.

b. Auscultate breath sounds for crackles, indicating pulmonary congestion, or decreased or absent breath sounds, indicating pneumothorax.

c. Promote coughing, deep breathing, and turning to keep airways patent, prevent atelectasis, and facilitate lung expansion. Use chest physiotherapy if congestion develops.

d. Suction as indicated; however, prolonged suctioning leads to hypoxia and possible cardiac arrest.

e. Titrate fluids carefully for first few days to reduce risk of pulmonary congestion from excessive fluid intake.

2. Monitor and support cardiac output through hemodynamic monitoring by blood pressure readings from intra-arterial line, central venous pressure (CVP) readings, left atrial line pressure, and pulmonary artery and capillary wedge pressures.

3. Also monitor for decreased urine output, cyanosis, and decreased level of responsiveness that reflect decreased cardiac output.

4. Be alert for signs of hypoxia — restlessness, headache, confusion, dyspnea, hypotension, and cyanosis.

5. Maintain adequate fluid volume and watch for signs of electrolyte imbalance, particularly hypokalemia, hyperkalemia, hyponatremia, hypocalcemia, hypercalcemia (see page 351).

6. Keep intake and output flow sheet to track fluid balance and the patient's fluid requirements, including I.V. fluids and flush solutions as intake and postoperative chest drainage (should not exceed 200 mL/hour for first 4 to 6 hours) as output.

7. Provide adequate pain control; differentiate between incisional pain and anginal pain. Be alert to possible myocardial infarction after surgery.

8. Examine sternotomy incision and leg incisions for drainage, hematoma, signs of infection.

9. Monitor electrocardiogram continuously and be prepared to treat arrhythmias.
   a. Institute cardiac pacing with temporary pacing wires from incision; wires usually pulled within 48 hours if rhythm is stable.
   b. Valvular and some other surgeries may cause swelling in the atrioventricular area, requiring pacing for 48 hours or more.

> ⚡ **EMERGENCY ALERT** Report dysrhythmia immediately and evaluate for cause — inadequate oxygenation, electrolyte imbalance, myocardial infarction, or mechanical irritation from invasive lines.

10. Assess for signs of cardiac tamponade, including hypotension; increasing CVP; increasing left atrial pressure; muffled heart sounds; weak, thready pulse; neck vein distention; decreasing urinary output; and possible diminished drainage in the chest-collection bottle; be prepared to assist with pericardiocentesis.
11. Be alert for excessive bleeding.
    a. Prepare to administer blood products, I.V. solutions, protamine sulfate, or vitamin K, as ordered.
    b. Prepare for possible return to surgery if bleeding persists (more than 300 mL/hour from chest tube) for 2 hours.
    c. Monitor hemoglobin level and be prepared to administer blood if hemoglobin falls below 8 g/dL.
12. Check cardiac enzyme levels daily — elevation may indicate a myocardial infarction.
13. Evaluate and treat fever as indicated. Most common cause of fever within first 24 hours is atelectasis.
    a. Evaluate for respiratory, urinary tract, or wound infection.
    b. If infective endocarditis is suspected because of persistent fever, draw blood cultures as directed.
14. Watch urine output, blood urea nitrogen, and serum creatinine levels to evaluate for renal insufficiency.
15. Encourage early ambulation to prevent embolic complications.
16. Promote perceptual and psychological orientation and watch for symptoms of postcardiotomy delirium (may ap-

pear after brief lucid period and may include delirium, transient perceptual distortions, visual and auditory hallucinations, disorientation, or paranoid delusions).

a. Encourage interaction with family and communication about patient's experience.

b. Maintain normal day or night pattern and limit environmental stimulation.

c. Reassure patient that psychiatric disturbance after surgery is usually transient.

Education and Health Maintenance

Note: Guidelines vary among health care providers and facilities; check with the patient's surgeon or cardiologist.

1. Instruct patient to increase activities gradually within limits and to avoid strenuous activities until after exercise stress testing.
2. Advise patient to take short rest periods, to avoid lifting more than 20 lb (9 kg), and to participate in activities that do not cause pain or discomfort.
3. Advise patient to increase walking time and distance each day. Stairs may be done once or twice per day the first week; increase as tolerated.
4. Tell the patient to avoid large crowds initially and to avoid driving until after the first postoperative checkup.
5. Tell the patient that sexual activities usually may be resumed 2 weeks after surgery. Instruct patient to avoid intercourse if tired or after a heavy meal and to consult health care provider if chest discomfort, difficulty breathing, or palpitations occur after intercourse.
6. Tell the patient that work may be resumed after first postoperative checkup, as advised by health care provider.
7. Tell the patient to expect some chest discomfort from incision.
8. Advise patient about low-salt and low-fat diet as indicated. Tell patient to report weight gain of more than 5 lb (2.3 kg) per week, which may indicate fluid retention.
9. Teach patient about medications, including one aspirin per day, antihypertensives, antilipid medications, and an-

tiarrhythmics, as indicated. Label all medications, and explain purposes and adverse effects.
10. Advise patient with prosthetic valves:
    a. Warfarin regimen may be continued indefinitely. Patients should watch for bleeding and avoid use of aspirin (and many other drugs) that interfere with action of warfarin.
    b. Pregnancy should be avoided.
    c. Antibiotic prophylaxis is needed before dental and surgical procedures.
11. Encourage compliance with rehabilitation and exercise program after exercise stress testing.
12. Inform the patient whom to contact (and how) in case of an emergency.
13. Refer the patient and family to such community support groups as the American Heart Association, *www.americanheart.org*.

CARDIOMYOPATHY

Cardiomyopathy refers to disease of the heart muscle. Primary cardiomyopathies have no known causes; secondary cardiomyopathies have a known or suspected basis. The cardiomyopathies fall into three major groups (dilated, hypertrophic, and restrictive), according to variations in structural and functional abnormalities that can occur.

In *dilated cardiomyopathy*, both right and left ventricles enlarge (dilate) significantly, reducing the heart's ability to pump blood efficiently to the body. Causes include alcohol abuse, chemotherapy, chemical agents, pregnancy (third trimester, postpartum), and infections.

In *hypertrophic cardiomyopathy (HCM)*, the ventricular septum is abnormally thickened. Other changes, such as patches of myocardial fibrosis, disorganization of myocardial fibers, and abnormalities of coronary microvasculature, also occur, leading to abnormal mitral valve function, filling, and contraction of the heart. This disorder has a genetic cause.

In *restrictive cardiomyopathy*, the heart muscle becomes infiltrated by various substances, resulting in severe fibrosis. The fibrotic muscle becomes stiff and nondistendible, causing inadequate ventricular filling. This disorder may be caused by myeloidosis and hemochromatosis (excessive iron deposition).

Complications of cardiomyopathy may include mural thrombus (caused by blood stasis in ventricles with dilated cardiomyopathy), severe heart failure, sudden cardiac death, and pulmonary embolism.

Assessment

1. Exertional dyspnea, chest pain
2. Arrhythmias—atrial/ventricular ectopic beats; sinus, atrial, and ventricular tachycardia
3. Decreased breath sounds caused by pericardial effusion in restrictive cardiomyopathy
4. Signs of heart failure (see page 424) and pulmonary edema (see page 766)
5. Heart murmur
6. Syncope

Diagnostic Evaluation

1. Electrocardiogram and 24-hour Holter monitoring detects arrhythmias.
2. Chest X-ray detects cardiomegaly.
3. Echocardiogram evaluates wall motion abnormalities.
4. Radionuclide imaging evaluates ventricular function.
5. Cardiac catheterization may be necessary to determine cause.

Collaborative Management
Pharmacologic Interventions

1. In dilated cardiomyopathy:
   a. Management of heart failure (see page 424)
   b. Oral anticoagulants, as indicated, especially in patients with atrial fibrillation.

DRUG ALERT Patients with dilated cardiomyopathy are susceptible to digoxin toxicity. Monitor the patient carefully for evidence of nausea, vomiting, "yellow vision" (yellow-green halos around visual images), and arrhythmias.

2. In HCM:
   a. Beta-adrenergic blockers to reduce the force of myocardial contraction, diminish obstructive pressure gradients, and decrease oxygen requirements.
   b. Calcium channel blockers, primarily to improve the heart's ability to relax, but also to help reduce the force of myocardial contraction, thereby providing symptom relief. Implemented when beta-adrenergic agents fail to control symptoms.
   c. Antiarrhythmics such as amiodarone to prevent lethal arrhythmias.

EMERGENCY ALERT Chest pain experienced by HCM patients is managed by rest and elevation of the feet (to improve venous return to the heart). Vasodilator therapy (nitroglycerin) may worsen chest pain by decreasing venous return to the heart and worsening obstruction of blood flow from the heart; agents that increase myocardial contractility (dopamine, dobutamine) should be avoided or used with extreme caution.

3. In restrictive cardiomyopathy:
   a. Therapy is palliative unless a specific underlying process is established.
   b. Fluid restrictions and diuretic therapy to control heart failure.
   c. Digoxin to control atrial fibrillation.
   d. Oral anticoagulants to prevent embolization.

Surgical Interventions

1. Heart transplantation must be considered in the terminal phase of dilated cardiomyopathy.
2. Myotomy and myectomy—surgical resection of a portion of the septum—may be needed to reduce muscle thickness and provide symptom relief in HCM.
3. Pacemakers and automatic internal defibrillators may be implanted to treat severe bradycardias and lethal tachycardias.
4. Percutaneous transluminal septal myocardial ablation—procedure to reduce the left ventricular outflow tract and thus reduce symptomatology.

Nursing Diagnoses
6, 19, 43

Nursing Interventions
Monitoring

1. Monitor heart rate, rhythm, temperature, and respiratory rate at least every 4 hours as condition indicates.
2. Institute continuous cardiac monitoring, as directed, and report arrhythmias.
3. Evaluate central venous pressure, pulmonary artery, and pulmonary capillary wedge pressures with a pulmonary artery catheter to assess progress and effect of drug therapy.
4. Calculate cardiac output, cardiac index, and systemic vascular resistance.
5. Observe for subtle changes in cardiac output, such as decreased blood pressure, change in mental status, or decreased urine output.
6. Monitor coagulation studies and observe for evidence of bleeding if anticoagulants used.
7. Monitor patient after cardiac catheterization (see page 180).

Supportive Care

1. Orient the patient to the unit, purpose of equipment, and plan of care. Explain all procedures and treatments.
2. Encourage the patient to ask questions and ventilate fears and concerns.
3. Make sure that the patient and visitors understand the importance of adequate rest. Advise about visiting hours and facility policy and whom to contact for information.
4. Provide uninterrupted rest periods and assist with ambulation as ordered.
5. Assist the patient in identifying stressors and reducing their effect. (This is especially important for patients with HCM because stress worsens the outflow obstruction.) Teach the use of diversional activities and relaxation techniques to relieve tension.

Education and Health Maintenance

1. Instruct the patient about taking medications such as digoxin.
   a. The patient should take the drug daily after taking a pulse. The patient should notify a health care provider if the pulse is below 60 beats/minute (or other specified rate).
   b. Tell the patient to immediately report signs of digoxin toxicity: anorexia, nausea, vomiting, or "yellow vision."
   c. Advise the patient that follow-up blood tests will be done to monitor serum drug levels.
2. Advise the patient to follow a low-sodium diet; teach him or her how to read food labels.
3. Advise the patient to immediately report signs of heart failure: weight gain, edema, shortness of breath, and increased fatigue.

COMMUNITY CARE CONSIDERATIONS

Make sure that family members know cardiopulmonary resuscitation because the patient is at risk for sudden cardiac arrest.

CARDIOMYOPATHY IN CHILDREN

Cardiomyopathy is an abnormality of the myocardium that impairs cardiac muscle contractility. Other heart structures are not usually involved and, in most cases, the cause is unknown. This condition is rare in children; the type known as dilated congestive cardiomyopathy is most commonly seen, but restrictive and hypertrophic may also occur. Complications of cardiomyopathy include intra-atrial or intraventricular thrombi, systemic or pulmonary emboli, severe malignant arrhythmias, and sudden death.

Assessment

1. History
   a. Fatigue, lethargy, exercise intolerance
   b. Poor weight gain

    c. Chest pain, syncope
    d. Family history of cardiomyopathy
    e. Recent viral infections, human immunodeficiency virus
    f. Collagen vascular disease
    g. Cocaine abuse, cardiotoxic drugs
    h. Sustained tachycardia
    i. Catecholamine surge; hyperthyroidism
2. Physical
    a. Tachycardia, dyspnea
    b. Poor growth
    c. Hepatosplenomegaly
    d. Arrhythmias, systolic murmur, prominent S_3 gallop

Diagnostic Evaluation
1. 12-lead electrocardiogram (ECG) is usually abnormal, with ST-segment changes, arrhythmias.
2. Chest X-ray shows cardiomegaly, congested lung fields.
3. Echocardiogram shows poor ventricular contractility, dilated left or right ventricle, asymmetric septal hypertrophy, increased left ventricular wall thickness with small left ventricular cavity.
4. Cardiac catheterization, not needed for initial diagnosis, but may be used for endomyocardial biopsy; assesses peripheral vascular resistance.

Collaborative Management
Therapeutic and Pharmacologic Interventions
1. Correct underlying cause of the disease if known, although cardiomyopathy is usually not a reversible disease.
2. Supplemental oxygen.
3. Activity restriction (usually self-imposed if younger child or infant). No participation in strenuous or competitive sports.
4. Pharmacologic treatment of dilated cardiomyopathy to treat systolic dysfunction:
    a. Inotropics: Digoxin
    b. Anticoagulants to prevent emboli
    c. Diuretics to relieve pulmonary and venous congestion
    d. Afterload reduction: Captopril, enalapril, lisinopril

e. Antiarrhythmics
5. Pharmacologic treatment for hypertrophic cardiomyopathy to treat diastolic dysfunction:
   a. Beta-adrenergic blockers
   b. Calcium channel blockers
6. Pharmacologic treatment for restrictive cardiomyopathy to treat diastolic dysfunction:
   a. Diuretics to decrease volume
   b. Anticoagulants

Surgical Interventions

1. Placement of automatic implantable defibrillator or biventricular pacing.
2. Cardiac transplantation is considered in severe disease unresponsive to other treatment.
3. Atrioventricular sequential pacing with hypertrophic cardiomyopathy.
4. Myomectomy or myotomy for hypertrophic cardiomyopathy.

Nursing Diagnoses
1, 10, 19, 43, 44, 51, 133

Nursing Interventions
Monitoring

1. Employ continuous vital sign and ECG monitoring; immediately report hypotension, tachycardia, tachypnea, or arrhythmias.
2. Monitor electrolytes; imbalances may depress cardiac output and cause increased arrhythmias.
3. Monitor intake and output, edema, and lung fields for crackles, all indicating heart failure (see page 424).
4. Monitor prothrombin time for patient receiving oral anticoagulants.

Supportive Care

1. Restrict level of activity.

2. Observe bleeding precautions for patients on anticoagulants (ie, no intramuscular injections, no rectal temperatures, urine and stool tests for blood).
3. Use mechanical ventilation to lessen the workload of the heart for severely ill and dyspneic children.
4. Provide frequent, small meals and high-calorie supplements such as milkshakes.
5. Consider supplemental tube feedings if nutritional requirements not met, or infuse hyperalimentation as ordered.
6. Answer questions about available treatment options, including ventilatory support and cardiac transplantation.
7. Organize a family meeting with family and members of the health care team to answer questions, review and explain treatments, and identify support systems.

Education and Health Maintenance
1. Teach the patient about interactions with other medications, adverse effects, and special precautions such as bleeding precautions for child on anticoagulant therapy.
2. Advise patient to report symptoms such as worsening shortness of breath, fatigability, irregular pulse, lightheadedness, and syncope.
3. Teach cardiopulmonary resuscitation to caregivers.
4. Advise patient on frequent follow-up for prothrombin times and other testing to monitor condition.

CARPAL TUNNEL SYNDROME

Carpal tunnel syndrome is an entrapment syndrome resulting from compression of the median nerve in the tendon sheath within the ventral surface of the wrist. Similarly, tarsal tunnel syndrome is a group of symptoms caused by pressure on the posterior tibial nerve in the medial aspect of the ankle and cubital tunnel syndrome is caused by pressure on the ulnar nerve at the medial epicondyle of the elbow. Compression symptoms due to entrapment include paresthesias, numbness, pain, weakness, and muscle atrophy. Compression results from repetitive motion of the wrist, trauma, local tenosynovitis, and mass, such as ganglion or neuroma. Repetitive motions causing carpal tunnel include use of computer, typing, and use of a jackhammer. Carpal tunnel syndrome is more common in those over age 50, in women, in pregnant women in the first trimester, and in those with rheumatoid arthritis. Complications include chronic pain and loss of function of the extremity.

Assessment

1. Progressive sensory changes including paresthesias and numbness of the thumb, index finger, and ring finger of the involved hand; leads to pain waking the patient up at night.
2. Motor changes beginning with clumsiness and progressing to weakness; edema and thenar atrophy may be noted.
3. Positive Tinel's sign: Increased paresthesias on tapping of tendon sheath (ventral surface of central wrist).
4. Positive Phalen test: Increased symptoms with acute palmar flexion for 1 minute.

Diagnostic Evaluation

1. Electromyogram shows weakened response to median nerve stimulation.

Collaborative Management

Therapeutic and Pharmacologic Interventions

1. Wrist splint in slight extension (cock-up splint) to relieve pressure aggravated by wrist flexion; worn at night, and during day if symptomatic.
2. Avoidance of flexion and twisting motion of the wrist.
3. Work or activity modification to relieve repetitive strain.
4. Nonsteroidal anti-inflammatory drugs (NSAIDs) such as ibuprofen 600 to 800 mg tid to relieve inflammation and pain.
5. Corticosteroid injection into tendon sheath to relieve inflammation.

Surgical Interventions

1. Surgery is indicated when conservative measures fail to relieve symptoms.

2. Procedure is release of carpal ligament and tendon to relieve pressure on median nerve.

Nursing Diagnoses
3, 33, 107, 136

Nursing Interventions
Also see *Orthopedic Surgery,* page 680.

Monitoring
1. Monitor level of pain, numbness, paresthesias, and functioning.
2. Monitor for adverse effects of NSAID therapy, especially in the elderly: GI distress or bleeding, dizziness, or increased serum creatinine.
3. After surgery, monitor neurovascular status of affected extremity: pulses, color, swelling, movement, sensation, or warmth.

Supportive Care
1. Apply wrist splint so wrist is in neutral position, with slight extension of wrist and slight abduction of thumb; make sure that it fits correctly without constriction.
2. Administer NSAIDs and assist with tendon sheath injections as required.
3. Apply ice or cold compress to relieve inflammation and pain.

Education and Health Maintenance
1. Teach patient the cause of condition and ways to alter activity to prevent flexion of wrists; refer to an occupational therapist as indicated.
2. Advise patient of NSAID therapy dosage schedule and potential adverse effects; instruct patient to report GI pain and bleeding.
3. Teach patient gentle range-of-motion exercises; refer to a physical therapist as indicated.

CATARACT

A *cataract* is a gradual and painless clouding or opacifying of the crystalline lens of the eye. Cataracts have various causes. *Senile cataracts* commonly develop in elderly patients because of degenerative changes in lens proteins. *Congenital cataracts* occur in neonates as genetic defects or possibly from measles in the mother. *Traumatic cataracts* may occur after injury sufficient to force vitreous humor into the lens capsule.

Risk factors for cataract development include diabetes; exposure to ultraviolet light or high-dose radiation; and drugs such as corticosteroids, phenothiazines, and some chemotherapy agents. If untreated, cataracts progress to blindness.

Assessment
1. Gradual painless vision loss, blurred or distorted vision, excessive glare from bright lights.
2. Pupil may appear milky or white.

Diagnostic Evaluation
1. Slit-lamp examination provides magnification and confirms diagnosis of an opacity
2. Other testing to rule out coexisting conditions of the eye: tonometry (to determine if there is increased intraocular pressure [IOP]), direct and indirect ophthalmoscopy (to rule out disease of retina), perimetry (to detect any loss of visual field)

Collaborative Management
Surgical Interventions
1. Surgery is the only cure and is recommended when vision causes problems in daily activities. Extracapsular extraction is usually done by cryosurgery or phacoemulsification under local anesthesia.
   a. Eyedrops are given to decrease response to pain and lessen motor activity of the eye.
   b. Medication is given to reduce IOP.
2. An intraocular lens implant is usually inserted at the time of surgery, designed for distance vision.

3. Congenital cataract is corrected within first 3 months followed by contact lens to correct vision.

4. Nonsteroidal anti-inflammatory agents, antibiotic ointments, and possibly corticosteroids may be necessary after lens implantation to reduce inflammation on other eye structures and prevent infection.

5. If patient is not candidate for lens implant, the lens and capsule are removed (intracapsular extraction), and eyeglasses and contact lenses are used to correct vision.

Nursing Diagnoses
3, 24, 33, 128, 135, 159

Nursing Interventions
Monitoring

1. Before surgery, monitor for worsening of visual acuity, glare, and ability to perform usual activities.

2. Monitor pain level postoperatively. Sudden onset may be caused by a ruptured vessel or suture and may lead to hemorrhage. Severe pain accompanied by nausea and vomiting may be caused by increased IOP.

3. Assess gradual adaptation to lens implant, contact lens, or glasses.

GERONTOLOGIC ALERT Be aware that elderly patients may have multiple sensory deficits, such as decreased hearing and reduced position sense, that increase the risk of falls and isolation when vision is affected.

Supportive Care and Education

1. Keep the patient comfortable and advise him not to touch his eyes.

PEDIATRIC ALERT Administer sedation to the infant for 24 hours postoperatively to prevent crying and vomiting, which may increase IOP and damage sutures.

2. If eye patch or shield is in place, advise using it for several days, as prescribed, to rest and protect eye, especially at night.

3. Caution the patient against coughing or sneezing, any rapid movement, or bending from the waist to prevent

increased IOP for first 24 hours. Instruct the patient to avoid heavy lifting or straining for up to 6 weeks, as directed by surgeon.

4. Advise patient to increase activities gradually; can usually resume normal activity the day after the procedure.
5. Teach proper instillation of eyedrops.
6. Encourage follow-up ophthalmologic examinations for corrective lenses and checking of IOP. Adjustment to eyeglasses to correct vision may take weeks to months.
   a. Tell the patient that glasses will cause the perceived image to be approximately one-third larger than that seen by the patient before cataract formation.
   b. Instruct the patient to look through the center of the corrective glasses and to turn head when looking to the side because peripheral vision is markedly distorted.
   c. Warn patient that it is necessary to relearn space judgment — walking, using stairs, reaching for articles on the table, or pouring liquids.
7. If contact lenses will be worn, teach the patient that magnification is only about 7% to 10% and peripheral vision is not distorted.
8. If the patient has a lens implant, magnification problems will be negligible. Both the operated eye and the unoperated eye can work together after cataract surgery with lens implantation.
   a. Advise use of sunglasses in bright lights because the pupil is not able to constrict completely after lens implant.
   b. Advise patient that eyeglasses may not be required for distance but may be needed for reading and writing.
9. Advise the patient not to get soap in the eyes.
10. Advise the patient to avoid tilting the head forward when washing hair, and to avoid vigorous head shaking, to prevent disruption of the lens until cleared by surgeon.

CELLULITIS

Cellulitis is an inflammation of the deep dermal and subcutaneous tissue of the skin caused by infection with group A beta-hemolytic streptococci, *Staphylococcus aureus, Haemophilus in-*

fluenzae, or other organisms. The organisms usually enter through a break in the skin integrity (eg, blunt trauma, needle stick, insect bite, or wound), and the resulting infection may spread rapidly through the lymphatic system. Untreated disease may lead to tissue necrosis and septicemia.

Necrotizing fasciitis is a severe soft tissue infection that spreads rapidly along fascia. It is usually caused by *Streptococcus* group A, known as flesh-eating bacteria.

Assessment
1. Tender, warm, erythematous, and swollen area that is not well demarcated
2. Tender, warm, erythematous streak extending proximally from the area, indicating lymph vessel involvement
3. Possibly fluctuant abscess or purulent drainage
4. Possibly fever, chills, headache, malaise

Diagnostic Evaluation
1. Gram stain and cultures identify causative organism from drainage.
2. Blood cultures may be helpful if septicemia develops.

Collaborative Management
Pharmacologic Interventions
1. Oral antibiotics (penicillinase-resistant penicillins, cephalosporins, or quinolones) may be adequate to treat small, localized areas of cellulitis of legs or trunk.
2. Parenteral antibiotics may be needed for cellulitis of the hands, face, lymphatic spread, or widespread involvement.
3. Diabetic patients and patients with peripheral vascular disease may require more intensive and longer-term therapy because of poor tissue penetration by antibiotic and slow healing. Monitor closely for worsening condition.

Surgical Interventions
1. Drainage and debridement may be required for suppurative areas (common with necrotizing fasciitis).

Nursing Diagnoses
3, 24, 49, 134

Nursing Interventions
Monitoring

1. Observe for expanding border, lymphatic streaking, fluctuant area (abscess), and report to health care provider.

EMERGENCY ALERT Monitor for signs of necrotizing fasciitis: pain out of proportion to appearance, fever, tachycardia, darkened tissue under skin, bullae, petechiae, foul odor, and drainage. Notify health care provider immediately.

2. Monitor for signs of antibiotic sensitivity: rash, pruritus, fever, urticaria, angioedema, shortness of breath, or stridor.

Supportive Care

1. Administer or teach self-administration of antibiotics as prescribed; teach dosage schedule and adverse effects.
2. Maintain I.V. infusion or venous access to administer I.V. antibiotics, if indicated.
3. Encourage comfortable position and immobilization of affected area.
4. Elevate affected extremity to promote drainage from area.
5. Use bed cradle to relieve pressure from bed covers.
6. Prepare patient for and assist with débridement as indicated.
7. Administer, or teach self-administration of, analgesics as prescribed; monitor for adverse effects.

Education and Health Maintenance

1. Make sure that the patient understands dosage schedule of antibiotics and the importance of complying with therapy to prevent complications.
2. Advise the patient to notify a health care provider immediately if condition worsens; hospitalization may be necessary.
3. Outpatient-treated cellulitis should be observed within 48 hours of starting antibiotics to determine adequacy of treatment.

4. Teach the patient with impaired circulation or sensation proper skin care and inspection.

CEREBRAL PALSY

Cerebral palsy refers to a group of incurable nonprogressive disorders resulting from central nervous system (CNS) damage that occurs before, during, or soon after birth, from such causes as infections, anoxia, or birth trauma. Although there are varying degrees and clinical manifestations of cerebral palsy, it is generally characterized by paralysis, weakness, or ataxia.

PEDIATRIC ALERT Significant prematurity (< 32 weeks) and very low birth weight (less than 1,500 g) are the most prevalent risk factors for cerebral palsy.

Three major clinical types of *cerebral palsy* are recognized: spastic (most common), dyskinetic or athetoid (25% of cases), and ataxic (10% of cases). In the spastic type, a defect in the cortical motor area or pyramidal tract causes abnormally strong tonus of certain muscle groups. Attempts at movement cause muscles to contract and block the motion, and permanent contractures develop without muscle training. In the dyskinetic type, lesions of the extrapyramidal tract and basal ganglia cause involuntary, uncoordinated, uncontrollable movements of muscle groups (athetosis). In the ataxic type, cerebellar involvement causes disturbances of balance, and gross or fine motor coordination is nearly impossible.

Cerebral palsy is a major cause of disability and the major complication is contractures, which limit mobility.

Assessment

1. Early manifestations (soon after birth) may include one or more of the following:
   a. Asymmetric movements.
   b. Listlessness or irritability.
   c. Difficulty in feeding, swallowing, or poor sucking with tongue thrust.
   d. Excessive, high-pitched, or feeble cry.
   e. Poor head control.
2. Late manifestations may include one or more of the following:

a. Failure to follow normal pattern of motor development. Delayed gross motor development is a universal manifestation of cerebral palsy.
b. Persistence of infantile reflexes.
c. Weakness.
d. Preference for one hand before the child is age 12 to 15 months.
e. Abnormal postures.
f. Delayed or defective speech.
g. Evidence of mental retardation.
3. Associated problems may include seizures, hearing and vision problems, speech and behavioral problems, or esophageal reflux.

Diagnostic Evaluation

1. Thorough evaluation of prenatal, perinatal, and postnatal factors; APGAR scores.
2. CT scanning and blood tests rule out presence of toxins, infectious processes, and neoplasms of CNS.
3. Psychological testing may be done to determine cognitive functioning.

Collaborative Management
Therapeutic Interventions

1. Orthopedic management of scoliosis, contractures, and dislocations with splints and surgery as needed.
2. Developmental enrichment programs including prevocational, vocational, and socialization skills; emotional and behavioral counseling.
3. Assist family to carry out supportive and participant roles in rehabilitation.

Pharmacologic Interventions

1. Antispasticity medications such as dantrolene or diazepam
2. Antireflux medications such as metoclopramide

Surgical Interventions

1. Selective dorsal rhizotomy may be performed in an attempt to decrease spasticity.

Nursing Diagnoses
8, 25, 28, 45, 62, 136

Nursing Interventions
Supportive Care
1. Carry out, and teach the parents to perform, appropriate exercises under the direction of the physical therapist.
2. Use splints and braces to facilitate muscle control and improve body functioning; make sure these fit properly. Assess skin integrity daily.
3. Use assistive devices, such as adapted grooming tools, writing implements, and utensils, to enhance independence.
4. Encourage self-dressing with easy pull-on pants, large sweatshirts, and other loose clothing.
5. Use play, such as board games, ball games, peg boards, and puzzles, to improve coordination.
6. Maintain good body alignment to prevent contractures.
7. Provide adequate rest periods.
8. Evaluate the child's developmental level and then assist with tasks within that level.
9. Provide for continuity of care at home, day care, therapy centers (physical, speech, and occupational), and the hospital.
10. During feeding, maintain a pleasant, distraction-free environment.
    a. Serve the child alone, initially. After the child begins to master the task of eating, encourage the child to eat with other children.
    b. Allow the child to hold the spoon, even if self-feeding is minimal.
    c. Use spoon and fork with special handles, plate and glass holders, and special feeding chair.
    d. Serve foods that stick to the spoon, such as thick applesauce or mashed potatoes.
    e. Encourage finger foods that the child can handle alone.
11. If the child must be fed, do so slowly and carefully. Be aware of any difficulty sucking and swallowing caused by poor muscle control.

12. Be alert for associated sensory deficits (hearing, speech, vision) that delay development and could be corrected. Report any squinting, failure to follow objects, or bringing objects very close to the face.

13. Evaluate the child's need for specific safety measures such as suction machine, safety helmet, or seizure precautions, and modify the environment as appropriate to ensure the child's safety.

14. Assist the parents to appraise the child's assets so they may capitalize on these positive features.

15. Provide positive feedback for effective parenting skills and positive approaches to caring for the child.

16. Assist parents to find local resources to help in the child's care, such as county social service agency, hospital social worker or discharge planner, local United Way, or Catholic Charities office.

Education and Health Maintenance

1. Instruct the parents in all areas of the child's physical care; their active participation in the rehabilitation program is the key to successful management of cerebral palsy.

2. Encourage regular medical and dental evaluations.
   a. The child should receive all regular immunizations.
   b. Dental visits should occur every 6 months, starting at age 2.

3. Advise parents that the child needs discipline to feel secure and relaxed.
   a. Set realistic limits within which the child can function successfully.
   b. Be firm but not rejecting.

4. Refer parents to agencies such as United Cerebral Palsy, *www.ucp.org*.

CERVICAL CANCER

See *Cancer, Cervical*.

CHOLECYSTECTOMY

Cholecystectomy is a very common surgical procedure involving removal of the gallbladder for acute and chronic cholecystitis. The procedure may be done through open laparotomy or laparoscopy (small incisions made to insert laparoscope and instruments used to manipulate and remove the gallbladder). The laparoscopic method decreases recovery time and risk of complications. After cholecystectomy, the bile ducts eventually dilate to accommodate the volume of bile once held by the gallbladder.

Potential Complications
1. Hemorrhage, infection, and bile duct injury
2. Pneumonia, atelectasis
3. Deep vein thrombosis and pulmonary embolism

Nursing Diagnoses
3, 51, 67, 135, 136

Collaborative Interventions
Preoperative Care
1. Make sure that the patient knows reason for cholecystectomy, what the procedure involves, and what to expect postoperatively.
2. Patient must have nothing by mouth from midnight the night before surgery, and must void before surgery.
3. Administer I.V. fluids to improve hydration status if the patient has been vomiting.
4. Administer antibiotics for acute cholecystitis, as ordered.

Postoperative Care
1. Assess vital signs, level of consciousness.
2. Administer prescribed pain medications or monitor patient-controlled analgesia.
3. Promote ambulation to prevent thromboembolus, facilitate voiding, decrease flatus and abdominal distention, and stimulate peristalsis.
4. Encourage splinting of incision when moving and coughing and deep breathing; encourage use of incentive spirometer.
5. Assess wound dressings and T-tube site for any drainage; note amount, color, and odor.

6. Assess bile drainage from T-tube; report any increase or decrease in drainage. Maintain T-tube patency and security.
7. Report right upper quadrant pain, abdominal distention, fever, chills, or jaundice indicating bile duct injury.
8. Administer antibiotics as prescribed.
9. Assess intake and output, including nasogastric (NG) and T-tube drainage.
10. Assess for nausea and vomiting, and administer antiemetics as prescribed. Ensure adequate replacement of fluids.
11. Discontinue suction of NG tube (if used), and monitor for bowel sounds when NG drainage decreases.
12. Encourage fluid intake and advance to regular diet as tolerated.
13. Clamp T-tube when ordered, and assess tolerance of food and color of stools.

Education and Health Maintenance

1. Tell the patient to keep the incision or wound sites dry for 5 to 7 days and to report any signs of redness, pain, or drainage.
2. Instruct the patient that usual activities can usually be resumed within 5 to 7 days after laparoscopic cholecystectomy or within 4 to 6 weeks of open cholecystectomy.
   a. Sexual activity may be resumed when pain has abated.
   b. Consult surgeon for specific instructions on heavy lifting, strenuous activity, showers and tub baths, and driving.
3. Advise patient to advance the diet as tolerated; fat can be ingested as tolerated because the bile ducts will dilate over a period of weeks to accommodate bile needed to digest fat.

CHOLELITHIASIS, CHOLECYSTITIS, CHOLEDOCHOLITHIASIS

Cholelithiasis is the presence of stones in the gallbladder. *Cholecystitis* is acute or chronic inflammation of the gallbladder. *Choledocholithiasis* is the presence of stones in the common bile duct.

Most gallstones result from supersaturation of cholesterol in the bile, which acts as an irritant, producing inflammation in the gallbladder, and which precipitates out of the bile, causing stones. Risk factors include gender (women are four times as likely to develop cholesterol stones as men), age (older than age 40), multiple parity, obesity, use of estrogens and cholesterol-lowering drugs, bile acid malabsorption with GI disease, genetic predisposition, and rapid weight loss. Pigment stones occur when free bilirubin combines with calcium. These stones occur primarily in patients with cirrhosis, hemolysis, and biliary infections.

Acute cholecystitis is caused primarily by gallstone obstruction of the cystic duct with edema, inflammation, and bacterial invasion. It may also occur in the absence of stones, as a result of major surgical procedures, severe trauma, or burns.

Chronic cholecystitis results from repeated attacks of cholecystitis, presence of stones, or chronic irritation. The gallbladder becomes thickened, rigid, and fibrotic, and functions poorly.

Complications of gallbladder disease include cholangitis; necrosis, empyema, and perforation of gallbladder; biliary fistula through duodenum; gallstone ileus; and adenocarcinoma of the gallbladder.

Assessment

1. Gallstones may be asymptomatic or cause biliary colic.
   a. Steady, severe aching pain or sensation of pressure in the epigastrium or right upper quadrant, which may radiate to the right scapular area or right shoulder.
   b. Begins suddenly and persists for 1 to 3 hours until the stone falls back into the gallbladder or is passed through the cystic duct.
2. Acute cholecystitis causes pain that persists more than 4 hours and increases with movement, including respirations.
   a. Also causes nausea and vomiting, low-grade fever, and possibly jaundice (with stones or inflammation in the common bile duct).

b. Right upper quadrant guarding and Murphy's sign (inability to take a deep inspiration when examiner's fingers are pressed below the hepatic margin) are present.

3. Chronic cholecystitis causes heartburn, flatulence, and indigestion. Repeated attacks of symptoms may occur, resembling acute cholecystitis.

Diagnostic Evaluation

1. Oral cholecystography, ultrasonography, and hepatobiliary scan (radiolabeled iminodiacetic acid) visualizes stones or inflammation

2. Endoscopic retrograde cholangiopancreatography and percutaneous transhepatic cholangiography visualize location of stones and obstruction

3. Elevated conjugated bilirubin levels caused by obstruction

Collaborative Management

Therapeutic and Pharmacologic Interventions

1. Supportive management includes rest, I.V. fluids, nasogastric (NG) suction, pain management, and possibly antibiotics.

2. Oral therapy with chenodeoxycholic acid, ursodeoxycholic acid, or a combination of both may decrease the size of existing cholesterol stones or dissolve small ones.
   a. Indicated for patients at high risk for surgery because of age or systemic disease.
   b. Major adverse effects include diarrhea, abnormal liver function tests, increases in serum cholesterol.
   c. Pigment stones cannot be dissolved.

3. Direct contact therapy, in which a local cholelitholytic agent is infused directly into the gallbladder by way of a percutaneous transhepatic biliary catheter.
   a. Indicated for symptomatic, high-risk patients whose gallbladder can be visualized on oral cholecystography.
   b. Adverse effects include pain from the catheter, nausea, transient elevations of liver function tests and white blood count.

Surgical Interventions

1. A cholecystostomy tube may be placed percutaneously into the gallbladder for decompression in preparation for surgery.
2. Cholecystectomy, open or laparoscopic
   a. Intraoperative cholangiography and choledochoscopy for common bile duct exploration
   b. Placement of a T-tube in the common bile duct to decompress the biliary tree and allow access into the biliary tree postoperatively
3. Intracorporeal lithotripsy may be performed after cholecystectomy to fragment retained stones in the common bile duct by pulsed laser or hydraulic lithotripsy applied through an endoscope directly to the stones. The stone fragments are removed by irrigation and aspiration or a basket through an endoscope or the T-tube.

Nursing Diagnoses
3, 23, 51, 92

Nursing Interventions
Also see *Cholecystectomy*, page 204.

Monitoring

1. Monitor temperature and white blood cell count for indications of infection or perforation.
2. Assess for signs of dehydration: dry mucous membranes, poor skin turgor, decreased urine output.

Supportive Care

1. Administer medications or monitor patient-controlled analgesia to control pain.
2. Assist the patient to position of comfort; maintain bed rest during acute illness.
3. Administer I.V. fluids and electrolytes as prescribed.
4. Administer antiemetics as prescribed to decrease nausea and vomiting.
5. Maintain NG decompression until nausea and vomiting subside.

6. Begin food and fluids as tolerated, after acute symptoms subside or postoperatively when bowel sounds return.
7. Observe and record amount of T-tube drainage, if applicable.

Education and Health Maintenance

1. Advise the patient to eat a low-fat diet to prevent contraction of gallbladder, which will aggravate symptoms.
2. Instruct the patient in care of any tubes or catheters that may be in place at discharge.
   a. Observe for bleeding or drainage around insertion site.
   b. Replace gauze dressing when it becomes wet or soiled.
   c. Report any change in drainage.
3. Review postoperative discharge instructions for activity, diet, medications, and postoperative follow-up.
4. Teach the patient to recognize and report symptoms of complications: pain, fever, jaundice, unusual drainage.
5. Encourage follow-up for further treatment as indicated.

CHRONIC OBSTRUCTIVE PULMONARY DISEASE

Chronic obstructive pulmonary disease (COPD) is a disease characterized by airflow limitation that is not fully reversible. Airflow limitation is usually progressive and associated with an inflammatory response in the lungs stimulated by irritants. COPD includes chronic bronchitis and pulmonary emphysema. Although sometimes included in COPD, *asthma* is a reversible disorder and is therefore considered elsewhere in this book.

Chronic bronchitis is chronic inflammation of the lower airways characterized by excessive secretion of mucus, hypertrophy of mucous glands, and recurring infection, progressing to narrowing and obstruction of airflow. Emphysema is the enlargement of air spaces distal to the terminal bronchioles, with breakdown of alveolar walls and loss of elastic recoil of the lungs (see *Figure C-3*). The two conditions may overlap, resulting in subsequent derangement of airway dynamics (eg, obstruction to airflow). In pulmonary emphysema, lung func-

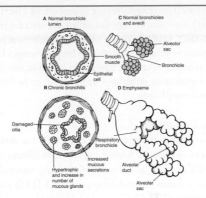

FIGURE C-3 Airway changes in COPD compared with normal.

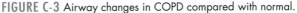

tion progressively deteriorates for many years before the illness becomes apparent.

The most common cause of COPD is cigarette smoking. Air pollution, occupational exposures, allergens, and infections may also act as irritants. Alpha$_1$-antitrypsin deficiency is an infrequent cause. Complications include respiratory failure, pneumonia or other overwhelming respiratory infection, right heart failure (cor pulmonale), arrhythmias, and depression.

Assessment

1. Signs and symptoms of chronic bronchitis (insidious onset):
   a. Productive cough lasting at least 3 months during a year for 2 successive years
   b. Thick, gelatinous sputum (greater amounts produced during superimposed infections)
   c. Dyspnea and wheezing as disease progresses
2. Signs and symptoms of emphysema (gradual in onset and steadily progressive):
   a. Dyspnea, decreased exercise tolerance
   b. Cough (may be minimal with mild sputum production, except with respiratory infection)

c. Increased anteroposterior diameter of chest (barrel chest) with diaphragm flattening (due to air trapping)

EMERGENCY ALERT Recognize early manifestations of respiratory infection — increased dyspnea and fatigue; changes in color, amount, and character of sputum; adventitious breath sounds, low-grade fever; nervousness; irritability — so treatment can be started early to prevent respiratory failure.

Diagnostic Evaluation

1. Pulmonary function tests, to demonstrate airflow obstruction — reduced forced expiratory volume in 1 second (FEV_1), FEV_1 to forced vital capacity ratio; increased residual volume to total lung capacity (TLC) ratio, possibly increased TLC
2. Chest X-rays to detect hyperinflation, flattened diaphragm, increased retrosternal space, decreased vascular markings, possible bullae (all in late stages)
3. Arterial blood gases, to detect decreased arterial oxygen pressure (PaO_2), pH, and increased arterial carbon dioxide pressure ($PaCO_2$)
4. Alpha$_1$-antitrypsin assay to detect this specific cause of emphysema
5. Sputum smears and cultures to identify pathogens

Collaborative Management
Therapeutic and Surgical Interventions

1. Smoking cessation to stop the progression and preserve lung capacity.
2. Low-flow oxygen to correct severe hypoxemia in a controlled manner and minimize carbon dioxide retention.

EMERGENCY ALERT Normally, carbon dioxide levels in the blood stimulate respiration. However, in patients with COPD, chronically elevated carbon dioxide impairs this mechanism, so low oxygen levels in the blood stimulate respiration. Giving a high oxygen concentration may remove the hypoxic drive, leading to hypoventilation, respiratory decompensation, and the development of a worsening respiratory acidosis.

3. Home oxygen therapy, especially at night to prevent nocturnal oxygen desaturation.

4. Pulmonary rehabilitation to reduce symptoms that limit activity.
5. Chest physical therapy, including postural drainage and breathing retraining.
6. Lung volume reduction surgery has been beneficial for some with emphysema.
7. Lung transplant in severe cases of alpha$_1$-antitrypsin deficiency.

Pharmacologic Interventions
See *Table C-1*, page 214.
1. Bronchodilators to reduce dyspnea and control bronchospasm delivered by metered-dose inhalers, other hand-held devices, or nebulization.
   a. Anticholinergics, such as ipratropium and tiotropium.

   DRUG ALERT Anticholinergic agents may worsen narrow-angle glaucoma, prostatic hypertrophy, and bladder neck obstruction.

   b. Short-acting beta agonists, such as albuterol and pirbuterol.
   c. Long-acting beta agonists, such as salmeterol and formoterol.
   d. Methylxanthines, such as theophylline, given orally, usually as sustained-release form for chronic maintenance therapy (less commonly used).
2. Inhaled corticosteroids may be useful for some with severe airflow limitation and frequent exacerbations.
3. Corticosteroids by mouth or I.V. in acute exacerbations
4. Antimicrobials to control secondary bacterial infections in the bronchial tree, thus clearing the airways
5. Alpha$_1$-antitrypsin replacement delivered by I.V. infusion

Nursing Diagnoses
1, 6, 34, 47, 51, 57, 64, 73, 75, 86, 135

TABLE C-1	Drugs Used for COPD
DRUG/ACTION	**ADVERSE REACTIONS/IMPLICATIONS**
Beta$_2$-adrenergic agonists	Sympathomimetic effects: nervousness, restlessness, tachycardia, insomnia, nausea, dizziness, cardiac dysrhythmias, sweating, flushing.
Anticholinergics	Anticholinergic and sympathomimetic effects (usually mild): nervousness, dizziness, headache, blurred vision, cough, nausea, hoarseness, dry mouth.
Methylxanthines	Adverse effects with serum level >20 μg/mL: nausea, vomiting, diarrhea, headache, insomnia, irritability, restlessness, loss of appetite, tachycardia, ventricular dysrhythmias possible. *Note:* Many drugs, cigarette smoking, and high-protein diet can affect serum concentration.
Corticosteroids	Oral and pharyngeal irritation and candidiasis are usually only adverse effects with respiratory inhalation; Cushing's syndrome possible with long-term, high-dose use.

Nursing Interventions

Monitoring

1. Monitor for adverse effects of bronchodilators — tremulousness, tachycardia, cardiac arrhythmias, central nervous system stimulation, hypertension.
2. Monitor condition after administration of aerosol bronchodilators to assess for improved aeration, reduced adventitious breath sounds, reduced dyspnea.
3. Monitor serum theophylline level, as ordered, to ensure therapeutic level and prevent toxicity.
4. Monitor oxygen saturation at rest and with activity.

EMERGENCY ALERT Watch for and report excessive somnolence, restlessness, aggressiveness, anxiety, or confusion; central cyanosis; and shortness of breath at rest, which frequently is caused by acute respiratory insufficiency and may signal respiratory failure.

Supportive Care

1. Eliminate all pulmonary irritants, particularly cigarette smoke. Smoking cessation usually reduces pulmonary irritation, sputum production, and cough. Keep the patient's room as dust-free as possible.
2. Use postural drainage positions to help clear secretions responsible for airway obstruction.
3. Teach controlled coughing.
4. Keep secretions liquid.
   a. Encourage high level of fluid intake (8 to 10 glasses; 2 to 2.5 L daily) within level of cardiac reserve.
   b. Give inhalations of nebulized saline to humidify bronchial tree and liquefy sputum. Add moisture (humidifier, vaporizer) to indoor air.
   c. Avoid dairy products if these increase sputum production.
5. Encourage the patient to assume comfortable position to decrease dyspnea.
6. Instruct and supervise patient's breathing retraining exercises. Teach lower costal, diaphragmatic, and abdominal breathing, using a slow and relaxed breathing pattern to reduce respiratory rate and decrease work of breathing.
7. Use pursed lip breathing at intervals and during periods of dyspnea to control rate and depth of respiration and improve respiratory muscle coordination.
8. Discuss and demonstrate relaxation exercises to reduce stress, tension, and anxiety.
9. Maintain the patient's nutritional status:
   a. Obtain nutritional history, weight, and anthropometric measurements.
   b. Encourage frequent small meals if the patient is dyspneic; even a small increase in abdominal contents may press on diaphragm and impede breathing.
   c. Offer liquid nutritional supplements to improve caloric intake and counteract weight loss.
   d. Avoid foods producing abdominal discomfort.

e. Advise good oral hygiene before meals to sharpen taste sensations.

f. Encourage pursed-lip breathing between bites (or give supplemental oxygen, as directed) if the patient is very short of breath; allow rest after meals.

g. Monitor body weight.

10. Reemphasize the importance of graded exercise and physical conditioning programs (enhances delivery of oxygen to tissues; allows a higher level of functioning with greater comfort).

11. Encourage use of portable oxygen system for ambulation for patients with hypoxemia and marked disability.

12. Encourage the patient to carry out regular exercise program to increase physical endurance.

13. Train the patient in energy conservation techniques.

14. Assess the patient for reactive behaviors (anger, depression, acceptance). Allow the patient to express feelings and retain (within a controlled degree) the mechanisms of denial and repression.

15. Be aware that sexual dysfunction is common in patients with COPD; encourage alternative displays of affection to loved one.

Education and Health Maintenance

1. Review with the patient the objectives of treatment and nursing management. Work with the patient to set goals (ie, stair climbing, return to work, and so forth).

COMMUNITY CARE CONSIDERATIONS

Early in the patient's course, the issues of living will, advanced directives, and resuscitation status need to be addressed. It is better to have these discussions with the patient before crisis situations.

2. Advise the patient to avoid respiratory irritants. Suggest that a high efficiency particulate air filter may have some benefit.

3. Warn patient to stay out of extremely hot or cold weather (and to avoid showering in very hot water) to avoid

aggravating bronchial obstruction and sputum production.

4. Instruct the patient to humidify indoor air in winter; maintain 30% to 50% humidity for optimal mucociliary function.

5. Warn the patient to avoid persons with respiratory infections, and to avoid crowds and areas with poor ventilation.

6. Stress the importance of obtaining influenza and pneumococcal vaccines to guard against these respiratory infections.

7. Teach the patient how to recognize and report evidence of respiratory infection *promptly* — chest pain, changes in character of sputum (amount, color, or consistency), increasing difficulty in raising sputum, increasing coughing and wheezing, increasing shortness of breath.

8. Tell the patient to use bronchodilators only as directed, and advise how to use metered-dose inhaler properly to maximize aerosol deposition in the bronchial tree. (See Box A-3, page 67.) If the patient cannot use inhaler effectively, suggest using a spacer device.

COMMUNITY CARE CONSIDERATIONS

Suggest a pulmonary rehabilitation program that is offered in most communities. Benefits include decrease in hospital admissions, decreased length of stay, and increase in the patient's sense of well-being. Contact local hospitals or the American Lung Association, *www.lungusa.org,* for further information.

CIRRHOSIS, HEPATIC

Cirrhosis of the liver is a chronic disease that causes cell destruction and fibrosis (scarring) of hepatic tissue. Fibrosis alters normal liver structure and vasculature, impairing blood and lymph flow and resulting in hepatic insufficiency and hypertension in the portal vein. Complications include hyponatremia, water retention, bleeding esophageal varices, coagulopathy, spontaneous bacterial peritonitis, and hepatic encephalopathy.

Cirrhosis is known in three major forms. In *Laënnec's (alcohol-induced) cirrhosis*, fibrosis occurs mainly around central veins and portal areas. This is the most common form of cirrhosis and results from chronic alcoholism and malnutrition. *Postnecrotic (micronodular) cirrhosis* consists of broad bands of scar tissue and results from previous acute viral hepatitis or drug-induced massive hepatic necrosis. *Biliary cirrhosis* consists of scarring of bile ducts and lobes of the liver and results from chronic biliary obstruction and infection (cholangitis), and is much rarer than the preceding forms.

Assessment

1. Early complaints include fatigue, anorexia, edema of the ankles in the evening, epistaxis, bleeding gums, and weight loss.
2. In later disease:
   a. Chronic dyspepsia, constipation or diarrhea
   b. Esophageal varices; dilated cutaneous veins around umbilicus (caput medusa); internal hemorrhoids, ascites, splenomegaly
   c. Fatigue, weakness, and wasting caused by anemia and poor nutrition
   d. Deterioration of mental function
   e. Estrogen–androgen imbalance causing spider angioma and palmar erythema; menstrual irregularities in women; testicular and prostatic atrophy, gynecomastia, loss of libido, and impotence in men
   f. Bleeding tendencies and hemorrhage
3. Enlarged, nodular liver

Diagnostic Evaluation

1. Elevated serum liver enzyme levels, reduced serum albumin
2. Liver biopsy detects cell destruction and fibrosis of hepatic tissue
3. Liver scan shows abnormal thickening and a liver mass

4. CT scan determines the size of the liver and its irregular nodular surface
5. Esophagoscopy determines the presence of esophageal varices
6. Percutaneous transhepatic cholangiography differentiates extrahepatic from intrahepatic obstructive jaundice
7. Paracentesis examines ascitic fluid for cell, protein, and bacteria counts

Collaborative Management
Therapeutic Interventions
1. Minimize further deterioration of liver function through the withdrawal of toxic substances, alcohol, and drugs.
2. Correct nutritional deficiencies with vitamins and nutritional supplements and a high-calorie and moderate- to high-protein diet.
3. Correct ascites and fluid and electrolyte imbalances.
   a. Restrict sodium and water intake, depending on amount of fluid retention.
   b. Bed rest to aid in diuresis.
   c. Abdominal paracentesis — to remove fluid and relieve symptoms of ascites (see *Box C-3*, page 220); ascitic fluid may be ultrafiltrated and reinfused through a central venous access.
4. Administer vitamin K for bleeding episodes.

Pharmacologic Interventions
1. Provide symptomatic relief measures such as pain medication and antiemetics.
2. Diuretic therapy, frequently with spironolactone, a potassium-sparing diuretic that inhibits the action of aldosterone on the kidneys.
3. I.V. albumin to maintain osmotic pressure and reduce ascites.
4. Administration of lactulose or neomycin through a nasogastric tube or retention enema to reduce ammonia levels during periods of hepatic encephalopathy.

BOX C-3 | **Assisting with Abdominal Paracentesis**

1. Explain procedure to patient; obtain paracentesis tray, local anesthetic, collection bottle, and laboratory specimen bottles; make sure that consent form has been signed; assess vital signs.
2. Have the patient void and then assist the patient into Fowler's position with back, arms, and legs supported. Drape patient with abdomen exposed.
3. Open sterile tray and assist in skin preparation and local anesthetic.
4. Assemble tubing, collection bottle, and specimen containers and have these available to connect to needle or trocar when the peritoneal cavity has been accessed.
5. Watch fluid drain slowly into collection bottle — usually limited to 1 to 2 qt (1 to 2 L).
6. Assess heart rate and respiratory status frequently during procedure; watch for pallor, cyanosis, and respiratory distress.
7. Apply dressing when needle is withdrawn and assist patient to comfortable position.
8. Check vital signs and monitor for bleeding at least every 30 minutes for 2 hours, then hourly for 4 hours, then every 4 hours for the first 24 hours.
9. Document the patient's condition during and after the procedure, the amount and color of fluid obtained, and the specimens sent to the laboratory.
10. Report any leakage or bleeding from paracentesis site, signs of shock, or scrotal edema.

Surgical Interventions

1. Transjugular intrahepatic portosystemic shunt may be performed in patients whose ascites prove resistant. This percutaneous procedure creates a shunt from the portal to systemic circulation to reduce portal pressure and relieve ascites.
2. Orthotopic liver transplantation may be necessary.

Nursing Diagnoses

1, 35, 51, 134, 135, 136

Nursing Interventions
Monitoring
1. Observe stools and emesis for color, consistency, and amount, and test each one for occult blood.
2. Be alert for symptoms of anxiety, epigastric fullness, weakness, and restlessness, which may indicate GI bleeding.
3. Observe for external bleeding: Ecchymosis, leaking needle stick sites, epistaxis, petechiae, and bleeding gums.
4. Monitor serum ammonia levels; restrict high-protein loads while serum ammonia is high to prevent hepatic encephalopathy.
5. Monitor fluid intake and output and serum electrolyte levels to prevent dehydration and hypokalemia (may occur with the use of diuretics), which may precipitate hepatic encephalopathy.
6. Assess daily weight and abdominal girth measurements for progression of ascites.
7. Assess level of consciousness and reorient the patient as needed.

DRUG ALERT Avoid giving opioids, sedatives, and barbiturates to a restless patient to avoid precipitating hepatic encephalopathy.

Supportive Care
1. Maintain some periods of bed rest with legs elevated to mobilize edema and ascites. Alternate rest periods with ambulation.
2. Encourage and assist with gradually increasing periods of exercise.
3. Encourage the patient to eat high-calorie, moderate-protein meals and supplementary feedings. Suggest small, frequent feedings.
4. Encourage oral hygiene before meals.
5. Administer or teach self-administration of medications for nausea, vomiting, diarrhea or constipation.
6. Note and record degree of jaundice of skin and sclera along with any skin trauma from scratching.
7. Encourage frequent skin care, bathing without soap, and massage with emollient lotions.

8. Keep the patient's fingernails short to prevent scratching from pruritus.
9. Keep the patient quiet and limit activity if signs of bleeding are evident.
10. Institute and teach measures to prevent trauma:
    a. Maintain safe environment.
    b. Blow nose gently.
    c. Use soft toothbrush.
11. Encourage eating foods with high vitamin C content.
12. Use small-gauge needles for injections and maintain pressure over injection site until bleeding stops.
13. Protect from sepsis through good handwashing and prompt recognition and management of infection.
14. Pad side rails and provide careful nursing surveillance to ensure the patient's safety.

Education and Health Maintenance

1. Stress the necessity of giving up alcohol completely; refer the patient to a substance abuse program.
2. Emphasize the importance of rest, a sensible lifestyle, and an adequate, well-balanced diet. Provide written dietary instructions.
3. Encourage the patient to weigh himself daily to monitor for fluid retention or depletion.
4. Discuss adverse effects of diuretic therapy.
5. Involve the person closest to the patient, because recovery usually is not easy and relapses are common.
6. Stress the importance of continued follow-up for laboratory tests and evaluation by the health care provider.

CLEFT LIP AND PALATE

Cleft lip and palate deformities cause a variety of structural facial malformations that are usually apparent at birth. These defects originate as a failure of embryonic development for unknown reasons, but chromosomal abnormalities, hereditary predisposition, and environmental toxins, such as maternal alcohol and smoking, may play a role.

Because the lip and palate develop independently, any combination of defects and degree of involvement can occur.

Cleft lip varies from a notch in the lip to complete separation of the lip into the nose, and may be unilateral or bilateral. It appears more frequently in boys. *Cleft palate* may involve the uvula, soft palate, or both the soft and hard palates through the roof of the mouth, and may also be unilateral or bilateral. It appears more frequently in girls. Complications of cleft lip and palate deformities include impaired speech and hearing, improper tooth placement, and recurrent otitis media.

Assessment

1. Physical appearance of cleft lip or palate
   a. Incompletely formed lip
   b. Opening in roof of mouth felt with examiner's finger on palpation
   c. Weight gain may be slow
2. Eating difficulty
   a. Suction cannot be created for effective sucking.
   b. Food returns through the nose.
   c. Weight gain may be slow.
3. Nasal speech

Diagnostic Evaluation

1. Prenatal ultrasound enables many cleft lips and some cleft palates to be identified.
2. MRI may be done to evaluate extent of abnormality before treatment.
3. Serial X-rays are taken before and after treatment.
4. Dental impressions are taken for expansion prosthesis in older child.
5. Photography to document the abnormality.
6. Genetic evaluation to determine recurrence.

Collaborative Management
Therapeutic Interventions

1. Interdisciplinary team approach from time of diagnosis usually into adolescence. The team should include plastic surgeon, otolaryngologist, pediatric dentist, prosthodontist, orthodontist, feeding specialist, speech pathologist, audiologist, geneticist, psychologist, and community

health nurse. Each team member has a role at various points in the child's care.

Surgical Interventions

1. The cleft lip is generally repaired before the palate defect.
   a. Immediate repair: Several hours to several weeks after birth is preferred by some surgeons.
   b. Intraoral or extraoral prosthesis to prevent maxillary collapse, stimulate bony growth, and aid in feeding and speech development; may be used before surgical repair.
   c. Later repair when infant is age 6 to 12 weeks is usually done; hemoglobin must be 10 g/dL, steady weight gain seen, and infant weighs more than 10 lb (4.5 kg).
2. Cleft palate repair may be done anytime between ages 6 months and 5 years, based on degree of deformity, width of oropharynx, neuromuscular function of palate and pharynx, and surgeon's preference.
   a. Repair at age 9 to 18 months may be preferred because speech patterns have not been set, yet growth of involved structures allows for improved surgical repair.
   b. If repair is delayed to age 4 or 5, a special denture palate is used to help occlude the cleft and aid in establishing speech patterns.

Nursing Diagnoses
82, 104, 119, 132, 135

Nursing Interventions
Monitoring

1. Observe for fever, irritability, redness, or drainage around cleft, and report these signs of infection promptly.
2. Monitor feeding pattern and weight both preoperatively and postoperatively.

Supportive Care
Preoperative Care

1. Administer gavage feedings if nipple feeding is to be delayed to prevent spread of a cleft lip.

2. If sucking is permitted, use a soft nipple with enlarged holes to facilitate feeding.

3. If sucking is ineffective because of inability to create a vacuum, try alternate oral feeding methods, such as regular nipple with enlarged holes or rubber-tipped Asepto syringe or dropper.

4. Feed baby in an upright, sitting position to decrease possibility of fluid being aspirated or returned through the nose, or back to the auditory canal. Avoid repeated removal of the nipple to avoid frustrating the infant. Bubble frequently to reduce air in stomach.

5. When feeding the infant with Pierre Robin syndrome (cleft palate, floppy tongue, and underdeveloped mandible), feed slowly and observe carefully for airway obstruction. If tongue is sutured to pull it forward, observe for slipping, laceration, and signs of infection.

6. Advance diet as appropriate for age and needs of baby.

7. Encourage the mother to begin feeding the baby as soon as possible to enhance bonding. Assist mother with breastfeeding if this is preferred.

8. Clean the cleft after each feeding with water and a cotton-tipped applicator.

9. Support parents. Demonstrate acceptance of both the baby and the parents' feelings. Parents may be grieving about the infant's cosmetic imperfections and may harbor ambivalent feelings about this baby. Reassure them that successful reparative surgery can be done.

10. Prepare family for home feedings by providing several days to practice feeding and to become familiar with the baby's feeding pattern. The infant must feed slowly in upright position, allowing time to clear the airway by sneezing.

11. Suggest that, about 1 week before scheduled admission for surgery, the mother begin using feeding techniques preferred by surgeon for postoperative feeding.

12. Prepare the parents emotionally for the postoperative appearance of the child.

    a. Explain the use of the Logan bow (a curved metal wire that prevents stress on the suture line) and restraints.

b. Encourage a parent to be with the child, especially when awakening from anesthesia, to offer security and comfort.

Postoperative Care

1. Postoperatively, apply elbow immobilizers to prevent child's hands from reaching the mouth while still allowing some freedom of movement. Jacket immobilizer may be used.
2. Protect the suture line from tension.
   a. Check Logan bow, butterfly-type adhesive, or bandage placed across top of lip to prevent lateral tension on cleft lip incision.
   b. Avoid wetting tape, or it will loosen.
   c. Observe for and report bleeding.
   d. Prevent the child from crying, blowing, sucking, talking, or laughing.
3. Position the child on back or propped on side (eg, on infant seat) to keep from rubbing lip on the sheets. If only cleft palate was repaired, child may lie on abdomen.
4. Provide for appropriate diversional activity (eg, hanging toys, mobiles, and so forth).
5. Monitor respiratory effort after cleft palate repair.
   a. Be aware that breathing with a closed palate is different from the child's customary way of breathing; the child must also contend with increased mucus production.
   b. Provide croup tent with mist to decrease occurrence of respiratory problems and provide moisture to mucous membranes that may become dry from mouth breathing.
6. Accomplish feeding without tension on the suture line for several days after lip repair.
   a. Use dropper or syringe with a rubber tip, and insert from the side to avoid suture line or to avoid stimulating sucking.
   b. Perform nasogastric lavage if needed.
   c. Advance slowly to nipple feeding as directed. The infant should be able to suck more efficiently with the lip repaired.

7. Clean suture line after every feeding; keep the mouth moist to promote healing and provide comfort.
8. After palate repair, feed the child in the manner used pre-operatively (cup, side of spoon, or rubber-tipped syringe). Never use straw, nipple, or plain syringe.
   a. Diet progresses from clear liquids to full liquids to soft foods.
   b. Soft foods are usually continued for about 1 month after surgery, at which time a regular diet is started, excluding hard food.
9. Administer prophylactic antibiotics as prescribed because the mouth and suture line are constantly contaminated.

Education and Health Maintenance

1. Instruct the parents on continued protection of the mouth after surgery. Child cannot put anything in mouth, including lollipops. Demonstrate how to rinse mouth after eating.
2. Continue to assess weight gain, feeding behavior, overall development, parent–child bonding and interaction.
3. Advise the parents on increased risk of ear infections and need to seek medical attention for colds, ear pain, fever, or other signs and symptoms. Routine ear examinations and hearing tests should be done to reduce the risk of hearing deficits.
4. Stress the importance of speech therapy and the parents practicing exercises with the child as directed by speech therapist.

COMMUNITY CARE CONSIDERATIONS

Speech difficulties require early identification and intervention. Monitor for reading and learning problems due to speech delays.

5. Help the parents realize that, although rehabilitation of the child is long and expensive, the child can live a normal life.

6. Advise the parents to discuss the child's problem with the school nurse, teacher, and other responsible adults who will have close contact with the child.
7. For additional information and support refer to The Cleft Palate Foundation, *www.cleftline.org*.

CLUBFOOT, CONGENITAL

Clubfoot (talipes equinovarus) is a congenital anomaly in which the foot is plantar flexed at the ankle and subtalar joints, the hind foot is inverted, and the midfoot and forefoot are adducted and inverted. Contractures of the soft tissues maintain the malalignments. Clubfoot occurs bilaterally in 50% of cases and other variations of foot and ankle deformities may occur congenitally, but are less common. The exact cause of clubfoot is unknown, but genetic factors; intrauterine infection; and bone, vascular, and nerve lesions have been suspected. Complications include "rocker bottom" deformity, disturbance in growth, and recurrent or residual deformity.

Assessment
1. Deformity is usually obvious at birth, with varying degrees of rigidity and ability to correct position.
2. Deformity becomes fixed with awkward gait.

Diagnostic Evaluation
1. Clinical presentation and physical examination are usually diagnostic.
2. X-ray determines bony anatomy and assesses treatment efficacy.

PEDIATRIC ALERT Children with clubfoot have a higher incidence of development dysplasia of the hip and neck abnormalities. Very rigid feet may be associated with other system abnormalities.

Collaborative Management
Therapeutic Interventions
1. Treatment should begin as soon after birth as possible, to establish a functional, pain-free foot that can be fit with standard footwear.

a. Serial manipulation with immobilization in a cast, done weekly for 6 weeks, then every 2 weeks.

b. After the initial period (approximately 3 months), evaluation will determine the need to continue with manipulation and casting, percutaneous tenotomy, or proceeding to corrective shoes or solid ankle orthotics.

c. About 50% of nonoperative treatment is successful.

2. Corrective footwear consists of a reverse last or outflare shoe with or without a Dennis-Browne bar or the more recent Wheaton brace or Bebax shoe.

Surgical Interventions

1. Usually performed between ages 4 and 9 months so child is free of postoperative immobilization before the beginning of walking.

2. Surgery consists of a medial plantar release, posterior release, lateral release, or reduction and fixation—depending on the extent of the deformity.

3. The child who presents late or has a recurrent or residual deformity may require an aggressive surgical procedure to stabilize the bony structures and balance the muscle and tendons by a combination of fusions, releases, lengthenings, and transfers.

4. Postoperative routines usually include a period of cast immobilization of up to 12 weeks followed by a brace or corrective shoe for a period of 2 to 4 years.

Nursing Diagnoses
3, 80, 88, 134

Nursing Interventions

Monitoring

1. Perform frequent neurovascular assessments after surgery, including color, warmth, sensation, capillary refill, pulses, and presence of pain.

Supportive Care

1. Discuss the deformity and expected treatment in terms the parents can understand. Respond to their questions and concerns.
2. Encourage parents to hold and play with child and participate in care.
3. Assess fit of cast, splint, orthotic device, or special shoes. Teach parents that, because of the rapid growth rate of the infant, device may need to be replaced to prevent blistering.
4. Assess and teach parents to assess for signs of excessive pressure on skin: redness, excoriations, foul odor from underneath cast, or pain.
5. Elevate the extremity to prevent edema.
6. Place ice packs over casts for the first 24 hours.
7. Stimulate movement of toes to promote circulation.
8. Assess for signs of discomfort such as irritability, crying, poor feeding and sleeping, tachycardia, or increased blood pressure.
9. Administer analgesics regularly for 24 to 48 hours after surgery.
10. Provide comfort measures such as soft music, pacifier, teething ring, or rocking.

Education and Health Maintenance

1. Teach the parents to remove cast by soaking in water and vinegar mixture at home before weekly manipulation and recasting. This avoids anxiety and possible abrasions from using cast saw.
2. Teach the parents when orthotic devices may be removed (usually for bathing). Stress that devices must be worn as prescribed.
3. Advise parents that infant's sleep may be disturbed initially because of wearing brace at night; may be irritable while awake because of fatigue.
4. Instruct parents on providing a safe environment for the ambulatory child.
5. Discuss the importance of long-term and frequent followup, and obtain social work consult to assist the parents

with special needs such as transportation, flexible appointment times, and financing orthotic equipment, as needed.

COLORECTAL CANCER
See *Cancer, Colorectal*.

CONGENITAL HEART DISEASE
See *Heart Disease, Congenital*.

CONGESTIVE HEART FAILURE
See *Heart Failure*.

CONJUNCTIVITIS
Conjunctivitis is inflammation or infection of the conjunctiva, the mucous membrane that lines the inner surface of the eyelids and the anterior portion of the eyeball. The disorder may be caused by bacteria, viruses, *Chlamydia*, fungi, allergens, chemical exposure, or trauma. Common bacteria are *Staphylococcus, Streptococcus pneumoniae*, and *Haemophilus influenzae*. Adenovirus is common. Also known as "pinkeye," this disorder is easily spread by contact with infectious material. It is usually self-limiting, but some organisms may cause extensive tissue damage and visual impairment.

Assessment
1. Itching, burning, feeling of foreign body in eye, and possible photophobia.
2. Redness, swelling, lacrimation, crusting of lids, and any discharge.
   a. Purulent discharge if infected by *Neisseria gonorrhoeae*.
   b. Abundant lacrimation with little discharge indicates viral infection.
3. Visual acuity is usually not affected.

EMERGENCY ALERT A painful red eye should be evaluated promptly for evidence of herpesvirus infection, which may cause corneal damage.

Diagnostic Evaluation

1. If indicated by purulent discharge, specimens for culture and sensitivity tests are collected to determine causative organism.
2. Fluorescein staining may be done to rule out ulceration or keratitis (corneal involvement).

Collaborative Management
Therapeutic Interventions

1. If foreign body is suspected, eye is irrigated with normal saline or prescribed solution to dislodge particles.
2. For common viral conjunctivitis, no treatment is usually indicated unless there is risk of secondary bacterial infection; then, topical antibiotic is given.

Pharmacologic Interventions

1. Topical antibiotic drops or ointment for bacterial conjunctivitis.
2. A topical or systemic antiviral may be given for herpes conjunctivitis.
3. For allergic conjunctivitis, anti-inflammatory, antihistamine, or mast cell stabilizer drops may be given.

PEDIATRIC ALERT One-dose antibiotic ointment (usually erythromycin or tetracycline) is given after delivery to prevent gonococcal or chlamydial conjunctivitis in neonates.

Nursing Diagnoses
3, 24, 136

Nursing Interventions
Education and Health Maintenance

1. Teach frequent handwashing, prompt disposal of contaminated tissues, and no sharing of washcloths and towels to prevent spread of infection.
2. Teach proper technique of instilling eyedrops or applying ointment.
3. Encourage use of warm compresses to remove crusting, or cold compresses to relieve redness and discomfort.

4. Encourage the patient to take medication for entire length of prescription.

CORONARY ARTERY DISEASE

Coronary artery disease (CAD) is characterized by the accumulation of plaque within the coronary arteries, which progressively enlarge, thicken, and calcify. This causes critical narrowing of the coronary artery lumen (75% occlusion), resulting in a decrease in coronary blood flow and an inadequate supply of oxygen to the heart muscle. Ischemia may be silent (asymptomatic but evidenced by ST depression of 1 mm or more on electrocardiogram [ECG]) or may be manifested by angina pectoris (chest pain). Risk factors for CAD include dyslipidemia, smoking, hypertension, male gender (women are protected until menopause), aging, non-white race, family history, obesity, sedentary lifestyle, diabetes mellitus, metabolic syndrome, elevated homocysteine, and stress.

Acute coronary syndrome is a complication of CAD due to lack of oxygen to the myocardium; manifestations include unstable angina, non-ST-segment elevation infarction, and ST-segment elevation infarction.

Other causes of angina include coronary artery spasm, aortic stenosis, cardiomyopathy, severe anemia, and thyrotoxicosis.

Assessment

Chest pain is provoked by exertion or stress and is relieved by nitroglycerin and rest.

1. *Character* — Substernal chest pain, pressure, heaviness, or discomfort. Other sensations include a squeezing, aching, burning, choking, strangling, or cramping pain.
2. *Severity* — Pain may be mild or severe and typically presents with a gradual buildup of discomfort and subsequent gradual fading away.
3. *Location* — Behind middle or upper third of sternum; the patient generally will make a fist over the site of the pain (positive Levine sign; indicates diffuse deep visceral pain), rather than point to it with fingers.

4. *Radiation* — Usually radiates to neck, jaw, shoulders, arms, hands, and posterior intrascapular area. Pain occurs more commonly on the left side than the right; may produce numbness or weakness in arms, wrist, or hands.

5. *Duration* — Usually lasts 2 to 10 minutes after stopping activity; nitroglycerin relieves pain within 1 minute.

6. *Precipitating factors* — Physical activity, exposure to hot or cold weather, eating a heavy meal, and sexual intercourse increase the workload of the heart and, therefore, increase oxygen demand.

7. *Associated manifestations* — diaphoresis, nausea, indigestion, dyspnea, tachycardia, and increase in blood pressure.

8. Signs of unstable angina:
   a. A change in frequency, duration, and intensity of stable angina symptoms.
   b. Angina pain lasts longer than 10 minutes, is unrelieved by rest or sublingual nitroglycerin, and mimics signs and symptoms of impending myocardial infarction (see page 640).

> ⚡ **EMERGENCY ALERT** Unstable angina may cause sudden death or result in myocardial infarction. Early recognition and treatment are imperative.

Diagnostic Evaluation

1. Resting ECG may show left ventricular hypertrophy, ST-T changes, arrhythmias, and possible Q waves.

2. Exercise stress testing with or without perfusion studies shows ischemia.

3. Cardiac catheterization shows blocked vessels.

4. Positron emission tomography may show small perfusion defects.

5. Radionuclide ventriculography shows wall motion abnormalities and ejection fraction.

6. Fasting blood levels of cholesterol, low-density lipoprotein, high-density lipoprotein, lipoprotein A, homocysteine, and triglycerides may be abnormal.

7. Coagulation studies, hemoglobin level, fasting blood sugar as baseline studies.

Collaborative Management
Therapeutic Interventions
1. Smoking cessation.
2. Control of hypertension below 140/90 mm Hg (below 130/80 mm Hg in diabetic patients, 130/85 mm Hg in patients with renal insufficiency or heart failure).
3. Diet low in saturated fat, control of weight, exercise.
4. Control of diabetes and hyperlipidemia.

Pharmacologic Interventions
1. Antianginal medications (nitrates, beta-adrenergic blockers, calcium channel blockers, and angiotensin converting enzyme inhibitors) to promote a favorable balance of oxygen supply and demand.
2. Antilipid medications to decrease blood cholesterol and triglyceride levels in patients with elevated levels.
3. Antiplatelet agents to inhibit thrombus formation.
4. Folic acid and B complex vitamins to reduce homocysteine levels.

Surgical Interventions
1. Percutaneous transluminal coronary angioplasty or intracoronary atherectomy, or placement of intracoronary stent. These procedures are performed through a catheter introduced through the femoral artery and into the coronary circulation to relieve obstruction. Drug eluting stents are becoming increasingly effective.
2. Coronary artery bypass grafting (see page 178).
3. Transmyocardial revascularization — laser is used to form channels in myocardium to encourage new blood flow.

Nursing Diagnoses
3, 6, 19, 108

Nursing Interventions
Monitoring
1. Monitor blood pressure, apical heart rate, and respirations every 5 minutes during an anginal attack.

2. Maintain continuous ECG monitoring or obtain a 12-lead ECG, as directed; monitor for arrhythmias and ST elevation.
3. Assess response to nitroglycerin, rest, or other treatment.
4. Assess for headache, orthostatic hypotension, and change in heart rate and rhythm related to antianginal therapy.
5. Evaluate for development of heart failure (due to treatment with beta-adrenergic blockers or calcium channel blockers).
   a. Obtain serial weights.
   b. Auscultate lung fields for crackles.
   c. Monitor for the presence of edema.
6. Monitor patient after cardiac catheterization (see page 180).

Supportive Care

1. Place patient in comfortable position and administer oxygen, if prescribed, to enhance myocardial oxygen supply.
2. Identify specific activities patient may engage in that are below the level at which anginal pain occurs.
3. Reinforce the importance of notifying nursing staff whenever angina pain is experienced.
4. Encourage supine position for dizziness caused by antianginals (usually associated with a decrease in blood pressure; preload is enhanced by this mechanism, thereby increasing blood pressure). Be sure to remove previous nitrate patch or paste before applying new paste or pad (prevents hypotension).

 DRUG ALERT Follow a 6- to 8-hour per day nitrate-free period, as directed, to avoid tolerance to nitrates.

5. Be alert to adverse reaction related to abrupt discontinuation of beta-adrenergic blocker and calcium channel blocker therapy. These drugs must be tapered to prevent a "rebound phenomenon": tachycardia, increase in chest pain, and hypertension.

Education and Health Maintenance

1. Explain to the patient the importance of anxiety reduction to assist in control of angina. (Anxiety and fear put

an increased stress on the heart, requiring the heart to use more oxygen.) Teach relaxation techniques.

2. Discuss measures to be taken when an anginal episode occurs.

   a. Place nitroglycerin under tongue at first sign of chest discomfort.

   b. Stop all effort or activity; sit, and take nitroglycerin tablet — relief should be obtained in a few minutes.

   c. Bite the tablet between front teeth and slip under tongue to dissolve if quick action is desired.

   d. Repeat dosage in a few minutes for total of three tablets if relief is not obtained.

> **EMERGENCY ALERT** Go to the nearest health care facility if chest pain persists more than 15 minutes, is unrelieved by three nitroglycerin tablets, or is more intense and widespread than the usual angina episodes (should not drive self).

   e. Keep a record of number of tablets taken — to evaluate any change in anginal pattern.

3. Review specific risk factors that affect CAD development and progression; highlight those risk factors that can be modified and controlled to reduce risk.

   a. Inform patient of methods of stress reduction, such as biofeedback and relaxation techniques.

   b. Review information on low-fat or low-cholesterol diet with patient and person who shops or cooks in home. Suggest available cookbooks (American Heart Association) that may assist in planning and preparing foods.

   c. Have dietitian visit patient to design a menu plan for patient.

   d. Inform patient of available cardiac rehabilitation programs that offer structured classes on exercise, smoking cessation, and weight control.

   e. Avoid excessive caffeine intake (coffee, cola drinks) that can increase the heart rate and produce angina.

   f. Do not use "diet pills," nasal decongestants, or any over-the-counter medications that can increase the heart rate or stimulate high blood pressure.

g. Avoid the use of alcohol or drink only in moderation (alcohol can increase hypotensive adverse effects of drugs).

h. Encourage follow-up for tight control of diabetes and hypertension.

4. Advise the patient on activity level to prevent angina.

a. Participate in a normal daily program of activities that do not produce chest discomfort, shortness of breath, and undue fatigue. Begin regular regimen of exercise as directed by health care provider.

b. Avoid activities known to cause anginal pain — sudden exertion, walking against the wind, extremes of temperature, high altitude, emotionally stressful situations; may accelerate heart rate, raise blood pressure, and increase cardiac work.

c. Refrain from engaging in physical activity for 2 hours after meals. Rest after each meal if possible.

d. Do not undertake activities requiring heavy effort (carrying heavy objects).

e. Try to avoid cold weather; dress warmly and walk more slowly. Wear scarf over nose and mouth when in cold air.

5. For more information, contact American Heart Association, *www.americanheart.org*.

COMMUNITY CARE CONSIDERATIONS

Make sure that patient has enough medication until next follow-up appointment or trip to the pharmacy. Warn against abrupt withdrawal of beta-adrenergic or calcium channel blockers to prevent rebound effect.

CRANIOTOMY

Craniotomy is the surgical opening of the skull to gain access to intracranial structures. Surgical approach may be supratentorial (above the tentorium, or dural covering that divides the cerebrum from cerebellum) or infratentorial (below the tentorium, including the brain stem). Procedures include craniotomy by means of bur holes or bony flap, craniectomy in which a portion of the skull is excised, cranioplasty in which a cranial defect is repaired, or transsphenoidal approach to the pituitary. Craniotomy is indicated for a variety of treatments, including removing a tumor or abscess, aspirating a hematoma, clipping an aneurysm, relieving increased intracranial pressure (ICP), stopping hemorrhage, or removing epileptogenic tissue.

Potential Complications
1. Intracranial hemorrhage or hematoma
2. Cerebral edema
3. Infections (postoperative meningitis, pulmonary, wound, and so forth)
4. Seizures
5. Cranial nerve dysfunction
6. Cerebral ischemia and brain damage

Nursing Diagnoses
3, 44, 88, 119, 122, 135, 136

Collaborative Interventions
Preoperative Care
1. Reinforce the surgeon's explanation of diagnostic findings, surgical procedure, and expectations.
2. Assist the patient with presurgical shampoo with an antimicrobial agent; explain the extent of head shave.
3. Administer corticosteroids to reduce cerebral edema.
4. Administer anticonvulsants to reduce risk of seizures.
5. Explain use of intraoperative antibiotics to reduce risk of infection, and urinary catheterization to assess urinary volume during operative period.
6. Administer mannitol and a diuretic such as furosemide immediately before the procedure, as ordered, to reduce cerebral edema.
7. Evaluate and record the patient's neurologic baseline and vital signs for postoperative comparison.
8. Explain immediate postoperative care, and where the physician will contact the family after surgery.

9. Provide supportive care to the patient with neurologic deficits.

Postoperative Care

1. Closely monitor level of consciousness, vital signs, pupillary response, and ICP, if indicated. Use Glasgow coma scale (see *Table C-2*).

   ⚡ **EMERGENCY ALERT** A change in the Glasgow coma scale of more than 2 points may signify deteriorating condition. Notify health care provider immediately if deterioration is suspected, and closely monitor all neurologic parameters.

2. Assess respiratory status by monitoring rate, depth, and pattern of respirations. Maintain a patent airway.

3. Teach the patient to avoid activities that can raise ICP, such as excessive flexion or rotation of the head and Val-

TABLE C-2	**The Glasgow Coma Scale**	
PARAMETER	**FINDING**	**SCORE**
Eye opening	Spontaneously	4
	To speech	3
	To pain	2
	Do not open	1
Best verbal response	Oriented	5
	Confused	4
	Inappropriate speech	3
	Unintelligible speech	2
	No verbalization	1
Best motor response	Obeys command	6
	Localizes pain	5
	Withdraws from pain	4
	Abnormal flexion	3
	Abnormal extension	2
	No motor response	1

Interpretation: best score = 15; worst score = 3; 7 or less generally indicates coma; changes from baseline are most important.

Nettina, S.M. (2006). *The Lippincott Manual of Nursing Practice* (8th ed.). Philadelphia: Lippincott Williams & Wilkins, page 475.

salva maneuver (coughing, straining at stool). Administer stool softeners as indicated.

4. Administer corticosteroids and other medications as prescribed to reduce ICP.

5. Manage arterial and central venous or pulmonary artery lines for accurate manipulation of blood pressure and fluid status.

6. Prepare to transport the patient for CT if patient status deteriorates.

7. Weigh the patient daily, and monitor intake and output.

8. Offer oral fluids only when patient is alert and swallow reflex and bowel sounds have returned.

9. Have suction equipment available at bedside. Suction only if necessary and carefully to prevent rise in ICP.

10. Elevate head of bed 15 to 30 degrees based on clinical response (want to reduce ICP but not compromise cerebral perfusion).

11. Use sterile technique for dressing changes, catheter care, and ventricular drain management to prevent infection.

12. Be aware of patients at higher risk of infection — those undergoing lengthy operations, those with ventricular drains left in longer than 48 to 72 hours, and those with operations of the third ventricle.

13. Assess surgical site for redness, tenderness, and drainage.

14. Watch for leakage of cerebrospinal fluid (CSF), which increases the danger of meningitis.

    a. Watch for sudden discharge of fluid from wound; massive leak requires surgical repair.

    b. Warn against coughing, sneezing, or nose blowing, which may aggravate leakage of CSF.

    c. Assess for moderate elevation of temperature and nuchal rigidity.

    d. Note patency of ventricular catheter system.

15. Control incisional and headache pain with analgesics as prescribed. Darken room if patient is photophobic.

16. To reduce periorbital edema, apply cold compresses and avoid positioning the patient to lay flat.

17. After supratentorial craniotomy, anticipate the use of post-operative anticonvulsants. Position the patient on back or unoperated side with one pillow under head.
18. After an infratentorial operation, keep the patient on side and off back with only a small firm pillow under head.

Education and Health Maintenance

1. Reinforce need to prevent increased ICP for several weeks by instructing patient not to bend over, strain at stool, lift heavy objects, engage in vigorous sexual activity, and have prolonged coughing.
2. Advise patient to report fever or any new or worsening neurologic deficits after surgery.
3. Advise patient to use proper care and precautions to prevent injury for specific neurologic deficits.

CROHN'S DISEASE

Crohn's disease (regional enteritis, granulomatous colitis, ileitis) is a chronic transmural inflammation of the GI tract that usually affects the small and large intestines. However, it can occur in any part of the alimentary canal. The intestinal tissue thickens, first by edema and later by formation of scar tissues and granulomas. Inflammation and ulcers form in the bowel mucosa, producing fissures, fistulae, and abscesses. The rectum is typically spared, and lesions may be discontinuous in the bowel (skip lesions). Cause is unknown, but is multifactorial with factors including viral or bacterial infection, immune disorder, defect in the intestinal barrier, dysfunctional repair of mucosal injury, genetic predisposition, dietary and environmental factors (chemical additives, milk products, heavy metals, low fiber), and cigarette smoking.

Complications include stricture and fistulae formation, dehydration, nutritional deficiencies, hemorrhage, bowel perforation, and intestinal obstruction. Incidence of colorectal cancer is higher in these patients.

Assessment

1. Signs and symptoms are characterized by exacerbations and remissions; onset may be abrupt or insidious.

2. Crampy intermittent pain.
    a. Inflammatory pattern results in milder abdominal pain, but with malnutrition due to malabsorption and weight loss, and possible anemia (hypochromic or macrocytic).
    b. Fibrostenotic pattern may present with partial small bowel obstruction: Diffuse abdominal pain, nausea, vomiting, and bloating.
    c. Perforating pattern is characterized by sudden profuse diarrhea, fever, localized tenderness (due to abscess), and symptoms of fistulae, such as pneumaturia and recurrent urinary tract infections.
3. Abdominal tenderness occurs, especially in right lower quadrant; right lower quadrant fullness or mass is palpable.
4. Chronic diarrhea caused by irritating discharge; usual consistency is soft or semiliquid. Bloody stools or steatorrhea (fatty stools) may occur. Fecal urgency and tenesmus occur.
5. Low-grade fever occurs if abscesses are present.
6. Arthralgias may also occur.

Diagnostic Evaluation

1. Increased white blood cell count and sedimentation rate; decreased hemoglobin; decreased albumin; and possibly decreased potassium, magnesium, and calcium due to diarrhea.
2. Stool analysis shows leukocytes but no pathogens.
3. Barium enema permits visualization of lesions of large intestine and terminal ileum; needs to be scheduled before upper GI to prevent interference by barium passing through colon.
4. Upper GI barium studies show classic "string sign" at terminal ileum that suggests constriction of a segment of intestine.
5. Colonoscopy to note cobblestone appearance of ulcerations and fissures, skip lesions, and rectal sparing; biopsy can be taken for definitive diagnosis.

Collaborative Management
Therapeutic Interventions

1. Diet low in residue, fiber, and fat, and high in calories, protein, and carbohydrates, with vitamin supplements (especially vitamin K)
2. During exacerbation, hyperalimentation to maintain nutrition while allowing the bowel to rest
3. During remission, regular balanced diet to maintain ideal body weight

Pharmacologic Interventions

1. 5-Aminosalicylic acid given orally or by enema or suppository releases mesalamine to have topical rather than systemic anti-inflammatory effect within the intestines.
2. Sulfasalazine is given orally to inhibit inflammatory process; effective only for colonic disease; adverse effects include nausea, vomiting, headache, rash, fever (about one-third is absorbed systemically).
3. Corticosteroids to reduce inflammation; rectally, orally or I.V., depending on severity of disease.
4. Antibiotics such as metronidazole to treat infection and try to induce remission.
5. Immunomodulators, such as 6-mercaptopurine, cyclosporine, and tacrolimus, are used in severe cases to improve healing of fistulas.
6. Infliximab is new monoclonal antibody given by injection that blocks action of tumor necrosis factor. It is indicated in moderate to severe disease not responsive to other treatments or those with draining fistulae.
7. Antispasmodics (dicyclomine) and bulking agents (psyllium) help reduce abdominal pain.
8. Antidiarrheal agents, such as loperamide, diphenoxylate and atropine, paregoric, codeine, to control diarrhea related to malabsorption of bile salts.
9. Fish oil may be used to maintain remission; adverse effects include diarrhea, flatulence, halitosis, and heartburn.

Surgical Interventions
1. Surgery is indicated only for complications. Roughly 70% of Crohn's disease patients eventually require one or more operations for obstruction, fistulae, fissures, abscesses, toxic megacolon, or perforation.
2. Surgical options include:
   a. Segmental bowel resection with anastomosis
   b. Subtotal colectomy with ileorectal anastomosis (spares rectum)
   c. Total proctocolectomy with end ileostomy for severe disease in colon and rectum

Nursing Diagnoses
3, 6, 27, 51, 78, 123

Nursing Interventions
Also see *Gastrointestinal or Abdominal Surgery*, page 381.

Monitoring
1. Monitor frequency and consistency of stools to evaluate volume losses and effectiveness of therapy.
2. Monitor dietary therapy; weigh the patient daily.
3. Monitor electrolytes, especially potassium. Monitor intake and output. Monitor acid–base balance because diarrhea can lead to metabolic acidosis.
4. Monitor for distention, increased temperature, hypotension, and rectal bleeding; all signs of obstruction caused by inflammation.
5. Observe and record changes in pain — frequency, location, characteristics, precipitating events, and duration.

Supportive Care
1. Offer understanding, concern, and encouragement — patient is often embarrassed about frequent and malodorous stools, and often fearful of eating.
2. Have patient participate in meal planning to encourage compliance and increase knowledge.
3. Encourage patient's usual support persons to be involved in management of the disease.

4. Provide small, frequent feedings to prevent distention of the gastric pouch. Diet is low in residue, fiber, and fat; high in calories, protein, vitamins, and minerals.
5. Provide fluids as directed to maintain hydration (1,000 mL/24 hours minimum intake to meet body fluid needs).
6. Clean rectal area and apply ointments as necessary to decrease discomfort from skin breakdown.
7. Facilitate supportive counseling, if appropriate.

Education and Health Maintenance

1. Instruct patient on prescribed medications to encourage compliance and understanding of management.
2. Review dietary changes with patient, such as increased fiber content and fluid intake and their importance in improving bowel function.
3. Instruct postoperative patient about wound care or ostomy care if applicable to promote healing and self-confidence.
4. Explain signs and symptoms of postoperative complications to report — elevated temperature, nausea or vomiting, abdominal distention, changes in bowel function and stool consistency, or hemorrhage.
5. Assess the need for home health follow-up and initiate appropriate referrals if indicated.
6. Refer for additional information and support to Crohn's & Colitis Foundation of America, *www.ccfa.org*.

CRYPTORCHIDISM

Cryptorchidism is a congenital disorder in which one or both testicles fail to descend through the inguinal canal to their normal position in the scrotum. The cause is unknown, but hormonal factors thought to be involved in the mechanism of testicular descent may play a role. Mechanical lesions or possibly endocrine disorders may also be involved.

Cryptorchidism primarily affects premature male neonates. If cryptorchidism is not corrected before puberty, impaired spermatogenesis and infertility result because abdominal temperatures are higher than in the scrotum. In addition, the risks of testicular torsion, associated hernias, emotional disturbances, and testicular malignancy are significantly increased.

Assessment
1. Physical examination discloses absence of one or both testicles within the scrotum.

Diagnostic Evaluation
1. Physical examination is reliable for diagnosis; ultrasonography also shows undescended testicle.

Collaborative Management
Pharmacologic Interventions
1. Administration of human chorionic gonadotropin has produced descent of the testicles in some children. Testicle may have descended spontaneously in many of these cases.

Surgical Interventions
1. Orchiopexy is performed to achieve permanent fixation of the testicle in the scrotum. Surgery should be performed when the child is between ages 6 and 15 months to prevent damage to the tissues and to lessen emotional concerns related to body image.
2. Plastic surgery may be performed in patients with an absent testicle.

Nursing Diagnoses
3, 24, 135

Nursing Interventions
Supportive Care
1. Encourage the parents to express their concerns about the condition and ask questions about surgery.
2. Monitor vital signs after surgery and make sure that child voids.
3. Prevent contamination of the suture line by changing diapers frequently, and keep operative site clean.
4. Administer antibiotics as prescribed to prevent infection.

5. Maintain traction on the testicle.
   a. A suture is placed in the lower portion of the scrotum and is attached to a rubber band that is fastened to the upper aspect of the inner thigh by a piece of adhesive.
   b. This traction anchors the testicle to the scrotum and is removed in 5 to 7 days.
6. Administer analgesics as needed.

Education and Health Maintenance
1. Encourage family to follow up to ensure proper fixation of testicle in scrotum.
2. Explain that sexual function should not be impaired with treatment.

CUSHING'S SYNDROME

Cushing's syndrome results from excessive secretion of one or all of the adrenocortical hormones: The glucocorticoid *cortisol* (predominant type), the mineralocorticoid *aldosterone*, and the *androgenital corticoids*. Types of Cushing's syndrome include:

Pituitary Cushing's syndrome (Cushing's disease) is the most common cause of Cushing's syndrome, and stems from hyperplasia of both adrenal glands caused by overstimulation by adrenocorticotropic hormone (ACTH), usually from pituitary adenoma. The syndrome affects mostly women between ages 20 and 40.

Adrenal Cushing's syndrome is associated with adenoma or carcinoma of the adrenal cortex. The disease may recur after surgery. Ectopic Cushing's syndrome results from autonomous ACTH secretion by extrapituitary tumors (such as the lung) producing excess ACTH. Iatrogenic Cushing's syndrome is caused by exogenous glucocorticoid administration.

Assessment
See *Figure C-4*.
1. Signs and symptoms of excess glucocorticoid (cortisol) secretion:
   a. Weight gain or obesity
   b. Heavy trunk; thin extremities

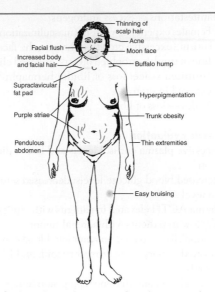

Thinning of scalp hair
Acne
Facial flush
Moon face
Increased body and facial hair
Buffalo hump
Supraclavicular fat pad
Hyperpigmentation
Purple striae
Trunk obesity
Pendulous abdomen
Thin extremities
Easy bruising

FIGURE C-4 Clinical manifestations of Cushing's syndrome.

C

    c. Fat pad (Buffalo hump) in neck and supraclavicular area

    d. Rounded face (moon face); plethoric, oily complexion

    e. Skin—fragile and thin; striae and ecchymosis, acne

    f. Musculoskeletal—muscle wasting caused by excessive catabolism; osteoporosis; characteristic kyphosis, backache

    g. Mental disturbances—mood changes, psychosis

    h. Increased susceptibility to infections

2. Manifestations of excess mineralocorticoid (aldosterone) secretion:

    a. Hypertension

    b. Hypernatremia, hypokalemia

    c. Weight gain

    d. Expanded blood volume

    e. Edema

3. Manifestations of excess androgens:
   a. Females experience virilism (masculinization) with hirsutism (excessive growth of hair on the face and midline of trunk); atrophied breasts; enlarged clitoris; masculinized voice; loss of libido; hermaphroditism (if exposed in utero)
   b. Males — loss of libido

Diagnostic Evaluation

1. Excessive plasma cortisol levels and loss of diurnal variation
2. Increased blood glucose levels; decreased serum potassium level
3. Plasma ACTH elevated in patients with pituitary tumors; very low in patients with adrenal tumor
4. Eosinophils decreased on complete blood count
5. Elevated urinary 17-hydroxycorticoids and 17-ketogenic steroids
6. Overnight dexamethasone suppression test, possibly with cortisol urinary excretion measurement, to check for:
   a. Unsuppressed cortisol level in Cushing's syndrome caused by adrenal tumors
   b. Suppressed cortisol level in Cushing's disease caused by pituitary tumor
7. Skull X-ray detects erosion of the sella turcica by a pituitary tumor; CT scan and ultrasonography locate tumor

Collaborative Management
Pharmacologic Interventions

1. In patients unable to undergo surgery, cortisol synthesis-inhibiting drugs may be used. These include:
   a. Mitotane, an agent toxic to the adrenal cortex (DDT derivative), known as "medical adrenalectomy." Adverse effects include nausea, vomiting, diarrhea, somnolence, and depression.
   b. Metyrapone is given to control steroid hypersecretion in patients who do not respond to mitotane.

    c. Aminoglutethimide is given to block cortisol produc-
tion. Adverse effects include GI disturbances, somnolence, and skin rashes.
2. Hormone replacement therapy is necessary postoperatively.
    a. Adrenalectomy patients require lifelong replacement
therapy with glucocorticoids and mineralocorticoids.
    b. After pituitary irradiation or hypophysectomy, the pa-
tient may require adrenal replacement plus thyroid,
posterior pituitary, and gonadal hormone replacement.
    c. After transsphenoidal adenomectomy, the patient needs
hydrocortisone replacement therapy for 12 to 18
months, and additional hormones if excessive loss of
pituitary function has occurred.
    d. Protein anabolic steroids may be given to facilitate pro-
tein replacement; potassium replacement is usually required.

Surgical Interventions

1. Pituitary surgery to treat pituitary Cushing's syndrome.
    a. Transsphenoidal adenomectomy or hypophysectomy.
    b. Transfrontal craniotomy may be necessary when a pi-
tuitary tumor has enlarged beyond the sella turcica.
2. Bilateral adrenalectomy is used to treat adrenal causes.
3. Radiation therapy may also be used to treat pituitary or
adrenal tumors.

Nursing Diagnoses

1, 8, 30, 36, 42, 134, 136

Nursing Interventions

Also see pages 239 and 381 for care of the surgical patient.

Monitoring

1. Monitor intake and output, daily weights, and serum glucose and electrolytes.
2. Monitor for signs of infection because risk is high with
excess glucocorticoids.

3. After hypophysectomy, monitor for diabetes insipidus (page 276), hypothyroidism (page 531), and other endocrine changes.

4. After adrenalectomy, monitor for adrenal crisis (page 3).

Supportive Care

1. Assess the skin frequently to detect reddened areas, skin breakdown or tearing, excoriation, infection, or edema.

2. Handle skin and extremities gently to prevent trauma; protect from falls by use of side rails.

3. Avoid using adhesive tape on the skin to reduce trauma on its removal.

4. Encourage the patient to turn in bed frequently or ambulate to reduce pressure on bony prominences and areas of edema.

5. Assist the patient with ambulation and hygiene when weak and fatigued. Use assistive devices during ambulation to prevent falls and fractures.

6. Help the patient to schedule exercise and rest. Advise the patient how to recognize signs and symptoms of excessive exertion.

7. Instruct the patient in correct body mechanics to avoid pain or injury during activities.

8. Provide foods low in sodium to minimize edema, and provide foods high in potassium (bananas, orange juice, tomatoes) and administer potassium supplement as prescribed to counteract weakness related to hypokalemia.

9. Report edema and signs of fluid retention.

10. Encourage the patient to verbalize concerns about illness, changes in appearance, and altered role functions.

 EMERGENCY ALERT Observe for evidence of depression, which may progress to suicide. Alert health care provider of mood changes, sleep disturbance, change in activity level, change in appetite, or loss of interest in visitors or other experiences.

11. Refer the patient for counseling, if indicated.

12. Explain to the female patient who has benign adenoma or hyperplasia that, with proper treatment, evidence of masculinization can be reversed.

Education and Health Maintenance

1. Teach the patient about lifelong hormone replacement therapy and the need for regular follow-up visits to determine if dosage is appropriate or to detect adverse effects.
2. Instruct the patient in proper skin care and stress prompt reporting of trauma or infection.
3. Teach the patient to monitor urine or blood glucose or report for blood glucose tests as directed to detect hyperglycemia.
4. Help the patient prevent hyperglycemia and obesity by teaching a low-calorie, low concentrated carbohydrate and fat diet and to increase activity as tolerated.
5. Advise the patient to follow a diet high in calcium (dairy products, broccoli) and encourage patient to perform weight-bearing activity to prevent osteoporosis caused by glucocorticoid replacement.

CVA

See *Stroke*.

CYSTIC FIBROSIS

Cystic fibrosis (CF) is an autosomal recessive disorder affecting the exocrine glands, in which their secretions become abnormally viscous and liable to obstruct glandular ducts. CF primarily affects pulmonary and GI function.

The disease is most common in whites (1 in every 3,200 births). The average life expectancy for the CF patient is currently age 30 to 40. Death may occur because of respiratory infection and failure. Other complications include esophageal varices, diabetes, chronic sinusitis, pancreatitis, rectal polyps, intussusception, growth retardation, and infertility.

EMERGENCY ALERT *Burkholderia cepacia* affects 5% to 10% of CF patients with a rapid decline in pulmonary function, fulminant septicemia, and necrotizing pneumonia leading to death. Mortality is high because it is a multiple drug resistant organism. Monitor respiratory status closely and report changes promptly. Adhere to infection control procedures.

Assessment

1. Usually present before age 6 months but severity varies and may present later.
2. Meconium ileus is found in neonate.
3. Usually present with respiratory symptoms, chronic cough, and wheezing.
4. Parents may report salty taste when skin is kissed.
5. Recurrent pulmonary infections.
6. Failure to gain weight or grow in the presence of a good appetite.
7. Frequent, bulky, and foul-smelling stools (steatorrhea); excessive flatus; pancreatitis and obstructive jaundice may occur.
8. Protuberant abdomen, pot belly, wasted buttocks.
9. Bleeding disorders.
10. Clubbing of fingers in older child.
11. Increased anteroposterior chest diameter (barrel chest).
12. Decreased exertional endurance.
13. Hyperglycemia, glucosuria with polyuria, and weight loss.
14. Sterility in males.

Diagnostic Evaluation

1. Sweat chloride test measures sodium and chloride level in sweat.
   a. Chloride level of more than 60 mEq/L is virtually diagnostic.
   b. Chloride level of 40 to 60 mEq/L is borderline and should be repeated.
2. Duodenal secretions: low trypsin concentration is virtually diagnostic.
3. Stool analysis:
   a. Reduced trypsin and chymotrypsin levels — used for initial screening for CF.
   b. Increased stool fat concentration.
   c. BMC (Boehringer-Mannheim Corp.) meconium strip test for stool includes lactose and protein content; used for screening.

4. Chest X-ray may be normal initially; later shows increased areas of infection, overinflation, bronchial thickening and plugging, atelectasis, and fibrosis.
5. Pulmonary function studies (after age 4) show decreased vital capacity and flow rates and increased residual volume or increased total lung capacity.
6. Diagnosis is made when a positive sweat test is seen in conjunction with one or more of the following:
   a. Positive family history for CF
   b. Typical chronic obstructive lung disease
   c. Documented exocrine pancreatic insufficiency
7. Genetic screening may be done for affected families.

Collaborative Management
Therapeutic Interventions
1. Chest physical therapy for bronchial drainage, especially during acute exacerbations.
   a. Postural drainage
   b. Coughing and deep-breathing exercises
   c. Active cycle breathing, autogenic training, and other breathing exercises
   d. Positive expiratory pressure valve and other techniques
   e. High-frequency chest compressions
2. Some centers employ bronchopulmonary lavage to treat atelectasis and mucoid impaction using large volumes of saline.
3. Increased carbohydrates, protein, and fat (possibly as high as 40%) for growth and repair, infection, the work of breathing, and energy expenditure for coughing, malabsorption, and physical activity.
4. Ensure adequate fluid and salt intake.

Pharmacologic Interventions
1. Antimicrobial therapy as indicated for pulmonary infection.
   a. Oral or I.V. antibiotics as required.
   b. Inhaled antibiotics, such as gentamicin or tobramycin, may be used for severe lung disease or colonization of

organisms. Recently, some practitioners advocate using nebulized antibiotics earlier in therapy.

2. Bronchodilators to increase airway size and assist in mucus clearance.
3. Pulmozyme recombinant human DNase (an enzyme) administered via nebulization to decrease viscosity of secretions.
4. Pancreatic enzyme supplements with each feeding.
   a. Favored preparation is pancrelipase.
   b. Occasionally, antacid is helpful to improve tolerance of enzymes.
   c. Favorable response to enzymes is based on tolerance of fatty foods, decreased stool frequency, absence of steatorrhea, improved appetite, and lack of abdominal pain.
5. Gene therapy, in which recombinant DNA containing a corrected gene sequence is introduced into the diseased lung tissue by nebulization, is in clinical trials.

Surgical Interventions

1. Lobectomy (resection of symptomatic lobar bronchiectasis) may be done to retard progression of lesion to total lung involvement.
2. Heart-lung, double-lung, or single-lung transplantation and liver transplantation have been tried for end-stage lung disease.

Nursing Diagnoses
1, 6, 27, 51, 73, 90, 135

Nursing Interventions
Monitoring

1. Monitor weight at least weekly to assess effectiveness of nutritional interventions.
2. Monitor respiratory status and sputum production, to evaluate response to respiratory care measures. Evaluate use of accessory muscles, breath sounds, child's perception of dyspnea, exercise and activity tolerance, and oxygen saturation in daytime and during sleep.

3. Monitor for signs and symptoms of pneumothorax, tachypnea, tachycardia, pallor, dyspnea, and cyanosis.
4. Monitor for hemoptysis, which, if it occurs, needs immediate treatment and may be life-threatening.

Supportive Care

1. To promote airway clearance, employ intermittent aerosol therapy three to four times per day when the child is symptomatic.
   a. Use before postural drainage.
   b. Administer bronchodilators and other medications, diluted in normal saline, in aerosol form to penetrate respiratory tract. Make sure that mask fits properly to deliver correct dose of medication.

   DRUG ALERT An improperly fitting mask could reduce the delivery of aerosolized medication by as much as 85%.

2. Perform chest physical therapy three to four times per day after aerosol therapy; perform more frequently if infection is present.
3. Help the child to relax to cough more easily after postural drainage.
4. Suction the infant or young child when necessary, if not able to cough.
5. Teach the child breathing exercises using pursed lips to increase duration of exhalation.
6. Provide good skin care and position changes to prevent skin breakdown in malnourished child.
7. Provide frequent mouth care to reduce chances of infection because mucus is present.
8. Restrict contact with people with respiratory infection.
9. Encourage diet composed of foods high in calories and protein and moderate to high in fat because absorption of food is incomplete.
10. Administer fat-soluble vitamins (A, D, E) in water-miscible solution in two to three times the normal dose, as prescribed, to counteract malabsorption. Vitamin K should be added when infection is present.
11. Administer pancreatic enzymes with each meal and snack. Dose is based on weight, growth rate, food intake, and

number and character of bowel movements. Withhold enzymes, as ordered, if child is only taking clear liquid diet or enteral feedings.

12. Increase salt intake during hot weather, fever, or excessive exercise to prevent sodium depletion and cardiovascular compromise.

13. To prevent vomiting, allow ample time for feeding because of irritability if not feeling well and coughing.

14. To reassure the child and promote self-esteem, explain each procedure, medication, and treatment to the child as appropriate for age.

15. Encourage older child to take responsibility for treatments and be involved in care plan.

16. Encourage regular exercise and activity to foster sense of accomplishment and independence and improve pulmonary function.

17. Provide opportunities for parents to learn all aspects of care for the child.

Education and Health Maintenance

1. Teach the parents about dietary regimen and special need for calories, fat, and vitamins. Encourage consultation with a dietitian, as needed.

2. Discuss need for salt replacement, especially on hot summer days or when fever, vomiting, and diarrhea occur.

3. Help the parents to become skilled at chest physical therapy and other pulmonary treatments.

4. Help the family to schedule care for the child within the framework of family life.

5. Help the parents to provide emotional support for their child. The child needs love, understanding, and security, not overprotection.

6. Inform the family about genetic counseling and support them through the process.

7. Emphasize to the parents the importance of regular medical follow-up care and immunizations.

8. Discuss the limitations and expectations for the child with the parents, and involve the school nurse and teachers.

9. Refer families for additional information and support to such agencies as Cystic Fibrosis Foundation, *www.cff.org*.

CYSTOCELE AND URETHROCELE

Cystocele is a downward displacement (protrusion) of the bladder into the vagina. *Urethrocele* is a downward displacement of the urethra into the vagina. These conditions may result from obstetric trauma to pelvic muscles, fascia, and ligaments during childbirth or hysterectomy. Impaired muscular support often becomes apparent years later, when genital atrophy associated with aging occurs. Some cases may result from a congenital defect. Complications include urinary incontinence and infection.

Assessment

1. Pelvic pressure or heaviness or backache aggravated by coughing, sneezing, standing for long periods, and obesity, which increase intra-abdominal pressure. Relieved by resting or lying down.
2. Urgency, frequency, incontinence, incomplete emptying.
3. Observe perineum while the patient bears down, or observe the patient in upright position for telltale bulge in vagina.

Diagnostic Evaluation

1. Pelvic examination identifies condition
2. Urine specimens for urinalysis and culture rule out infection

Collaborative Management
Therapeutic and Pharmacologic Interventions

1. Vaginal pessary to insert into vagina to temporarily support pelvic organs.
   a. Prolonged use may lead to necrosis and ulceration.
   b. Should be removed and cleaned every 1 to 2 months.
2. Estrogen therapy after menopause may decrease genital atrophy.

Surgical Interventions

1. If cystocele is large and interferes with bladder functioning, may perform anterior vaginal colporrhaphy (repair of anterior vaginal wall).
2. Complications of surgery include urinary retention, bleeding (requires vaginal packing).

Nursing Diagnoses

3, 135, 136, 161, 166

Nursing Interventions

Supportive Care

1. Encourage periods of rest with legs elevated to relieve strain on pelvis.
2. Advise use of mild analgesics as necessary.
3. Teach the patient Kegel pelvic floor exercises to regain muscle tone and control incontinence.
   a. Practice while voiding by stopping the flow of urine for 3 to 5 seconds, then releasing for 5 seconds.
   b. Patient can then tighten pelvic floor muscle at any time, repeat 10 times, three times per day; increase as able.
4. Encourage the patient to void frequently, respond to the urge to void promptly.
5. Warn patient to avoid straining to prevent incontinence.
6. Encourage the patient to drink fluids to decrease concentration of bacterial flora in the bladder.
7. Provide postoperative care:
   a. Encourage voiding every 2 to 4 hours to reduce pressure so that no more than 5 oz (148 mL) will accumulate in bladder.
   b. Catheterize as necessary.
   c. Administer perineal care to the patient after each voiding and defecation.
   d. Employ a heat lamp to help dry the incision line and enhance the healing process.
   e. Use available sprays for anesthetic and antiseptic effects.

f. Apply an ice pack locally to relieve congestion and discomfort.

Education and Health Maintenance
1. Teach patient to avoid straining, remain active, avoid weight gain, and perform Kegel exercises to minimize pelvic relaxation in older years.
2. Encourage the patient to recognize and report symptoms of urinary tract infection (dysuria, frequency, foul-smelling urine).

C

D

DELIRIUM, DEMENTIA, AND AMNESIC DISORDER

Delirium, dementia, and amnesic disorder are classified by the *Diagnostic and Statistical Manual of Mental Disorders*, 4th edition, Text Revision (*DSM-IV-TR*), as cognitive impairment disturbances, in which psychological or behavioral dysfunction results from temporary or permanent neuronal damage. Without treatment and supportive care, injury, depression, and caregiver strain may result.

Delirium is an acute disturbance of consciousness and a change in cognition that develops over a brief period. It can be caused by numerous pathophysiologic conditions such as head trauma; hypertensive encephalopathy; seizures; brain tumors; hypothyroidism; hypoxemia; hypothermia or hyperthermia; intoxication, abstinence and withdrawal states; poisoning due to metals, toxins, or drugs; diabetic ketoacidosis; hypoglycemia; acid-base imbalances; hepatic encephalopathy; thiamine deficiency; and psychosocial stressors such as relocation, sensory deprivation or overload, sleep deprivation, and immobilization. Delirium is reversible if the underlying cause is treated.

Dementia is a chronic disturbance involving multiple cognitive deficits, including memory impairment. Primary dementias are degenerative disorders that are progressive, irreversible, and not attributable to any other condition. Primary dementias include dementia of the Alzheimer's type and vascular (formerly multi-infarct) dementia. Secondary dementias are also permanent and accompany many disorders, such as infections (acquired immunodeficiency syndrome, chronic meningitis, syphilis); degenerative disorders (Parkinson's disease); head trauma; brain tumors; inflammatory conditions; toxins; and metabolic disorders.

Amnesic disorder is characterized by memory impairment in the absence of other significant cognitive impairments. Amnesia is most commonly caused by head trauma. Other causes include stroke, neoplasms, anoxic or hypoglycemic states, herpes simplex encephalitis, epileptic seizures, electroconvulsive therapy, or substance abuse. Amnesia is often reversible.

Assessment

1. Delirium
   a. Acute onset, usually brief course (1 week)
   b. Fearfulness, anxiety, irritability
   c. Auditory, visual, tactile hallucinations; illusions
   d. Impaired short-term memory
   e. Slurred speech, confabulation
   f. Fluctuating levels of awareness
   g. Confusion and disorientation
   h. Altered sleep-wake cycle
   i. Electroencephalogram changes
2. Dementia
   a. Slow, insidious onset; progresses over years
   b. Labile mood; personality traits accentuated
   c. Impaired short-term memory followed by impaired long-term memory
   d. Progressive aphasia and confabulation
   e. Deterioration of cognitive abilities (judgment, abstract thinking)
   f. Personality changes
3. Amnesic disorder
   a. Sudden onset; may be transient or chronic
   b. Apathy, agitation, emotional blandness
   c. Impaired short- and long-term memory; impaired ability to learn new information; remote memory is better preserved
   d. Confabulation

Diagnostic Evaluation

1. Basic laboratory examination determines underlying cause, including complete blood count with differential, chemistry panel (including blood urea nitrogen, creatinine, electrolytes, glucose, and ammonia), arterial blood gas

values, chest X-ray, toxicology screen, thyroid function tests, and serologic tests for syphilis.
2. Other tests include CT, MRI, lumbar puncture, and positron emission tomography.
3. Mental status examination (Folstein scale, Mini-Mental; Blessed Dementia Scale)
4. Physical examination, vital signs, and review of medications

Collaborative Management
Therapeutic Interventions
1. Safe, structured environment to prevent disorientation, accidents, or violence toward self, others, or property
2. Treatment of specific causes of delirium or amnesia
3. Family involvement in therapy

Pharmacologic Interventions
1. Benzodiazepines, such as lorazepam, are used for abstinence withdrawal states.
2. Neuroleptics, such as risperidone and haloperidol, are used for agitation or psychosis.
3. Combined I.V. administration of haloperidol and lorazepam for agitated and psychotic symptomatology.
4. Antidepressants for depression.
5. Optimal hypertension management in vascular dementia.
6. Cholinesterase inhibitors for Alzheimer's dementia (see page 11).

Nursing Diagnoses
2, 8, 10, 36, 70, 90, 136, 139, 146, 159

Nursing Interventions
Monitoring
1. Monitor food and fluid intake; weigh patient weekly.
2. Monitor functional capacity and self-care ability.
3. Closely observe the patient if he or she is smoking.

Supportive Care

1. Speak slowly and use short, simple words and phrases.
2. Consistently identify yourself, and address the person by name at each meeting.
3. Focus on one piece of information at a time. Review what has been discussed with the patient.
4. If the patient has vision or hearing disturbances, have the patient wear prescription eyeglasses or a hearing aid.
5. Maintain a well-lighted environment.
6. Use clocks, calendars, and familiar personal effects in the patient's view (with Alzheimer's dementia, reorientation is not recommended).
7. If the patient becomes verbally aggressive, identify and acknowledge how he or she is feeling.
8. If the patient becomes aggressive, shift the topic to a safer, more familiar one. Respond calmly and do not raise your voice.
9. If the patient becomes delusional, acknowledge his or her feelings and reinforce reality. Do not attempt to challenge the content of the delusion.
10. Remove objects that might be used to harm self or others.
11. Identify stressors that increase agitation.
12. Distract the patient when an upsetting situation develops.
13. Use clothing with elastic and Velcro closures. Label clothes with the patient's name, address, and telephone number.
14. Remain with the patient during mealtime to determine the level of need for assistance or cueing in the ability to eat.
15. Initiate a bowel and bladder training program early in the disease process to maintain continence and prevent constipation or urinary retention.
16. Give the patient a card with simple instructions (address and phone number) in case he or she gets lost. Also provide a medical alert bracelet.
17. Encourage participation in simple, familiar group activities, such as singing, reminiscing, and painting.

18. Encourage participation in simple activities that promote the exercise of large muscle groups.

Education and Health Maintenance

1. Instruct the family about the disease process.
2. Instruct the family about safety measures to be used when the patient is at home or in the hospital.

COMMUNITY CARE CONSIDERATIONS

Assess the patient's home for safety: Remove throw rugs, label rooms, and keep the house well lit, including night-lights. Advise installing complex safety locks and alarm devices on doors to outside or basement; install safety bars in bathroom. Assess community for safety and, if the patient tends to wander, alert neighbors about wandering behavior; alert police and have current pictures taken.

3. Refer family members to community-based groups (adult day-care centers, senior assessment centers, home care, respite care, and family support groups).
4. For additional information and support, refer to Alzheimer's Association, *www.alz.org*.

DEPRESSIVE DISORDERS

Depressive disorders include major depressive disorder and dysthymic disorder. These are categorized as mood disorders, in which a disturbance of mood (sustained emotion) is overly intense and prolonged; in severe cases, it ultimately interferes with interpersonal or occupational functioning. Depression is much more than just sadness; it affects the way one feels about the future and can alter basic attitudes about the self. A depressed person can feel so much despair as to express hopelessness and may contemplate suicide.

The cause of depressive disorders is not fully understood, but factors that play a role include genetic predisposition, biochemical factors, the perception of loss and other life experiences, medications, and some illnesses.

Assessment

1. Major depressive disorder occurs over a 2-week period and impairs social and occupational functioning. Five or more of the following signs and symptoms occur nearly every day for most waking hours:
   a. Depressed mood
   b. Anhedonia — inability to express pleasure
   c. Significant weight loss or gain (more than 5% of body weight per month)
   d. Insomnia or hypersomnia
   e. Increased or decreased motor activity
   f. Anergia (fatigue or loss of energy)
   g. Feelings of worthlessness or inappropriate guilt (may be delusional)
   h. Decreased concentration or indecisiveness
   i. Recurrent thought of death or suicidal ideation (with or without plan)
2. Depression is further classified by severity, psychotic features, chronicity, seasonality, catatonic features, melancholic features, atypical features, and postpartum onset.
3. Dysthymic disorder occurs over a 2-year period (1 year for children and adolescents) with depressed mood and many of the features of depression, but still retaining social and occupational functioning.

Diagnostic Evaluation

1. Rating scales determine presence and severity of depression:
   a. Zung Self-Rating Scale
   b. Raskin Severity of Depression Scale
   c. Hamilton Depression Scale
   d. Beck Depression Inventory
2. Laboratory studies:
   a. Thyroid function tests and thyrotropin-releasing hormone stimulation test detect underlying hypothyroidism, which may cause depression.
   b. Dexamethasone suppression test evaluates depression that may be responsive to antidepressant or electroconvulsive therapy (ECT).

c. 24-hour urinary 3-methoxy-4-hydroxyphenylglycol levels may be slightly lower in patients with unipolar depression than in those with bipolar depression.
3. Polysomnography detects an increase in the overall amount of rapid eye movement (REM) sleep and shortened REM latency period in patients with major depression.
4. Additional diagnostic tests that evaluate physical conditions include CT or MRI, complete blood count, chemistry panel, serologic test for syphilis, test for human immunodeficiency virus, electroencephalogram, vitamin B_{12} and folate levels, and toxicology studies.

Collaborative Management
Therapeutic Interventions
1. Inpatient treatment may be required for those who are suicidal, are severely disabled, require a complex diagnostic evaluation, or who require ECT.
2. Goals of treatment for depression are symptom reduction, improved function, and recurrence prevention.
3. Psychotherapy modes include psychodynamic therapy, cognitive-behavioral therapy, and family therapy.
4. Additional somatic therapies include ECT and ultraviolet light therapy for seasonal affective disorder.

Pharmacologic Interventions
1. Antidepressant therapy (see *Table D-1*): tricyclic antidepressants; selective serotonin reuptake inhibitors (SSRI); monoamine oxidase inhibitors (MAOI); and unicyclic, bicyclic, tetracyclic, and other agents.
2. Treatment with an antidepressant may trigger a manic episode in patients with bipolar disorder.

Nursing Diagnoses
8, 34, 38, 48, 78, 136, 152, 159

Nursing Interventions
Monitoring
1. Monitor patient's response to antidepressant therapy; some medications may lower seizure threshold.

TABLE D-1	Commonly Used Antidepressants

DRUG/DOSAGE	ADVERSE REACTIONS
Selective Serotonin Reuptake Inhibitors (SSRIs) • Fluoxetine (Prozac) 10-40 mg qd • Paroxetine (Paxil) 20-50 mg qd • Sertraline (Zoloft) 50-150 mg qd; elderly and children 25 mg and up • Fluvoxamine (Luvox) 50-300 mg; elderly and children 25 mg and up • Citalopram (Celexa) 20-60 mg qd • Escitalopram (Lexapro) 10-20 mg qd	Sexual dysfunction, headache, nervousness, tremor, insomnia, drowsiness, dizziness, nausea, diarrhea, constipation, anorexia, dry mouth
Tricyclic Antidepressants (TCAs) • Amitriptyline (Elavil) 75-300 mg/day divided into two to three doses; elderly and children 10 mg am, 20 mg pm • Desipramine (Norpramin) 75-300 mg/day in one or two divided doses • Imipramine (Tofranil) 75-300 mg qd at hs; elderly and children 30-40 mg hs • Nortriptyline (Pamelor) 75-150 mg/day divided in two to four doses; elderly and children 30-50 mg/day in divided doses	Anticholinergic effects: dry mouth, constipation, urinary retention, blurred vision; Autonomic effects: orthostatic hypotension, increased blood pressure, sweating, palpitations; Cardiac effects: tachycardia, T wave flattening, prolonged QT interval; other: sedation, twitch, extrapyramidal movements
Other Agents • Mirtazapine (Remeron) 15-45 mg qd at hs (tetracyclic agent) • Nefazodone (Serzone) 200-600 mg/day divided into two doses (phenylipiperazine agent)	Somnolence, anticholinergic effects, weight gain, agranulocytosis Headache, nervousness, insomnia, drowsiness, dizziness, dry mouth, postural hypotension

(continued)

D

Commonly Used Antidepressants *(continued)*

DRUG/DOSAGE	ADVERSE REACTIONS
Other Agents *(continued)* • Bupropion (Wellbutrin) 225-450 mg/day divided into three doses; SR 150 mg bid (unicyclic agent)	Agitation, insomnia, tremor, dizziness, headache, dry mouth, risk of seizure
• Venlafaxine (Effexor) 37.5-225 mg/day divided into two to three doses (bicyclic agent) or venlafaxine XR once daily	Nervousness, dizziness, somnolence, insomnia, anorexia, constipation, dry mouth, sexual dysfunction, headache, hypertension

DRUG ALERT Be aware that antidepressants take 2 to 4 weeks before beneficial effects occur. Serotonin syndrome may result from adding a second antidepressant before withdrawal of the first; signs include insomnia, confusion, agitation, hyperreflexia, involuntary movements, and hypotension.

2. If indicated, implement appropriate level of observation based on a focused suicide assessment (eg, constant observation or 15-minute checks); explain observation precautions to the patient.

Supportive Care
1. Initiate interaction with the patient at a regularly scheduled time.
2. Be clear and honest about your own feelings related to the patient's behavior.
3. Encourage verbal expression of feelings.
4. Validate feelings that are appropriate to the situation.
5. Explore with the patient what is producing and maintaining the feeling of depression.
6. Assess real, significant losses the patient has experienced.
7. Identify cultural and social factors that may contribute to how the patient copes with loss and feelings.

8. Assess the patient's support network.
9. Assess the patient's current suicide risk.
10. Remove harmful objects from the patient's possession, and assess environmental safety of the patient's room and unit.
11. Encourage the patient to negotiate a no self-harm or no suicide agreement with the staff.
12. Provide additional structure by keeping the patient involved in therapeutic and psychorehabilitative activities.
13. Collaborate with occupational and physical therapists to determine patient's functional capacity to accomplish activities of daily living (ADLs).
14. If patient is unable to accomplish ADLs independently, provide hygienic activities in collaboration with patient.
15. Acknowledge and reinforce the patient's efforts to maintain appearance; do not rush the patient when self-care is slow.
16. Reinforce what the patient can do rather than what he or she cannot do without assistance.
17. Remain with the patient during mealtime to determine the level of need for assistance or cueing in the ability to eat.
18. Determine the patient's past and current sleep patterns and sleep hygiene. Reinforce patient's successful sleep strategies.
19. Consider decreasing the amount of daytime sleep by encouraging the patient to participate in an activity.
20. Discuss alternative methods for facilitating sleep:
    a. Avoid caffeine and nicotine.
    b. Avoid emotionally charged or upsetting discussions before bedtime.
    c. Avoid exercise 30 to 60 minutes before bed.
    d. Increase physical activity within functional limits.
    e. Use relaxation techniques.
    f. Try a warm bath or warm milk.

Education and Health Maintenance

1. Instruct patient and family members about biologic symptoms of depression.

2. Instruct patient and family members about purpose of antidepressant medication, desired and adverse effects and their management, and how to recognize early signs and symptoms of relapse:
   a. Do not drink alcoholic beverages if taking tricyclic antidepressants or drugs that cause sedation.
   b. Avoid sympathomimetic drugs and foods containing caffeine, tryptophan, or tyramine if taking MAOI because they may precipitate a hypertensive crisis (eg, cheese, beer, Chianti wine, sherry, coffee, cola drinks, liver, raisins, bananas, avocados, fava beans).
3. Provide patient and family members with written material about coping with depression.
4. Provide patient and family members with information about appropriate community-based programs and support groups such as National Foundation for Depressive Illness, *www.depression.org.*

ALTERNATIVE INTERVENTION

St. John's wort is a popular herbal preparation used to treat depression. Warn patient that it should not be taken with an SSRI or MAOI and that its concentration may vary.

DERMATITIS, ATOPIC

Atopic dermatitis (eczema) is a chronic pruritic, inflammatory skin disorder affecting 10% to 20% of all children. It involves an abnormal immune response to environmental triggers in genetically susceptible individuals. It usually starts in infancy or young childhood and may last into adulthood. There is a familial or personal tendency toward other atopic disorders (eg, asthma, food allergies, allergic rhinitis).

Assessment
1. Infantile (age 2 months to 2 years)—half of patients have spontaneous resolution by age 2 or 3
   a. Intense itching, erythema, papules, vesicles, oozing, and crusting

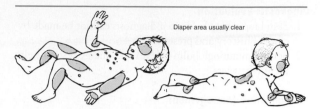

FIGURE D-1 Infantile atopic eczema occurs primarily on the face, but may develop on symmetrical areas of the body. (From Sauer, GC. *Manual of Skin Diseases.* 6th ed. Philadelphia, JB Lippincott, 1991)

D

    b. Begins on cheeks, forehead, or scalp and extends to the trunk or extremities in scattered, usually symmetric patches

    c. Perioral and perinasal and diaper areas are spared (see *Figure D-1*).

2. Childhood (age 4 to 10) — may resolve completely; stop, then recur in adulthood; or progress with little relief

    a. Dry, papular, circumscribed, scaly patches

    b. Chronic rash with lichenification

    c. Involves face, neck, antecubital and popliteal fossae, wrists, and ankles

3. Adult (puberty to old age)

    a. Main areas of involvement include flexor folds, face, neck, upper arms, back, dorsa of hands and feet, fingers, and toes.

    b. Dry, thick, confluent papular lesions and lichenified plaques. Weeping and crusting may occur as result of irritation or infection.

4. Classified into three stages based on appearance of lesions:

    a. *Acute* — moderate to intense erythema, vesicles, wet surface, and severe itching

    b. *Subacute* — faint erythema and scaling, dry surface, indistinct borders, pruritus

    c. *Chronic* — thickened lesions with prominent skin markings, dry surface, well-defined borders, moderate to intense itching

Diagnostic Evaluation

1. Skin biopsy may be done if diagnosis cannot be made by clinical history and presentation.
2. Serum immunoglobulin E level and allergy testing help identify triggers.

Collaborative Management

Therapeutic Interventions

1. Open, wet dressings for 1 to 3 days during acute stage to reduce inflammation.
2. Prevent drying of skin in subacute and chronic stages through decreased bathing, use of mild soap and hydrophilic lotions, use of emollients, tar preparations in baths, and increased environmental humidity.
3. Avoid known allergens and skin irritants.
4. Follow a hypoallergenic diet trial for severe, recalcitrant atopic dermatitis.
5. Consider referral for allergy testing in difficult-to-control cases.

Pharmacologic Interventions

1. Topical corticosteroids applied three times per day

   DRUG ALERT Long-term use of topical corticosteroids can cause striae, atrophy of skin, acne, telangiectasia, and possible adrenal suppression.
2. Oral antipruritics such as hydroxyzine
3. Oral antibiotics to manage secondary infection
4. Topical immunomodulators such as tacrolimus or pimecrolimus. They do not cause skin atrophy and can be used on the face.

Nursing Diagnoses

24, 33, 63, 135

Nursing Interventions

Supportive Care

Perform or teach the family to perform the following:

1. Apply lightweight, nonfibered cloth dressings (such as sheeting) saturated in lukewarm water to lesions for 20 minutes, three to four times per day during acute stage.
2. Discourage hot tub baths with harsh soap; instead, use lukewarm water and mild soap such as Neutrogena. Rinse well and pat dry with towel.
   a. If bath water stings, add 1 cup of table salt.
   b. Prepare tar bath as directed for soaking 15 to 20 minutes daily, preferably in the evening. Tar can stain skin and clothes and cause photosensitivity of skin.
   c. If bathing must be avoided, clean skin with a hydrophilic lotion such as Cetaphil. Apply without water until foamy, then remove it with soft cotton cloth.
3. Monitor for response to treatment — reduced inflammation and dryness; cutaneous atrophy, telangiectasia, and acne; or sedation caused by antipruritics.
4. Apply an unscented emollient cream or ointment (not lotion), such as Eucerin or Lubriderm, to the skin within 3 minutes of bathing.

PEDIATRIC ALERT Employ interventions to prevent food allergies: avoid introduction of solid foods until age 6 months; cow's milk until age 12 months, eggs until age 24 months, and peanuts, tree nuts, fish, and shellfish until age 36 months.

5. Report any discharge, oozing, or crust formation that may indicate secondary infection, and administer antibiotics as directed. Loosen crusts with water or wet dressings.

Education and Health Maintenance

1. Teach about possible exacerbating factors:
   a. Excessive heat or cold, windy weather, and rapidly changing temperatures
   b. Wearing wool or occlusive synthetic fabrics
   c. Strenuous athletic activity that provokes sweating
   d. Emotional stress
   e. Soaps, bubble baths, detergents, cleaning preparations, and other chemicals
2. Recommend use of a humidifier, especially in the winter.
3. Refer families and others for additional information and support to National Eczema Society, *www.eczema.org*.

DIABETES INSIPIDUS

Diabetes insipidus (DI) is failure of the body to conserve water because of lack of antidiuretic hormone (ADH; vasopressin), which is secreted by the kidneys, or because of inability of the kidneys to respond to ADH. The condition may be temporary or chronic and results from one of several causes. Deficiency of ADH (central DI), which may be congenital or acquired, is caused by defects in the central nervous system, head trauma, infection, brain tumor, or is idiopathic. Decreased renal sensitivity to ADH (nephrogenic DI) is usually attributable to chronic renal disease or suppression of ADH secondary to excessive ingestion of fluids (primary polydipsia). Complications are dehydration and hypernatremia.

Assessment

1. Sudden onset of excessive thirst and polyuria
2. In infants:
   a. Excessive crying—quieted with water more than milk feeding
   b. Rapid weight loss—caloric loss due to water preference over feedings
   c. Constipation
   d. Growth failure—failure to thrive
   e. Sunken fontanelle with dehydration
3. In children:
   a. Excessive thirst and drinking; child may even drink from toilet bowls or pet dishes
   b. Polyuria with nocturia and enuresis
   c. Pale, dry skin with reduced sweating

Diagnostic Evaluation

1. Urinalysis shows decreased specific gravity, decreased osmolality, and decreased sodium.
2. Elevated serum sodium.
3. Serum ADH is low in conjunction with high serum osmolality (greater than 295 mOsm).
4. Water deprivation test (potentially dangerous) to distinguish central DI from nephrogenic DI.

   a. Fluids are restricted, and the urinary volumes and concentrations are monitored hourly, along with the patient's weight.
   b. Test is terminated if patient loses more than 3% to 5% of body weight. Posttest serum sodium and osmolality are high; urine osmolality remains lower.
   c. Test is completed by giving a dose of ADH, which should stop the abnormal diuresis. If it does not, the child may have nephrogenic DI.
5. MRI or CT scan may be done to examine hypothalamic-pituitary region (high incidence of associated anterior pituitary disorders).

Collaborative Management
Pharmacologic Interventions
1. In central DI, daily replacement of vasopressin using desmopressin acetate (DDAVP), a synthetic analogue. Available as a metered nasal spray or a measured insufflation (nasal) tube. In children with cleft lip and palate, sublingual administration has been shown to be effective.
2. In nephrogenic DI, thiazide diuretics are given to reduce serum osmolality.

Nursing Diagnoses
23, 34, 51

Nursing Interventions
Monitoring
1. Monitor intake and output and urine specific gravity to adjust medication dosage if needed.
2. Monitor for signs of water intoxication while on DDAVP therapy.

EMERGENCY ALERT Watch for and report signs of water intoxication caused by excess free water and hyponatremia — drowsiness, listlessness, headache, confusion, anuria, and weight gain. Withhold DDAVP to prevent seizures, coma, and death.

3. Monitor infant's length, weight, and developmental milestones periodically.

Supportive Care

1. Assess for and teach parents assessment of dehydration.
2. Administer I.V. fluids as ordered if acutely dehydrated.
3. Maintain and teach parents to maintain liberal intake of fluids in child. Free access of water should be available. Reduced output may require restriction of fluids if overdosage of DDAVP is suspected.
4. Calculate rough estimate of total daily fluid requirements based on body size to assess fluid replacement versus excess: 100 mL/kg for first 22 lb (10 kg) body weight, 50 mL/kg for second 22 lb (10 kg) body weight, and 20 mL/kg for each additional 2.2 lb (1kg).
5. Stress to parents or caregivers the importance of providing nutritional requirements with fluids to meet caloric demands for growth.
   a. For infant feeding, make sure that adequate formula is ingested between bottles of plain water.
   b. For older child, provide liquid nutritional supplements.
   c. Consult with dietitian about need for vitamins or other supplements.
6. Administer and teach proper administration of DDAVP. Proper management should eliminate symptoms. Ensure adequate evening dose to prevent nighttime water craving and enuresis.
7. Suggest use of diapers at night and plastic padding on bed until condition is adequately managed, or ensure easy access to toilet or commode for older child during night.

Education and Health Maintenance

1. Teach family about administration of medication.
   a. Demonstrate insufflation method for infants and young children; inhalation for older children and adults.
   b. Nostrils should be as clear as possible before administration of dose.
   c. Advise that medication must remain cool or refrigerated.
   d. If dose is thought to be swallowed, *do not* readminister because of potential for overdosing. Split the dose into both nares if swallowing is occurring.

2. Advise use of medical alert bracelets.
3. Advise parents to notify school personnel about the child's condition and symptoms the need attention.
4. Advise routine follow-up; treatment may be temporary or lifelong, depending on cause.

DIABETES MELLITUS, TYPE 2

Diabetes mellitus (DM) is a metabolic disorder characterized by hyperglycemia that results from defective insulin production, secretion, or utilization. The classification of diabetes includes:

In *type 1 DM*, the pancreas produces little or no endogenous insulin (see page 287).

In *type 2 DM*, disease results from a defect in insulin manufacture and release from the beta cells and from insulin resistance in the peripheral tissues. It has a strong genetic component and is commonly associated with obesity. Onset is usually in adulthood; however, cases are increasingly occurring in teenagers and older children.

In *impaired fasting glucose*, fasting blood glucose is 100 mg/dL or greater, but less than 126 mg/dL, and no symptoms are present.

In *impaired glucose tolerance*, glucose is 140 to 199 mg/dL on a glucose tolerance test. It may be a risk factor for hypertension, coronary artery disease, and hyperlipidemia.

In *gestational diabetes*, carbohydrate intolerance occurs during pregnancy but usually disappears after delivery. It occurs in 4% of all pregnancies, and these women are at higher risk for developing diabetes later. Risk of fetal morbidity is increased.

Complications include hypoglycemia; diabetic ketoacidosis, which occurs primarily in type 1 DM during times of severe insulin deficiency or illness (see page 293); hyperosmolar hyperglycemic nonketotic syndrome, which affects patients with type 2 DM (see page 499); and chronic complications, occurring both in type 1 and type 2 DM (see *Table D-2*, pages 280 and 281).

| TABLE D-2 | Chronic Complications of Diabetes Mellitus |

COMPLICATION	MANIFESTATIONS
Macroangiopathy	
Cerebrovascular disease	Hypertension, change in mental status, hemiparesis, aphasia, other focal neurologic symptoms
Coronary artery disease	May be asymptomatic with only electrocardiogram changes; or pain in neck, jaw, or epigastric area
Peripheral vascular disease	Decreased lower-leg hair, decreased pedal pulses, poor capillary refill, pale and cool extremity, pain on walking
Microangiopathy	
Retinopathy	Floaters, flashing lights, blurred vision indicate hemorrhage or retinal detachment; may progress to blindness
Nephropathy	Asymptomatic; microalbuminuria is first sign, followed by proteinuria, elevated blood urea nitrogen and creatinine
Peripheral Neuropathy	
	Decreased light touch, vibratory, and temperature sensation; loss of foot proprioception, followed by ataxia and gait disturbance; diminished ankle reflex; development of Charcot joint disease
Autonomic Neuropathy	
Gastroparesis	Nausea, vomiting, early satiety, bloating, poor glucose absorption
Diarrhea	Often occurs without warning during night or after meals, may cause incontinence

Chronic Complications of Diabetes Mellitus
(continued)

COMPLICATION	MANIFESTATIONS
Autonomic Neuropathy *(continued)*	
Sexual dysfunction	Men may experience absence of early-morning erection; females may have vaginal dryness and dyspareunia
Orthostatic hypotension	Syncope, weakness, visual impairment with postural changes; decrease in systolic pressure of 30 mm Hg or diastolic pressure of 10 mm Hg with change from lying to standing

Assessment
1. Onset is usually insidious with type 2 DM.
2. Symptoms of hyperglycemia include polyuria, polydipsia, polyphagia, weight loss, fatigue, and blurred vision.
3. Signs of altered tissue response include poor wound healing and recurrent infections, particularly of the skin.

Diagnostic Evaluation
1. Elevated serum glucose levels
   a. Fasting blood glucose (sugar, FBS) greater than or equal to 126 mg/dL on two occasions confirms DM.
   b. Random blood glucose greater than or equal to 200 mg/dL in presence of classic symptoms (polyuria, polydipsia, polyphagia, and weight loss) confirms DM.
   c. 2-hour postprandial blood sample evaluates glucose metabolism, assists with control.
2. Glucose tolerance test may be indicated.
   a. FBS is obtained before ingestion of 50 to 200 g glucose load, and blood samples are taken at 30 minutes, 1, 2, 3 and, possibly, 4 and 5 hours.
   b. Diagnostic for DM if the 2-hour result greater than or equal to 200 mg/dL.

3. Glycosylated hemoglobin measures glycemic control over 60- to 120-day period; fructosamine assay measures control over 20 days and is more accurate in patients with hemoglobin variants.

Collaborative Management
Therapeutic Interventions
1. Weight reduction is a primary goal for type 2 DM.
2. Dietary control with caloric restriction of carbohydrates and saturated fats to maintain ideal body weight and control blood glucose and lipid levels.
3. Regular exercise promotes utilization of carbohydrates, assists with weight control, enhances the action of insulin, and improves cardiovascular fitness.

Pharmacologic Interventions
1. Oral hypoglycemic agents for patients with type 2 DM who do not achieve glucose control through diet and exercise (see *Table D-3*). Single-agent or combination therapy may be used to achieve optimal glucose control.
   a. Second-generation sulfonylureas stimulate secretion of insulin by beta cells, decrease hepatic glucose production, and increase peripheral sensitivity to insulin.
   b. Biguanides may be used alone or in combination with sulfonylureas to increase production of insulin, and decrease hepatic glucose production and triglyceride levels.
   c. Alpha-glucosidase inhibitors work locally in the small intestine to slow carbohydrate breakdown and glucose absorption.
   d. Repaglinide and nateglinide increase insulin release by selectively closing potassium channels (which results in opening of insulin-releasing calcium channels) in the beta cells of the pancreas.
   e. Thiazolidinediones resensitize tissues to insulin, decrease hepatic gluconeogenesis, and increase insulin-dependent muscle glucose uptake.
2. Insulin therapy for those who do not respond to diet, exercise, and oral agents:

TABLE D-3 Oral Antidiabetic Agents

AGENT	DOSAGE AND INSTRUCTIONS
Second-Generation Sulfonylureas	
Glyburide (Micronase, Diabeta)	1.25-20 mg in single or divided dose with meals
Glyburide, micronized (Glynase)	0.75-12 mg in single or divided doses
Glipizide: (Glucatrol)	2.5-15 mg in single dose before breakfast
(Glucatroi XL)	5-20 mg in single dose before breakfast
Glimepiride (Amaryl)	1-8 mg in single dose with first main meal
Biguanides	
Metformin (Glucophage)	1,000-2,550 mg in two to three divided doses with meals
Metformin (Glucophage XR)	500-2,000 mg with evening meal
Alpha-Glucosidase Inhibitors	
Acarbose (Precose)	150-300 mg in three divided doses with meals; if less than 132 lb (60 kg), maximum dose 50 mg three times per day
Miglitol (Glyset)	150-300 mg in three divided doses with meals
Meglitinide Analog	
Repaglinide (Prandin)	1-16 mg in two to four divided doses within 30 minutes of starting meal
Amino Acid Derivative	
Nateglinide (Sterlix)	120-360 mg in three divided doses within 30 minutes of starting meal

(continued)

Oral Antidiabetic Agents (continued)

AGENT	DOSAGE AND INSTRUCTIONS
Thiazolidinediones Rosiglitazone (Avandia)	4-8 mg in one or two divided doses
Pioglitazone (Actos)	15-45 mg once daily in single dose

a. Hypoglycemia and rebound hyperglycemia (Somogyi effect) may result.

b. Regimens are based on glycemic control, provider preference, and patient motivation. They include NPH insulin only once or twice per day; NPH and regular (or lispro) combination to better control postprandial glucose elevations; intensive insulin therapy with multiple injections related to meals and physical activity; sliding scale therapy; continuous subcutaneous (S.C.) insulin infusion (insulin pump therapy); and combination oral agent and insulin therapy.

Nursing Diagnoses
1, 6, 24, 52, 134, 136

Nursing Interventions
Monitoring
1. Closely monitor glucose levels by fingerstick or serum specimens to detect hyperglycemia and hypoglycemia. Be aware that capillary blood values are usually lower than venous samples.

COMMUNITY CARE CONSIDERATIONS

Insulin injection and self-glucose monitoring in the home are considered clean procedures — have patient wash his or her hands before the procedure. Alcohol cleansing is usually unnecessary.

2. Monitor and report signs and symptoms of hypoglycemia.

    a. Adrenergic—sweating, tremor, pallor, tachycardia, palpitations, and nervousness from the release of adrenaline when blood glucose falls rapidly

    b. Neurologic—headache, lightheadedness, confusion, irritability, slurred speech, lack of coordination, and staggering gait from depression of central nervous system as glucose progressively falls

3. Monitor for microvascular, macrovascular, and neuropathic complications by performing repeated physical assessments and laboratory screening of kidney function, lipid levels, and glycohemoglobin (complications more likely to occur with glycohemoglobin > 10).

Supportive Care

1. Advise patient about the importance of an individualized meal plan in meeting weekly weight loss goals, and assist with compliance.
2. Assess patient for cognitive or sensory impairments, which may interfere with ability to accurately administer insulin.
3. Demonstrate and explain thoroughly the procedure for insulin self-injection. Help patient to achieve mastery of technique by taking a step-by-step approach.

GERONTOLOGIC ALERT Assess elderly patients for sensory deficits, such as impaired vision, hearing, and fine touch, and tremors, which may affect learning and ability to self-administer insulin. Suggest use of an insulin pen or magnifying glass to assist with drawing up insulin. Discourage the practice of prefilling syringes because insulin may be absorbed by the plastic syringe, thereby altering the dosage.

4. Review dosage and time of injections in relation to meals, activity, and bedtime based on patient's individualized insulin regimen.
5. Instruct patient in the importance of accuracy in insulin preparation and meal timing to avoid hypoglycemia.
6. Treat hypoglycemia promptly with 10 to 15 g fast-acting carbohydrates.

    a. Give orally one-half cup (4 oz [120 mL]) juice, three glucose tablets, four sugar cubes, or five to six pieces of hard candy.

b. Provide glucagon 1 mg S.C. or I.M. if the patient cannot ingest a sugar treatment. A family member or care provider can administer injection.

c. Give I.V. bolus of 50 mL 50% dextrose solution if the patient fails to respond to glucagon within 15 minutes.

7. Nutrition bars specifically designed for patients with diabetes should be used after immediate treatment of hypoglycemia to prolong the effect if a full meal cannot be eaten.

DRUG ALERT If patient is taking an alpha-glucosidase inhibitor, use a monosaccharide such as glucose tablets to treat hypoglycemia because sucrose will not be absorbed.

8. Explain the importance of exercise in maintaining or reducing body weight.

9. Advise patient to assess blood glucose level before strenuous exercise and to eat a carbohydrate snack before exercising to avoid hypoglycemia.

10. Advise patient that prolonged strenuous exercise may require increased food at bedtime to avoid nocturnal hypoglycemia.

11. Instruct patient to avoid strenuous exercise whenever blood glucose levels exceed 250 mg/day and urine ketones are present, to prevent lactic acidosis.

12. Advise patient to inject insulin into the abdominal site on days when arms or legs are exercised.

13. Assess feet and legs for skin temperature, sensation, soft tissue injuries, corns, calluses, dryness, hammertoe or bunion deformation, hair distribution, pulses, and deep tendon reflexes.

14. Maintain skin integrity by protecting feet from breakdown.
    a. Use of heel protectors, special mattresses, or foot cradles for patients on bed rest
    b. Avoidance of drying agents to skin (eg, alcohol)
    c. Application of skin moisturizers to maintain suppleness and prevent cracking, and fissures

15. Advise patient who smokes to stop smoking or reduce if possible, to reduce vasoconstriction and enhance peripheral blood flow.

Education and Health Maintenance

1. For newly diagnosed patients or those undergoing stressful circumstances that preclude more in-depth education, focus on skills management related to insulin or oral agents, hypoglycemia treatment, blood glucose monitoring, and basic dietary information.

2. For ongoing education, include advanced skills and rationales for treatment and management. Focus on lifestyle management issues, such as sick-day management (see page 295), exercise adjustments, travel preparations, foot care guidelines, intensive insulin management, and dietary considerations for dining out.

ALTERNATIVE INTERVENTION

D

Cinnamon has shown some benefit in lowering blood glucose level and is safe in reasonable quantities. Chromium supplements may cause hypoglycemia when combined with antidiabetic medications.

3. For additional information and support, refer to agencies such as American Diabetes Association, Inc., *www.diabetes.org*.

DIABETES MELLITUS, TYPE 1

Diabetes mellitus (DM) is a disorder of glucose intolerance caused by a deficiency in insulin production and action resulting in hyperglycemia and abnormal carbohydrate, protein, and fat metabolism. More than 98% of cases of diabetes in children are type 1 DM. In this disorder, the pancreas produces little or no endogenous insulin, which must be treated with insulin injections to control the diabetes and prevent ketoacidosis. Type 1 DM may be caused by autoimmunity, viral, and genetic components.

Diabetic ketoacidosis (DKA), also known as diabetic coma, is the most important acute complication (see page 293). It accounts for 70% of diabetes-related deaths in children younger than age 10. However, if treated promptly, DKA is reversible. Chronic complications of diabetes include skeletal and joint abnormalities, growth failure and delayed sexual maturation caused by underinsulinization; and retinopathy, neuropathy, nephropathy, and cardiac disease as the child gets older.

Assessment

1. Onset rapid (usually over a few weeks)
2. Major symptoms include increased thirst and appetite, frequent urination, enuresis, weight loss, and fatigue
3. Minor symptoms include dry skin, skin infections, poor wound healing, and (in adolescent girls) candidal vaginitis
4. Manifestations of DKA (See *Diabetic Ketoacidosis*, page 293.)

Diagnostic Evaluation

1. For type 1 DM: random blood glucose 200 mg/dL or greater; or fasting blood glucose 126 mg/dL or greater

Collaborative Management
Pharmacologic and Therapeutic Interventions

1. Fluid therapy in DKA to treat dehydration and replace sodium and potassium.
2. Insulin therapy — to reduce hyperglycemia and inhibit lipolysis and ketogenesis (see *Table D-4*).
   a. Dosage needs are based on the child's size, diet, and level of activity. Dosages are adjusted through daily monitoring of blood glucose levels.
   b. DKA treatment — low-dose continuous I.V. infusion of regular insulin only. *Note:* Lispro insulin is not approved for I.V. administration.
   c. Insulin pump therapy, consisting of a continuous subcutaneous (S.C.) infusion of insulin that can be programmed to give bolus and basal rates, may be used by some children.
3. Research is ongoing to develop alternative routes for insulin administration; most promising is intranasal insulin.
4. Balanced diet with controlled carbohydrates and adequate protein and fat to meet energy and growth requirements.

TABLE D-4	Types of Insulin and Their Effects		
TYPE OF INSULIN	**ONSET (MINUTES)**	**MAXIMAL ACTIVITY (HOURS)**	**DURATION (HOURS)**
Aspart (Novolog)	< 15	1-3	3-5
Lipsro (Humalog)	10-30	1-2	2-4
Regular	30-60	2-4	6-8
Semi-Lente	30-60	2-4	10-12
NPH	120	4-12	24
Lente	120	8-10	24
Ultralente	4-8 hours	14-20	36
Glargine (Lantus)	≥ 60	N/A	≥ 24

D

Nursing Diagnoses
24, 44, 51, 80, 123, 135

Nursing Interventions
Monitoring
1. Monitor intake and output, blood pressure, serum electrolyte results, and daily weights while patient is on I.V. fluid replacement.
2. Monitor for potential cerebral edema (diminished level of consciousness) when fluid replacement is initiated for DKA.
3. Monitor for tachycardia with dehydration and arrhythmias related to potassium imbalances.
4. Monitor urine for ketones if the child is ill or if glucose is above 240 mg/100 mL.
5. Observe for hypoglycemia caused by overtreatment of insulin.
6. Review blood glucose diaries for level of control and need for insulin adjustments.

7. Monitor insulin injection sites:
   a. Watch for signs of lipohypertrophy (localized tissue buildup from giving injections in the same site).
   b. Observe for signs of irritation; avoid injection site for several weeks if these occur.
   c. Observe skin for signs of hypersensitivity reaction to insulin and notify doctor immediately.

Supportive Care

1. Administer I.V. fluids as ordered during periods of dehydration from vomiting and osmotic diuresis.
2. Consult with a dietician to provide for energy needs of the patient with a diet consisting of 55% carbohydrate, 30% fat, and 15% protein.
3. Develop a systematic plan for giving insulin injections that emphasizes rotation of sites. Give serial injections S.C., about 1 inch (2.5 cm) apart (see *Figure D-2*).
   a. Arms: begin below the deltoid muscle and end one handbreadth above the elbow. Begin at the midline and progress outward laterally, using the external surface only.
   b. Thighs: begin one handbreadth below the hip and end one handbreadth above the knee. Begin at the midline and progress outward laterally, using only the outer, anterior surface.

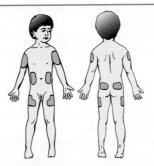

FIGURE D-2 Insulin injection sites.

     c. Abdomen: avoid the beltline and 1 inch (2.5 cm) around the umbilicus.

     d. Buttocks: use the upper outer quadrant of the buttocks.

4. Help child control fear of injections through interactive play and participation in the procedure.

5. Be aware of factors that influence insulin therapy, especially exercise and infection.

     a. Exercise tends to lower blood glucose level; encourage normal activity, regulated in amount and time.

     b. Infection or illness increases insulin requirement (insulin still administered during illness). Be alert for signs of infection and dehydration.

6. Teach child and parents the chosen method for blood glucose monitoring.

     a. Blood glucose measurements are usually made four times per day, before meals and at bedtime. May be more frequent during hypoglycemic episodes or other problem situations.

     b. Help child to understand how disease is controlled by teaching the child to test own blood, record results, and report information to health care provider and parents.

7. Have glucagon available if hypoglycemic reaction occurs. Administer 0.5 to 1 mg I.M. or S.C. and assess response.

8. Explain to child that he or she did not cause the disease; young children often blame themselves for "bad" things that happen to them. Help the child understand that good management is the key to participating in all usual activities. The perspective should be that he or she is a "child with diabetes," not a "diabetic child."

Education and Health Maintenance

1. Teach parents about influence of exercise, emotional stress, and other illnesses on both insulin and diet needs.

2. Teach parents to recognize the symptoms of insulin shock and DKA and review related emergency management.

3. Teach family the causes, signs and symptoms, and treatment for hypoglycemia.

D

a. Watch for a pattern of activity or time of day that precedes hypoglycemic reactions, and work with the family to alter behavior to prevent reactions.

b. If prescribed, teach the child and family how to use glucagon in an emergency.

COMMUNITY CARE CONSIDERATIONS

Suggest a simple, convenient source of sugar that can be easily carried by the child or parents in a pocket, purse, or backpack to have available for hypoglycemic symptoms. Glucose tablets or gel provide a measured source of fast-acting glucose.

4. Instruct parents about prevention of infection.
   a. Attend to regular body hygiene with special attention to foot care.
   b. Report breaks in the skin; treat promptly.
   c. Wear only properly fitted shoes; do not wear vinyl or plastic, which lack ventilation. Take measures to prevent calluses and blisters.
   d. Dress the child appropriately for the weather.
   e. Make sure that the child receives regular dental check-ups and maintenance every 6 months.
   f. Follow routine immunizations according to the recommended schedule.
5. Have the child carry a medical alert card or bracelet.
6. Have the family discuss the child's disease with the school nurse and with other responsible adults who are in close contact with the child.
7. Advise parents that vials of insulin should be kept on one's person when traveling because baggage may be subjected to extreme temperatures and pressures incompatible with the stability of insulin. If necessary, a thermos can be used to keep the insulin at appropriate temperature.
8. For additional information and support, refer to agencies such as Juvenile Diabetes Research Foundation International, *www.jdfcure.org*.

DIABETIC KETOACIDOSIS

Diabetic ketoacidosis (DKA) is an acute complication of diabetes mellitus (usually type 1) characterized by hyperglycemia, ketonuria, acidosis, and dehydration. Insulin deficiency prevents glucose from being used for energy, forcing the body to metabolize fat. DKA commonly occurs from failure to increase the insulin dose during periods of stress (eg, infection, surgery, pregnancy). It may also occur in previously undiagnosed or untreated patients with diabetes.

PEDIATRIC ALERT DKA accounts for 70% of diabetes-related deaths in children younger than age 10.

Assessment

1. Early manifestations include polydipsia, polyuria, fatigue, malaise, drowsiness, anorexia, nausea, vomiting, abdominal pain, and muscle cramps.
2. Later signs include Kussmaul (deep) respirations, acetone breath (fruity, sweet odor), hypotension, weak pulse, stupor, and coma.

Diagnostic Evaluation

1. Serum glucose: usually elevated over 300 mg/dL, may be as high as 1,000 mg/dL.
2. Serum and urine ketone bodies are present.
3. Serum bicarbonate and pH are decreased because of metabolic acidosis, and partial pressure of arterial carbon dioxide is decreased as a respiratory compensation mechanism.
4. Serum sodium and potassium may be low, normal, or high because of fluid shifts and dehydration, despite total body depletion.
5. Serum blood urea nitrogen, creatinine, hemoglobin, and hematocrit are elevated because of dehydration.

EMERGENCY ALERT Severity of DKA cannot be determined by serum glucose levels; acidosis may be prominent with glucose level of 200 mg/dL or less.

6. Urine glucose is present in high concentration and specific gravity is increased, reflecting osmotic diuresis.

Collaborative Management
Therapeutic and Pharmacologic Interventions

1. I.V. fluids to replace losses from osmotic diuresis and vomiting.

 EMERGENCY ALERT Too-rapid infusion of I.V. fluids in cases of severe dehydration can cause cerebral edema and death.

2. Short-acting I.V. insulin drip to increase glucose utilization and decrease lipolysis.
   a. Premature discontinuation of I.V. insulin can result in prolongation of DKA.
   b. Failure to institute subcutaneous (S.C.) insulin injections before discontinuation of I.V. insulin can result in extended hyperglycemia.
3. Replace electrolytes.
   a. Sodium chloride and phosphate as required.
   b. Potassium chloride to begin as soon as urine output and renal function are established; total body deficit is likely despite normal blood level.
   c. Bicarbonate may be given for severe or refractory acidosis.

Nursing Diagnoses
23, 86

Nursing Interventions
Monitoring

1. Monitor for symptoms of hypokalemia, including fatigue, anorexia, nausea, vomiting, muscle weakness, decreased bowel sounds, paresthesia, arrhythmias, flat T waves, and ST-segment depression.
2. Monitor intake and output every hour for fluid balance.
3. Monitor urine specific gravity to assess fluid changes.
4. Monitor capillary blood glucose frequently; however, may not be accurate at higher levels.
5. Monitor serum glucose, bicarbonate, and pH levels periodically.
6. Monitor blood pressure and heart rate frequently, depending on patient's condition; check skin turgor and temperature.

Supportive Care

1. Reassure the patient about improvement of condition and that correction of fluid imbalance will help reduce discomfort.
2. Replace fluids and electrolytes as ordered through peripheral I.V. line, usually starting with 0.9% normal saline and changing to 5% glucose in 0.45% saline when glucose falls below 250 mg/dL.
3. Administer regular (regular is the only insulin approved for I.V. administration) insulin drip through peripheral or central I.V. Flush the entire I.V. infusion set with solution containing insulin and discard the first 50 mL because plastic bags and tubing may absorb some insulin, thereby reducing insulin concentration of initial solution.

EMERGENCY ALERT Any interruption in insulin administration may result in reaccumulation of ketone bodies and worsening acidosis. Glucose will normalize before acidosis resolves so I.V. insulin is continued until bicarbonate levels normalize and S.C. insulin takes effect and the patient starts eating.

Education and Health Maintenance

1. To prevent further episodes of DKA, teach patient to identify and report early signs and symptoms of DKA.
2. Help patient to identify and avoid precipitating events to DKA.
3. Instruct the patient in sick-day guidelines.
   a. Never omit dose of insulin when sick.
   b. When blood glucose is greater than 240 mg/dL, test urine for ketones.
   c. Drink 6 to 8 oz (177 to 237 mL) of fluid every hour.
   d. If unable to eat, drink fluids with carbohydrates.

DIARRHEA IN CHILDREN

Diarrhea is the rapid movement of fecal matter through the intestine resulting in and producing more frequent loose, watery, or excessive loss of water and electrolytes that occurs with passage of unformed stools. It is a symptom of many conditions and may be caused by many diseases. Organisms causing diarrhea in infants and young children include viruses (rotaviruses [most common], echoviruses, adenoviruses, and human reovirus-like agent); bacteria (*Escherichia coli, Salmonella, Shigella, Yersinia enterocolitica,* and *Campylobacter fetus*); fungi (*Candida*); and parasites (*Giardia*). Diarrhea may also result from other disorders such as celiac disease, food allergies, mechanical obstruction, inflammatory disorders, GI irritants, and congenital anomalies.

Acute diarrhea is characterized by a sudden change in frequency and quality of stools. It is usually self-limiting but can result in dehydration. Chronic diarrhea lasts more than 2 weeks. Uncontrolled diarrhea may lead to severe dehydration, acid-base derangements with acidosis, and shock.

COMMUNITY CARE CONSIDERATIONS

Infants and young children in day-care centers may be at increased risk for diarrhea caused by *Shigella, Salmonella,* rotavirus, endopathogenic *E. coli,* and giardiasis. This is known as "day-care diarrhea," and hand-washing is the major preventive measure.

Assessment
1. Loose and fluid consistency stools that are greenish or yellow-green and may contain mucus, pus, or blood. Frequency varies from 2 to 20 per day. Stools are expelled with force and may be preceded by pain.

 PEDIATRIC ALERT Severe diarrhea with sudden onset in an infant carries a high risk of mortality. Bloody diarrhea should be evaluated immediately.

2. Indications of dehydration (see *Table D-5*).
3. Fever (low-grade to 106° F [41.1° C]), anorexia, and vomiting may occur.
4. Behavioral changes:
    a. Crying or legs drawn up to abdomen usually indicates pain
    b. Irritability and restlessness
    c. Weakness
    d. Extreme prostration
    e. Stupor and seizures
    f. Flaccidity

TABLE D-5	Assessment of Dehydration in Infants and Children		
SIGN	**MILD**	**MODERATE**	**SEVERE**
Blood pressure	=	=	=/–
Pulses	=	=/–	–
Heart rate	=	+	+
Fontanelle	Flat	Slightly –	–
Mucosa	Dry lips, thick saliva	Dry lips and buccal mucosa	Very dry lips and mucosa
Eyes	=	Sunken	Deeply sunken
Turgor	=	–	Tenting
Cap refill	< 1.5 sec.	1.5-3 sec	> 3 sec.
Output	Slightly –	<1 mL/kg/hour	<1 mL/kg/hour
Mental status	=	=/listless	= to comatose
Thirst	Slight +	Moderate +	Very thirsty or cannot indicate

Key: = normal   – decreased   + increased

Diagnostic Evaluation

1. No testing may be done if diarrhea and dehydration are mild.
2. For moderate to severe dehydration:
   a. Serum electrolytes, blood urea nitrogen, and creatinine are performed to evaluate fluid and electrolyte balance and kidney function.
   b. Serum carbon dioxide (CO_2), arterial pH, and arterial CO_2 may be abnormal because of acid-base imbalance.

3. For moderate to severe diarrhea:
   a. Complete blood count can determine plasma volume by hematocrit; white blood cell (WBC) count and differential can detect infection.
   b. Blood cultures can rule out septicemia.
   c. Serologic studies can detect viruses.
   d. Stool for WBC to rule out invasive bacterial disease, stool and rectal swab cultures, stool for ova and parasites to detect cause.
   e. Stool pH, reducing substances — decreased pH may indicate various noninfectious causes; acid stool containing sugar is characteristic of disaccharide intolerance.
   f. Breath hydrogen test can determine carbohydrate malabsorption and bacterial overgrowth.

Collaborative Management
Therapeutic Interventions
1. Prevent spread of disease: suspect disease to be communicable until proven otherwise. Use enteric isolation precautions; follow standard precautions when handling laboratory specimens.
2. Maintain hydration and electrolyte balance through oral or I.V. fluids. Oral electrolyte rehydrating solution may be used for mild to moderate diarrhea.
   a. For oral rehydration, give 100 mL/kg over 4 hours with additional fluid after each liquid bowel movement.
   b. I.V. fluid is given at rate of approximately 20 mL/kg over 2 days to prevent hypotonic hypervolemia.

Pharmacologic Interventions
1. Specific antimicrobial therapy against causative organism (vancomycin, metronidazole).
2. Antidiarrheal medications are rarely used in children younger than age 5. They have little effect and may cause toxicity and can mask signs and symptoms of more serious illness.

Nursing Diagnoses
6, 23, 51, 134, 135

Nursing Interventions
Monitoring
1. Monitor volume and rate of I.V. fluid therapy.
   a. Check flow rate and amount absorbed hourly and totally.
   b. Follow prescribed volume carefully when oral feedings are given in conjunction with I.V. fluid.
   c. Observe for signs of fluid overload, including edema, increased blood pressure, bounding pulse, labored respirations, and crackles in lung fields.
2. Check I.V. site for infiltration or improper flow so site can be changed as necessary.
3. Weigh the infant or child daily to guide fluid needs and patient status.
4. Monitor urine output and keep accurate intake and output record, including vomitus and liquid stools.

Supportive Care
1. Provide frequent mouth care and nonnutritive sucking with a pacifier if food and fluids are being restricted. Continue to bubble infant to expel air swallowed while crying or sucking.
2. Give oral rehydrating solution based on number of stools and degree of dehydration.
   a. Resume previous diet once fluid and electrolytes are replaced. If diarrhea was severe, advance slowly from clear liquids to half-strength formula to regular diet. Older child may advance more rapidly.
   b. If infant or young child is well hydrated, regular formula should be used.
   c. As diet is advanced, note vomiting or increase in stools and report it immediately.
   d. Breast-feeding may be resumed once electrolytes are replaced.

3. Provide parenteral nutrition if nutrition is compromised for more than 2 days with severe vomiting.
4. To prevent spread of infection, ensure adherence to good hand-washing and gown technique protocols for all persons having contact with enteric secretions.
5. Dispose of diapers carefully, following facility policy.
6. Implement measures to prevent skin irritation or breakdown.
   a. Avoid commercial baby wipes, which contain alcohol and may sting inflamed or excoriated diaper area. Use mild soap and water or place infant in tub of water for cleaning.
   b. Prevent scratching or rubbing of irritated area.
   c. Use protective barrier creams, such as zinc oxide or karaya powder; soak off or pat dry after a diaper change.
   d. Leave diaper area open to air until thoroughly dried.
7. Explain to family that intermittent abdominal cramps may be painful, and provide support. Drawing up legs to abdomen indicates pain.
8. Provide some means of pleasant stimulation, entertainment, or diversion, especially while child remains in bed.

Education and Health Maintenance
1. Teach good hygiene measures to older child and parents.

2. After the cause of the diarrhea is determined, it may be necessary to teach proper hygiene, formula or food preparation, handling, and storage.
   a. Use handwashing before bottle and food preparation.
   b. Use disposable bottles, or sterilize or use dishwasher for reusable bottles.
   c. Refrigerate reconstituted formula and all other fluids between uses. Milk may become contaminated within 1 hour if left out at room temperature; juice becomes contaminated within several hours.
   d. Discard small amounts of food or fluid from containers already used.
3. Explain the fecal-oral mode of transmission of infectious diarrheal illnesses.
4. Explain the early symptoms of a diarrheal illness and of dehydration, which requires notification of the health care provider.

D

DISSEMINATED INTRAVASCULAR COAGULATION

Disseminated intravascular coagulation (DIC) is an acquired thrombotic and hemorrhagic syndrome involving abnormal activation of the clotting cascade together with accelerated fibrinolysis. This causes widespread clotting in small blood vessels with consumption of clotting factors and platelets, so that bleeding and thrombosis occur simultaneously.

For unknown reasons, DIC occurs as a complication of a variety of underlying disorders or events, such as overwhelming infections (bacterial sepsis), massive tissue injury (burns, trauma, fractures, major surgery, fat embolism); obstetric complications (abruptio placentae, eclampsia, retention of dead fetus); vascular and circulatory collapse; shock; hemolytic transfusion reaction; and malignancies, particularly of the lung, colon, stomach, and pancreas.

Clotting may lead to pulmonary embolism; cerebral myocardial, splenic or bowel infarction; acute renal failure; tissue necrosis or gangrene. Hemorrhage may lead to cerebral hemorrhage, which is the most common cause of death in DIC.

Assessment
1. Abnormal clotting: coolness and mottling of extremities; acrocyanosis (cold, mottled extremities with clear demarcation from normal tissue); dyspnea, adventitious breath sounds; altered mental status; decreased urine output; and pain of extremities, abdomen, chest, and so forth, related to infarction.
2. Abnormal bleeding: oozing, bleeding from sites of procedures, I.V. catheter insertion sites, suture lines, mucous membranes, orifices; hematuria; internal bleeding leading to changes in vital organ function, and altered vital signs.

Diagnostic Evaluation
1. Platelet count—diminished
2. Prothrombin time and partial thromboplastin time and thrombin time—prolonged
3. Fibrinogen level—decreased
4. Antithrombin III—decreased
5. D-dimer fibrin degradation products—increased
6. Fibrin split products—increased
7. Arterial blood gas levels, blood urea nitrogen, creatinine and other laboratory tests to monitor functioning of vital organs

Collaborative Management
Therapeutic Interventions
1. Treat underlying disorder.
2. Supportive measures, including fluid replacement, oxygenation, maintenance of blood pressure and renal perfusion.

Pharmacologic Interventions
1. Replacement therapy for serious hemorrhaging:
   a. Fresh frozen plasma to replace clotting factors
   b. Platelet transfusions
   c. Cryoprecipitate to replace clotting factors
2. Heparin therapy (controversial) to inhibit clotting component of DIC

Nursing Diagnoses
44, 88, 136

Nursing Interventions

Monitoring
1. When administering blood products, monitor for signs and symptoms of transfusion reactions (see *Table D-6*).
2. Monitor cardiac rhythm, level of consciousness (LOC), respiratory status, and urine output for dysfunction of vital organs caused by ischemia.
3. Evaluate fluid status and bleeding by frequently measuring vital signs, central venous pressure, and intake and output.
4. Monitor for signs of vascular occlusion and report immediately:
   a. Brain—decreased LOC, sensory and motor deficits, seizures, coma
   b. Eyes—visual deficits

TABLE D-6	Acute Blood Transfusion Reactions
TYPE OF REACTION	**CLINICAL MANIFESTATIONS**
Allergic	Flushing, pruritus, rash, urticaria, bronchospasm, anaphylaxis
Febrile, nonhemolytic	Sudden chills and fever, headache, flushing, anxiety
Septic	Rapid onset of chills, high fever, vomiting, diarrhea, hypotension
Circulatory overload	Elevated central venous pressure, distended jugular veins, dyspnea, cough, crackles at lung bases
Hemolytic	Chills, fever, lower back pain, headache, anxiety, flushing, tachycardia, tachypnea, hypotension, hemoglobinuria, renal failure

c. Bone — bone pain
d. Pulmonary — chest pain, dyspnea, tachypnea, tachycardia
e. Extremities — coolness, mottling, numbness
f. Coronary — chest pain, arrhythmia
g. Bowel — pain, tenderness, distention, decreased bowel sounds

▓ **EMERGENCY ALERT** Be aware that all seriously ill patients are at risk for DIC; monitor closely.

Supportive Care

1. Institute bleeding precautions — avoid use of plain razor, hard toothbrush or floss, intramuscular injections, tourniquets, rectal procedures or suppositories; administer stool softeners as necessary to prevent constipation.
2. Monitor pad count and amount of saturation during menses; administer hormones to suppress menstruation, as ordered.
3. Avoid dislodging clots. Apply pressure to sites of bleeding for at least 20 minutes; use topical hemostatic agents. Use tape cautiously.
4. Maintain bed rest.
5. If internal bleeding is suspected, assess bowel sounds and abdominal girth.
6. To promote tissue perfusion, keep patient warm, avoid systemic or topical vasoconstrictive agents, and change patient's position frequently. Perform range-of-motion exercises.

Patient Education and Health Maintenance

1. Reassure the patient and family by explaining the syndrome and its management. Answer all questions.

DISSOCIATIVE DISORDERS

See *Anxiety, Somatoform, and Dissociative Disorders.*

DIVERTICULAR DISEASE

Diverticular disease has three clinical forms: prediverticular disease, diverticulosis, and diverticulitis. In prediverticular disease, the colonic musculature is weakened and degenerated, and the bowel lumen is narrowed. In diverticulosis, there are multiple diverticula, or saccular dilatations at weak points of the colonic wall where nutrient blood vessels penetrate (see *Figure D-3*). In diverticulitis, one or more of the pouches become inflamed and may perforate the thin diverticular wall because of a fecalith plug and accumulating bacteria. If the diverticulum perforates, local abscess or peritonitis may occur. Uninflamed or minimally inflamed diverticula may erode adjacent arterial branches, causing acute massive rectal bleeding.

The cause of diverticular disease is unclear, but a low-residue diet is a contributing factor. Diverticulosis occurs more often in persons older than age 60. Complications include hemorrhage, bowel obstruction, fistula formation, and septicemia.

D

Assessment

1. Prediverticular disease — intermittent or chronic abdominal pain, worsening after eating or before bowel movements; constipation or diarrhea; may be asymptomatic

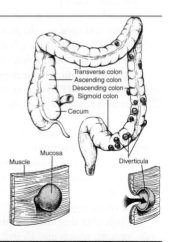

FIGURE D-3 Diverticula are most common in the sigmoid colon; they diminish in number and size as the colon approaches the cecum. Diverticula are rarely found in the rectum.

Transverse colon
Ascending colon
Descending colon
Sigmoid colon
Cecum
Mucosa
Muscle
Diverticula

2. Diverticulosis — crampy abdominal pain, bowel irregularity, periodic abdominal distention, possible sudden massive hemorrhage; may be asymptomatic
3. Mild diverticulitis — bouts of soreness, mild lower abdominal cramps, bowel irregularity, mild nausea, gas, low-grade fever
4. Severe diverticulitis — crampy left lower quadrant pain, low-grade fever and chills, signs of peritonitis or massive hemorrhage if rupture, stool in the urine or vagina if fistula
5. Peritonitis and sepsis
   a. Increasing abdominal pain, rigidity
   b. Guarding, rebound tenderness
   c. Abdominal distention, nausea and vomiting
   d. Fever, hypotension

Diagnostic Evaluation

1. White blood cell count and differential may show leukocytosis with shift to the left; hemoglobin and hematocrit may be low with chronic or acute bleeding.
2. X-rays of abdomen, ultrasonography, and CT scan may show free air under diaphragm with perforation into the abdominal cavity.
3. Sigmoidoscopy, and possible colonoscopy, rules out carcinoma and confirms diagnosis.
4. After infection subsides, barium enema to visualize diverticular sacs, narrowing of colonic lumen, partial or complete obstruction, or fistulae.

 EMERGENCY ALERT Barium enema is contraindicated in acute diverticulitis because bowel rupture may result.

Collaborative Management
Therapeutic Interventions

1. In prediverticular disease, a high-fiber diet with additional bran or psyllium products to counteract tendency toward constipation.
2. In diverticulosis:
   a. High-fiber diet with possible avoidance of large seeds or nuts, which may clog diverticular sac.

b. Bran supplements, psyllium preparations, or stool softeners to avoid constipation.
c. For abdominal pain, switch to a liquid or low-residue diet and stool softeners to relieve symptoms, minimize irritation, and slow progression to diverticulitis.

3. In diverticulitis, bed rest, liquid or low-residue diet, and stool softeners are indicated. I.V. therapy, nasogastric intubation, and NPO status are indicated if peritonitis or massive bleeding occur.

Pharmacologic Interventions

1. Broad-spectrum antibiotic to control infection with diverticulitis
2. Analgesics and anticholinergics to control pain and spasms in diverticulitis
3. Vasopressin and blood replacement for massive bleeding

Surgical Interventions

1. Bowel resection and possible temporary colostomy if there is little response to medical treatment, or if severe complications develop
2. Laparoscopic sigmoid resection with anastomosis in uncomplicated cases

Nursing Diagnoses

3, 16, 24, 27, 123, 135

Nursing Interventions
Monitoring

1. Monitor for signs of peritonitis: increased pain, nausea and vomiting, guarding, distention, and rebound tenderness.
2. Monitor vital signs for shock caused by hemorrhage: tachycardia, thready pulse, and decreased blood pressure.
3. Monitor dietary intake, fiber content, bowel sounds, and stool consistency to determine bowel status.

Supportive Care

1. Maintain NPO status and nasogastric suction for acute stage and GI bleeding. Provide I.V. fluid and prepare for blood transfusion as directed.
2. When condition is stable, encourage patient to follow prescribed high-residue diet to provide bulk and more consistency to the stool. Refer to nutritionist as indicated.
3. Advise patient to add fiber gradually, as tolerated, and avoid foods that aggravate symptoms.
4. Encourage patients to drink fluids to promote bowel stimulation if he or she is constipated.
5. Advise patient to establish regular bowel habits to promote regular and complete evacuation.
6. Observe color, consistency, and frequency of stools and record.

Education and Health Maintenance

1. Explain the disease process to the patient and its relationship to diet.
2. Inform the patient that bran products will add bulk to the stool and can be taken with milk or sprinkled over cereal.
3. Have the patient continue periodic medical supervision and repeat complete blood count to follow up for anemia; report problems and untoward symptoms.

DOWN SYNDROME

Down syndrome (trisomy 21) is a genetic disorder that usually results from formation of three copies of chromosome 21 instead of the normal two because of impaired chromosome separation during meiosis. If the fertilized embryo survives, it has 47 chromosomes instead of 46. Two other causes of Down syndrome, translocation of chromosome 21 and mosaicism involving two cell lines that develop after conception, are rare.

This disorder is the most common identifiable cause of mental retardation and is often associated with heart defects and other congenital anomalies. Down syndrome occurs in 1 of every 700 births. Incidence increases with parental age; risk at maternal age 25 is 1 in 1,350; at age 35, 1 in 384; and at age 45, 1 in 28.

The most common life experience of a child with Down syndrome is to live with the family, participate in infant stimulation and preschool programs, and attend school while receiving some support for special education. Adults with Down syndrome can function in supported employment programs, and live in small groups. Their life expectancy depends on the presence of medical complications; where there are no complications, it is slightly shorter than average.

Assessment

1. Physical signs of Down syndrome are usually apparent at birth:
   a. Brachycephaly (flattened head)
   b. Upward slanting eyes with prominent epicanthal folds
   c. Brushfield spots (small white spots on iris of each eye)
   d. Flat nasal bridge
   e. Small mouth with protruding tongue
   f. Small, low-set ears
   g. Clinodactyly (small little finger that curves inward)
   h. Simian crease (single transverse palmar crease)
2. Other clinical manifestations:
   a. Hypotonia
   b. Dry, scaly skin
   c. Heart defects (eg, atrial or ventricular septal defects, tetralogy of Fallot) — 40% of patients
   d. GI malformations (eg, pyloric stenosis, duodenal atresia, tracheoesophageal fistula) — 12% of patients
   e. Hypothyroidism — 10% to 20% of patients
   f. Visual defects — refractive errors (70%), strabismus (50%), nystagmus (35%), cataracts (3%)
   g. Hearing defects (60% to 90% of patients) — mild to moderate conductive hearing loss, chronic middle ear infections, enlarged adenoids, sleep apnea
   h. Atlanto-occipital and atlanto-axial subluxation (dislocation of upper spine caused by joint laxity) — 15% of patients
   i. Gait abnormalities — 15% of patients

    j. Short stature — 100% of patients

    k. Obesity — 50% of patients

    l. Malocclusions — 60% to 100% of patients

    m. Mental retardation (mild to moderate) — 100% of patients

Diagnostic Evaluation

1. Amniocentesis may be done for prenatal diagnosis; recommended for pregnant women older than age 34 even with negative family history.
2. Chromosome analysis may be done to rule out other chromosomal aberrations.
3. Echocardiogram to check for heart defects — usually done during neonatal period on all infants with Down syndrome.
4. Radiographic studies to demonstrate congenital GI abnormalities.
5. An interdisciplinary and multispecialty team is essential to evaluate physiologic and psychosocial functioning.
6. Vision screening to demonstrate deficits.
7. Auditory brain stem response assesses hearing in infants; sound field testing is done for children older than age 1.
8. Spinal X-rays at age 2 and then every 5 years during childhood, to document alignment of skull and vertebrae for possible correction to avoid compression and neurologic damage.
9. Hip X-rays can document dislocation or subluxation in gait abnormalities.
10. Thyroid-stimulating hormone, thyroxine assays in neonatal screening to detect hypothyroidism; done biannually thereafter.

Collaborative Management

Therapeutic Interventions

1. Hypotonia in infants requires physical therapy. Adaptive equipment gives extra support to head and neck when handling neonate.
2. Physical therapy to correct gait abnormalities.
3. Special education and training for mental retardation.

Pharmacologic Interventions
1. Thyroid hormone replacement in hypothyroidism
2. Possible use of human growth hormone to correct short stature (controversial)

Surgical Interventions
1. Correction of congenital heart defects, GI malformations
2. Myringotomy tubes, adenoidectomy for recurrent ear infections
3. Correction of severe upper spine dislocation through fusion of cervical vertebrae and occiput
4. Orthopedic procedures sometimes required to correct gait abnormalities

Nursing Diagnoses
1, 25, 33, 79, 89, 119, 131, 132, 136

Nursing Interventions
Monitoring
1. Monitor hypotonic infant for feeding and head control.
2. Assess for potential cardiac defects:
   a. Color, pulse, and respiratory rate changes at rest and with stress.
   b. Early tiring or frequent interruptions in feeding.
3. Observe for coughing or vomiting, with or after feeding, indicating GI defects.
   a. Bile-stained vomitus suggests lower tract problem; partially digested contents suggest upper tract problem.
   b. Observe bowel movements and for abdominal distention.
4. Monitor growth on Down syndrome growth chart.
5. Monitor for failure to thrive.
   a. Check feedings for length of feeding, feeding schedule, loss of feeding by vomiting or poor seal on nipple.
   b. Monitor type of formula and caloric content.

Supportive Care
1. Allow the parents access to the infant at all possible times to promote bonding when parents appear ready.

D

2. Focus on the positive aspects of the infant and serve as a role model for handling and stimulating.

3. Be aware of the grieving process (loss of the "normal child") that families experience when a diagnosis is made, and be aware that spouses can be at different stages.

4. Accept all questions and reactions nonjudgmentally, and offer verbal and written explanations.

5. Provide the family a quiet place to discuss their questions with each other and someone knowledgeable about the condition (primary care provider, clinical nurse specialist) to support them in grieving, understanding of the condition, and their ability to cope.

6. Offer the family the option to take advantage of counseling (eg, with a social worker or psychologist).

PEDIATRIC ALERT Children with developmental disabilities and chronic illness are at greater risk of experiencing divorce, child abuse, and neglect than the general population.

7. For those parents concerned with their ability to care for a child, explore with them their options of adoption or institutionalization in a nonjudgmental manner.

8. Demonstrate proper feeding positioning with head elevated and encourage the parents to always hold the infant during feedings with head elevated and supported in arms.

   a. Investigate alternative positions and nipples for feeding caused by weak sucking reflex and large, protruding tongue.

   b. Elevate the head for at least 1 hour after meals.

   c. Allow adequate time for feeding and increase frequency of feedings if infant tires easily.

   d. Offer support and guidance for breast-feeding.

9. When handling the infant, provide adequate support with a firm grasp because infant may be floppy because of poor muscle tone.

10. Position the infant so that, if vomiting should occur, aspiration will be prevented.

    a. Prop infant with a diaper roll so position will be maintained.

b. Change position frequently because this infant is not usually active.
11. Continuously check environment for safety needs for this child.

COMMUNITY CARE CONSIDERATIONS

Teach caregivers to base safety needs on the developmental rather than chronological age of the child.

12. Demonstrate and encourage play with the child at the appropriate level to provide stimulation, and work toward achieving developmental milestones.
13. Use appropriate behavior modification techniques, such as extinction, time-out, and reward to achieve cooperation and success.

Education and Health Maintenance

1. Remind the parents to recognize the child's routine health care needs and maintain regular follow-up with a primary care provider:
   a. Immunizations
   b. Regular dental checkups beginning at age 2
   c. Visual and hearing examinations — should be seen by an ophthalmologist at age 1
2. Teach parents to provide a therapeutic home environment.
   a. Maintain regular sleeping, eating, working, and playing routines.
   b. Divide tasks and expectations into small, manageable parts. Give only one or two instructions at a time.
   c. Set firm but reasonable limits on behavior and carry through with consistent discipline.
   d. Provide energy outlet through physical activity, vocal outlet, and outdoor play.
3. Advise parents to teach habits to older children that are essential to later vocational life, such as getting to places on time, cooperating, focusing on the task at hand, and establishing acceptable interpersonal relationships.

4. Tell family about genetic counseling, which supplies information on risk in subsequent pregnancies (parents) or risk to offspring (patient).
5. Refer to local parent support group or National Down Syndrome Society, *www.ndss.org*.

DYSRHYTHMIAS

Cardiac dysrhythmias are disturbances in regular heart rate or rhythm caused by change in electrical conduction or automaticity. Dysrhythmias may arise from the sinoatrial node (sinus bradycardia or tachycardia) or anywhere within the atria or ventricles (known as ectopic beats). Some may be benign and asymptomatic, whereas others are life-threatening.

Assessment
1. May cause light-headedness, shortness of breath, fatigue, and palpitations, or may be asymptomatic.
2. Objectively, there may be change in heart rate or rhythm by palpation of the pulse and auscultation of the heart.
3. 12-lead electrocardiogram (ECG) and rhythm strip, or continuous cardiac monitoring will show features of dysrhythmia.
4. Analysis of ECG strip (see *Figure D-4*):
   a. Determine the rate for bradycardia or tachycardia.
   b. Determine the rhythm for regularity.
   c. Assess P waves for their relationship to QRS complex and their similarity to each other.
   d. Measure the PR interval for prolongation.
   e. Assess the QRS complexes for their appearance, length, and similarity to each other.
   f. Assess T waves for presence after each QRS and their configuration.
5. Assess that pulse reflects ECG reading, as well as other vital signs and level of consciousness to see if cardiac output is affected by dysrhythmia.

 EMERGENCY ALERT Be prepared to begin cardiopulmonary resuscitation (CPR) if pulselessness develops despite ECG reading.

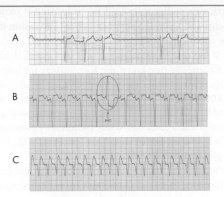

FIGURE D-4 Rhythm strips. (**A**) Atrial fibrillation with slow ventricular response (controlled). (**B**) Normal sinus rhythm with premature ventricular contraction. (**C**) Ventricular tachycardia.

D

Collaborative Management

1. Recognition and treatment of underlying cause such as hypoxia, metabolic acidosis, electrolyte imbalance, myocardial ischemia or infarction, valvular disease, heart failure, digoxin toxicity, illicit drug overdose, or other cardiac or systemic disorders.
2. Paroxysmal atrial tachycardia — adenosine, a beta-adrenergic blocker, or a calcium channel blocker administered I.V.; cardioversion may be effective.
3. Atrial fibrillation — treatment to slow rate and prevent clot formation; digoxin and other antiarrhythmics are used; cardioversion if atrial fibrillation is of recent onset; anticoagulation may be given.
4. Atrial flutter — calcium channel blocker, digoxin, quinidine, or beta-adrenergic blocker; cardioversion if drugs unsuccessful.
5. Premature ventricular contractions — treated when they occur at a rate exceeding six per minute, occur as two or more consecutively, fall on T wave, or are of varying configurations; lidocaine is drug of choice; procainamide or bretylium may also used.

6. Ventricular tachycardia (VT) — lidocaine if patient is conscious and not decompensated; cardioversion if lidocaine ineffective and patient remains alert; precordial blow if unconscious and event was witnessed; defibrillation if consciousness and pulse lost; surgery for long-term management; magnesium sulfate for torsades de pointes.

> **⚡ EMERGENCY ALERT** Torsades de pointes is an atypical VT characterized by a QT interval greater than 0.06 seconds, varying R-R, and polymorphous QRS complexes. It may be caused by quinidine toxicity. Lidocaine is to be avoided because this will prolong the QT. Treatment is magnesium sulfate 1 g I.V.

7. Ventricular fibrillation — defibrillation if patient remains unresponsive, begin CPR and administer epinephrine to reverse lactic acidosis and make the heart more responsive to defibrillation.

8. Atrioventricular (AV) block — no treatment necessary for first-degree AV block, second-degree block treated if cardiac output falls, third-degree block usually treated; atropine temporarily until pacemaker can be inserted.

E

EATING DISORDERS

The two major eating disorders are *anorexia nervosa* and *bulimia nervosa*. Anorexia nervosa is characterized by self-induced weight loss greater than 15% of minimally normal weight for age and height. Periods of starvation may be mixed with binging and purging. This leads to a semistarvation state with glucose and protein sparing, fat utilization, endocrine changes, and fluid and electrolyte disturbances. Psychological components include a distorted body image, fear of gaining weight, and loss of self-esteem.

In contrast to anorexia, bulimia is marked by recurrent episodes of binge eating at least twice per week for 3 months. The patient feels a lack of control over eating behavior during these episodes, and later tries to prevent weight gain by self-induced vomiting, excessive use of laxatives, diuretics, fasting, or excessive exercise. Self-induced vomiting may result in electrolyte imbalance (hypokalemia, hyponatremia, hypochloremia, elevated bicarbonate) or esophageal tears or gastric rupture. Starvation and its physiologic effects may not be evident as they are in anorexia nervosa. Bulimia is linked to a personal or family history of obesity, substance abuse, depression, anxiety, or mood disorders.

Many patients with an eating disorder are between ages 14 and 24, in the middle and upper socioeconomic levels, and 90% are women. Anorexia and bulimia may occur simultaneously or alternately.

Assessment

1. In anorexia look for:
   a. Cold intolerance, constipation, and abdominal pain
   b. Amenorrhea for 3 consecutive months, decreased libido
   c. Dry skin, thinning scalp hair, lanugo hair

    d. Anxiety, increased exercise activity, inhibited or de-structive social interactions, sleep disturbance

    e. Bradycardia, hypotension, hypothermia

    f. Loss of adipose tissue and weight loss of greater than 15% of ideal body weight

    g. Perfectionistic or obsessive-compulsive behavior with high performance expectations

    h. Depression, diminished sexual interest

2. In bulimia look for:

    a. Depression, anxiety, personality disorder, abnormal eating behaviors, history of family dysfunction

    b. Calluses or skin changes on hands and fingers

    c. Loss of dental enamel, swollen lymph nodes, enlarged parotids, and bad breath or mouthwash smell on breath because of self-induced vomiting

    d. Endocrine changes such as amenorrhea

    e. Weight is usually maintained within normal range, or may be significantly elevated or decreased

Diagnostic Evaluation

1. Decreased chloride, potassium, phosphate, magnesium, zinc, albumin levels may occur.

2. Increased blood urea nitrogen, creatinine, liver function tests, bicarbonate, amylase.

3. Hormone studies may show decreased luteinizing hormone, follicle-stimulating hormone, estrogen, testosterone (in men), and thyroid hormone, and decreased response to luteinizing hormone–releasing hormone.

4. Complete blood count may show decreased white blood cells and hematocrit, indicating starvation's effect on immunity and anemia.

5. Electrocardiogram should be done to detect arrhythmias or other signs of electrolyte imbalance.

6. Urinalysis may show ketonuria.

Collaborative Management
Therapeutic and Pharmacologic Interventions

1. Develop a nutritional plan to accomplish weight goal (gain or loss) and achieve normal eating habits.

2. Assist in setting up a reasonable exercise and activity program once patient is eating and weight gain is seen.
3. Provide psychological counseling and support:
   a. Assist anorexic or bulimic patient to develop insight into behavior and a more realistic body image.
   b. Assist patient to develop effective coping strategies and problem-solving mechanisms.
   c. Inpatient treatment is recommended if weight is below 75% ideal weight; marked orthostatic hypotension, bradycardia less than 40 beats/minute, sustained tachycardia greater than 100 beats/minute, inability to maintain core body temperature near normal, suicidal, or no response to outpatient therapy.
4. Enteral or parenteral feeding may be necessary if prescribed diet cannot be maintained by anorexic patient and physical status warrants.
5. Antidepressants may be tried as well as other pharmacologic agents for associated psychiatric problems.

E

Nursing Diagnoses
12, 30, 51, 78, 152

Nursing Interventions
Monitoring
1. Monitor daily dietary intake and weights.
2. Monitor intake and output and serum electrolytes.
3. Monitor urine for ketones.
4. Assess patient's risk for suicide and maintain level of surveillance called for by the situation.

Supportive Care
1. Assess the patient's bowel function. Promote fluids and activity to prevent constipation in anorexia.
2. Assist the patient to select well-balanced diet and maintain appropriate eating habits. Small, frequent meals or snacks of high-calorie foods and beverages with liquid nutritional supplements may be helpful in severe anorexia.
3. Provide positive reinforcement for improved intake and weight control.

4. Establish a trusting relationship and provide for the patient's safety and security needs.
5. Be alert for lying and manipulation the patient may display to preserve control.
6. Involve the patient in the treatment plan, offering choices to increase the patient's sense of control. Set limits to give a sense of external control.
7. Encourage patient to verbalize feelings about body image, self-concept, fears, and frustrations.
8. Stress the importance of counseling, stress management, assertiveness training, problem solving, and other therapies.
9. Teach the patient the risks associated with abnormal eating behavior and benefits of maintaining healthful nutritional and exercise habits.
10. Encourage the patient to set realistic goals for weight and appearance.

Education and Health Maintenance

1. Teach principles of nutrition and healthful diet and eating habits. Discuss food matter-of-factly to avoid feeding into the patient's preoccupation with food.
2. Teach the impact of starvation on both physiologic and psychological functioning.
3. Involve the patient's family and significant others in the treatment plan as appropriate.
4. Describe the dangers of using laxatives and diuretics in weight control, such as electrolyte imbalances, dehydration, and bowel atony.
5. Stress the importance of maintaining follow-up and counseling.
6. For additional information, refer to National Association of Anorexia Nervosa and Associated Disorders, *www.anad. org*.

ECZEMA

See *Dermatitis, Atopic*.

ENCEPHALITIS

Encephalitis is an inflammation of cerebral tissue typically accompanied by meningeal inflammation, caused by an infection or other source. It can present as acute viral encephalitis, most frequently caused by herpesvirus and most commonly occurring in children. Cytomegalovirus (CMV) and *Toxoplasma* are common causes in patients with acquired immunodeficiency syndrome. It may also present as postinfectious encephalitis, which follows a viral or bacterial infection, usually of the respiratory or GI tract. It may also present as an arthropod-borne infection such as West Nile virus. The disease, which is commonly fatal, causes lymphocytic infiltration of the brain, which leads to cerebral edema, basal ganglia degeneration, and diffuse nerve cell destruction. Complications include motor and sensory deficits, amnesia syndrome, syndrome of inappropriate antidiuretic hormone (SIADH), coma, and death.

E

Assessment

1. Fever, headache, nausea and vomiting, mental status changes
2. Meningeal signs — nuchal rigidity (stiff neck), photophobia
3. Seizures, motor deficits, personality changes
4. Signs of brain stem involvement, such as nystagmus, extraocular nerve palsies, hearing loss, dysphagia, and respiratory dysfunction
5. Patients with hypothalamic-pituitary involvement may develop diabetes insipidus (page 276) hypothermia, or SIADH.

Diagnostic Evaluation

1. Lumbar puncture evaluates cerebrospinal fluid (CSF) for increased cell count; polymerase chain reaction analysis of CSF for viral antibodies.
2. Electroencephalogram may reveal abnormalities.

3. Gadolinium-enhanced magnetic resonance imaging can detect different patterns of inflammation to differentiate type of encephalitis.
4. Blood cultures rarely identify causative organism, but brain-tissue biopsy may indicate presence of microorganism.
5. West Nile virus serologic testing on blood or CSF.

Collaborative Management
Pharmacologic Interventions
1. Antiviral agent acyclovir given I.V. for 10 days to 3 weeks for herpes simplex virus
2. Ganciclovir and foscarnet I.V. for CMV encephalitis
3. Anticonvulsants to treat seizures, corticosteroids to reduce cerebral edema, and sedatives and analgesics as supportive therapy

Nursing Diagnoses
35, 49, 88, 136

Nursing Interventions
Monitoring
1. Monitor pupils and vital signs frequently for increased intracranial pressure (ICP; irregular pupils, widening pulse pressure, tachycardia, irregular breathing, hyperthermia).
2. Monitor the patient's response to medications and observe for adverse reactions.
3. Monitor neurologic status closely. Watch for subtle changes, such as behavior or personality changes, weakness, or cranial nerve involvement. Notify health care provider if changes occur.
4. Monitor fluid intake and output to ensure adequate hydration.

Supportive Care
1. Maintain quiet environment and provide care gently, to avoid excessive stimulation and agitation, which may cause increased ICP.

2. Maintain seizure precautions: pad side rails of bed and have airway and suction equipment available at bedside.
3. Maintain standard precautions and additional isolation according to your facility's policy to prevent transmission.
4. Administer antipyretics and other cooling measures as indicated.
5. Provide fluid replacement through I.V. lines as needed.
6. Reorient patient frequently.
7. Provide supportive care if coma develops; may last several weeks.
8. Encourage significant others to interact with patient even while in coma and to participate in care to promote rehabilitation.

Education and Health Maintenance

1. Encourage follow-up for evaluation of deficits and rehabilitation potential.
2. Educate others about prevention of mosquito-borne illnesses.
3. Encourage vaccination for measles, mumps, and rubella to prevent encephalitis due to those viruses.

ENDOCARDITIS, INFECTIVE

Infective endocarditis (IE; bacterial endocarditis) is an infection of the inner lining of the heart (endocardium) caused by direct invasion of bacteria or other organisms leading to deformity of the valve leaflets. When the endocardium becomes inflamed, a fibrin clot (vegetation) forms, which may become colonized by pathogens during transient episodes of bacteremia resulting from invasive procedures (venous or arterial cannulation, dental work causing gingival bleeding, GI or genitourinary tract surgery, liver biopsy, sigmoidoscopy, and so forth), urinary tract infections, and wound or skin infections.

Common organisms include *Streptococcus viridans* (after dental work or upper respiratory infection), *Staphylococcus aureus* (after cardiac surgery or parenteral drug abuse), *Enterococcus* (usually occurs in elderly people with genitourinary tract infection), and fungi such as *Candida albicans* and *Aspergillus*, and *Rickettsia*.

Increased risk for IE exists with rheumatic heart disease, congenital defects, abnormally vascularized valves, and mechanical or biological heart valves.

IE may be acute or subacute, depending on the microorganisms involved. Acute IE manifests rapidly with danger of intractable heart failure and occurs more commonly on normal heart valves. Additional complications include uncontrolled or refractory infection, embolic episodes (ischemia or necrosis of extremities and organs), and conduction disturbances.

Subacute IE manifests a prolonged chronic course with a lesser chance of complications and occurs more commonly on damaged or defective valves.

Assessment

1. Fever, chills, sweats, anorexia, weight loss, weakness, cough, back and joint pain, headache
2. Characteristic skin and nail manifestations:
   a. Petechiae of conjunctiva and mucous membranes
   b. Splinter hemorrhages in nail beds
   c. Osler's nodes — painful red nodes on pads of fingers and toes; usually late sign of subacute infection
   d. Janeway's lesions — light pink macules on palms or soles, nontender, may change to light tan within several days, fade in 1 to 2 weeks; usually an early sign of IE
3. New pathologic or changing murmur — no murmur with other signs or symptoms may indicate right heart infection
4. Additional findings may include splenomegaly, altered mental status, aphasia, hemiplegia, cortical sensory loss, Roth's spots on fundi, pulmonary involvement
5. Emboli: can travel to the lungs, kidneys, spleen, heart, brain, abdomen, and extremities

Diagnostic Evaluation

1. Laboratory tests include sedimentation rate (increased), complete blood count (mildly elevated white blood cell count), a series of blood cultures from well-cleaned

venipuncture site to isolate bacteria or fungi, and additional blood tests to evaluate kidney function.
2. Baseline electrocardiogram is usually normal.
3. Echocardiography identifies vegetations and assesses location and size of lesions.
4. Serum levels of antibiotics.

Collaborative Management
Pharmacologic Interventions
1. I.V. antimicrobial therapy based on sensitivity of causative agent, usually penicillin G, nafcillin, vancomycin, rifampin, or an aminoglycoside, alone or in combination for 4 to 6 weeks. Obtain audiogram before antibiotic therapy, and repeat blood cultures after 48 hours to assess efficacy of drug therapy.
2. Antipyretics and analgesics.

Surgical Interventions
1. Surgery is necessary in the event of:
   a. Acute destructive valvular lesion — excision of infected valves or removal of prosthetic valve
   b. Hemodynamic impairment
   c. Recurrent emboli
   d. Infection that cannot be eliminated with antimicrobial therapy
   e. Drainage of abscess or empyema — for patient with localized abscess or empyema
   f. Repair of peripheral or cerebral mycotic aneurysm

Nursing Diagnoses
6, 19, 49, 51, 88, 134, 136

Nursing Interventions
Monitoring
1. Monitor for signs of decreased cardiac output and heart failure, such as third heart sound, decreasing blood pressure, increasing pulse, pulsus alternans, decreased pulse pressure, jugular vein distention, and crackles of lung fields.

2. Monitor intake and output; observe skin turgor, urine specific gravity, and mucous membranes for adequate hydration; and check daily weights to ensure adequate fluid balance.
3. Monitor temperature every 2 to 4 hours and record on graph.
4. Watch for signs of embolic episodes, such as altered mentation, aphasia, loss of muscle strength, loss of vision, hemoptysis, hematuria, and complaints of pain; report promptly.
5. Monitor for therapeutic antibiotic blood levels and response to therapy. Patient should have a general "sense of well-being" 5 to 7 days after initiation of therapy.

DRUG ALERT Rapid infusion of vancomycin (less than 1 hour) may cause "red neck" syndrome (intense rash over upper half of body) due to histamine release. Slow the rate of infusion and the rash will clear.

6. Monitor for signs of renal toxicity caused by antibiotic therapy, such as changes in urinalysis, blood urea nitrogen, and creatinine.

Supportive Care
1. Reposition patient frequently to prevent skin breakdown and pulmonary complications associated with bed rest.
2. Observe basic principles of asepsis, good handwashing techniques, and continuity of patient care by primary nurse.
3. Employ meticulous I.V. care for long-term antibiotic therapy.
4. Provide cooling measures, such as cool compresses and cooling blanket as directed.
5. Provide blankets and temperature-controlled comfortable environment if patient has shaking chills; change bed linens as necessary.
6. Promote adequate hydration, both oral and I.V., because diaphoresis and increased metabolic rate may cause dehydration.

7. Promote adequate nutrition with small meals and snacks throughout the day to meet the body's needs in fighting infection.
8. Encourage diversional activities appropriate for patient's age, such as television, reading, and quiet games.
9. Coordinate home care nursing and I.V. therapy for outpatient antibiotic treatment, as indicated.

Education and Health Maintenance
For all patients at risk for IE:

1. Discuss endocarditis, the mode of entry of infection, and early signs and symptoms.
2. Indicate that antibiotic prophylaxis is recommended for people with:
   a. Congenital heart defects, prosthetic or biological heart valves, idiopathic hypertrophic subaortic stenosis
   b. History of endocarditis
   c. Mitral valve prolapse with insufficiency
   d. Rheumatic heart disease and valvular dysfunction
   e. Cardiomyopathy
3. Identify procedures most likely to cause bacteremia (dental procedures causing gingival bleeding, surgery on or instrumentation of GI tract, certain genitourinary procedures, rigid bronchoscopy, and tonsillectomy).
4. Identify individual steps necessary to prevent infection.
   a. Good oral hygiene, regular tooth brushing, and flossing
   b. Notification to health care personnel of any history of congenital heart disease or valvular disease
   c. Importance of carrying emergency identification with information of medical history at all times
   d. Take temperature if infection is suspected and notify health care provider of elevation
   e. Early treatment of illness that could lead to bacteremia — injuries, sore throats, and furuncles
5. Encourage susceptible people to receive pneumococcal and influenza vaccines.
6. Teach women in childbearing years the risks of using intrauterine devices for birth control (source of infection)

E

and that antibiotic therapy is not necessary for women who have normal deliveries.

For people who have had endocarditis, regarding possible relapse:

1. Discuss importance of keeping follow-up appointments after hospital discharge (infection can recur in 1 to 2 months).
2. Teach person to inspect soles for Janeway's lesions indicative of possible relapse.
3. Advise family to allow child to resume activities gradually, and to ensure adequate rest periods throughout the day.

ENDOMETRIOSIS

Endometriosis is an abnormal proliferation of uterine endometrial tissue outside the uterus. Although it most commonly occurs in the pelvic area, ectopic endometrial tissue may occur elsewhere in the body; an intact uterus is not needed for endometriosis to occur. This ectopic tissue is sensitive to ovarian hormones and bleeds during menstruation, resulting in accumulated blood and inflammation and subsequent adhesions and pain. It also regresses during periods of amenorrhea (ie, pregnancy and menopause) and with hormonal contraceptive and androgen use.

Endometriosis is most common in women ages 25 to 45 but may occur at any age. It is more likely to occur in women with shorter menstrual cycles and longer duration of flow; in siblings; in whites more than blacks; and in women who do not exercise and are obese. Complications include infertility and rupture of endometrial cysts.

Assessment

May be asymptomatic or cause pain based on site of implantation:

1. Pelvic pain — especially during or before menstruation
2. Flank pain, hematuria, dysuria — if bladder involved
3. Painful defecation — if sigmoid colon or rectum involved
4. Dyspareunia (painful sexual intercourse)
5. Rupture of endometrial cysts mimics ruptured appendix

6. Abnormal uterine bleeding and infertility commonly occur

Diagnostic Evaluation

1. Pelvic and rectal examinations may reveal tender, fixed nodules or ovarian mass or uterine retrodisplacement.
2. Laparoscopy views ectopic implants and determines extent of disease.
3. Other studies, including ultrasound, CT, and barium enema, determine extent of organ involvement.

Collaborative Management
Pharmacologic Interventions

Drug treatment may include one or more of the following:

1. Progestins — create a hypoestrogenic environment
2. Gonadotropin-releasing hormone antagonist (leuprolide) injections over a 6-month period — create hypoestrogenic environment
3. Hormonal contraceptives — use small amount of estrogen, maximum amount of progestin and androgen effect to decrease ectopic implant size
4. Danazol — synthetic androgen suppresses endometrial growth; contraindicated in pregnancy; adverse effects limit use

Surgical Interventions

1. Laparoscopic surgery — preferred procedure to remove implants and lyse adhesions; not curative; high recurrence rate
2. Carbon dioxide laser laparoscopy — for minimal to moderate disease; vaporizes tissue; may be done at same time as diagnosis; good pregnancy rate
3. Laparotomy — for severe endometriosis or persistent symptoms
4. Presacral neurectomy — to decrease central pelvic pain; preserves fertility
5. Hysterectomy — if fertility is not desired and symptoms are severe; ovaries are usually removed

Nursing Diagnoses
3, 13, 84

Nursing Interventions
Supportive Care
1. Teach the use of analgesics for exacerbations.
2. Encourage the patient to use a heating pad for painful areas, as needed.
3. Teach the patient relaxation techniques to control pain, such as deep breathing, imagery, and progressive muscle relaxation.
4. Encourage the patient to try position changes for sexual intercourse if experiencing dyspareunia.
5. Include the patient in treatment planning; answer questions about drug and surgical treatment so she can make informed choices.
6. Encourage adequate rest and nutrition.
7. Provide emotional support and encourage the patient to discuss treatment of infertility with her health care provider.

Education and Health Maintenance
1. Instruct the patient about the adverse effects of prescribed medication.
   a. Leuprolide may cause nausea, vomiting, constipation, headache, hot flashes, sweats, edema, dizziness, and difficulty urinating.
   b. Danazol may cause voice changes, increased facial hair, acne, weight gain, decreased breast size, and vasomotor reactions.
2. Refer the patient to support groups such as Endometriosis Association, *www.endometriosis.org*.

ESOPHAGEAL ATRESIA AND TRACHEOESOPHAGEAL FISTULA

Esophageal atresia is failure of the esophagus to form a continuous passage from the pharynx to the stomach during embryonic development. *Tracheoesophageal fistula* (TEF) is an abnormal connection between the trachea and esophagus.

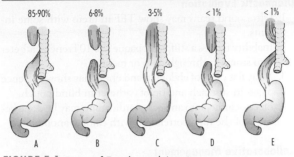

85-90%   6-8%   3-5%   < 1%   < 1%

A   B   C   D   E

FIGURE E-1 Types of Esophageal Atresia.

E

Esophageal atresia is classified into five types (see *Figure E-1*). Type A is most common (80% to 90% of cases) and will be discussed further in this entry. The proximal segment of the esophagus has a blind end, whereas the distal segment connects with the trachea by way of a fistula. In type B atresia, which comprises most of the remaining cases, both proximal and distal segments of the esophagus are blind, with no connection to the trachea.

In TEF, the child cannot swallow effectively, and saliva or formula may be aspirated into the airway; air entering the lower esophagus through the fistula may cause gastric distention and respiratory distress. Aspiration pneumonia and dehydration are the greatest complications. Other congenital defects occur in 50% of infants with esophageal atresia.

Assessment

1. Excessive secretions, constant drooling, large amount of secretions from nose
2. Intermittent unexplained cyanosis
3. Laryngospasm caused by aspiration of accumulated saliva in blind pouch
4. Abdominal distention
5. Violent response after first or second swallow of feeding; infant coughs and chokes as fluid returns through nose and mouth; cyanosis occurs

Diagnostic Evaluation

1. Ultrasound scans may show TEF in utero with some infants.
2. Inability to pass a stiff, radiopaque size 10 French catheter into stomach through nose or mouth.
3. X-ray flat plate of abdomen and chest may show presence of gas in stomach and tip of catheter in blind pouch.
4. Electrocardiogram and echocardiograms may be done because of the high correlation with cardiac anomalies.

Collaborative Management

Therapeutic and Pharmacologic Interventions

1. Immediate treatment consists of giving nothing by mouth, propping infant at 30-degree angle, and giving histamine-2 receptor blockers to prevent reflux of gastric contents; #10 nasogastric tube inserted into proximal esophagus for continuous or gentle intermittent suction to prevent aspiration. Gastrostomy tube may also be placed for suction of gastric contents.
2. Supportive therapy includes meeting nutritional requirements, hydration, antibiotics, oxygen, and respiratory support for aspiration pneumonia; and maintaining a thermally neutral environment to reduce energy expenditure.

Surgical Interventions

1. Prompt primary repair: division of fistula followed by esophageal anastomosis of proximal and distal segments if infant is greater than 2,000 g (4.4 lb) and is without pneumonia.
2. Short-term delay (subsequent primary repair): to stabilize infant and to prevent deterioration when the infant cannot tolerate immediate surgery.
3. Staging: initially, fistula division and gastrostomy are performed with later secondary esophageal anastomosis. Approach may be used with a very small, premature neonate or a very sick neonate, or when severe congenital anomalies exist.

4. Circular esophagomyotomy may be performed on proximal pouch to gain length and allow for primary anastomosis at initial surgery.

5. Cervical esophagostomy (artificial opening in neck that allows for drainage of the upper esophagus) may be done when ends of esophagus are too widely separated; esophageal replacement with segment of intestine is done at age 18 to 24 months.

6. Postoperative complications (5% to 10% of cases):
   a. Leak at anastomosis site
   b. Recurrent fistulas
   c. Esophageal strictures
   d. Gastroesophageal reflux and esophagitis
   e. Tracheomalacia
   f. Feeding problems with the older child

Nursing Diagnoses
3, 6, 51, 73, 119, 123, 132, 135

E

Nursing Interventions
Monitoring

1. Preoperatively be alert for indications of respiratory distress: retractions, circumoral cyanosis, restlessness, nasal flaring, and increased respiration and heart rate.

2. Monitor vital signs frequently for changes in blood pressure and pulse, which may indicate dehydration or fluid volume overload.

3. Record intake and output, including esophageal and gastric drainage. Weigh diapers.

4. Monitor for abdominal distention.

5. Monitor for signs or symptoms that may indicate additional congenital anomalies or complications.

6. Postoperatively, assess for leak at the anastomosis causing mediastinitis and pneumothorax. Look for saliva in chest tube, hypothermia or hyperthermia, severe respiratory distress, cyanosis, restlessness, and weak pulses.

7. Continue to monitor for complications during the recovery process:

   a. Stricture at the anastomosis: difficulty in swallowing, vomiting or spitting up of ingested fluid, refusing to eat, and fever (secondary to aspiration and pneumonia)

   b. Recurrent fistula: coughing, choking, and cyanosis associated with feeding; excessive salivation; difficulty in swallowing associated with abnormal distention; repeated episodes of pneumonitis; and general poor physical condition (no weight gain)

   c. Atelectasis or pneumonitis: aspiration, respiratory distress

Supportive Care
Preoperative

1. Position the infant with head and chest elevated 20 to 30 degrees to prevent or reduce reflux of gastric juices into the tracheobronchial tree. Turn the infant frequently to prevent atelectasis and pneumonia.

2. Perform intermittent oral suctioning and maintain indwelling double-lumen tube with constant suction or gentle intermittent suction to remove secretions from proximal esophagus. Irrigate with air only.

   a. Make sure that indwelling tube is kept patent and changed as needed and at least once every 12 to 24 hours (by the health care provider); alternate nostrils. Prevent necrosis of nostrils from pressure by catheter.

3. If gastrostomy placed before definitive surgery, maintain tube to straight gravity drainage and irrigate with air only.

4. Place the infant in an Isolette or under a radiant warmer with high humidity.

   a. Aids in liquefying secretions and thick mucus

   b. Maintains the infant's temperature in thermoneutral zone and ensures environmental isolation to prevent infection

5. Administer oxygen as needed.

6. Maintain NPO and administer parenteral fluids and electrolytes, as directed, to prevent dehydration.

7. Be available and recognize need for emergency care or resuscitation.

8. Explain procedures and necessary events to parents as soon as possible. Orient them to facility and neonatal intensive care unit environment.
9. Allow the family to hold and assist in caring for infant.
10. Offer reassurance and encouragement to family frequently. Provide for additional support by social worker, clergy, or counselor as needed.

Postoperative

1. Maintain airway patency. Suction frequently, at least every 1 or 2 hours; may be needed every 5 to 10 minutes.
   a. Ask the surgeon to mark a suction catheter to indicate how far the catheter can be safely inserted without disturbing the anastomosis.
   b. Observe for signs of obstructed airway.
   c. Wean from respirator when airway potency is maintained and respiratory effort is good.
2. Administer chest physiotherapy as directed.
   a. Change the infant's position by turning; stimulate crying to promote full expansion of lungs.
   b. Elevate head and shoulders 20 to 30 degrees.
   c. Use mechanical vibrator 2 to 3 days postoperatively (to minimize trauma to anastomosis), followed by more vigorous chest physical therapy after the third day.

EMERGENCY ALERT Avoid hyperextending the neck, which places stress on the operative site.

3. Continue use of Isolette or radiant warmer with humidity.
4. Continue to have emergency equipment available, including suction machine, catheter, oxygen, laryngoscope, and endotracheal tubes in varying sizes.
5. Administer I.V. solutions until gastrostomy feedings can be started.
6. Administer analgesics as indicated.
7. Begin gastrostomy feedings as soon as ordered because adequate nutrition is an important factor in healing.
   a. Gastrostomy is generally attached to gravity drainage for 2 or 3 days postoperatively. When gastric drainage

decreases, gastrostomy may be clamped or left open to air to let gastric secretions flow into the duodenum.

    b. Give the infant a pacifier to suck during feedings, unless contraindicated.

    c. Prevent air from entering the stomach and causing gastric distention and possible reflux.

    d. Begin oral feedings 10 to 14 days after surgery but continue gastrostomy feedings until the infant can tolerate full feedings orally.

8. Maintain patency of chest drainage.

    a. If a break occurs in closed drainage system, immediately clamp tubing close to the infant to prevent pneumothorax.

9. If infant has had cervical esophagostomy:

    a. Keep the area clean of saliva with soap and water and place an absorbent pad over the area.

    b. As soon as possible, allow the infant to suck a few milliliters of milk at the same time gastrostomy feeding is being done.

    c. Advance the infant to solid foods as appropriate if esophagostomy is maintained for a few months.

10. When oral feedings are begun, use demand feedings rather than strictly scheduled feeding.

    a. Use upright sitting position and burp frequently.

    b. Do not allow the infant to become overtired at feeding time. Note heart rate.

11. Try to make each feeding a pleasant experience for the infant. Use a consistent approach and patience. Encourage parental involvement.

12. Encourage parents to cuddle and talk to the infant.

13. Provide for visual, auditory, and tactile stimulation as appropriate for the infant's physical condition and age.

14. Help to develop a healthy parent-child relationship through flexible visiting, frequent phone calls, and encouraging physical contact between child and parents.

Education and Health Maintenance

1. Teach all procedures to be done at home. Watch return demonstration of the following:

a. Gastrostomy feedings and care
b. Esophagostomy care with feeding technique
c. Suctioning
d. Identifying signs of respiratory distress

2. Help the parents understand the psychological needs of the infant for sucking, warmth, comfort, stimulation, and affection. Suggest that activity be age-appropriate.

3. Encourage the parents to continue close medical follow-up and help them learn to recognize possible problems:
   a. Eating problems may occur, especially when solids are introduced.
   b. Repeated respiratory tract infection should be reported.
   c. Occurrence of stricture at site of anastomosis weeks to months later may be indicated by difficulty in swallowing, spitting of ingested fluid, and fever.
   d. Dilatation of esophagus may be necessary to treat stricture at the site of the anastomosis.
   e. Signs of fistula leakage are dusky color or choking with feeding.

4. Help the parents understand the need for good nutrition and the need to follow the diet regimen suggested by the health care provider.

5. Reassure parents that an infant's raspy cough is normal and will gradually diminish as the infant's trachea becomes stronger over 6 to 24 months (most infants have some tracheomalacia).

6. Teach parents to protect the child from swallowing foreign objects.

7. Refer parents for additional information to EA/TEF Child and Family Support Connection, *www.eatef.org*.

ESOPHAGEAL CANCER

See *Cancer, Esophageal*.

ESOPHAGEAL VARICES, BLEEDING

Esophageal varices are dilated tortuous veins that occur in the submucosa of the lower esophagus, and sometimes extend to the stomach or the upper esophagus. Varices usually result from portal hypertension, which commonly results from obstruction of the portal venous circulation and cirrhosis of the liver.

Mortality is high because of further deterioration of liver function with hepatic coma, and complications, such as massive recurrent hemorrhage, aspiration pneumonia, sepsis, and renal failure.

Assessment

1. Hematemesis — vomiting of bright red blood
2. Melena — passage of black, tarry stools
3. Possible bright red rectal bleeding caused by bowel hypermotility
4. Blood loss may be sudden and massive, causing shock

Diagnostic Evaluation

1. Upper GI endoscopy identifies the cause and site of bleeding.
2. Liver function tests, including elevated ammonia level.

Collaborative Management

Therapeutic and Pharmacologic Interventions

1. Blood products and I.V. fluids to restore circulation and blood volume; give vitamin K to enhance clotting.
2. Octreotide is a synthetic hormone given I.V. that mimics the action of somatostatin to reduce splanchnic blood flow and increase clotting and hemostasis.
3. Administration of vasopressin I.V. to reduce portal venous pressure and control variceal bleeding; however, it has profound vasoconstrictor effects.
4. Gastric lavage to remove blood from the GI tract, vasoconstrict esophageal and gastric blood vessels, and enhance visualization for endoscopic examination.
5. Esophageal balloon tamponade (using Sengstaken-Blakemore or Minnesota tube), whereby balloons are inflated in the distal esophagus and the proximal stomach to collapse the varices and induce hemostasis.
6. Parenteral feedings after bleeding is controlled to allow the esophagus to rest.

Surgical Interventions

1. Endoscopic sclerotherapy, whereby a sclerosing agent is injected directly into the varix by way of a flexible fiberoptic endoscope to control bleeding and reduce frequency of subsequent variceal hemorrhages. Repeated treatments may be required.
2. Ligation of varices ties off blood vessels at the site of bleeding; may be done endoscopically (variceal banding).
3. Esophageal transection and devascularization to separate bleeding site from portal system.
4. Shunts to bypass liver, thereby lowering portal pressure.
   a. *Portal-systemic (portacaval) shunt:* portal vein is anastomosed to the inferior vena cava to reduce variceal blood flow and pressure.
   b. *Splenorenal shunt:* shunt is made between the splenic vein and the left renal vein after splenectomy; done when the portal vein cannot be used because of thrombosis or other problems.
   c. *Interposition mesocaval shunt:* superior mesenteric vein is grafted to the inferior vena cava.
5. Transjugular intrahepatic portosystemic shunting: an invasive, but nonsurgical procedure to lower portal pressure.

Nursing Diagnoses
6, 19, 88, 119, 136

Nursing Interventions
Also see *Gastrointestinal or Abdominal Surgery,* page 381.

Monitoring

1. Monitor vital signs, hemodynamic parameters, oxygen saturation, skin condition, and urine output for signs of hypovolemia and shock.
2. Monitor infusion of blood products.
3. If the patient is receiving vasopressin, monitor for possible complications, including hypertension, bradycardia, esophageal ulceration or perforation, aspiration pneumonitis, abdominal cramps, chest pain, worsening variceal

hemorrhage, water intoxication, and cardiac ischemia in patients with preexisting cardiac disease.

4. If the patient is receiving octreotide, monitor for blood glucose abnormality, particularly in patients with diabetes; may also affect thyroid and growth hormone levels.

5. If the patient is receiving esophageal balloon therapy, monitor for possible complications, including esophageal necrosis, perforation, aspiration, asphyxiation, or stricture.

6. Check all GI secretions and feces for occult and frank blood.

Supportive Care

1. Try to prevent straining, gagging, or vomiting; these increase pressure in the portal system and increase risk of further bleeding.

2. Make sure that gastric decompression is maintained.

3. Keep head of bed elevated to avoid gastric regurgitation and aspiration of gastric contents.

4. Inspect nares for skin irritation around nasogastric tube; clean and lubricate frequently to prevent bleeding.

5. Remain with the patient or maintain close observation and place call bell within the patient's reach. Explain treatment and reassure patient and family about positive aspects of patient's condition.

6. Provide alternate means of communication if tubes or other equipment interferes with the patient's ability to talk.

7. Use protective restraints to prevent dislodging of tubes in confused, combative patient.

8. Provide one-to-one care for patient with esophageal balloon tamponage (see *Box E-1*).

EMERGENCY ALERT For patients receiving esophageal balloon therapy, observe for respiratory distress and keep a pair of scissors taped to the head of the bed. The tube should be cut (to deflate both balloons) and removed if the patient experiences signs of acute respiratory distress because of the balloon slipping into the oropharynx.

BOX E-1	Esophageal Balloon Tamponade

The following are nursing responsibilities:

- Maintain gentle traction to balloon when it has been inserted and placement verified with X-ray; a foam cube may be placed at the nares and the tube may be taped to a face guard or football helmet.
- Maintain gastric suction and irrigate the tube hourly.
- Insert a nasogastric tube above the esophageal balloon if a Sengstaken-Blakemore tube is used, or apply suction to the esophageal port if a Minnesota tube is used, to remove secretions or blood that pool above the esophageal balloon that could be aspirated.
- Label each port of the esophageal tube (gastric balloon, gastric aspirate, esophageal balloon with Y connector to manometer, and esophageal aspirate) to prevent accidental deflation or irrigation.
- Maintain esophageal balloon pressure at 25 to 35 mm Hg to tamponade the bleeding but avoid necrosis of tissue; double clamp as necessary.
- Maintain constant vigilance to patient's needs while balloons are inflated.
- Be alert for signs of obstructed airway and esophageal rupture and report immediately: presence of chest pain and change in skin color, pulse, blood pressure, respirations, breath sounds, and level of consciousness.
- Have scissors at bedside for immediate deflation, if necessary.

E

Education and Health Maintenance

1. Discuss signs and symptoms of recurrent bleeding and the need to seek emergency medical treatment if these occur.
2. Instruct the patient to avoid behaviors that increase portal system pressure: straining, gagging, or Valsalva maneuvers.
3. Warn the patient against effects of high-protein diets and alcohol consumption in causing further complications.
4. Encourage the patient to get help for alcoholism through an organization such as Alcoholics Anonymous.

ESOPHAGITIS AND GASTROESOPHAGEAL REFLUX

In *gastroesophageal reflux disease* (GERD), gastric contents flow back into the esophagus due to incompetent lower esophageal sphincter (LES). GERD may result from impaired gastric emptying from gastroparesis or partial gastric outlet obstruction; or motility disorders such as achalasia, scleroderma, or esophageal spasm. *Esophagitis* is acute or chronic inflammation of the esophageal mucosa caused by repeated or prolonged contact with acidic gastric contents, or other irritants. This condition may result from severe GERD; medications such as potassium chloride pills, quinidine, ascorbic acid, and bisphosphonates; infections by viruses (herpes simplex or cytomegalovirus [CMV]) or fungi (*Candida*); ingestion of corrosive alkalis or acids; or motility disorders (achalasia, scleroderma, esophageal spasm).

Complications include stricture; ulceration and possible fistula; aspiration pneumonia; and Barrett's esophagus (presence of columnar epithelium above gastroesophageal junction), which increases risk of adenocarcinoma.

Assessment

1. Signs and symptoms of gastroesophageal reflux:
   a. Heartburn, most commonly occurring 30 to 60 minutes after meals and with reclining positions
   b. Complaints of spontaneous regurgitation of sour or bitter gastric contents into the mouth
   c. Generalized dysphagia may also occur
   d. Patient may also present with substernal chest pain, hoarseness, sore throat, or chronic cough
2. Signs and symptoms of esophagitis:
   a. Patient may report dysphagia (difficulty or discomfort in swallowing) and odynophagia (sharp substernal pain on swallowing), which may limit oral intake
   b. Substernal chest pain may occur
   c. Oral thrush may be visible in patients with *Candida* esophagitis; oral ulcers are common with herpes simplex esophagitis

d. Burns of oral mucosa may be visible with alkali or acid burns
3. Characteristics of pill-induced esophagitis — severe retrosternal chest pain, odynophagia, and dysphagia several hours after swallowing a pill

Diagnostic Evaluation

1. Endoscopy visualizes inflammation, lesions, strictures, or erosions; obtain biopsy specimen; and dilate strictures, if necessary.
2. Barium swallow (esophagography) diagnoses mechanical and motility disorders.
3. Esophageal manometry measures esophageal sphincter tone.
4. Acid perfusion test evaluates response after ingestion of dilute hydrochloric acid and saline. Onset of symptoms is considered positive.
5. Ambulatory 24-hour pH monitoring determines the amount of gastroesophageal acid reflux. A pH monitoring capsule may be placed in the esophagus that transmits information to a receiver. The Bravo pH capsule is contraindicated in patients who have pacemakers, implanted defibrillators, and neurostimulators.

E

Collaborative Management
Therapeutic Interventions

1. Have patient follow a bland antireflux diet: avoid garlic, onion, fatty foods, chocolate, coffee (even decaffeinated), citrus juices, colas, peppermint, and tomato products, all of which reduce LES pressure.
2. Raise head of bed 6 to 8 inches (15 to 20 cm).
3. Remain upright for 3 hours after eating.
4. Avoid overeating.
5. Cease smoking to help increase LES pressure.
6. Reduce or eliminate alcohol intake.
7. Avoid tight-fitting clothes, which increase intra-abdominal pressure.

Pharmacologic Interventions

1. Antacids as needed to treat heartburn; provide symptomatic relief but does not heal esophageal lesions.
2. Histamine-2 receptor antagonists, such as ranitidine, cimetidine, and famotidine, to decrease gastric acid secretions.

 EMERGENCY ALERT With chemical esophagitis — maintain airway, give I.V. fluids and analgesics. Nasogastric lavage and oral antidotes are not used because they risk causing further damage. Surgery may be indicated.

3. Proton pump inhibitor (PPI) such as omeprazole or lansoprazole to suppress gastric acid; helpful in healing esophagitis.

DRUG ALERT Carbamazepine, diazepam, diclofenac, digoxin, iron, ketoconazole, metoprolol, propranolol, and warfarin may interact with some PPIs.

4. In candidal esophagitis, antifungals are given topically, orally, or I.V.
5. Antiviral therapy: in CMV esophagitis, ganciclovir; in herpetic esophagitis, acyclovir.
6. To prevent pill-induced esophagitis, may give sucralfate; drug provides a protective coating against gastric acids.

Surgical Interventions

1. Surgery is indicated for patients who do not respond to other approaches. Consists of Nissen fundoplication; upper portion of stomach is wrapped around the distal esophagus and sutured, creating a tight LES.
2. There are several endoscopic procedures that reduce reflux symptoms by tightening the LES.
3. For strictures, mechanical dilatation may be necessary several times.

Nursing Diagnoses
3, 24

Nursing Interventions
Also see *Gastrointestinal or Abdominal Surgery*, page 381.

Supportive Care and Education

1. Teach the patient all lifestyle modifications, and encourage their use throughout treatment, no matter what medications are prescribed.
2. Teach the patient about prescribed medications and adverse effects.
3. Advise patient that many prescription and over-the-counter drugs may exacerbate symptoms, including anticholinergics (may further impair functioning of LES), antihistamines, antidepressants, antihypertensives, antispasmodics, and some neuroleptics and antiparkinson drugs. These agents decrease saliva production, which may decrease acid clearance from the esophagus.
4. Advise the patient to sit or stand when taking any solid medication (pills, capsules); emphasize the need to follow the drug with at least 3 oz (90 mL) of liquid.
5. Teach the patient and family what foods and activities to avoid.
6. Encourage a weight-reduction program, if the patient is overweight, to decrease intra-abdominal pressure.

EYE INJURIES

Eye injuries refer to damage to the eyes resulting from a wide variety of causes, including blunt injuries (contusion); laceration or perforation; foreign bodies; orbital fracture; hyphema; ruptured globe; and burns. Complications include infection, retinal detachment, increased intraocular pressure (IOP), cataract formation, and disfigurement. Blunt trauma is considered here; refer to *Table E-1*, pages 346 and 347, for other types of eye trauma.

Assessment

1. History of injury
2. Blunt trauma may present as:
   a. Tissue swelling, discoloration
   b. Bleeding into tissues and eye structures
   c. Blurred or double vision
   d. Loss of portion of visual field

TABLE E-1 Other Types of Eye Injuries

TYPE	TREATMENT
Hyphema Presence of blood in anterior chamber in front of the iris, caused by torn ciliary body and iris. Blood may be reabsorbed in 72 hours; if not, secondary glaucoma and loss of vision in affected eye may result.	Keep patient on bed rest; provide eye shield. Monitor blood level in anterior chamber; continued bleeding may require paracentesis of anterior chamber.
Orbital Fracture Fracture and dislocation of walls of the orbit, orbital margins, or both.	Injury may heal on its own if there is no displacement of other structures. Otherwise may require surgery.
Foreign Body May occur on the cornea (25% of all ocular injuries) and conjunctiva. Intraocular particles may penetrate sclera, cornea, or globe.	Requires immediate medical attention. Removal by irrigation, cotton-tipped applicator, magnet, or possibly surgery.
Laceration, Perforation Cutting or penetration of tissue may occur. May affect any part of eye—eyelid, conjunctiva, cornea, sclera, globe.	Requires immediate medical attention. Topical or systemic antibiotics may be given. Surgical repair depends on severity of injury.
Ruptured Globe Concussive injury to globe with tearing of ocular contents (usually the sclera). May be caused by sharp penetrating object or high-velocity projectile.	Requires immediate medical attention. Antibiotics or steroids may be given. Surgery includes vitrectomy, scleral buckle, enucleation.

Other Types of Eye Injuries (continued)

TYPE	TREATMENT
Burns Caused by chemicals such as lye, cleaning fluids, acid; thermal burns from fire or intense heat; ultraviolet burns from excessive sunlight, sunlamp, or welding.	Requires immediate medical attention. Determine causative agent; irrigate affected area until pH is 7.0 (neutral). Administer antibiotics and protective patch. Leave blisters intact. Severe scarring may require keratoplasty.
Corneal Abrasion Loss of epithelial layers of cornea; may result from overwear of contact lenses. Corneal ulcer (keratitis) is inflammation and loss of entire depth of cornea.	Topical antibiotics and patching; abrasion usually heals in 24 to 48 hours; ulcer may require frequent around-the-clock drops or I.V. antibiotics and corticosteroids.

E

Diagnostic Evaluation
1. Visual acuity tests detect altered vision.
2. Ophthalmoscopy detects changes in cornea, vitreous, choroid, and retina.
3. Tonometry evaluates IOP.

Collaborative Management
Therapeutic Interventions
1. Measures to reduce tissue swelling.
2. Analgesics as needed.
3. Surgery may be indicated to repair retinal detachment or other eye or orbital structures.

Nursing Diagnoses
3, 24, 35, 135

Nursing Interventions

Also see *Ocular Surgery*, page 677.

Supportive Care and Education

1. Apply cool compresses to relieve discomfort and swelling.
2. Provide eye patch and instill medications, as ordered.
3. Maintain safe environment if visual acuity is affected.
4. Be alert for and report signs of complications, including increased swelling or pain, worsening visual acuity, development of fever or drainage, and neurologic deterioration.
5. Encourage follow-up ophthalmologic examinations.

F

FIBROMYALGIA

Fibromyalgia is a syndrome characterized by fatigue, diffuse muscle pain and stiffness, sleep disturbance, and the presence of tender points on physical examination. There is no known etiology, but theories have suggested a variety of possible pathophysiologic mechanisms, such as neural-hormonal disturbance, antecedent physical trauma, viral infection, immune dysregulation, psychiatric disturbances, and heightened sensitivity to pain. Complications include disability and inability to maintain functional roles.

Assessment

1. Fatigue, poor or nonrestorative sleep
2. Generalized muscle aches and stiffness
3. Irritable bowel syndrome
4. Tension headaches
5. Paresthesias, sensation of swollen hands
6. Presence of pain in 11 of 18 defined tender point sites
   a. Anterior: low cervical, second rib, lateral epicondyle, knee
   b. Posterior: occiput, trapezius, supraspinatus, gluteal, greater trochanter
7. Complete history and physical examination to rule out other disorders

Diagnostic Evaluation

1. Complete blood count, blood chemistries, erythrocyte sedimentation rate, thyroid-stimulating hormone, and arthritis panel rule out other disorders.
2. X-rays and imaging studies are all normal.

Collaborative Management
Therapeutic Interventions

1. Cardiovascular fitness training

2. Electromyogram biofeedback
3. Cognitive behavioral therapy
4. Hypnotherapy
5. Electrical stimulation or acupuncture

Pharmacologic Interventions
1. Nonsteroidal anti-inflammatory drugs, acetaminophen, or tramadol to relieve pain.
2. Antidepressants to help control chronic pain and depression.
3. Muscle relaxants, such as cyclobenzaprine, to relieve muscle tension and spasm.
4. Sleep agents and antianxiety agents may be considered.

Nursing Diagnoses
13, 34, 84

Nursing Interventions
Monitoring
1. Monitor pain level and effectiveness of treatment plan.
2. Assess functional ability.

Supportive Care
1. Encourage regular use of analgesics and antidepressants as directed.
2. Encourage regular exercise routine, including stretching, aerobic activity, and muscle-strengthening exercises.
3. Suggest referrals to physical therapist or pain specialists for additional pain control modalities as needed.
4. Suggest regular nighttime ritual to promote sleep.
5. Discourage staying up late and erratic sleep habits.
6. Encourage relaxation periods or short nap during day as needed for fatigue.
7. Advise limiting caffeine intake during day and especially after 4 p.m.
8. Encourage patient to look at fibromyalgia as a chronic condition that can be controlled.
9. Help patient plan schedule and pace activities to accomplish routine activities.

Education and Health Maintenance

1. Teach patient and family that fibromyalgia is a real disorder that causes pain and fatigue despite the normal test results and lack of "ill appearance."
2. Explain proper use of analgesics and potential adverse effects.
3. Encourage regular activity as much as possible while avoiding physical and emotional stress.
4. Advise patient to discuss all types of alternative and complimentary therapy with health care provider.
5. Encourage regular follow-up with primary care provider, rheumatologist, and physical therapist as indicated.
6. For additional help and information, refer to The Arthritis Foundation, *www.arthritis.org*.

FLUID AND ELECTROLYTE IMBALANCE

Approximately 60% of an adult's and 75% of an infant's body weight is made up of fluid (water and electrolytes). Fluid is contained in the intracellular space and extracellular space. Intracellular fluid (ICF) is largely distributed to skeletal muscle cells, but is contained inside all cells. Extracellular fluid (ECF) is contained in the intravascular space, interstitial space (fluid outside of cells and blood vessels such as lymph), and the transcellular spaces (cerebrospinal, synovial, intraocular, pleural, and other fluids). Fluid shifts between the intracellular and extracellular compartments to maintain equilibrium. Loss of fluid from the body or abnormal shift of fluid into the interstitial space (called third spacing) may disrupt the equilibrium.

Electrolytes are positively (cations) and negatively (anions) charged particles, which make up body fluids, but may exist in different concentrations in the ICF and ECF. The major cations are sodium, potassium, calcium, and magnesium. The major anions are chloride, bicarbonate, and phosphorus. Electrolytes are measured in milliequivalents per liter, a measure of electrical activity as compared to hydrogen, rather than weight. Sodium is normally present in high concentration in the ECF, and potassium is present in high concentration in the ICF. This equilibrium is maintained through high-energy

F

pumps in the cell membranes. Fluid movement between compartments takes place because of opposing forces: hydrostatic pressure (outward pushing pressure exerted by fluid on the blood vessel walls) and osmotic pressure (inward pulling pressure exerted by plasma proteins).

Common fluid and electrolyte imbalances are fluid volume deficit (hypovolemia), fluid volume excess (hypervolemia), sodium deficit (hyponatremia), sodium excess (hypernatremia), potassium deficit (hypokalemia), and potassium excess (hyperkalemia). Bicarbonate imbalances occur as it attempts to buffer major acid-base (pH) changes in the ECF. Bicarbonate deficit (acidosis) and bicarbonate excess (alkalosis) are reflected by arterial blood gas (ABG) measurements as well as serum carbon dioxide (CO_2; a potential acid) and anion gap measurements.

Underlying causes of fluid and electrolyte imbalances include vomiting, nasogastric suction, diarrhea, GI obstruction, ascites, burns, wounds, fever, diaphoresis, tachypnea, polyuria, renal failure, heart failure, excessive free water intake, and starvation (see *Table F-1*).

GERONTOLOGIC ALERT Elderly people are at risk for fluid and electrolyte imbalances because of several physiologic changes of aging — decreased total body fluid, reduced renal function, and decreased sensitivity of hormonal regulatory responses.

(Also see related entries, such as *Hypoparathyroidism*, *Renal Failure*, *Diarrhea in Children*, and *Heat Exhaustion*.)

Assessment
See *Table F-2*, pages 355 and 356 for signs and symptoms of common fluid and electrolyte imbalances.

GERONTOLOGIC ALERT Gradual, subtle signs of fluid and electrolyte imbalance may be absent in elderly patients. The first signs may be dramatic changes in vital signs and level of consciousness.

Diagnostic Evaluation
1. Serum osmolality will be increased with hypovolemia; decreased with hypervolemia.
2. Hemoglobin and hematocrit will be increased with hypovolemia; decreased with hypervolemia.

TABLE F-1	Causes of Fluid and Electrolyte Imbalances

IMBALANCE	CAUSE
Hypovolemia	Inadequate water intake; loss through vomiting, diarrhea, GI obstruction, fever or sweating, hemorrhage, burns; third-space fluid shifting
Hypervolemia	Excessive fluid administration; compensatory mechanism failure through renal failure, heart failure; hyperaldosteronism
Hyponatremia	Use of diuretics; loss of GI fluids; renal disease; adrenal insufficiency; gain of excess water through hypotonic I.V. infusions and parenteral tube feedings, water abuse, use of oxytocin, syndrome of inappropriate antidiuretic hormone
Hypernatremia	Water deprivation; hypertonic tube feedings or I.V. infusions; diabetes insipidus; heat stroke; watery diarrhea; excessive corticosteroid, sodium bicarbonate, or sodium chloride administration
Hypokalemia	Vomiting, diarrhea, gastric suction; prolonged corticosteroid or ACTH therapy; diuretic therapy; diabetic ketoacidosis (DKA); shift of potassium into cells as in the healing phase of burns, recovery from DKA
Hyperkalemia	Excessive potassium-containing solutions (stored blood, I.V. fluids, salt substitutes, oral potassium replacement); release from cells in burns and crush injury; severe kidney disease; adrenal insufficiency
Bicarbonate deficit (primary)	Diarrhea in infants, DKA, starvation, severe infections, shock, anoxia

(continued)

F

Causes of Fluid and Electrolyte Imbalances
(continued)

IMBALANCE	CAUSE
Bicarbonate excess (primary)	Loss of chloride through vomiting, gastric suction, excessive use of diuretics; excessive ingestion of alkali (milk, antacids)
Hypocalcemia	Hypoparathyroidism, malabsorption, pancreatitis, massive transfusions, renal failure
Hypercalcemia	Hyperparathyroidism, malignancy, immobilization, digoxin toxicity
Hypomagnesemia	Alcoholism, hypoparathyroidism, hyperaldosteronism, renal failure, malabsorption, DKA, refeeding after starvation
Hypermagnesemia	Renal failure, adrenal insufficiency, excess I.V. magnesium administration

3. Blood urea nitrogen and creatinine will be increased with hypovolemia, and with electrolyte imbalances caused by renal failure.
4. Urine osmolality and specific gravity will be increased with hypovolemia and hypernatremia; decreased with hypervolemia and hyponatremia.
5. Serum electrolytes (chemistry values) elevated or decreased as indicated; chloride is directly related to sodium, phosphorus is inversely related to calcium; note that laboratory values reflect electrolyte concentrations in the ECF only.
6. Electrocardiogram (ECG) changes:
   a. Hypokalemia—flattened T waves, prominent U waves, ST depression, prolonged PR interval
   b. Hyperkalemia—tall, tented T waves, widened QRS, shortened QT, ventricular arrhythmias
   c. Hypocalcemia—prolonged QT interval

TABLE F-2	Signs and Symptoms of Fluid and Electrolyte Imbalance
IMBALANCE	**SIGNS AND SYMPTOMS**
Hypovolemia	Oliguria, concentrated urine, weight loss, dry skin and mucous membranes, lassitude, sunken fontanelles in infants, lack of tear formation, furrowed tongue, flattened neck veins, weak and rapid pulse, increased pulse pressure, light-headedness, orthostatic hypotension, decreased central venous pressure (CVP)
Hypervolemia	Weight gain, distended neck veins, dyspnea, edema, rales, bounding pulse, increased CVP
Hyponatremia	Headache, abdominal cramps, apprehension, confusion, fingerprinting on sternum, increased lacrimation and salivation seen in children, oliguria, hypotension, muscle twitching, seizures
Hypernatremia	Thirst, oliguria, weakness, dry and sticky mucous membranes, flushed skin, hypotension, tachycardia, hallucinations
Hypokalemia	Weakness, lethargy, anorexia, abdominal distention, decreased bowel sounds, muscle tenderness
Hyperkalemia	Confusion, nausea, diarrhea, irritability, paresthesias, abdominal cramps, cardiac arrhythmias and arrest
Bicarbonate deficit	Increasing rate of respiration to Kussmaul respirations (deep, rapid); weakness; flushed, warm skin; disorientation to stupor to coma
Bicarbonate excess	Depressed respirations, paresthesias, increased muscle tone, hyperactive reflexes, tetany

(continued)

F

Signs and Symptoms of Fluid and Electrolyte Imbalance *(continued)*

IMBALANCE	SIGNS AND SYMPTOMS
Hypocalcemia	Numbness and tingling of hands, feet and circumoral region; Trousseau's and Chvostek's signs; corpopedal spasm; seizures; hyperactive reflexes; irritability; bronchospasm
Hypercalcemia	Muscle weakness, constipation, anorexia, nausea and vomiting, polyuria, hypoactive reflexes, lethargy, bradycardia
Hypomagnesemia	Neuromuscular irritability, Chvostek's signs, insomnia, mood changes, anorexia, vomiting
Hypermagnesemia	Flushing, hypotension, drowsiness, hypoactive reflexes, depressed respirations, cardiac arrest, coma

    d. Hypercalcemia — shortened QT interval, heart block
    e. Hypermagnesemia — prolonged PR interval and QRS

Collaborative Management

Therapeutic and Pharmacologic Interventions

1. Correction of underlying cause or reduction of its effect with such treatments as antiemetics, antidiarrheals, and skin grafting or wound coverage for burns.
2. Increased oral fluids, particularly rehydrating preparations containing electrolytes, when at increased risk for loss.
3. I.V. fluid replacement when necessary. Initial infusion replaces ECF to prevent or treat shock; subsequent infusion over 8 to 12 hours replenishes ICF.
    a. Isotonic solutions (lactated Ringer's and 0.9 sodium chloride) are preferred in hypovolemia when the patient is hypotensive.

    b. Hypotonic solutions (0.45 sodium chloride) are initi-
ated when the patient becomes normotensive to promote renal excretion of metabolic wastes.

    c. Dextrose 5% in water may be used for hypernatremia
or dehydration, but is not used alone in hypovolemia
because it dilutes electrolytes.

    d. A fluid challenge may be done before giving large vol-
umes of fluid if the patient is oliguric, to rule out acute
tubular necrosis; 3 to 7 oz (90 to 207 mL) is infused
over 15 minutes to see if urine output will increase; if
it does, renal function is preserved and fluids can be
given.

4. Replacement of electrolytes as needed, either orally or
I.V.

    a. Potassium chloride 10 to 80 mEq/L I.V. fluid; pediatric
dose 3 mEq/kg/day

    b. Oral potassium in the range of 16 to 24 mEq/day for
prevention of hypokalemia, 40 to 100 mEq/day for treatment of hypokalemia

    c. Sodium easily replaced through dietary sources if oral
intake possible

    d. Calcium replacement through diet, oral preparations,
and I.V. (See *Hypoparathyroidism*, page 523.)

    e. Magnesium replacement through diet, oral salts, par-
enterally, or I.V. (cautiously)

5. Diuretic therapy to treat hypervolemia; may cause hypokalemia and hyponatremia.

6. Diet therapy usually as prevention of imbalance or as adjunct therapy.

    a. Low-sodium diet with hypervolemia, hypernatremia,
and third spacing syndromes

    b. Increased potassium diet with hypokalemia, use of di-
uretics

    c. Low-potassium and low-phosphorus diet with renal fail-
ure

7. Hyperkalemia with potassium greater than 7 and ECG
changes should be treated emergently.

    a. I.V. calcium gluconate will antagonize the effects of
potassium on the heart for about 30 minutes.

F

    b. I.V. sodium bicarbonate or regular insulin along with dextrose will temporarily shift potassium into cells.

    c. Cation exchange resins are given orally or by enema to remove potassium.

8. Peritoneal or hemodialysis may be necessary in severe cases of hyperkalemia and other imbalances complicated by renal failure.

Nursing Diagnoses
19, 23, 35, 42, 92, 108, 136

Nursing Interventions
Monitoring

1. Monitor intake and output, including GI drainage, every 8 hours, or hourly if signs of shock.
2. Weigh daily, realizing that 2.2 lb (1 kg) body weight loss or gain indicates 1 L fluid deficit or excess.
3. Monitor vital signs, central venous pressure, and other hemodynamic parameters continuously every 4 to 8 hours based on condition.
4. Monitor ECG for arrhythmias and changes indicative of electrolyte imbalance.
5. Monitor serial chemistry, urine specific gravity, and ABG as indicated to guide treatment.
6. Monitor for dyspnea, adventitious breath sounds, and dependent edema if at risk for hypervolemia.
7. Monitor level of consciousness for subtle changes, which may indicate electrolyte imbalances secondary to I.V. fluid or medication therapy.

Supportive Care

PEDIATRIC ALERT Infants are at highest risk for fluid and electrolyte imbalance due to their greater proportion of total body fluid, their greater water turnover rate, their high surface area, immaturity of the kidneys, and their inability to independently respond to fluid losses.

1. Encourage the patient with edema to rest with legs elevated higher than heart, or turn and reposition a bed-

bound patient frequently to reduce venous pooling and improve circulation and reabsorption of fluid.

2. When administering enteral feedings with high osmolarity, supplement with free water as directed to prevent hypernatremia.

3. Use caution when administering I.V. potassium replacement.

   a. Dilute in dextrose solutions and do not exceed 10 mEq/hour infusion in routine situations; in emergency situations, higher concentrations may be given at faster rates through a central venous access.

   b. Stop potassium infusion if less than 20 mL/hour urine output for 2 consecutive hours; hyperkalemia may result when kidney excretion is impaired.

4. Administer oral potassium after meals or with full glass of water to reduce GI upset.

5. Be alert for changes in the patient's diuretic prescription and electrolyte profile that may necessitate change in potassium dosage.

DRUG ALERT Hypokalemia results more quickly with loop diuretic therapy, such as furosemide, than with thiazide diuretics. Hyperkalemia may result from potassium supplementation in patients taking potassium-sparing diuretics such as spironolactone.

6. For serious hyperkalemia, give cleansing enema and then administer cation exchange resin by way of a large, soft, rubber rectal tube inserted 8 inches (20 cm). Clamp the tube for retention of at least 30 to 60 minutes, then irrigate the colon with tap water and let drain. Repeat as directed based on ECG and serial serum electrolyte levels.

Education and Health Maintenance

1. Advise patient to bring all medications to follow-up appointments and to discuss all over-the-counter drugs with his or her health care provider because many drugs may interfere with fluid and electrolyte balance, including antacids, calcium supplements, diuretics, and some analgesics.

2. Advise patient to have a reasonable intake of fluid (primarily free water), making adjustments for losses through increased sweating, illness, and other losses.
3. Advise patient to read labels to determine sodium content of foods and to use salt substitutes carefully because they may contain a large amount of potassium.
4. Teach the patient to avoid foods high in potassium if at risk for hyperkalemia, including fruits (especially raisins, bananas, apricots, oranges), vegetables (especially tomatoes), legumes, whole grains, milk, and meat.

FRACTURE

A *fracture* is a break in the continuity of bone. A fracture occurs when the stress placed on a bone is greater than the bone can absorb. The stress may be mechanical (trauma) or related to a disease process (pathologic). Muscles, blood vessels, nerves, tendons, joints, and body organs may be injured when fracture occurs. In elderly people, osteoporosis is a major fracture risk, particularly for hip and vertebral compression fractures. In children, fracture may cause disturbance to the epiphysis (growth plate); identification and proper management are imperative to prevent cessation or disruption in growth.

A fracture may be complete (involving the entire cross-section of the bone), incomplete, closed (simple), open (compound, graded by the amount of soft tissue injury accompanying fracture), or plastic deformation (bending of bone with microscopic fracture in children), or pathologic (through an area of diseased bone). In addition, fractures are described as greenstick (one side of the bone is broken and the other side is bent), buckle (causing a bulge), transverse (straight across), oblique (at an angle), spiral, epiphyseal (through the growth plate), comminuted (splintered), depressed (fragment driven inward), compression (bones such as vertebrae collapse on themselves), avulsion (portion of bone pulled off with a ligament or tendon), or impacted (portion of bone wedged into another).

Complications of fractures include problems associated with immobility (muscle atrophy, joint contracture, pressure sores), growth problems (in children), infection, shock, venous stasis and thromboembolism, pulmonary emboli and fat emboli, and bone union problems.

PEDIATRIC ALERT Up to age 2, most fractures are the result of injury by another person. Suspect child abuse with fractures in neonates and infants.

Assessment

1. Pain — usually progressive, localized, deep throbbing, persistent, unrelieved by immobilization and medications; increased on passive stretch, movement
2. Swelling, tenderness, deformity, and ecchymosis
3. Crepitus (grating sensation) and loss of function
4. Signs of shock with fractures causing overt hemorrhage through open wound or with femoral fracture or pelvic fracture

EMERGENCY ALERT Change in behavior or cerebral functioning may be an early indicator of cerebral anoxia from shock or pulmonary or fat emboli.

Diagnostic Evaluation

1. X-ray and other imaging studies, such as bone scan, determine integrity of bone.
2. Complete blood count, serum electrolytes if blood loss and extensive muscle damage have occurred; may show decreased hemoglobin and hematocrit.
3. Arthroscopy detects joint involvement.
4. Angiography if associated with blood vessel injury.
5. Nerve conduction and electromyograms detect nerve injury.

Collaborative Management

See *Table F-3*, pages 362 to 365.

Therapeutic Interventions

1. Emergency management includes splinting fracture above and below site of injury, applying cold, and elevating limb to reduce edema and pain.

(Text continues on page 366.)

TABLE F-3	Fractures of Specific Sites

SITE AND MECHANISM	NURSING INTERVENTIONS
Clavicle • Fall on shoulder	1. Maintain immobilization with clavicular strap, figure 8 bandage, or sling. 2. Pad axilla to prevent nerve damage from pressure of immobilizer. 3. Teach shoulder exercises through full range of motion as prescribed, to prevent frozen shoulder.
Proximal Humerus • Fall on outstretched arm • Osteoporosis is predisposing factor	1. Maintain sling and swathe or Belpeaw bandage for comfort. 2. Place a soft pad under the axilla to prevent skin maceration. 3. Encourage shoulder range-of-motion exercises after specified period of immobilization to prevent frozen shoulder.
Shaft of Humerus • Direct fall, blow to arm, or auto injury • Twisting injury in infants and toddlers (may be due to child abuse) • Damage to radial nerve may occur	1. Maintain sling and swathe, splint or hanging cast as indicated. 2. Hanging cast must remain unsupported to maintain traction. Patient should sleep in upright position to maintain 24-hour traction. 3. Encourage exercise of fingers immediately after application of cast. 4. Teach pendulum exercises of arm as directed to prevent frozen shoulder.
Elbow and Forearm • Fall on elbow, outstretched hand, or direct blow (sideswipe injury) • Common in children	1. Maintain patency of drainage tube, if used to decrease hematoma formation and swelling. 2. If radial pulse weakens or disappears, report immediately to prevent irreversible ischemia. 3. Elevate arm to control edema. 4. Encourage finger and shoulder exercises.

Fractures of Specific Sites *(continued)*

SITE AND MECHANISM	NURSING INTERVENTIONS

Wrist
- Colles' fracture is common (½ to 1 inch [1.3 to 2.5 cm] above the wrist with dorsal displacement of lower fragment)
- Caused by fall on outstretched palm
- Often associated with osteoporosis

1. Elevate arm above level of heart for 48 hours after reduction to promote venous and lymphatic return and reduce swelling.
2. Watch for swelling of fingers and check for constricting bandages or cast.
3. Teach finger exercises to reduce swelling and stiffness.

Hand
- Caused by numerous injuries

1. Provide aggressive care and encouragement with rehabilitation plan to regain maximal hand function.

Hip (Proximal Femur)
- Occur frequently in older adults, women with osteoporosis, and with falls

1. Identify hip fracture by shortening and external rotation of affected leg.
2. Maintain Buck's traction until surgery.
3. Provide constant monitoring and nursing care to reduce the risk of complications (eg, pneumonia, thrombophlebitis, fat emboli, dislocation of prosthesis, infection, and pressure sores).
4. Administer aspirin, warfarin, or low-dose subcutaneous heparin as ordered.
5. Following surgery, keep affected leg in abduction and neutral rotation.
6. Teach quadriceps setting exercises to prevent muscle atrophy of affected leg.

F

(continued)

Fractures of Specific Sites *(continued)*

SITE AND MECHANISM	NURSING INTERVENTIONS
Femoral Shaft • Falls from height, motor vehicle accidents with high impact	1. Marked concealed blood loss may occur; watch for signs of shock initially and anemia later. 2. Examine skin under the ring of the Thomas splint, if used for traction, for signs of pressure. 3. Provide nursing care to prevent complications (see above) while in traction or following surgery.
Knee • Direct blow to knee area; involve distal shaft of femur, articular surfaces, or patella	1. Elevate extremity by raising foot gatch of bed. 2. Evaluate for effusion—report and loosen pressure dressing if pain is severe; prepare for joint aspiration. 3. Teach quadriceps setting exercises and limited weight bearing as directed.
Tibia and Fibula/Ankle • Generally result from forceful twisting of ankle; often associated with ligament disruption • Also high incidence of open fractures of tibial shaft because tibia lies superficially beneath the skin • Tibial fractures in children often involve growth plate	1. Elevate lower leg to control edema. 2. Avoid dependent position of extremity for prolonged periods. 3. Prepare patient for long immobilization period, because union is slow (12 to 16 weeks, longer for open and comminuted fractures). 4. Prepare patient for extensive physical therapy for stiff ankle joint after immobilization.

Fractures of Specific Sites *(continued)*

SITE AND MECHANISM	NURSING INTERVENTIONS

Foot
- Metatarsal fracture caused by crush injuries of foot

1. Encourage partial weight bearing as allowed.
2. Elevate foot to control edema.

Thoracic and Lumbar Spine
- Trauma from falls, contact sports, or motor vehicle accidents or excessive loading may cause fracture of vertebral body, lamina, spinous and transverse processes
- Usually stable compression fractures

1. Treatment is usually bed rest on firm mattress followed by ambulation with back-strengthening exercises. Use log roll technique to change positions.
2. Monitor bowel and bladder dysfunction.
3. Teach proper body mechanics and back-preservation techniques.
4. Encourage weight reduction.
5. Teach patient with osteoporosis the importance of safety measures to avoid falls.

F

Pelvis
- Sacrum, ilium, pubic, ischium, coccyx fractures may occur from motor vehicle accidents, crush injuries, and falls
- Most are stable fractures that do not involve the pelvic ring and have minimal displacement

1. Monitor for shock and internal injuries and support vital functions as indicated.
2. Do not attempt to insert urethral catheter until patency of urethra is known; observe urine output for blood, indicating genitourinary injury.
3. Maintain bed rest as directed, then allow progressive weight bearing and light activity as tolerated.

2. Control bleeding and provide fluid replacement to prevent shock, if necessary.
3. Traction used for fractures of long bones.
   a. Skin traction — force applied to the skin using foam rubber, tapes, and so forth
   b. Skeletal traction — force applied to the bony skeleton directly, using wires, pins, or tongs placed into or through the bone
4. External fixation to stabilize complex and open fracture with use of a metal frame and pin system.

Pharmacologic Interventions

1. Local anesthetic, opioid analgesic, muscle relaxant, or sedative is given to assist the patient during closed reduction procedure.
2. Closed reduction may also be done with general anesthesia.
3. Analgesics are given as directed to control pain postoperatively.

Surgical Interventions

1. Reduction to restore bone continuity
   a. Closed reduction: bony fragments are brought into apposition (ends in contact) by manipulation and manual traction — restores alignment. Cast or splint is applied to immobilize extremity and maintain reduction.
   b. Open reduction with internal fixation: bone fragments are directly visualized. Internal fixation devices are used to hold bone fragments in position until solid bone healing occurs; they may be removed when bone is healed. After wound closure, splints or casts may be used for additional stabilization and support.
2. Endoprosthetic replacement
   a. Replacement of a fracture fragment with an implanted metal device
   b. Used when fracture disrupts nutrition of the bone or treatment of choice is bony replacement

Nursing Diagnoses
3, 8, 36, 62, 96, 123, 127, 135, 136, 141

Nursing Interventions
Also see *Orthopedic Surgery*, page 680.

Monitoring

1. Monitor for hemorrhage and shock in patients with severe fractures.
   a. Check vital signs as frequently as clinical condition indicates, observing for hypotension, elevated pulse, cold clammy skin, restlessness, and pallor.
   b. Watch for evidence of hemorrhage on dressings or in drainage containers.
2. Monitor for sudden or progressive changes in respiratory status that may indicate pulmonary embolus.
3. Monitor neurovascular status for compression of nerve, diminished circulation, or development of compartment syndrome.

> **EMERGENCY ALERT** Monitoring the neurovascular integrity of the injured extremity is essential. Development of compartment syndrome (palpable tightness of muscle compartment and elevated measured tissue pressure causing anoxia) leads to permanent loss of function in 6 to 8 hours. This condition must be identified and managed promptly.

4. Monitor for development of thrombophlebitis with pain and tenderness in calf, increased size, and warmth of calf.
5. Monitor for development of infection.

Supportive Care

1. Administer fluids and blood products as directed to maintain circulating volume in hemorrhage and shock.
2. Position the patient to enhance respiratory effort.
3. Encourage coughing and deep breathing to promote lung expansion and diminish pooling of pulmonary secretions.
4. Administer oxygen as directed.
5. Reduce swelling.

    a. Elevate injured extremity (unless compartment syndrome is suspected; may contribute to vascular compromise).

    b. Apply cold to injury if prescribed.

6. Assist with casting as directed.

    a. Apply adequate padding over extremity before casting material applied; pad edges of cast well.

    b. If plaster is applied, be aware that drying may take 24 to 48 hours, so minimize handling and use palms, not fingertips, to handle the cast.

    c. Warn patient that the plaster cast will generate heat as it hardens.

    d. Follow and teach cast care instructions as in *Box F-1*.

7. Relieve pressure caused by immobilizing device as prescribed (such as bivalving cast, rewrapping elastic bandage, or splinting device).

8. Relieve pressure on skin to prevent development of pressure ulcer; employ frequent repositioning, skin care, special mattresses.

9. Prevent development of thromboembolism.

    a. Encourage active and passive ankle exercises.

BOX F-1   Cast Care

- Keep the casted part elevated on a pillow for the first few days to decrease swelling.
- Avoid touching the cast until it is fully dry to avoid denting it (several hours for fiberglass, 24 to 48 hours for plaster); cast will release heat as it hardens.
- Move the body part below the cast at least every 4 hours for the first 24 hours to promote circulation.
- Do not put anything inside the cast; if itching occurs, blow cool air into it with a hair dryer.
- Keep the cast dry; securely cover with plastic bag to shower; do not swim or submerge in water.
- Try to remain active and develop a plan to carry out usual activities, but do not participate in any activities that increase risk for injury to the casted or other extremities.
- Report any blueness, coldness, numbness, or loss of movement of the body part.

    b. Use elastic stockings and sequential compression devices as prescribed.

    c. Elevate legs to prevent stasis, avoiding pressure on blood vessels.

    d. Encourage mobility; change position frequently; encourage ambulation.

    e. Administer anticoagulants as directed.

GERONTOLOGIC ALERT Older adults with fractures, trauma, immobility, obesity, or history of thrombophlebitis are at high risk for developing thromboembolism.

10. Evaluate the patient for proper body alignment and pressure from equipment (casts, traction, splints, appliances) that may cause pain.

11. Encourage nonpharmacologic measures for pain reduction, such as cutaneous stimulation, distraction, guided imagery, transcutaneous electrical nerve stimulation, and biofeedback.

12. Administer prescribed medications as indicated. Encourage use of less potent drugs as severity of discomfort decreases.

13. Clean, debride, and irrigate open fracture wound as prescribed as soon as possible, to minimize risk of infection. Use sterile technique during dressing changes.

14. Administer antibiotic therapy as directed.

15. Assist with activities of daily living as needed.

16. Teach the family ways to assist the patient while promoting independence in self-care.

17. Perform active and passive exercises to all nonimmobilized joints.

18. Encourage patient participation in frequent position changes, maintaining supports to fracture during position changes.

19. Minimize prolonged periods of physical inactivity, encouraging ambulation when prescribed.

20. Teach and encourage isometric exercises to diminish muscle atrophy and prevent development of disuse syndrome.

21. Make sure that traction lines and weights are hanging freely and in proper position.

F

22. Help the patient move through phases of posttraumatic stress (outcry, denial, intrusiveness, working through, completion).
23. Encourage the patient to participate in decision making to reestablish control and overcome feelings of helplessness.
24. Teach relaxation techniques to decrease anxiety.
25. Refer the patient to support group or psychotherapy as needed.

Education and Health Maintenance

1. Explain basis for fracture treatment and need for patient participation in therapeutic regimen.
2. Promote adjustment of usual lifestyle and responsibilities to accommodate limitations imposed by fracture.
3. Instruct the patient to actively exercise joints above and below the immobilized fracture at frequent intervals.
   a. Isometric exercises of muscles covered by cast — start exercise as soon as possible after cast application.
   b. Increase isometric exercises as fracture stabilizes.

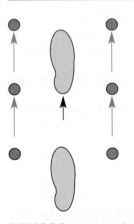

4. Step on the good leg again as you move the crutches forward.

3. Swing the good leg forward (be careful not to go too far).

2. Move both crutches forward about the length of one step.

1. Stand with both crutches slightly forward and apart.

FIGURE F-1 Crutch Walking (nonweight-bearing).

4. After removal of immobilizing device, have the patient start active exercises and continue with isometric exercises.
5. Instruct the patient on exercises to strengthen upper extremity muscles if crutch walking is planned.
6. Instruct the patient in methods of safe ambulation — walker, crutches, cane. (See *Figure F-1*.)
7. Emphasize instructions concerning amount of weight bearing that will be permitted on fractured extremity.
8. Discuss prevention of recurrent fractures; review safety considerations, avoidance of fatigue, proper footwear.
9. Encourage follow-up medical supervision to monitor for bone union problems, especially in children and the elderly.
10. Teach the patient to recognize and report symptoms needing attention, such as numbness, decreased function, increased pain, or elevated temperature.
11. Encourage the patient to follow an adequate balanced diet to promote bone and soft tissue healing.

F

G

GALLBLADDER SURGERY

See *Cholecystectomy*.

GALLSTONES

See *Cholelithiasis, Cholecystitis, Choledocholithiasis*.

GASTRIC CANCER

See *Cancer, Gastric*.

GASTROESOPHAGEAL REFLUX

See *Esophagitis and Gastroesophageal Reflux*.

GASTROESOPHAGEAL REFLUX IN CHILDREN

Gastroesophageal reflux (GER) is a malfunction of the distal end of the esophagus, which acts as an antireflux barrier. This barrier is controlled primarily by pressure at the lower esophageal sphincter (LES). Failure of this barrier allows acidic stomach or duodenal contents to flow back up into the esophagus. Not all infants with GER are symptomatic; however, it becomes a problem when feeding difficulty, poor weight gain, and respiratory problems become apparent. The cause of GER is commonly unknown, but may be due to immaturity, delayed neuromuscular development obstruction, or increased abdominal pressure.

Recurrent GER may lead to complications such as chronic esophagitis, recurrent pulmonary disease, aspiration pneumonia, failure to thrive, anemia, apnea, and apparent life-threatening event.

Assessment

1. In an infant:
   a. Unexplained vomiting occurs immediately after feeding, especially when placed in supine position

  b. Usually regurgitation rather than projectile vomiting
  c. Onset usually after age 2 months
  d. Weight loss or failure to gain weight; rumination
  e. Dehydration
  f. Recurrent pulmonary symptoms
  g. Irritability, excessive crying
  h. Sleep disturbances
  i. Arching, stiffening

EMERGENCY ALERT Referral to specialist is indicated for infants younger than age 2 months with continuous regurgitation of feedings.

  2. In an older child:
  a. Substernal burning, upper abdominal discomfort, pressure or "squeezing" feeling
  b. Persistent pulmonary problems, chronic cough, nocturnal asthma (particularly after a large meal)
  c. Dysphagia and odynophagia (painful swallowing)
  d. Anemia
  e. Hematemesis or melena (blood in stools)

Diagnostic Evaluation

  1. History of infant's or child's feeding habits and weight gain.
  2. Upper GI series rule out anatomic abnormality.
  3. Esophageal pH monitoring documents frequency and duration of reflux.
  4. Technetium scintigraphy (milk scan) documents reflux and defines gastric emptying and aspiration.
  5. Endoscopy with biopsy determines structural or functional lesions of esophagus, stomach, or duodenum.
  6. Swallow study and evaluation by speech therapist detects oral motor dysfunction.

Collaborative Management
Therapeutic Interventions

  1. Positional therapy: although studies have shown that infants have less reflux while prone, the risk of sudden infant death syndrome (SIDS) usually outweighs the benefits of prone positioning for sleep.

a. Can place infant at 30 degrees elevation (with straight plane body alignment); avoid swing, bouncers, and infant seats, which allow the infant to slump, causing increased intra-abdominal pressure.

b. Can place infant in a prone position while awake and is being observed.

c. Older children can be positioned with head elevated and lying on the left side; avoid lying down for several hours after large meals.

EMERGENCY ALERT Placing an infant in the prone position to nap with its head elevated is no longer recommended because of the association with SIDS.

2. Feeding

a. Infant — continue breast-feeding or may thicken feedings, using dry rice cereal or commercial thickening agent to reduce vomiting; small, frequent feedings followed by proper positioning

b. Older child — nothing to eat 2 hours before bedtime; possible avoidance of certain foods; should remain upright while awake

3. Other lifestyle changes include preventing obesity and restrictive clothing; avoiding spicy foods, esophageal irritants (chocolate, caffeine, peppermint, second-hand smoke), carbonated beverages; and allowing gum chewing to promote esophageal clearance.

Pharmacologic Interventions

(If therapeutic interventions fail; usually not recommended in children younger than age 2)

1. Antacids, taken immediately after meals.

2. Histamine-2 blockers, such as cimetidine and ranitidine, given I.V. or orally.

3. Prokinetic agents, such as metoclopramide, may be tried.

4. Proton pump inhibitors, such as omeprazole, are usually reserved for children with very resistant GER and esophagitis.

5. Sucralfate, a surface-protecting agent, may be used.

Surgical Interventions

1. Surgery may be necessary if conservative management does not improve condition, or if recurrent severe respiratory disease and apnea or refractory esophagitis with stricture occur. Surgical options include:
   a. Fundoplication, a wrapping of the fundus around the LES.
   b. Antroplasty or pyloroplasty.
   c. Temporary gastrostomy may be performed in children with neurologic abnormalities for feeding or to decompress the stomach, avoiding gastric distention.

Nursing Diagnoses
3, 6, 51, 80, 119, 123

Nursing Interventions
Monitoring

1. Use cardiac and apnea monitors for infants and children with severe reflux.
   a. Observe for apnea episodes lasting longer than 20 seconds or accompanied by cyanosis, pallor, or bradycardia.
   b. Document apnea episodes, associated symptoms, and recovery efforts.
2. Monitor weight frequently to evaluate infant's progress.
3. Monitor vital signs and intake and output (weigh diapers); assess skin turgor for signs of dehydration.
4. Monitor serum electrolytes and chemistry values.

 EMERGENCY ALERT Monitor for refeeding syndrome due to rapidly shifting levels of magnesium, calcium, and phosphorous in a malnourished child; check at least daily, more often if abnormal.

5. Monitor for adverse effects of pharmacologic treatment if initiated. Metoclopramide may cause parkinsonian reaction, tardive dyskinesia, irritability, insomnia, and lowered seizure threshold.
6. Monitor for dumping syndrome after surgery; usually occurs 30 minutes after a meal and includes symptoms such

G

as diaphoresis, palpitations, weakness, syncope, abdominal fullness, nausea, and diarrhea.

Supportive Care

1. Observe careful positioning with infants at all times.
2. Thicken formula for each feeding; enlarge nipple hole so formula can be more easily extracted.
   a. Add 1 tablespoon of rice cereal per ounce of formula.
   b. Watch for fatigue during feeding; more energy is needed to suck thickened formula.
   c. Get a speech therapy consultation for difficulty swallowing or sucking.
3. Provide comfort measures to reduce crying before and after meals to avoid increased intra-abdominal pressure and swallowing of air.
4. Use a pacifier for nonnutritive sucking after eating only when infant is seated upright because use of pacifier in prone position increases reflux.
5. Provide frequent, small feedings and bubble infant frequently holding infant over shoulder during and after feeding.
6. Accurately record infant feeding activity.
   a. Amount of food taken; whether retained
   b. Emesis: estimated amount, type, occurrence in relation to feeding
   c. Any change in behavior as a result of feeding technique
7. If infant is breast-fed and is not gaining weight, teach the mother to express milk and thicken it with cereal.
8. Make sure that older children avoid caffeine-containing food and beverages (such as chocolate and cola) to reduce gastric acid production. Discourage eating 2 to 4 hours before bedtime.

Education and Health Maintenance

1. Teach the parents how to handle and care for the infant. Make sure that they have proper equipment for propping the infant; inform parents that it is not necessary to keep infant upright at all times.

2. Help the parents to understand that reflux is often self-limiting; symptoms often disappear within 12 months.

3. If a temporary gastrostomy is done, teach parents about tube use and care.

4. Encourage follow-up for monitoring weight gain and development.

5. Instruct the parents and caregivers in cardiopulmonary resuscitation training before discharge of infant, if indicated.

6. Provide written and verbal instructions about prescribed medications and when to call the health care provider.

COMMUNITY CARE CONSIDERATIONS

Make sure that caregivers know the signs of dehydration, including decrease in wet diapers, listlessness, reduced appetite, and sunken fontanelle.

7. Instruct the parents not to expose child to secondhand smoke (exacerbates GER).

8. Evaluate support systems, need for community resources, financial assistance, and so forth.

GASTROINTESTINAL BLEEDING

Gastrointestinal bleeding is a symptom of many upper or lower GI disorders. It may be obvious (in emesis or stool) or occult (hidden). Such bleeding may result from trauma anywhere along the GI tract; erosions or ulcers; esophageal or gastric varices; esophagitis, gastritis, inflammatory bowel disease; bacterial infection; diverticulosis; neoplasms; ischemic bowel or aortoenteric fistula; Mallory-Weiss syndrome; or anal disorders, such as hemorrhoids or fissures. Alcohol and drugs, such as nonsteroidal anti-inflammatory drugs (NSAIDs), corticosteroids, anticoagulants, and aspirin, may lead to GI bleeding. Untreated GI bleeding may progress to hemorrhage, shock, and death.

G

Assessment

1. Changes in bowel patterns or in stool color (dark black, red, or streaked with blood); hematemesis
2. Nausea, abdominal pain or tenderness, or rectal pain
3. Intermittent melena or "coffee-ground" emesis to large amount of melena with clots or bright red hematemesis
4. Rapid pulse, drop in blood pressure, and signs of shock may occur with significant blood loss
5. Pallor, weakness, dizziness, and shortness of breath may occur as anemia develops
6. Stool or emesis will test positive for occult blood
7. Characteristics of blood help determine site of origin
   a. Bright red hematemesis — vomited from high in esophagus
   b. Bright red flow or coating stool — from rectum or distal colon
   c. Dark red blood mixed with stool — higher up in colon and small intestine
   d. Shades of black ("coffee-ground") emesis — vomited from esophagus, stomach, and duodenum
   e. Tarry stool (melena) — occurs when excessive blood accumulates in the stomach

Diagnostic Evaluation

1. Complete blood count detects decreased hematocrit and hemoglobin; coagulation studies evaluate prothrombin time.
2. Endoscopy visualizes the GI mucosa and source of bleeding and also determines the risk of rebleeding.
3. Imaging studies may be necessary to detect source of bleeding.
4. Stool test for occult blood.

Collaborative Management

Therapeutic and Surgical Interventions

1. If life-threatening bleeding occurs, treat shock and administer I.V. fluid and blood replacement.
2. Nasogastric (NG) intubation with lavage to clear blood; bloody aspirate after 2 to 3 qt (2 to 3 L) of tap water lavage,

BOX G-1	Inserting a Nasogastric Tube

- Place the patient in a sitting or high Fowler's position; place a towel around chest.
- Remove the patient's dentures; place emesis basin and tissues within the patient's reach.
- Have the patient blow nose to clear nostrils, if able, and inspect the nostrils with a penlight, observing for any obstruction.
- Wash your hands. Put on disposable gloves.
- Measure the patient's NEX (nose, earlobe, xiphoid) to determine length of the tube to reach the stomach.
- Coil the first 3 to 4 inches (7 to 10 cm) of the tube around your fingers to create a curve. Lubricate with water-soluble lubricant. Avoid occluding the tube's holes with lubricant.
- Tilt the patient's head back before inserting tube into nostril, and gently pass tube into the posterior nasopharynx, directing downward and backward toward the ear.
- When tube reaches the pharynx, the patient may gag; allow patient to rest for a few moments.
- Have the patient tilt head slightly forward. Offer several sips of water through a straw, or permit patient to suck on ice chips, unless contraindicated. Advance tube as patient swallows.
- Gently rotate the tube 180 degrees to redirect the curve and continue to advance tube gently each time the patient swallows.
- If obstruction appears to prevent tube from passing, do not use force. Rotating tube gently may help. If unsuccessful, remove tube and try other nostril.
- If there are signs of distress such as gasping, coughing, or cyanosis, immediately remove tube.
- Continue to advance the tube when the patient swallows, until the mark reaches the patient's nostril.
- Anchor the tube to the patient's nose and confirm placement by injecting air while auscultating the epigastric area or obtain X-ray as directed.

G

indicates active bleeding requiring definitive therapy. (See *Box G-1*.)

3. Electrocoagulation or injection of a sclerosant or epinephrine by way of endoscopy may be the treatment of choice to stop site of bleeding. Instilling topical thrombin to clot blood at the bleeding site may also be done.

> **DRUG ALERT** Because of the action of topical thrombin, it is used only on the surface of bleeding tissue and is never injected into the bloodstream, where intravascular clotting could take place.

4. Surgery (resection and anastomosis) may be necessary to treat some causes of bleeding.

Pharmacologic Interventions

1. For upper GI bleeding, I.V. histamine-2 blockers may be used to block the acid-secreting action of histamine. Antacids or cytoprotective agents such as sucralfate may also be used.
2. If peptic ulcer disease is the cause, an antiulcer drug is prescribed, along with lifestyle change and dietary modifications.
3. Discontinue any medications such as NSAIDs that may be causing bleeding.

Nursing Diagnoses

19, 23, 51

Nursing Interventions

Also see *Shock*, page 865.

Monitoring

1. Monitor intake and output, vital signs, and central venous pressure (CVP) to evaluate fluid status.
2. Observe for changes indicating shock, such as tachycardia, hypotension, decreasing CVP, increased respirations, decreased urine output, and changes in mental status.
3. Monitor stools and NG drainage for blood.

Supportive Care

1. Maintain patient on NG tube and NPO status to rest GI tract and evaluate bleeding.
2. Administer I.V. fluids and blood products as ordered to maintain volume and treat anemia. Provide oxygen therapy as directed.

3. Begin liquids when patient is no longer NPO. Advance diet as tolerated. Diet should be high calorie, high protein. Frequent, small feedings may be indicated.
4. Weigh daily to monitor nutritional status.

Education and Health Maintenance

1. Discuss the cause and treatment of GI bleeding with patient.
2. Instruct patient to report signs and symptoms of GI bleeding: melena, emesis that is bright red or "coffee ground" color; rectal bleeding; weakness, fatigue, and shortness of breath.
3. Instruct patient on how to test stool or emesis for occult blood if applicable.
4. Encourage compliance with abstinence if alcohol use caused bleeding, and refer to support group such as Alcoholics Anonymous.

GASTROINTESTINAL OR ABDOMINAL SURGERY

Gastrointestinal surgeries are operative procedures performed to aid in the treatment of many types of GI disorders. Procedures include total gastrectomy (complete excision of stomach with esophageal-jejunal anastomosis), subtotal or partial gastrostomy (Billroth I — gastric remnant anastomosed to duodenum; Billroth II — gastric remnant anastomosed to jejunum), gastrostomy (Janeway or Spivak), herniorrhaphy (repair of hernia), hernioplasty (reconstruction of hernia with mesh graft sewn over defect), appendectomy, various types of small and large bowel resections (proximal or distal anastomosis, temporary or permanent ostomy, Hartmann's pouch), low-anterior resection (resection of rectum with colorectal or coloanal anastomosis), abdominoperineal resection (removal of rectum and anus with permanent colostomy), subtotal and total colectomies with anastomosis, and total colectomies with a variety of ostomy procedures (ileostomy, colostomy, Kock pouch).

An *ostomy surgery* takes place when a stoma is created. A stoma is a part of the small or large intestine that is brought above the abdominal wall to serve as the outlet for discharge of intestinal contents. The term *stoma* is often used interchangeably with *ostomy*.

Abdominal surgery is any procedure performed on the abdomen, which may include renal, urologic, adrenal, gynecologic, or male reproductive procedures.

Cholecystectomies, hernia repairs, and appendectomies are routinely done through *laparoscopy,* and additional procedures are being done through this approach. Advantages include shorter hospital stay and recuperation time, less cost, less pain, and better cosmetic outcome.

Potential Complications
1. Paralytic ileus or obstruction
2. Peritonitis or sepsis
3. Anastomotic leakage, which may result in peritonitis
4. For ostomy surgery:
   a. Mucocutaneous separation (between skin and stoma)
   b. Stomal ischemia
   c. Stomal stricture or stenosis
   d. Stomal prolapse
   e. Peristomal hernia
   f. Peristomal skin breakdown
5. General postoperative complications: hemorrhage, infection, thromboembolism, pneumonia, atelectasis, wound dehiscence, and evisceration

Nursing Diagnoses
3, 16, 24, 30, 51, 67, 123, 135, 136, 156

Collaborative Interventions
Preoperative Care
1. Explain all diagnostic tests and procedures to promote the patient's cooperation and relaxation.
2. Describe the reason for and type of surgical procedure, as well as postoperative care (eg, I.V., patient-controlled analgesia [PCA] pump, nasogastric [NG] tube, surgical drains, incision care, possibility of ostomy).

3. Explain the rationale for deep breathing and teach the patient how to turn, cough, deep breathe, use the incentive spirometer, and splint the incision. These measures will minimize postoperative complications.

4. Administer I.V. fluids or hyperalimentation before surgery, as ordered, to improve fluid and electrolyte balance and nutritional status. Before an ostomy procedure, give large quantities of replacement fluids, as ordered, to accommodate expected increased output during the postoperative phase.

5. Send blood samples, as ordered, for preoperative laboratory studies and monitor results.

6. Explain that bowel cleansing will be initiated 1 or 2 days before surgery for better visualization. Preparation may include diet modifications, such as liquid or low residue; oral laxatives; suppositories; enemas; or polyethylene glyco-electrolyte solution (CoLyte, GoLYTELY).

7. Administer antibiotics, as ordered, to decrease bacterial growth in the colon.

8. Coordinate consultation with the enterostomal therapy nurse if patient is scheduled for an ostomy, to initiate early understanding and management of postoperative care. Tell the patient that the enterostomal therapist or surgeon will mark the abdomen to ensure proper positioning of the stoma.

9. Explain that the patient may not have anything by mouth after midnight the night before surgery. Medications may be withheld, if ordered.

Postoperative Care

1. Assess vital signs frequently for signs of shock or infection — hypotension, tachycardia, decreased central venous pressure, fever, and increased respirations.

2. Assess abdomen and report increased pain, distention, rigidity, and rebound tenderness, which may indicate paralytic ileus, internal bleeding, or infection. Abdominal distention also causes reduction in blood flow to a stoma through mesenteric tension.

3. Administer prescribed analgesics and provide instructions if using PCA pump, to keep patient comfortable.
   a. Assess the effectiveness of the pain medications. If ordered, Phenergan can potentiate the effectiveness of opioid.
   b. Provide diversion and teach relaxation techniques as needed.
4. Encourage and assist patient with turning, coughing, deep breathing, and incentive spirometry every 2 hours.
   a. Assess breath sounds for decrease (atelectasis) or crackles (pneumonia).
   b. Assist patient to dangle legs at bedside the night of surgery and attempt ambulation the first postoperative day, unless ordered otherwise.
5. Apply antiembolism stockings and pneumatic compression device to reduce risk of thromboembolism; administer subcutaneous heparin as ordered.
6. Maintain NG tube, if ordered. To maintain patency, irrigate the tube with 1 oz (30 mL) normal saline every 2 hours and as needed. If there are large amounts of NG output, I.V. replacement may be necessary.

 EMERGENCY ALERT Because of the type of abdominal surgery and location of the suture line, the health care provider may order not to irrigate or manipulate the NG tube.

7. Monitor intake and output frequently to determine fluid retention, dehydration, or shock. Include all drains in evaluating output.
8. Weigh patient daily to ensure fluid balance and adequate calorie intake.
9. Assess bowel sounds frequently. Maintain NPO status until return within several days after surgery.
10. Advance diet as ordered, after presence of bowel sounds indicates GI tract has regained motility. The usual diet progression is ice chips, sips of water, clear liquids, full liquids, and soft or regular diet.
11. Assess wound for signs of erythema, swelling, and purulent drainage, which may indicate infection.

a. Change surgical dressings every 24 hours and as needed to protect skin from drainage and to decrease risk
of infection.

b. Apply gauze on skin to protect against leaking from
drains or stomas.

12. Once the patient's indwelling catheter is removed, ensure voiding and monitor for signs of urinary tract infection.

13. Assess ostomy patient's stoma every shift for color and
record findings. Swelling will decrease gradually and the
stoma may bleed slightly when rubbed.

a. Normal color — pink-red

b. Dusky — dark red; purplish hue (ischemic sign)

c. Necrotic — brown or black; may be dry (notify health
care provider to determine extent of necrosis)

14. Select a pouching system based on type of ostomy and
condition of stoma and skin (see *Figure G-1*, page 386).

a. Apply pouching system with ⅟₁₆- to ⅛-inch (0.2 to
0.3 cm) clearance to prevent stomal constriction, which
contributes to edema.

b. Empty pouch when one-third to one-half full to avoid
overfilling, which interferes with pouch seal.

15. Treat peristomal skin breakdown as needed.

a. Dust with skin barrier powder.

b. Seal powder with water or skin sealant.

c. Allow skin to dry before applying a pouching system.

16. Be alert for pruritic erythematous rash with possible white
patches, which indicates candidiasis secondary to excess
moisture. An antifungal powder will be used instead of
skin barrier.

17. Encourage early ambulation but, while in bed, turn patient frequently or encourage position changes to prevent
skin breakdown at pressure areas.

18. Monitor for passage of stool from rectum or ostomy (see
Figure G-2, page 387). Note frequency, amount, and consistency.

a. Administer a stool softener or laxative, as ordered, to
promote comfort with elimination.

G

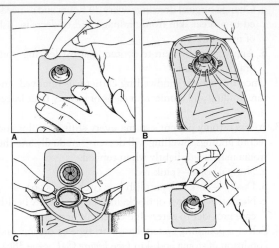

FIGURE G-1 Two-piece fecal pouching system. **(A)** A wafer with flange (1½″, 1¾″, 2¼″, 2¾″, 4″) is applied after cleaning and drying of peristomal skin. **(B)** A transparent or opaque drainable pouch is positioned over stoma at desired angle. **(C)** Pouch may be removed without removal of wafer. **(D)** Stoma may be assessed without removing wafer.

    b. Encourage diet with adequate fiber and fluid content for natural laxative effect.

    c. Encourage and assist with ambulation to promote peristalsis.

Education and Health Maintenance

1. Review signs and symptoms of wound infection so early intervention may be instituted.
2. Explain signs and symptoms of other postoperative complications to report — elevated temperature, nausea or vomiting, abdominal distention, changes in bowel function and stool consistency, and dysuria and frequency.
3. Instruct the patient about turning, coughing, deep breathing, use of incentive spirometer, and ambulation. Discuss

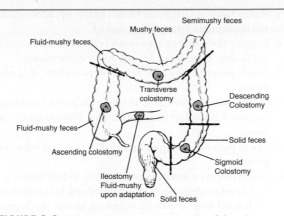

FIGURE G-2 A diagrammatic representation of the placement of fecal ostomies and nature of discharge at these sites.

purpose and continued importance of these maneuvers during the recovery period.

4. Instruct the patient to gradually resume daily activities; no heavy lifting (greater than 10 lb [4.5 kg]), pushing, pulling, or driving for 6 weeks with major abdominal surgery.

5. Review dietary changes, such as increased fiber content and fluid intake, and their importance in improving bowel function.

6. Inform ostomy patient about gas-forming foods, such as beans and cabbage; instruct patient to avoid them when appropriate. It takes about 6 hours for gas to travel from mouth to colostomy. Advise patient to avoid foods that stimulate elimination, such as nuts, seeds, and certain fruits.

G

COMMUNITY CARE CONSIDERATIONS

A person who has undergone a total gastrectomy needs lifelong parenteral administration of vitamin B_{12} to prevent pernicious anemia.

7. Assess the need for home health follow-up, and initiate the appropriate referrals if indicated.
8. Instruct the patient about wound care or ostomy care, if applicable, to promote healing and self-confidence.
9. Teach patient colostomy irrigation procedure, if appropriate.
10. Involve the enterostomal therapist in ostomy teaching and reinforce information, including lifestyle modifications.
11. Teach patient about periostomy skin care and odor and gas control.
12. Teach ostomy patient about activities of daily living.
    a. Advise resumption of normal bathing habits (tub or shower) with or without pouching system on. Suggest waterproof tape on edges of pouching system because it may be helpful with bathing or swimming.
    b. Inform patient that clothing modifications are usually minimal. Girdles and panty hose can be worn.
    c. Suggest carrying an ostomy supply kit during work or travel in case of an emergency.
    d. Remind the patient with an ostomy that participation in sports is possible; however, caution must be exercised with contact sports. During vigorous sports, a belt or binder may provide extra security.
13. Help ostomy patient achieve sexual well-being:
    a. Encourage patient and significant other to express feelings about the ostomy.
    b. Discuss ways to conceal pouch during intimacy, if desired (eg, pouch covers, special ostomy underwear). Tell patient that a small-capacity pouch (mini-pouch or cap) may be used for a short period.
    c. Recommend different positions for sexual activity to decrease stoma friction and skin irritation.
    d. Review that an ostomy in a woman does not prevent a successful pregnancy.
    e. Recommend counseling as needed.
14. For additional help and information, refer to United Ostomy Association, *www.uoa.org*.

GLAUCOMA

Glaucoma is a condition marked by high intraocular pressure (IOP) that damages the optic nerve. Glaucoma occurs in two major forms: *acute (angle-closure)* and *chronic (open-angle)*. Acute glaucoma results when the angle between the iris and the cornea becomes narrowed, restricting or blocking the drainage of aqueous humor through the trabecular network and canal of Schlemm. This causes IOP to increase suddenly. Acute angle-closure may result from trauma, stress, or any process that pushes the iris forward against the inside of the cornea when there is already an anatomically shallow anterior chamber. It is an acute, painful condition that can cause permanent eye damage within several hours. Angle closure can also exist in subacute and chronic forms.

Chronic (open-angle) glaucoma results from the gradual deterioration of the trabecular network that, as in the acute form, blocks drainage of aqueous humor and causes IOP to increase. Untreated, this results in degeneration of the optic nerve and visual field loss. Chronic glaucoma is the most common form of glaucoma, and its incidence increases with age. Genetics and conditions, such as diabetes and hypertension, also play a role. Glaucoma may also occur in neonates and children because of a congenital abnormality or acquired obstruction.

Assessment

1. Acute glaucoma:
   a. Severe pain, occurring in and around the eyes due to increased IOP; may be transitory attacks
   b. Cloudy, blurred vision; rainbow of color around lights
   c. Hazy cornea due to edema; may be profuse lacrimation and ciliary injection
   d. Nausea and vomiting may occur
   e. Pupil is mid-dilated and fixed

> **EMERGENCY ALERT** Acute angle-closure glaucoma is a medical emergency and requires immediate treatment. Untreated, it can result in blindness in less than 1 week.

2. Chronic glaucoma:
   a. Mild, bilateral discomfort (tired feeling in eyes)

b. Slow loss of peripheral vision — central vision remains unimpaired; in later stages, progressive loss of visual field
c. Increased IOP causes halos to appear around lights

PEDIATRIC ALERT Glaucoma presents in infants and children as haziness of the cornea, photophobia, excessive tearing, and decreased visual acuity.

Diagnostic Evaluation

1. Tonometry shows elevated IOP in acute and chronic disease.
2. Gonioscopy studies the angle of the anterior chamber of the eye in acute disease.
3. Ophthalmoscopy may show a pale optic disk (acute disease) or signs of clipping and atrophy of the disk (chronic disease). Dilation of the pupil is avoided if the anterior chamber is shallow.

COMMUNITY CARE CONSIDERATIONS

All people older than 35 and those at risk for developing glaucoma (family history, diabetes, previous eye trauma or surgery) should have periodic examination and tonometry by an ophthalmologist. Early detection and treatment will prevent blindness.

Collaborative Management
Pharmacologic Interventions

1. In acute glaucoma, emergency drug management is initiated to decrease eye pressure.
   a. Parasympathomimetics (carbachol, pilocarpine) may be used as miotics to cause the pupil to contract and draw the iris away from the cornea, thus enlarging the angle and allowing aqueous humor to drain; give topically.
   b. Carbonic anhydrase inhibitors (acetazolamide, methazolamide), given orally to depress aqueous humor production.

c. Beta-adrenergic blockers (betaxolol, timolol), given topically, may reduce aqueous humor or facilitate its drainage.

d. Hyperosmotics (mannitol, glycerol) increase blood osmolarity and diurese the aqueous humor; given I.V.

2. In chronic glaucoma, a combination of miotic agent and carbonic anhydrase inhibitor is usually given. Follow-up is continued at 3- to 6-month intervals to control IOP.

Surgical Interventions

1. Surgery is indicated for acute glaucoma if IOP is not maintained within normal limits by pharmacotherapy and if there is progressive visual field loss with optic nerve damage.

2. Types of surgery for acute glaucoma include:
   a. Peripheral iridectomy (small portion of iris excised so aqueous humor can bypass pupil)
   b. Trabeculectomy (part of trabecular meshwork and iris removed) may be necessary if peripheral anterior adhesions have developed because of repeated glaucoma attacks
   c. Laser iridectomy creates multiple incisions in the iris to create openings for aqueous flow

3. Types of surgery for chronic glaucoma include:
   a. Laser trabeculoplasty—creates multiple surface burns to increase outflow of aqueous humor; treatment of choice if IOP unresponsive to medical regimen
   b. Iridencleisis—opening between anterior chamber and conjunctiva to bypass blocked meshwork and allow aqueous humor to be absorbed into conjunctival tissues
   c. Cyclodiathermy or cyclocryotherapy—super-cooled probe or electrical current used to interfere with ability to secrete aqueous humor by ciliary body
   d. Corneoscleral trephine (rarely done)—a permanent drainage opening is made at the junction of the cornea and sclera through the anterior chamber

G

Nursing Diagnoses
3, 24, 33, 44

Nursing Interventions
Monitoring
1. Monitor for any pain or visual changes.
2. Monitor the patient's compliance with medications and follow-up care.

Supportive Care and Education
1. Administer antiemetics as directed to prevent vomiting, which will increase IOP.
2. Administer medications I.V., orally, or topically, as directed, and explain the importance of medications, the proper procedure for administration of drops, and possible adverse reactions.
   a. Mannitol may cause transient blurred vision, rhinitis, thirst, nausea, headache, and transitory circulatory overload.
   b. Carbonic anhydrase inhibitors may cause drowsiness, anorexia, paresthesia, tinnitus, electrolyte loss, and possible liver dysfunction.
   c. Pilocarpine may cause burning and redress of eye, headache, poor vision in dim light, and retinal detachment.
   d. Beta-adrenergic blockers (topical) may cause eye irritation, headache, decreased corneal sensitivity, blurred vision, bradycardia, palpitations, bronchospasm, and hypotension.
3. After surgery:
   a. Elevate head of the bed 30 degrees to promote drainage of aqueous humor after a trabeculectomy.
   b. Administer medications (steroids and cycloplegics) as directed after peripheral iridectomy to decrease inflammation and to dilate the pupil.
   c. Use an eye patch or shield in children for several days to protect the eye; in adults, patch is usually removed within several hours.

4. Alert the patient to avoid, if possible, circumstances that may increase IOP:
   a. Prolonged coughing or vomiting
   b. Emotional upsets—worry, fear, anger
   c. Exertion such as snow shoveling, pushing, heavy lifting

PEDIATRIC ALERT Advise parents not to overfeed infant with glaucoma, which may cause vomiting and increased IOP.

5. Instruct the patient to seek immediate medical attention if signs and symptoms of increased IOP should recur: severe eye pain, photophobia, and excessive lacrimation.

GLOMERULONEPHRITIS, ACUTE

Acute glomerulonephritis (poststreptococcal glomerulonephritis) is an inflammation of the glomeruli that occurs when antigen–antibody complexes become trapped in the glomerular capillary membranes. Eventual scarring and loss of glomerular filtering surface may lead to renal failure. The disease occurs 1 to 3 weeks after onset of an upper respiratory infection (typically, pharyngitis from group A beta-hemolytic streptococci), skin infection, or systemic infection (hepatitis B, endocarditis).

Acute glomerulonephritis occurs at all ages. Complications are rare but include hypertension, heart failure, uremia, anemia, endocarditis, hypertensive encephalopathy, and end-stage renal disease.

Assessment

1. Oliguria, hematuria, tea-colored urine
2. Edema—periorbital or generalized and dependent; weight gain
3. Hypertension (in more than 50% of patients)—usually mild, but can be moderate or severe
4. Malaise, mild headache, anorexia, and vomiting
5. Diuresis starts 1 to 2 weeks after onset

Diagnostic Evaluation

1. Urinalysis
   a. Hematuria (microscopic or gross)

    b. Proteinuria (3+ to 4+)

    c. Sediment: red cell casts, white blood cells, renal epithelial cells

    d. Specific gravity: moderately elevated

2. 24-hour urine for creatinine clearance decreased

3. Blood studies

    a. Blood urea nitrogen (BUN) and creatinine elevated

    b. Albumin decreased

    c. Serum complement, C3 usually decreased

    d. Antistreptolysin-O titer increased

3. Chest X-ray may show pulmonary congestion

4. Needle biopsy of the kidney to show obstruction of glomerular capillaries and confirm diagnosis

Collaborative Management

Therapeutic Interventions

1. Restrict fluid intake; potassium and sodium intake, if hyperkalemia, edema, or signs of heart failure.

2. Moderate protein restriction with oliguria and elevated BUN; more drastic restriction if acute renal failure develops.

PEDIATRIC ALERT Protein is usually not restricted from the diet in children because of growth needs.

3. Increased carbohydrates to provide energy and reduce protein catabolism.

Pharmacologic Interventions

1. Antihypertensives and diuretics to control hypertension and edema.

2. Cation-exchange resin to control hyperkalemia secondary to renal insufficiency, if necessary.

3. Histamine-2 blockers to prevent stress ulcers in acute illness.

4. Phosphate-binding agents to reduce phosphate and elevate calcium levels.

5. Antibiotics, if infection is still present.

Nursing Diagnoses

22, 42, 69, 88, 104

Nursing Interventions
Monitoring
1. Monitor vital signs and intake and output during acute phase of the disease; check urine for protein and blood as directed.
2. Carefully monitor fluid balance with central venous pressure or pulmonary artery pressure readings as indicated; weigh the patient daily.
3. Monitor for signs and symptoms of heart failure: distended neck veins, tachycardia, gallop rhythm, enlarged and tender liver, increasing edema, and crackles at bases of lungs.
4. Monitor neurologic status for signs of encephalopathy or seizure activity secondary to hypertension.

EMERGENCY ALERT Hypertensive encephalopathy is a medical emergency; treatment must reduce blood pressure without impairing renal function. Monitor vasodilator therapy closely.

Supportive Care
1. Encourage bed rest during the acute phase until the urine clears and BUN, creatinine, and blood pressure normalize. Rest also facilitates diuresis.
2. For children on fluid restriction, offer small amount of desired fluids in appropriate size cup at regular intervals during day. Give fluids after, rather than with, meals.
3. Suggest age-appropriate nonexertional diversional activities while on bed rest.
4. Ensure adequate fluid replacement once diuresis phase begins through oral fluid intake.

Education and Health Maintenance
1. Advise that family members need to recognize and seek treatment of any future infections or sore throats.
2. Advise that tonsillectomy or oral surgery is not recommended for several months after glomerulonephritis to prevent endocarditis.
3. Explain that the patient must have follow-up evaluations of blood pressure, urinalysis, and BUN concentrations to check for exacerbation of the disease. Microscopic hematuria and proteinuria may persist for many months.

G

4. Explain that prognosis is good, with 90% of patients regaining normal renal function within 60 days.
5. Instruct the patient to report signs of decreasing renal function and to obtain treatment immediately.

GOUT

Gout is a disorder of purine metabolism characterized by elevated uric acid levels with deposition of urate crystals in joints and other tissues. High uric acid levels result from decreased excretion of uric acid (90% of cases) or overproduction of the acid (10% of cases) due to a wide variety of causes. The disorder may progress from an asymptomatic stage through acute gouty arthritis, to chronic tophaceous gout. Complications include erosive deforming arthritis, uric acid kidney stones, and urate nephropathy caused by hyperuricemia.

Assessment

1. Acute gouty arthritis
   a. Generally affects one joint — often the first metatarsophalangeal joint (podagra).
   b. Other joints can be affected, such as ankle, tarsals, or knee. Upper extremities less commonly involved.
   c. Warm erythema and swelling of tissue surrounding the affected joint; fever may occur.
   d. Pain — sudden onset, severe intensity.
   e. Duration of symptoms is self-limiting; lasts approximately 3 to 10 days without treatment.
2. Chronic tophaceous gout
   a. Tophi (deposits of uric acid) in and around joints, cartilage and soft tissues, such as pinnae, olecranon bursa, and Achilles tendon
   b. Arthritis more chronic in nature, with discrete attacks less common; can produce bone erosions and subsequent bony deformities that can resemble rheumatoid arthritis

Diagnostic Evaluation

1. Synovial fluid for analysis.

   a. Identification of monosodium urate crystals under polarized microscopy
   b. Synovial white blood cell count can range from 2,000 to 100,000/µl
   c. Culture rules out infection
2. Elevated serum uric acid level, but does not correlate with severity of gout.
3. Elevated erythrocyte sedimentation rate.
4. Uric acid level decreased on 24-hour urine specimen with underexcretion; increased with overproduction.
5. X-rays of affected joints show changes consistent with gout.

Collaborative Management
Therapeutic Interventions
1. Avoidance of obesity and excess alcohol, which predispose gout attacks
2. Low-purine diet (obtains small reduction of serum uric acid levels)

Pharmacologic Interventions
1. Nonsteroidal anti-inflammatory drugs to relieve pain and swelling of acute attacks.
2. Colchicine to prevent as well as treat acute attacks
   a. I.V. for acute attacks
   b. Orally at onset of attack, given hourly until pain relief or first signs of toxicity (diarrhea)
3. Corticosteroids given intra-articularly if attack is confined to a single joint; or orally in short tapering course if other treatments contraindicated or if attack involves several joints.
4. Urate-lowering agents to prevent renal disease progression of gout.
   a. Uricosurics such as probenecid interfere with tubular reabsorption of uric acid.
   b. Allopurinol interferes with conversion of hypoxanthine and xanthine to uric acid.
   c. Give cautiously to patients with renal disease.

G

Nursing Diagnoses
3, 24, 62, 134

Nursing Interventions
Monitoring
1. Monitor skin surrounding affected joint because it is prone to break down.
2. Monitor for adverse effects of allopurinol, including skin rash (including exfoliative rashes), hypersensitivity syndrome (fever, eosinophilia, leukocytosis, worsening renal failure, hepatocellular injury, rash), and bone marrow depression.

Supportive Care
1. Administer and teach self-administration of pain-relieving medications as directed.
2. Encourage adequate fluid intake to assist with excretion of uric acid and decrease likelihood of stone formation.
3. Reinforce importance of taking prescribed medications consistently because interruption of therapy can precipitate acute attacks.
4. Elevate and protect affected joint during acute attack.
5. Assist with activities of daily living.
6. Encourage exercise and maintenance of routine activity in chronic gout, except during acute attacks.
7. Protect draining tophi by covering and applying antibiotic ointment as needed.
8. Avoid thiazide diuretics, low-dose aspirin, and the antitubercular agent pyrazinamide, which may increase uric acid levels in these patients.

Education and Health Maintenance
1. Instruct the patient and family in nature of disease.
   a. Generally, acute attacks are followed by periods of remission.
   b. Once need for chronic treatment has been determined, it will generally be lifelong.
2. Encourage the patient to avoid alcohol, which can precipitate acute attack.

3. Instruct the patient to avoid rapid weight loss by fasting or crash diets. Explain that rapid weight loss results in production of chemicals that compete with uric acid for excretion from the body, causing increased uric acid levels.
4. Advise patient to seek prompt treatment of acute attacks to reduce joint damage associated with repeated attacks.
5. Teach patient to recognize and report signs and symptoms of allopurinol hypersensitivity syndrome.
6. Review foods containing purines (eg, sardines, anchovies, shellfish, organ meats) if low-purine diet has been advised.

GRAVES' DISEASE

See *Hyperthyroidism*.

GROWTH HORMONE INSUFFICIENCY

Growth hormone insufficiency is an impaired secretion of growth hormone (GH) by the anterior pituitary gland either by lack of pituitary production of GH or the lack of hypothalamic stimulation of the pituitary to produce GH. This results in abnormal protein, fat, and carbohydrate metabolism. A child with this condition has short stature but normal body proportions. GH inefficiency may be organic due to tumors, intracranial cysts, head trauma, infection, radiation therapy, or idiopathic. Turner syndrome is a genetic syndrome that causes GH to be bioinactive due to binding problems. Complications include hypoglycemia, causing seizures and death in the neonate. See *Box G-2*, page 400, for other causes of short stature.

Assessment

1. Hypoglycemia, prolonged jaundice, small penis (in the neonate)
2. Growth velocity usually less than the fifth percentile for chronological age
3. Delayed skeletal maturation — bone age at least 1 year behind chronological age
4. "Pudgy," where the weight age (50% for weight) exceeds the height age (50% for height)

BOX G-2	Causes of Short Stature

- Familial short stature
- Constitutional delay
- Dwarfism
- Turner syndrome
- Russel-Silver syndrome
- Prader-Willi syndrome
- Down syndrome
- Cystic fibrosis
- Hypothyroidism

- Growth hormone deficiency
- Glucocorticord excess (iatrogenic or intrinsic)
- Chronic cardiopulmonary and metabolic diseases
- Pituitary surgery or radiation

5. Delayed eruption of primary and secondary teeth (not as severe as in hypothyroidism)
6. Delayed or absent sexual development
7. School nurse who measures the child on an annual basis is the best source for detecting a growth disorder (Height percentiles should accompany absolute measurements. Changes in percentiles on consecutive measurements indicate need for a closer evaluation of growth.)
8. Increased body fat mass, reduced exercise capacity, decreased strength, hyperlipidemia, reduced bone density, and impaired cardiac function may develop in young adulthood

Diagnostic Evaluation
1. Rule out organic, nonendocrine causes of short stature (eg, chronic illness, nutritional deficiencies, genetic disorders, psychosocial factors).
2. Calculate growth velocity to determine if growth pattern parallels or deviates from the growth curve.
3. Assess bone age by X-ray to ascertain age of physical development; usually delayed.
4. Thyroid function tests may be done to rule out hypothyroidism.
5. GH secretion laboratory indicators: insulin-like growth factor I and IGF binding protein 3 are decreased.
6. Subnormal secretion of GH in provocative testing.

7. Insulin-induced hypoglycemia; in the neonate with hypoglycemia, GH release is reduced at time of documented hypoglycemia.
8. Abnormal response to orginine infusion, L-dopa, clonidine, or glucagon.
9. Chromosome testing of females.

PEDIATRIC ALERT Blood for evaluation of cortisol and GH level must be drawn before treatment for hypoglycemia; otherwise, the laboratory result will not accurately reflect these levels. Accurate diagnosis and early detection will prevent future episodes of hypoglycemia and its potentially fatal complications in the neonate.

10. MRI may be done to rule out central nervous system lesions.

Collaborative Management
Pharmacologic Interventions
1. Replacement of deficiency uses recombinant DNA-derived GH (somatrem) given as subcutaneous (S.C.) injection.
2. Typical pediatric dose is 0.2 to 0.3 mg/kg/week divided in six or seven doses weekly until final height is achieved. In patients with Turner syndrome, 0.375 mg/kg is used.
3. Replacement therapy is being recommended for adults with GH deficiency, depending on the degree of deficiency. Dosing is from 0.006 mg/kg/day to 0.0125 mg/kg/day after epiphyseal fusion has occurred.
4. Complications of therapy include leukemia, recurrence of tumor, pseudotumor cerebri, slipped capital femoral epiphysis, and diabetes.

Nursing Diagnoses
12, 24, 25, 159

Nursing Interventions
Supportive Care
1. Teach the child and parents, through written and verbal instructions, how to inject GH. Give demonstration and encourage return demonstration. Review mixing technique, storage, and stability of preparation used.

G

2. Encourage rotation of sites in the subcutaneous tissue of the upper arms or thighs to prevent skin irritation or hypertrophy.
3. Document growth every 3 to 6 months while on therapy.
4. Encourage the child to verbalize feelings regarding short stature. Help the child understand that friendships and social value are based on personality traits rather than physical height.
5. Suggest involvement in activities that do not use height as an advantage, such as music, art, and gymnastics.
6. Help child and parents to identify age-appropriate behaviors and develop a plan for maintaining consistent behaviors both in the home and socially.
7. Make sure parents have realistic expectations of child; encourage use of positive feedback rather than punishment.

Education and Health Maintenance

1. Teach that growth catch-up to peers usually occurs when peers have stopped growing. After initial startup of treatment, growth rate should be 4 to 5 inches (10 to 13 cm) in the first year, then 3 to 3½ inches (7 to 9 cm) per year.
2. Stress that treatment is not to make child tall—it is to optimize final height outcome.
3. Review medication dosage and injection techniques periodically. Teach family to report possible signs of adverse effects of therapy—severe headache, hip or knee pain, and increased thirst and urination.
4. Tell the family to think of GH as a replacement rather than a medication; therefore, it should always be given regardless of illness or other medication therapies.
5. Encourage regular follow-up for growth evaluation and maintenance of therapy.
6. If needed, involve the school nurse in the care and follow-up of the child.

GUILLAIN-BARRÉ SYNDROME

Guillain-Barré syndrome (polyradiculoneuritis) is an acute inflammatory polyneuropathy of the peripheral sensory and motor nerves and nerve roots. Affected nerves are demyelinated with possible axonal degeneration. Although its exact cause is unknown, Guillain-Barré syndrome is believed to be an autoimmune disorder that may be triggered by viral infection, *Campylobacter* diarrheal illness, immunization, or other precipitating event. The syndrome is marked by acute onset of symmetric progressive muscle weakness, most often beginning in the legs and ascending to involve the trunk, upper extremities, and facial muscles. Paralysis may develop. Complications may include respiratory failure, cardiac arrhythmias, and complications of immobility; about 30% of people still have residual weakness after 3 years.

Assessment

1. Acute onset (hours to weeks) of progressive, usually ascending muscle weakness and fasciculation, possibly leading to paralysis (maximal weakness is reached within 2 weeks)
2. Paresthesia and painful sensations
3. Possible hypoventilation due to chest muscle weakness
4. Difficulty with swallowing, chewing, speech, and gag, indicating fifth (trigeminal) and ninth (glossopharyngeal) cranial nerve involvement
5. Reduced or absent deep tendon reflexes, position and vibratory perception
6. Autonomic dysfunction with orthostatic hypotension and tachycardia

G

Diagnostic Evaluation

1. Lumbar puncture obtains cerebrospinal fluid samples, which reveal low cell count and high protein levels.
2. Nerve conduction studies, which show decreased conduction velocity of peripheral nerves due to demyelination.
3. Abnormal laboratory studies may point to prior infection or illness.

Collaborative Management
Therapeutic Interventions
1. Plasmapheresis may be tried to temporarily reduce circulating disease-related antibodies to reduce the severity and duration.
2. High-dose immunoglobulin therapy may reduce severity.
3. Continuous cardiac monitoring to monitor for arrhythmias, indicating thoracic spinal nerve involvement.
4. If respiratory paralysis develops, intubation, mechanical ventilation, and support of vital functions.
5. Analgesics and muscle relaxants may be needed.

Pharmacologic Interventions
1. Analgesics and muscle relaxants to control painful sensations and fasciculations

Nursing Diagnoses
3, 6, 8, 45, 51, 62, 70, 75, 84

Nursing Interventions
Monitoring
1. Monitor respiratory status through vital capacity measurements, rate and depth of respirations, and breath sounds.
2. Monitor level of muscle weakness as it ascends toward respiratory muscles. Watch for breathlessness while talking, a sign of respiratory fatigue.
3. Monitor the patient for signs of impending respiratory failure; heart rate > 120 beats/minute or < 70 beats/minute; respiratory rate > 30 breaths/minutes; prepare to intubate.
4. Monitor gag reflex and swallowing ability.

Supportive Care
1. Position patient with the head of bed elevated to provide for maximum chest excursion.
2. Avoid giving opioids and sedatives that may depress respirations.
3. Position patient correctly and provide range-of-motion exercises.

4. Provide good body alignment, range-of-motion exercises, and change of position to prevent complications such as contractures, pressure sores, and dependent edema.

5. Ensure adequate nutrition without the risk of aspiration; use parenteral nutrition, gastrostomy feeding, oral supplements as indicated.

6. Auscultate for bowel sounds; if bowel sounds are absent, hold feedings to prevent gastric distention.

7. Encourage physical and occupational therapy exercises to help the patient regain strength during rehabilitation phase.

8. Provide assistive devices as needed (cane or wheelchair) to maximize independence and activity.

9. During rehabilitation period, encourage a well-balanced, nutritious diet using small, frequent feedings with vitamin supplement if indicated. Weigh weekly. Encourage patient to consume fluids and fiber-rich foods to prevent constipation.

10. If verbal communication is possible, discuss the patient's fears and concerns. Reassure the patient that complete recovery is probable.

11. If the patient cannot speak, use mechanical speech aids or a communication board. Provide an adaptive patient call system as needed.

12. Encourage speech therapy during rehabilitation phase.

13. Provide adjunct pain management therapies such as therapeutic touch, massage, diversion, and imagery.

14. Provide choices in care to give the patient a sense of control.

Education and Health Maintenance

1. Advise patient and family that the acute phase of the syndrome lasts 1 to 4 weeks, then the patient stabilizes and rehabilitation can begin; however, convalescence may be lengthy, from 3 months to 2 years.

2. Teach patient about breathing exercises or use of an incentive spirometer to reestablish normal breathing patterns.

3. Instruct patient to wear good supportive and protective shoes while out of bed to prevent injuries due to weakness and paresthesia.

4. Instruct patient to check feet routinely for injuries because trauma may go unnoticed due to sensory changes.

5. Urge patient to maintain normal weight; additional weight will further stress motor function.

6. Encourage scheduled rest periods to avoid fatigue.

7. Refer patient and family to agencies such as The Guillain-Barré Syndrome Foundation International, *www. gsfi.com*.

H

HEADACHE

Headache is one of the most common human ailments. Primary headache syndromes include *tension headaches, migraines,* and *cluster headaches*. Headache may also be a symptom of underlying disorder, such as meningitis, increased intracranial pressure, temporal arteritis, sinus infection, and head injury. Acute, severe headache may signal cerebral bleeding in subdural hematoma. Tension headaches result from irritation of sensitive nerve endings in the head, jaw, and neck caused by prolonged muscle contraction, and often are related to prolonged or abnormal posture, or teeth clenching. Migraine pain and other symptoms are the result of vasospasm, then dilation of intracranial and extracranial arteries; their cause appears to be a genetically based hyperreactivity to the neurotransmitter serotonin. Cluster headaches are less common and occur more in men, and their pathogenesis involves increased release of histamine, which causes vasodilation.

Assessment

1. *Tension headache:* dull bandlike pain and pressure in the back of the head and neck, across forehead, bitemporal areas; dull, persistent ache; tender spots of head or neck.
2. *Migraine headache:* gradual onset of severe unilateral, throbbing pain that may become bilateral; lasts 4 to 72 hours.
   a. May be preceded by sensory, motor, or mood alterations known as aura, including scintillating scotoma, hemianopsia, and paresthesia.
   b. Nausea, vomiting, and photophobia may occur.
   c. May be triggered in women by hormonal fluctuations (menses, pregnancy).
3. *Cluster headache:* pain is severe, unilateral, involving the face, always occurs on the same side, and occurs suddenly at the same time of day, sometimes at night. Attacks

last 20 minutes to 2 hours. Several attacks may occur in 1 day.

  a. Occurs in clusters of 2 to 8 weeks followed by periods of remission.

  b. Associated with unilateral excessive tearing, redness of the eye, nasal congestion, facial swelling, flushing, and sweating.

4. *Sinus headache*: pain is usually felt over sinus areas — above the eyes, along the side of the nose, and in the cheeks. May be accompanied by fever, nasal drainage, erythema, and swelling and tenderness of the sinus areas with acute sinusitis.

5. *Temporal arteritis*: unilateral or bilateral pain is particularly severe at night with tender temporal areas.

Diagnostic Evaluation

1. Skull and sinus X-rays rule out headache-related lesions or sinusitis.

2. CT scanning or MRI rule out lesions or hemorrhage.

3. Erythrocyte sedimentation rate is elevated in temporal arteritis.

Collaborative Management
Therapeutic Interventions

1. Nonpharmacologic management includes relaxation techniques, such as distraction, imagery, and progressive muscle relaxation, as well as biofeedback to control pain.

2. Avoidance of tyramine-containing foods (eg, cheese or chocolate) to prevent migraines, as well as identification of other triggers, such as skipping meals, intake of certain spices and preservatives, and withdrawal from caffeine.

3. Inhalation of 100% oxygen to abort a cluster headache.

Pharmacologic Interventions

1. Aspirin, acetaminophen, and nonsteroidal anti-inflammatory drugs for mild to moderate pain of primary headache syndromes and headache as a symptom of other disorders, unless contraindicated

2. Antihistamines and decongestants for sinus headaches
3. Drugs to treat vascular headaches at their onset, including methysergide, a serotonin antagonist; ergotamine, a vasoconstrictor; or 5-HT agonist drugs such as sumatriptan
4. Beta-adrenergic blockers, calcium channel blockers, or antidepressants as prophylaxis against recurrent migraines
5. Corticosteroids for temporal arteritis
6. Opioid analgesics, muscle relaxants, and antianxiety agents for severe pain of headache

DRUG ALERT Vasoconstrictors and 5-HT agonists are contraindicated in patients with uncontrolled hypertension, coronary artery disease, hemiplegic migraine, and peripheral vascular disease.

Nursing Diagnoses
3, 33, 78, 92

Nursing Interventions
Supportive Care
1. Reduce environmental stimuli, such as light, noise, and movement.
2. To relieve tension headaches:
   a. Suggest light massage of tight muscles in neck, scalp, and back.
   b. Apply warm, moist heat to areas of muscle tension.
   c. Teach progressive muscle relaxation.
3. Administer abortive and preventive medications as directed.
   a. Administer sumatriptan by subcutaneous (S.C.) injection if ordered, and warn patient of transient feeling of dizziness, tingling, or pressure that may occur.
   b. Administer opioids as directed but maintain patient safety if patient becomes drowsy.
   c. Avoid routine and frequent analgesic administration, which may cause rebound headaches.
4. Encourage the patient to lie down and attempt to sleep. Encourage adequate rest once headache is relieved to recover from fatigue of the pain.

H

5. Encourage adequate nutrition, rest and relaxation, and avoidance of stress and overexertion to better cope with headaches.
6. Review coping mechanisms and strengthen positive ones.

Education and Health Maintenance

1. Teach proper administration of medications:
   a. Sumatriptan, given S.C. with autoinjector for quick relief, or given orally
   b. Oral and nasal formulations of other 5-HT agonists
   c. Ergotamine given through metered-dose inhaler
   d. Take pain medications at onset of headache and repeat as prescribed.
2. Teach patient about the adverse effects of headache medications. Reportable adverse effects include:
   a. Numbness, coldness, paresthesias, and pain of extremities with ergot derivatives
   b. Chest pain, wheezing, swelling of lips, or flushing with sumatriptan
   c. Light-headedness and hypotension with beta-adrenergic blockers and calcium channel blockers (Warn the patient using beta-adrenergic blockers to arise slowly, adhere to prescribed dosage, and avoid abrupt withdrawal of the drug.)

ALTERNATIVE INTERVENTION

Feverfew is an herbal product that may be used for migraine headaches. It has been considered as generally safe, but may cause adverse effects such as mouth ulcers and GI upset. Patients with migraines who take a 5-HT agonist should not take St. John's wort, an herbal product for depression, because the combination causes an increased risk of a severe reaction.

3. Warn the patient not to drink alcohol, skip meals, or change sleep pattern (all can trigger migraine headaches).
4. Teach the patient with migraine to avoid foods high in tyramine, such as aged cheese, red wine, liver, and chocolate.

HEAD INJURY

Head injury, also known as *traumatic brain injury* (TBI), is the disruption of normal brain function due to trauma (blunt or penetrating injury). Neurologic deficits result from shearing of white matter, ischemia and mass effect from hemorrhage, and cerebral edema of surrounding brain tissue. Types of brain injuries include *concussion, cerebral contusion, brain stem contusion, epidural hematoma, subdural hematoma,* and *diffuse axonal injury.* Associated injuries include facial and skull fractures, vertebral or carotid artery dissection, spinal cord injury, and soft tissue injuries.

TBI is classified from mild to severe according to Glasgow Coma Scale (GCS) score (see page 240). Mild TBI is characterized by GCS of 13 to 15 with loss of consciousness up to 15 minutes; moderate TBI is characterized by GCS of 9 to 12 with loss of consciousness up to 6 hours; and severe TBI is characterized by GCS of 3 to 8 with loss of consciousness longer than 6 hours. Complications include infections, such as meningitis or ventriculitis, complications of immobility, hydrocephalus, posttraumatic seizure disorder, permanent neurologic deficits, coagulopathy, sympathetic storming, diabetes insipidus (DI), syndrome of inappropriate antidiuretic hormone (SIADH), cerebral salt-wasting, lasting emotional and behavioral changes, mental retardation, and persistent vegetative state.

Assessment

1. Disturbance in level of consciousness (LOC) from slightly drowsy (concussion) to unconscious
   a. Acute subdural hematoma may present as persistent unconsciousness or deteriorating LOC progressing to decerebrate or decorticate posturing (see *Figure H-1,* page 412).
   b. Chronic subdural hematoma may present gradually with irritability and seizures.
2. Headache, vertigo, agitation, restlessness
3. Cerebrospinal fluid (CSF) leakage at ears and nose, which may indicate skull fracture

H

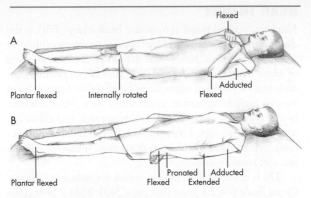

FIGURE H-1 **(A)** Decorticate posturing (loss of motor control by cerebral cortex). **(B)** Decerebrate posturing (brain stem dysfunction).

4. Contusions about eyes (raccoon eyes) and ears (battle sign) indicating skull fractures
5. Irregular respirations
6. Cognitive deficit
7. Pupillary abnormality
8. Sudden onset of neurologic deficits
9. Otorrhea (may indicate leakage of CSF from ear) indicating posterior fossa skull fracture
10. Rhinorrhea (may indicate leakage of CSF from nose) indicating anterior fossa skull fracture

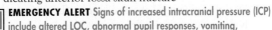 **EMERGENCY ALERT** Signs of increased intracranial pressure (ICP) include altered LOC, abnormal pupil responses, vomiting, widened pulse pressure, bradycardia, and hyperthermia. Notify a health care provider immediately.

EMERGENCY ALERT Regard every patient who has a brain injury as having a potential spinal cord injury. Many patients are under the influence of alcohol at the time of injury, which may mask the nature and severity of the injury.

Diagnostic Evaluation
1. CT identifies and localizes lesions, cerebral edema, and bleeding.

2. Skull and cervical spine X-rays identify fracture and displacement.
3. Complete blood count, coagulation profile, electrolyte levels, serum osmolarity, arterial blood gases, and other laboratory tests monitor for complications.
4. Neuropsychological tests during rehabilitation phase determine cognitive deficits.

Collaborative Management
Therapeutic and Pharmacologic Interventions
1. Maintenance of airway, breathing, and circulation.
   a. Intubate for GCS < 8 (comatose)
   b. Placement of nasogastric tube with intubation to prevent aspiration
   c. Oxygen as needed to maintain a partial pressure of arterial oxygen (PaO_2) > 100 mm Hg; maintain a partial pressure of arterial carbon dioxide ($PaCO_2$) between 35 and 45 mm Hg (avoid use of hyperventilation)
   d. Maintain systolic blood pressure > 90 mm Hg through use of vasopressors and albumin
   e. Maintain normovolemia; treat symptomatic anemia with packed red blood cells and iron supplements
   f. Treat symptomatic arrhythmias
2. Management of increased ICP with osmotic diuretics, corticosteroids, mechanical hyperventilation, or barbiturates to induce coma.
3. Antibiotics to prevent infection in open skull fractures or penetrating wounds.
4. Management of sympathetic storming with medications, such as oxycodone (opiate), propranolol (beta-adrenergic blocker), clonidine (alpha-adrenergic antagonist), dantrolene (muscle relaxant), gabapentin (antiepileptic), and bromocriptine (dopamine-receptor agonist). Response to medications is very individual. Sympathetic storming may be triggered by suctioning, turning, hyperthermia, or loud noises.
5. Treatment of hypernatremia (due to DI, dehydration, diaphoresis) with fluid replacement, and possible desmopressin (DDAVP) therapy.

H

6. Treatment of hyponatremia (due to cerebral salt-wasting or SIADH) by monitoring daily fluid status, fluid restriction, oral salt replacement, and I.V. saline 0.9% or 3% (240 to 500 mL) over 3 to 5 hours.

Surgical Interventions

1. Surgery may be necessary for evacuation of intracranial hematomas, debridement of penetrating wounds, elevation of skull fractures, subdural tapping to remove fluid, or repair of CSF leaks.
2. Shunting to relieve persistent fluid build-up with subdural hematoma.

Nursing Diagnoses

15, 35, 51, 62, 75, 88, 135, 136

Nursing Interventions

Monitoring

1. Maintain ICP monitoring, as indicated, and report abnormalities.
2. Maintain a neurologic flow sheet to track changes in cranial nerve, sensory, motor, and reflex function.
3. Monitor results of serial serum and urine electrolyte and osmolality studies; potassium and sodium imbalances are common.
4. Monitor hemodynamic measurements to guide fluid replacement; monitor urinary output. Excessive, dilute urine may indicate DI; decreased, concentrated urine indicates SIADH.
5. Monitor for anemia (decreased hemoglobin and hematocrit) and infection (elevated white blood cells).
6. Monitor respiratory rate, depth, and pattern of respirations; report any abnormal pattern, such as Cheyne-Stokes respirations or periods of apnea.

EMERGENCY ALERT Monitor for signs of sympathetic storming: diaphoresis, tachycardia, tachypnea, hypertension, hyperthermia, agitation, and dystonia. Report immediately and try to identify and eliminate triggers.

7. Maintain constant vigilance of agitated patient confined to bed and avoid use of restraints if possible.

Supportive Care

1. Maintain a patent airway; assist with intubation and ventilatory assistance if needed.
2. To facilitate respirations, turn the patient every 2 hours and encourage coughing and deep breathing.
3. Replace I.V. fluids as indicated. Avoid rapid change in electrolytes, which may precipitate cerebral edema.
4. Apply firm pressure over puncture site for subdural tap, and observe for drainage on dressing.
5. Suction the patient as needed; hyperventilate the patient before suctioning to prevent hypoxia.
6. Institute measures to prevent increased ICP or other neurovascular compromise: avoid neck flexion, avoid hip flexion (which may reduce venous drainage), and prevent straining; spread out care evenly over 24-hour period so patient is not overstimulated at any time.
7. Feed the patient as soon as possible after a head injury and administer histamine-2 blockers to prevent gastric ulceration and hemorrhage from gastric acid hypersecretion.
8. If the patient is unable to swallow, provide hyperalimentation, then enteral feedings after bowel sounds have returned. Caloric needs of the head-injured patient increase by 100% to 200%. Consult a dietitian to institute nutritional support within the first 2 to 3 days after injury to support the recovery process.
9. Elevate the head of the bed after feedings, and check residuals to prevent aspiration. Also check glucose level and give insulin as directed to prevent hyperglycemia.

PEDIATRIC ALERT Remain nonjudgmental in cases of suspected child abuse and ensure that it is reported to the appropriate agency, and that the parents are referred for counseling.

10. During rehabilitation, recognize the dysphagic patient and encourage oral feeding of soft or pureed foods. Refer the patient to a speech or physical therapist as indicated for feeding difficulties.

11. Provide stimulation of all sensory avenues. Orient the patient to time and place.
12. Observe the patient for fatigue or restlessness from overstimulation.
13. Involve the family in sensory stimulation program; refer the patient for cognitive retraining if appropriate.
14. Warn the family regarding restlessness and combativeness that may occur during recovery from brain injury.
15. Pad side rails, and wrap hands in mitts if the patient is agitated.
16. Investigate for physical sources of restlessness, such as uncomfortable position, signs of urinary tract infection, or pressure ulcers.
17. Provide adequate light and reorient frequently if the patient is hallucinating.
18. Perform passive range-of-motion exercises to release muscle tension from inactivity.
19. Avoid sedatives to avoid medication-induced confusion and altered states of cognition.
20. Refer the family to social worker and community support services such as respite care.

COMMUNITY CARE CONSIDERATIONS

Observe for signs of postconcussion syndrome (PCS), which include headache, decreased concentration, irritability, dizziness, insomnia, restlessness, diminished memory, anxiety, easy fatigability, and alcohol intolerance. Be aware that persistence of these symptoms can interfere with relationships and employability of the patient. Encourage the patient and family to report these symptoms and obtain additional support and counseling as needed. PCS may persist as long as 1 or 2 years.

Education and Health Maintenance

1. Review with the family the signs of increased ICP.
2. Teach the family therapeutic use of touch, massage, and music to calm the agitated patient.
3. Make the family aware of guidelines for return to sports (refer to National Athletic Trainers Association at *www.nata.org*).

4. Refer the patient and family to agencies such as Brain Injury Association of America, *www.biausa.org.*

HEART DISEASE, CONGENITAL

Congenital heart disease (CHD) refers to a variety of structural malformations that may be in the chambers, valves, or great vessels arising from the heart, either singularly or in combination with each other or other congenital defects. The defects are present at birth but not necessarily diagnosed at that time. They are picked up by signs of respiratory distress, cyanosis, failure to gain weight, and heart murmurs. Most children with CHD can be successfully managed with medications and surgery.

In general, CHD results from abnormal embryonic development or the persistence of fetal structure beyond the time of normal involution. Factors associated with the development of CHD may include infection during the first trimester of pregnancy (rubella); chromosomal defects; maternal type 1 diabetes, and drug or alcohol use during pregnancy. Children with CHD are more likely to have associated syndromes, such as Marfan, Down, Turner, Noonan, Williams, and DiGeorge. Complications include heart failure (see *Heart Failure*, page 424), infective endocarditis, sudden death, and stroke caused by embolus.

Congenital cardiac anomalies are generally classified into three categories that may or may not cause cyanosis: obstruction to blood flow (acyanotic), increased pulmonary blood flow (acyanotic), and decreased pulmonary blood flow (cyanotic).

Types of CHD

1. Obstructive lesions (normal pulmonary blood flow)
   a. Aortic stenosis (AS)
   b. Pulmonic stenosis (PS)
   c. Coarctation of the aorta (CoA)
   d. Interrupted aortic arch (IAA)
2. Increased pulmonary blood flow
   a. Patent ductus arteriosus (PDA)
   b. Atrial septal defect (ASD)

H

    c. Ventricular septal defect (VSD)

    d. Atrioventricular canal (AVC)

    e. Partial anomalous pulmonary venous return (PAPVR)

3. Decreased pulmonary blood flow

    a. Tetralogy of Fallot (TOF)

    b. Tricuspid atresia (TA)

    c. Transposition of great arteries (TGA)

    d. Total anomalous pulmonary venous return (TAPVR)

    e. Truncus arteriosus

    f. Hypoplastic left heart syndrome (HLHS)

    g. Double outlet right ventricle (DORV)

See *Table H-1* for description and management of these conditions.

Diagnostic Evaluation

1. Chest X-ray may show cardiomegaly.
2. Electrocardiogram may show hypertrophy and axis deviation.
3. Echocardiography, Doppler study, and color flow mapping show characteristic changes.
4. Cardiac catheterization may be done for further evaluation.

Nursing Diagnoses

1, 3, 6, 15, 19, 22, 25, 51, 57, 130, 132, 135

Nursing Interventions

Monitoring

1. Assess and document growth and development parameters (including weight, length, head circumference, motor coordination, muscular development, cognitive abilities, and psychosocial skills).
2. Monitor exercise tolerance.
    a. Observe child at play and watch for squatting (characteristic position assumed by cyanotic child when resting after exertion).

(Text continues on page 422.)

TABLE H-1   Congenital Heart Abnormalities

DESCRIPTION	MANAGEMENT

Aortic stenosis

Obstruction to left ventricular outflow, causing hypertrophy, left-sided heart failure, myocardial ischemia, and pulmonary edema

- Stabilize neonate with prostaglandin E1 infusion (to maintain patent ductus arteriosus [PDA]), intubation, ventilation, and blood pressure support.
- Cardiac catheterization may be performed for balloon valvuloplasty or angioplasty.
- In older children with less severe symptoms, condition is monitored closely and exercise is restricted.
- Surgical valvotomy, commissurotomy, myotomy, or aortic valve replacement for definitive therapy.
- Lifelong endocarditis prophylaxis is given.

Pulmonic stenosis

Obstruction of blood flow from right ventricle causing hypertrophy and right-sided heart failure

- Stabilize neonate as above.
- Catheterization for balloon pulmonary valvuloplasty or Blalock-Taussig shunt between subclavian and pulmonary artery to supply pulmonary blood flow.
- In older child with less severe symptoms, monitor right ventricle pressure and function and assess exercise tolerance; intervene with balloon valvuloplasty, surgical valvotomy, or valvectomy when necessary.
- Lifelong endocarditis prophylaxis is given.

Coarctation of the aorta

Narrowing of aorta, resulting in increased pressure and workload of left ventricle and development of collateral vessels

- Stabilize neonate as above.
- Provide anticongestive therapy with digoxin and furosemide and lifelong endocarditis prophylaxis.
- Balloon angioplasty if at risk for surgery.
- Surgical intervention as soon as diagnosis made via subclavian flap repair or end-to-end anastomosis; Dacron patch may be used for older child.

(continued)

H

Congenital Heart Abnormalities *(continued)*

DESCRIPTION   **MANAGEMENT**

Patent ductus arteriosus

Blood continues to flow from the aorta to the lower pressure pulmonary artery resulting in pulmonary overcirculation and overloaded left ventricle

- Indomethacin is given to the symptomatic neonate to stimulate closure; close monitoring; diuretic therapy.
- Catheterization for coil occlusion of small PDA or other procedures for large PDA; surgery for PDA ligation.
- Endocarditis prophylaxis for 6 months following intervention.

Atrial septal defect

Blood flow from the left atrium to the lower pressure right atrium causes right ventricular overload and increased pulmonary blood flow

- Monitor and reassess for closure; anticongestive therapy with digoxin and furosemide if necessary.
- Catheterization for use of atrial occlusion device or surgery in early childhood via suturing or patch repair.
- Endocarditis prophylaxis for 6 months following intervention.

Ventricular septal defect (VSD)

Blood flow from the left ventricle to lower pressure right ventricle resulting in increased pulmonary artery pressure and pulmonary overcirculation

- Anticongestive therapy and supplemental nutrition for cases of large VSD.
- Oxygen is avoided because it is a pulmonary vasodilator.
- Catheterization for occlusion device or surgical intervention in one or two stages before first birthday, followed by endocarditis prophylaxis for 6 months.

Congenital Heart Abnormalities (continued)

DESCRIPTION	MANAGEMENT

Tetralogy of Fallot

Consists of large VSD, aortic override, pulmonary stenosis, and right ventricular hypertrophy resulting in deoxygenated blood being shunted out through aorta

- Supplemental oxygen; monitor growth and development.
- Treat hypercyanotic spells (tachypnea, irritability, cyanosis, loss of consciousness) by placing child in knee-chest position; administer oxygen, beta-adrenergic blockers, and phenylephrine (to increase systemic vascular resistance).
- One-stage surgical repair, if possible.
- Lifelong endocarditis prophylaxis and monitor for arrhythmias.

Tricuspid atresia

Absence of tricuspid valve forces blood from right atrium to flow across an atrial septal opening to left atrium and eventually into right ventricle through a ventricular septal opening

- Stabilize neonate (see aortic stenosis).
- Surgical intervention in neonate if pulmonary circulation is not balanced; two-stage repair at age 6-9 months and 18-36 months.
- Lifelong endocarditis prophylaxis.

Hypoplastic left heart

Consists of mitral stenosis or atresia, hypoplastic left ventricle, aortic stenosis or atresia, hypoplastic ascending aorta with coarctation, forcing right ventricle to support both pulmonary and systemic circulation

- Stabilize neonate (see aortic stenosis).
- Catheterization for balloon atrial septostomy to allow unrestricted flow between ventricles.
- Surgical intervention is a three-stage procedure that is palliative; cardiac transplantation is curative.
- Lifelong endocarditis prophylaxis.

H

b. Be alert for infant who may stop feeding to rest or may fall asleep during feeding. Assess pulse and respirations during feeding.

3. Monitor skin and mucous membranes for color and temperature changes.

   a. Color changes vary from pink, dusky, mottled, to cyanotic.

   b. Mucous membranes are vascular and indicate color changes quickly.

   c. Circumoral cyanosis is good indicator of central cyanosis.

4. Assess for clubbing of fingers, especially the thumbnails — may occur in cyanotic children by age 2 or 3 months.

5. Monitor for increased respiratory rate, grunting, retractions, nasal flaring, irregularity of respirations, and weak cry.

   a. Infants — respirations exceeding 60 breaths per minute indicate respiratory difficulty.

   b. Young children — respirations exceeding 40 breaths per minute indicate respiratory difficulty.

6. Monitor pulses in all extremities.

▣ **PEDIATRIC ALERT** Radial and dorsalis pedis pulses are difficult to feel in the neonate. Femoral pulsations are easily felt in the inguinal region and can be compared with brachial pulsations.

7. Monitor heart rate and rhythm and auscultate for any murmurs.

8. Monitor vital signs (apical pulse, blood pressure, respirations). Record extremity used for blood pressure measurement. Make sure that blood pressure cuff is the appropriate size for the child.

9. Monitor serum drug levels of digoxin and watch for signs of digoxin toxicity — bradycardia, nausea, vomiting, and anorexia.

10. Monitor fluid status by daily weights and intake and output; weigh diapers if necessary.

Supportive Care

1. To facilitate breathing, position the infant or child at a 45-degree angle (orthopneic position) to decrease pres-

sure of the viscera on the diaphragm and increase lung volume.

   a. Tilt the infant's or child's head back slightly.

   b. Pin diapers loosely; provide loose-fitting pajamas for older children.

   c. Feed slowly to avoid risk of aspiration. Observe for abdominal distention, which may increase respiratory difficulty.

2. Suction the nose and throat if the child is unable to adequately cough up secretions.

3. Provide oxygen therapy as indicated; offer face mask or nasal cannula to older child.

4. Restrict fluids as ordered and maintain strict intake and output.

5. To improve cardiac output, organize nursing care to provide periods of uninterrupted rest.

   a. Avoid unnecessary activities, such as frequent, complete baths and clothing changes; avoid excessive handling.

   b. Prevent excessive crying in infant; anticipate needs.

   c. Avoid temperature excesses; maintain normothermia.

6. Check heart rate for 1 minute and withhold digoxin if less than 90 beats per minute in an infant.

7. Provide diversional activities for child that require limited expenditures of energy; provide passive play.

8. Try to prevent constipation with stool softeners or glycerin suppositories as ordered.

9. Provide small, frequent feedings; provide foods easy to chew and digest.

   a. Feeding should generally be completed within 45 minutes or sooner if the infant tires. Use soft nipples with large holes.

   b. Provide foods that have high nutritional value. Include foods high in iron and potassium levels, if needed.

   c. Provide supplemental nasogastric feedings for weight gain as needed.

10. Maintain adequate hydration in the cyanotic child who is vomiting, has diarrhea or fever, or is exposed to high

H

environmental temperatures because polycythemia predisposes to thrombosis.

11. To avoid infection, prevent exposure to children with upper respiratory infections, diarrhea, wound infections, and other contagious disorders.

12. Report temperature elevation, diarrhea, vomiting, and upper respiratory symptoms promptly.

Education and Health Maintenance

1. Instruct the family in necessary measures to maintain the child's health.
   a. Complete immunization.
   b. Adequate diet and rest.
   c. Prevention and control of infections.
   d. Regular medical and dental checkups. The child should be given prophylactic antibiotics to prevent infective endocarditis when undergoing certain dental or genitourinary procedures.
   e. Regular cardiac checkups.

2. Teach the family about the cardiac defect, its treatment, and any complications.
   a. Recognize and report signs and symptoms of complications, heart failure (see page 424), infection, and dehydration.
   b. Emergency precautions related to hypoxic attacks, pulmonary edema, cardiac arrest (if appropriate).
   c. Special home care equipment, monitors, and oxygen.

3. Encourage the parents and other people (eg, teachers, peers, and so forth) to treat the child in as normal a manner as possible.

4. Initiate home nursing referral and refer the family to appropriate resources, for example, social worker, organized support groups, and the American Heart Association, *www.americanheart.org*.

HEART FAILURE

Heart failure, also known as *congestive heart failure*, is a clinical syndrome that results from the progressive process of remodeling, in which mechanical and biochemical forces alter the size, shape, and function of the ventricle's ability to pump enough oxygenated blood to meet the body's metabolic requirements. Compensatory mechanisms of increased heart rate, vasoconstriction, and hypertrophy eventually fail, leading to the characteristic syndrome of heart failure: elevated ventricular or atrial pressures, sodium and water retention, decreased cardiac output, and circulatory and pulmonary congestion. Systolic dysfunction occurs when there is difficulty emptying the left ventricle because of impaired myocardial contractility; diastolic dysfunction occurs when the left ventricle is unable to relax and fill sufficiently to accommodate enough oxygenated blood returning from the pulmonary circuit. Systolic dysfunction leads to increased systemic vascular resistance and increased afterload. Diastolic dysfunction leads to pulmonary vascular congestion.

Causes of heart failure include disorders of heart muscle that reduce cardiac contractility, such as myocarditis, cardiomyopathy, and myocardial infarction; congenital or acquired valvular disease; hypertension; and arrhythmias.

Complications of heart failure include refractory heart failure leading to death, cardiac arrhythmias, myocardial failure, pulmonary infarction, pneumonia, and emboli.

Assessment

1. Manifestations of left-sided heart failure (forward failure):
   a. Shortness of breath, dyspnea on exertion, paroxysmal nocturnal dyspnea (caused by reabsorption of dependent edema that has developed during the day), orthopnea, cough (may be dry, unproductive; often occurs at night), fatigability, insomnia, and restlessness
   b. Pulmonary edema (see page 766)
2. Manifestations of right-sided heart failure (backward failure):
   a. Edema of ankles and feet (pitting edema is obvious only after retention of at least 10 lb [4.5 kg] of fluid), unexplained weight gain, upper abdominal pain (caused by liver congestion), anorexia and nausea (caused by hepatic and visceral engorgement), nocturia, and weakness

H

    b. Distended jugular veins; pleural effusion, ascites, and other abnormal fluid accumulations

3. Physical assessment findings:
   a. Cardiomegaly—detected by displaced position of maximal impulse
   b. S_3 gallop by auscultation in systolic dysfunction; S_4 gallop in diastolic dysfunction
   c. Rapid heart rate
   d. Pulsus alternans (alternating weak and strong beats)

4. History of precipitating stressor that may have overwhelmed compensatory mechanisms:
   a. Infection, fever
   b. Surgery, anesthesia
   c. Transfusions, I.V. infusions
   d. Pregnancy
   e. Anemia, hemorrhage
   f. Physical and emotional stress
   g. Excessive sodium intake

5. Functional classification by New York Heart Association
   a. Class I: ordinary activity does not cause undue fatigue, palpitations, dyspnea, or chest pain.
   b. Class II: ordinary physical activity causes fatigue, palpitations, dyspnea, or angina.
   c. Class III: less than ordinary activities cause fatigue, palpitations, dyspnea, or angina.
   d. Class IV: symptoms occur even at rest.

Diagnostic Evaluation

1. 12-lead electrocardiogram (ECG) shows ventricular hypertrophy and strain.
2. Chest X-ray shows cardiomegaly and possible pleural effusion and pulmonary vascular congestion.
3. Echocardiography (two-dimensional) with Doppler flow study detects hypertrophy, dilation of chambers, and abnormal contraction.
4. Arterial blood gas analysis may be done to detect hypoxemia.

5. Liver function tests may be elevated with hepatic congestion; digoxin level, serum electrolytes, and kidney function tests may also be done to monitor condition.

6. Brain natruretic peptide — produced by cardiac cells as pressure increases; increasingly elevated as heart failure worsens.

7. Cardiac catheterization may be done to evaluate ischemia.

Collaborative Management
Pharmacologic Interventions

1. Diuretics eliminate excess body water and decrease ventricular pressures. A low-sodium diet and fluid restrictions complement this therapy and potassium supplements may be given.

2. Positive inotropic agents, such as digoxin, improve myocardial contractility and increase the heart's ability to pump more effectively; dopamine, dobutamine, and milrinone may be used in severe heart failure.

3. Vasodilators decrease cardiac workload by dilating peripheral vessels, thus reducing ventricular filling pressures (preload) and volumes, and reducing impedance to left ventricular ejection and thus improving stroke volume; drugs include nitrates, hydralazine, and prazosin.

4. Angiotensin-converting enzyme (ACE) inhibitors, such as captopril and enalapril, inhibit angiotensin II — a potent vasoconstrictor — thus decreasing left ventricular afterload, which reduces heart rate and cardiac workload, thereby increasing cardiac output; may also reduce remodeling of the ventricle.

5. Angiotension II receptor blockers work similar to ACE inhibitors.

6. Beta-adrenergic blockers, such as metoprolol and carvedilol, decrease myocardial workload.

7. Spironolactone, an aldosterone antagonist, reduces sodium retention, sympathetic nervous system activation, and cardiac remodeling.

8. Nesiritide is a new drug in a new class — human B-type natriuretic peptides — that works similarly to vasodila-

tors to improve symptoms in decompensated heart failure. It is administered I.V. and may cause hypotension.

Therapeutic and Surgical Interventions

The following procedures may be helpful for circulatory support in late-stage heart failure:

1. Intra-aortic balloon pump.
2. Enhanced external counterpulsation — pneumatic cuffs are wrapped around the calves, thighs, and buttocks and inflated in rhythm with the patient's ECG.
3. Continuous positive airway pressure — decreases sleep apnea, which worsens heart failure, slows ventricular remodeling, improves hemodynamics, and reduces ventricular irritability.
4. Cardiac resynchronization therapy or biventricular pacing — help improve synchronous ventricular contractions.
5. Left ventricular assist device — see page 180.
6. Partial left ventriculectomy or reduction ventriculoplasty or Batista procedure — a triangular section of the weakened heart muscle is removed to reduce ventricular wall tension.
7. Endoventricular circular patch plasty or the Dor procedure — removal of diseased portion of septum of the left ventricle with a synthetic or autologous tissue patch, thus providing a more normal shape and size of the heart, which improves hemodynamics.
8. Acorn cardiac support device — a polyester mesh, custom-fitted jacket is surgically placed on the epicardial surface, which provides diastolic support and, over time, decreases or halts remodeling.

Nursing Diagnoses

1, 6, 19, 42, 57, 108

Nursing Interventions
Monitoring

1. Monitor for lowering of systolic pressure, narrowing of pulse pressure, and pulsus alternans, indicating progression of left-sided heart failure.

> **EMERGENCY ALERT** Watch for sudden unexpected hypotension, which can cause myocardial ischemia and decrease perfusion to vital organs.

2. Auscultate heart sounds frequently, noting appearance of a new gallop or irregular heartbeat.
3. Observe for signs or symptoms of reduced peripheral tissue perfusion: cool temperature of skin, pallor, and poor capillary refill of nail beds.
4. Auscultate lung fields every 4 hours for crackles and wheezes in dependent lung fields. Mark with water-soluble ink the level on the patient's back where adventitious breath sounds are heard; use markings for comparative assessment over time.
5. Observe for increased rate of respirations (may indicate falling arterial pH) and Cheyne-Stokes respirations (may occur in elderly because of a decrease in cerebral perfusion).
6. Monitor intake and output and daily weight to determine adequate kidney perfusion and fluid balance.
7. Monitor potassium levels while patient is on diuretic therapy, and observe for symptoms of hypokalemia: fatigue, anorexia, nausea and vomiting, muscle weakness, and arrhythmias.
8. Monitor digoxin levels as indicated, and watch for signs of digoxin toxicity, including fatigue, muscle weakness, anorexia, nausea, and yellow-green halos around objects.

Supportive Care

1. Place the patient at physical and emotional rest to reduce cardiac workload. Offer careful explanations and answers to the patient's questions. Avoid situations that tend to promote anxiety or agitation.
   a. Provide rest in semirecumbent position or in armchair in air-conditioned environment. (Recumbency also promotes diuresis by improving renal perfusion.)
   b. Provide a bedside commode, to reduce effort of toileting.
   c. Assist the patient with self-care activities early in the day to avoid fatigue.

H

2. Position the patient to minimize dyspnea.
   a. Raise the head of the bed 8 to 10 inches (20 to 25 cm) to reduce venous return to the heart and lungs and alleviate pulmonary congestion.
   b. Support lower arms with pillows to reduce the burden on the shoulder muscles.
   c. Have an orthopneic patient sit on the side of the bed with feet supported by a chair; head and arms resting on an over-the-bed table; and lumbosacral area supported with pillows.
   d. Reposition the patient every 2 hours (or encourage the patient to change position frequently) to help prevent atelectasis and pneumonia.
3. Administer oxygen as directed.
4. Encourage deep-breathing exercises every 1 to 2 hours to avoid atelectasis.
5. Use pressure-reducing devices to prevent pressure sores (poor blood flow and edema increase susceptibility).
6. Offer small, frequent feedings to avoid excessive gastric filling, abdominal distention, and reduced lung capacity. To prevent hypokalemia from diuretic therapy, encourage foods or juices high in potassium, such as apricots, bananas, and tomatoes.
7. Caution patient to avoid added salt in food and foods with high sodium content.
8. Increase the patient's activities gradually. Alter or modify activities to keep within the limits of cardiac reserve.
9. Relieve nighttime anxiety and provide for rest and sleep. Give appropriate sedation to relieve insomnia and restlessness.

ALTERNATIVE INTERVENTION

Ask the patient if taking such herbal products as coenzyme Q10 or hawthorn, known for their cardiac effects. Discuss these with the health care provider; hawthorn may interact with digoxin.

Education and Health Maintenance

1. Explain the disease process to the patient; the term "failure" may have terrifying implications. Explain the difference between "heart attack" and heart failure.
2. Teach the signs and symptoms of recurrence.
   a. Advise the patient to weigh self at same time daily to detect any tendency toward fluid retention and to report a weight gain of more than 2 or 3 lb (0.9 to 1.4 kg) in a few days.
   b. Advise the patient to report swelling of ankles, feet, or abdomen; persistent cough; tiredness; loss of appetite; and frequent urination at night.
3. Review the patient's medication regimen.
   a. Teach the patient to take and record pulse rate and blood pressure.
   b. If the patient is taking oral potassium solution, it may be diluted with juice and taken after a meal.
   c. Explain major adverse effects and signs of toxicity that should be reported.
4. Review the patient's activity program. Instruct the patient to increase walking and other activities gradually, provided these do not cause fatigue and dyspnea. In general, the patient can continue at whatever activity level can be maintained without the appearance of symptoms.
5. Encourage a weight-reduction program until optimal weight is reached.
6. Advise the patient to avoid extremes in heat and cold, which increase the work of the heart; air conditioning may be essential in a hot, humid environment.
7. Urge the patient to keep regular appointments with a health care provider or clinic.
8. Educate the patient to restrict dietary sodium, as indicated.
   a. Teach the patient that sodium is present in antacids, cough remedies, laxatives, pain relievers, estrogens, and other drugs. Advise the patient to examine all labels to ascertain sodium content.
   b. Teach the patient to rinse the mouth well after using tooth cleansers and mouthwashes—some of these con-

tain large amounts of sodium. Tell patient to avoid use
of water softeners.
c. Encourage patient to use flavorings, spices, herbs, and
lemon juice.
d. If the patient is taking spironolactone or has renal disease, warn against use of salt substitutes that contain
potassium chloride.

HEART FAILURE IN CHILDREN

Heart failure, also called *congestive heart failure*, occurs when
cardiac output is inadequate to meet the metabolic demands
of the body. The heart rate increases as a compensatory mechanism to increase cardiac output, and vasoconstriction occurs
to try to maintain blood pressure. Eventually, the chronic increase in preload and afterload contribute to chamber dilation and hypertrophy, worsening heart failure.

Underlying causes of heart failure include congenital heart
disease, rheumatic heart disease, endocarditis, myocarditis,
and noncardiovascular causes, such as chronic pulmonary disease, various metabolic diseases, and anemia.

Complications of heart failure include pneumonia, pulmonary edema, pulmonary emboli, refractory heart failure,
and myocardial failure.

Assessment

1. Manifestations of left-sided heart failure (congestion occurs mainly in the lungs from backing up of blood into
pulmonary veins and capillaries)
   a. Dyspnea, tachypnea, orthopnea
   b. Nonproductive, irritative cough
   c. Retractions, nasal flaring, grunting, cyanosis
2. Manifestations of right-sided heart failure (mainly signs
and symptoms of elevated pressures and congestion in systemic veins and capillaries)
   a. Hepatomegaly or abdominal discomfort
   b. Peripheral, orbital, scrotal edema
   c. Weight gain, oliguria
3. Manifestations of impaired myocardial function in both
left- and right-sided heart failure

a. Tachycardia, restlessness
b. Weak cry, easy fatigability
c. Weak peripheral pulses, delayed capillary refill, cool extremities
d. Pallor, diaphoresis
e. Feeding difficulties or anorexia
f. S_3 gallop

Diagnostic Evaluation

1. Characteristic physical examination
2. Chest X-ray shows cardiomegaly and pulmonary congestion.

Collaborative Management

Pharmacologic Interventions

See *Heart Failure*, page 424.

Nursing Diagnoses

1, 6, 19, 42, 51, 57, 135

Nursing Interventions

Monitoring

1. Monitor digoxin levels as indicated and watch for signs of digoxin toxicity: anorexia, bradycardia, nausea, and vomiting.
2. Monitor serum electrolytes. Hypokalemia may cause weakened myocardial contractions and may precipitate digoxin toxicity.

> **EMERGENCY ALERT** Hypokalemia can contribute to the development of digoxin toxicity even in the presence of low serum digoxin levels. Hypomagnesemia and hypercalcemia may also aggravate digoxin toxicity.

3. Monitor the child's response to diuretic therapy.
4. Monitor vital signs and oxygen saturation frequently.
5. Observe for signs and symptoms of reduced peripheral tissue perfusion: cool temperature of skin, facial pallor, and poor capillary refill of nail beds.

H

6. Monitor intake and output and daily weight to determine kidney perfusion and fluid balance. Weigh diapers if necessary.

Supportive Care

1. Carefully calculate digoxin dosage *daily,* based on child's daily weight; digoxin is given to infants and children in very small amounts. Have another nurse double-check dose.

    a. Count apical pulse for 1 full minute before administering; hold dose and notify health care provider if heart rate less than 90 beats/minute or prescribed level.

    b. Check last potassium level; withhold digoxin if potassium is below 3.5 mEq/L.

DRUG ALERT Be aware of the heart rate at which the health care provider wants digoxin to be withheld (usually 90 to 100 beats per minute for infants). Also, hold digoxin if PR interval is prolonged on electrocardiogram or cardiac monitor.

    c. Report vomiting (which may occur after administration of digoxin) to determine if health care provider desires dose to be repeated.

    d. Observe for the development of premature ventricular contractions when digoxin is initially started; report this to health care provider.

2. Administer afterload-reduction medications cautiously.

    a. Check blood pressure before and after administering.

    b. Withhold medication according to blood pressure parameters ordered by health care provider.

    c. Notify health care provider if two consecutive doses are withheld.

    d. Watch for hypotension.

3. Weigh the child at least daily to observe response to diuretic therapy (same time of day, same scale, same attire).

4. Encourage foods, such as fruit juices, bananas, and tomatoes, which have a high potassium content, to prevent potassium depletion associated with many diuretics.

5. Sodium restriction is usually not needed; however, excess should be avoided.

6. Avoid excessive fluid intake; monitor intake and output.

7. Administer oxygen therapy as directed to improve tissue oxygenation and relieve respiratory distress. Place in upright position, infant seat.
8. Anticipate the infant's needs to prevent excessive crying and reduce energy expenditure.
9. Provide diversional activities for child that requires limited expenditure of energy.
10. To reduce danger of infection that could overwhelm compensatory mechanisms, avoid exposure to other children with upper respiratory infections, diarrhea, and so forth, and ensure that everyone practices good hand washing.
11. Report changes, such as temperature elevation, diarrhea, vomiting, and upper respiratory symptoms, promptly.
12. To support nutritional needs, provide high-calorie foods that the child enjoys in small amounts because he or she may have a poor appetite due to liver enlargement.
13. Feed the infant frequently and in small amounts with high-calorie formula.
    a. Supplement oral feedings with gavage feeding if the infant is unable to take an adequate amount of formula by mouth. Consider tube feeding during sleeping hours.
14. To reduce anxiety, correct misinterpretations about treatment and allow parents and child to ask questions and express concerns.

Education and Health Maintenance

1. Teach signs and symptoms of heart failure, and advise when to seek help. Teach cardiopulmonary resuscitation.
2. Teach home medications, including adverse effects, withholding parameters, and toxic effects. Reinforce need to maintain schedule.
3. Explain dietary or activity limitations, restrictions, or supplementations.
4. Explain methods to prevent infection.
5. Initiate a community health nursing referral if indicated.
6. Stress need for continued follow-up care.

HEART SURGERY

See *Cardiac Surgery*.

H

HEAT EXHAUSTION AND HEAT STROKE

Heat exhaustion is the inadequacy or the collapse of peripheral circulation caused by volume and electrolyte depletion. Untreated heat exhaustion may progress to *heat stroke*, which is a life-threatening medical emergency. A combination of hyperpyrexia (105° F [40.6° C]) and neurologic symptoms, heat stroke is caused by failure of the heat-regulating mechanisms of the body. The patient with heat stroke should be admitted to an intensive care unit; death may occur from complications, such as heart failure, cardiovascular collapse, hepatic failure, renal failure, disseminated intravascular coagulation, and rhabdomyolysis.

Assessment

1. With heat exhaustion, expect the patient to be alert without significant cardiorespiratory or neurologic compromise.
   a. Symptoms include headache, fatigue, dizziness, muscle cramping, and nausea.
   b. Skin is usually pale, ashen, and moist.
   c. Hypotension, orthostatic changes.
   d. Tachycardia, tachypnea.
   e. Temperature may be normal, slightly elevated, or as high as 104° F (40° C).
2. In heat stroke, initially, the patient may exhibit bizarre behavior or irritability. This may progress to confusion, combativeness, delirium, and coma.
   a. Other central nervous system disturbances include tremors, seizures, fixed and dilated pupils, and decerebrate or decorticate posturing.
   b. Temperature greater than 105° F [40.6° C].
   c. Hypotension, tachycardia, tachypnea.
   d. Skin may appear flushed and hot. In early heat stroke, skin may be moist, but, as heat stroke progresses, skin becomes dry as the body loses its ability to sweat.

Diagnostic Evaluation

1. Laboratory tests show hemoconcentration (increased hematocrit) and hyponatremia (if sodium depletion is the primary problem) or hypernatremia (if water depletion is the primary problem).
2. Electrocardiogram may show arrhythmias without evidence of infarction.
3. Arterial blood gas analysis shows metabolic acidosis in heat stroke.
4. As condition progresses, laboratory tests reflect renal failure and other complications.

Collaborative Management

Therapeutic Interventions

1. Rapid body cooling is treatment of choice in exhaustion or stroke. In heat stroke, the core (internal) temperature should be reduced to 102° F (39° C) as rapidly as possible.

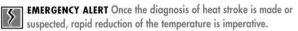 **EMERGENCY ALERT** Once the diagnosis of heat stroke is made or suspected, rapid reduction of the temperature is imperative.

2. In heat stroke, oxygen therapy is begun to supply tissue needs that are exaggerated by the hypermetabolic condition. Use 100% nonrebreather mask or intubate the patient if necessary to support a failing cardiorespiratory system.
3. Fluid replacement is begun to support circulation and facilitate cooling.
   a. Oral rehydrating solutions, such as Gatorade, may be used in heat exhaustion if patient is fully conscious and vital signs are stable.
   b. Otherwise, initial I.V. therapy is lactated Ringer's or normal saline solution until electrolyte results are confirmed.
   c. With heat stroke, at least one I.V. line should be a central line.
   d. Amount of fluid replacement is based on the patient's response and laboratory results.

H

> **GERONTOLOGIC ALERT** Vigorous fluid replacement in the elderly or those with underlying cardiovascular disease may cause pulmonary edema.

4. Cardiopulmonary resuscitation may be necessary at any time if cardiorespiratory arrest occurs.

Pharmacologic Interventions

1. Diuretics to promote diuresis.
2. Anticonvulsants to control seizures.
3. Potassium for hypokalemia and sodium bicarbonate to correct metabolic acidosis, depending on laboratory results.
4. Antipyretics are not useful in treating heat stroke. They may contribute to the complications of coagulopathy and hepatic damage.
5. Intense shivering may be controlled by diazepam (Valium). Shivering will generate heat and increase the metabolic rate.
6. Patients with depleted clotting factors may be treated with platelets or fresh frozen plasma.

Nursing Diagnoses

23, 49, 87, 88

Nursing Interventions

Monitoring

1. In heat exhaustion, monitor for changes in cardiac rhythm and vital signs. Take vital signs at least every 15 minutes until the patient is stable.
2. In heat stroke, monitor and record the core temperature continually during cooling process to avoid hypothermia; also, hyperthermia may recur spontaneously within 3 or 4 hours.
3. Monitor vital signs continuously, including cardiac rhythm, central venous pressure, blood pressure, pulse, and respiratory rate, for possible ischemia, infarction, and arrhythmias.
4. Perform neurologic assessment every 30 minutes.

5. Monitor urinary output at least hourly to detect acute tubular necrosis.
6. Monitor for development of seizures and provide a safe environment in case of seizures.

Supportive Care

1. Move the patient to a cool environment and remove his or her clothing.
2. Place the patient in a supine position with the feet slightly elevated.
3. If the patient complains of nausea or vomiting, do not give fluids by mouth.
4. Provide fans and cool sponge baths as cooling methods.
5. In heat stroke, spray tepid water on the skin as electric fans blow continuously over the patient to augment heat dissipation.
   a. Apply ice packs to neck, groin, axillae, and scalp (areas of maximal heat transfer).
   b. Soak sheets or towels in ice water and place on the patient, using fans to accelerate evaporative cooling rate.
6. If the temperature fails to decrease, initiate core cooling: iced saline lavage of stomach, cool fluid peritoneal dialysis, cool fluid bladder irrigation, or cool fluid chest irrigations.
7. Place the patient on a hypothermia blanket.
8. Discontinue active cooling when the temperature reaches 102° F (39° C). In most cases, this will reduce the chance of overcooling because the body temperature will continue to decrease after cessation of cooling.

Education and Health Maintenance

1. Advise the patient to avoid immediate reexposure to high temperatures; the patient may remain hypersensitive to high temperatures for a considerable length of time.
2. Emphasize the importance of maintaining an adequate fluid intake, wearing loose clothing, and reducing activity in hot weather.

H

3. Advise athletic patient to monitor fluid losses, replace fluids, and use a gradual approach to physical conditioning, allowing sufficient time for acclimatization.

COMMUNITY CARE CONSIDERATIONS

Identify persons at increased risk for heat exhaustion and heat stroke so preventive measures can be taken. Risk factors include underlying conditions, such as cardiovascular disease, alcohol abuse, malnutrition, diabetes, skin diseases, and major burn scarring; very young or very old age; drugs, such as anticholinergics, phenothiazines, diuretics, antihistamines, antidepressants, and beta-adrenergic blockers; and behaviors, such as working outdoors, wearing inappropriate clothing, inadequate fluid intake, and living in poor environmental conditions.

HEMOPHILIA

Hemophilia is an X-linked congenital bleeding disorder that primarily affects males with females as carriers. It is marked by a deficiency of specific blood clotting factors in the intrinsic phase of the coagulation cascade that prevents formation of a stable fibrin clot.

There are three forms: a person with hemophilia A, or classic hemophilia, has a deficiency of factor VIII (80% to 85% of patients), and a person with hemophilia B, or Christmas disease, has a deficiency of factor IX (15% to 20% of patients). Factor XI deficiency or hemophilia C is rare.

Poor clotting may result in death from exsanguination after any serious hemorrhage in intracranial, airway, or other highly vascular areas, and a number of complications can arise from bleeding into body structures (degenerative joints, intestinal obstruction, compartment syndrome). Infection with the human immunodeficiency virus (HIV) is also a complication for many who received contaminated platelet transfusions before 1985. However, as a result of advances in replacement therapy (viral inactivation of human plasma, derived factor concentrates, and new recombinant factor VIII concentrate), a normal life span is now possible for many persons with hemophilia.

Assessment

1. Hemophilia is seldom diagnosed in infancy unless excessive bleeding is observed from the umbilical cord or after circumcision. It is usually diagnosed after the child becomes active.
2. Severity of disease depends on the plasma level of the coagulation factor involved.
   a. A patient with less than 1% of normal level of coagulation factor often demonstrates severe clinical bleeding with a tendency for spontaneous bleeds.
   b. A patient in the 1% to 5% range may be free of spontaneous bleeding and may not manifest severe bleeding until after trauma.
   c. A patient in the 6% to 30% range is mildly afflicted and usually leads a normal life and bleeds only on severe injury or surgery.
3. Signs and symptoms of abnormal bleeding include:
   a. History of prolonged bleeding episodes such as after circumcision.
   b. Easily bruised.
   c. Prolonged bleeding from the mucous membranes of the nose and mouth from lacerations.
   d. Spontaneous soft tissue hematomas.
   e. Hemorrhages into the joints (hemarthrosis) — especially elbows, knees, and ankles, causing pain, swelling, limitation of movement, contractures, and atrophy of adjacent muscles.
   f. Spontaneous hematuria.
   g. GI or rectal bleeding.
   h. Black, tarry stools.
   i. Cyclic bleeding episodes may occur, with periods of slight bleeding followed by periods of severe bleeding.
   j. Intracranial hemorrhage from head trauma.

Diagnostic Evaluation

1. Prothrombin time and bleeding time: normal
2. Partial thromboplastin time: prolonged
3. Prothrombin consumption: decreased
4. Thromboplastin: increased

5. Factor VIII or IX assays: abnormal
6. Gene analysis may be done to detect carrier state, for prenatal diagnosis.

Collaborative Management
Therapeutic Interventions

1. Physical therapy may be required to prevent contractures and muscle atrophy in hemarthrosis; this includes exercise, whirlpool baths, and application of ice. Casting may be necessary.
2. Orthopedic appliances may be employed to prevent injury to affected joints and help to resolve hemorrhages.

Pharmacologic Interventions

1. Bleeding is resolved by replacement of deficient coagulation factors (VIII or IX) through I.V. administration of type-specific coagulation concentrates during bleeding episodes. No viral inactivated concentrate exists for factor XI, so fresh frozen plasma is given for hemophilia C.
2. People with mild and moderate factor VIII-deficient hemophilia may respond to desmopressin, which causes the release of factor VIII from endothelial stores.
3. Antifibrinolytics, such as aminocaproic acid and tranexamic acid, are given as adjunctive therapy for mucosal bleeding to prevent clot breakdown by salivary proteins.
4. Activated prothrombin complex concentrates that have activated factors VII, X, and IX are used when inhibitors (autoantibodies) to infused factor VIII and IX replacements have developed. In the case of factor VIII inhibitors, porcine factor VIII may also be given.

 DRUG ALERT About 20% of patients will develop an inhibitor or autoantibody to the factor replacement. Huge doses of the factor would be needed to control bleeding; however, activated prothrombin complex has been developed to bypass the inhibitor.

5. Nonsteroidal anti-inflammatory drugs (NSAIDs) are used to decrease inflammation and arthritis-like pain associated with chronic hemarthroses. NSAIDs must be used with caution because some types and higher doses inter-

fere with platelet adhesion. Short courses of corticosteroids may be necessary to relieve inflammation.
6. Research into gene therapy is being done to enable the patient to produce factor VIII or XI.

Surgical Interventions
1. Orthopedic surgery (synovectomy) may be done to remove damaged synovium in chronically involved joints, through open procedure, arthroscopy, or instillation of a radionucleotide.

Nursing Diagnoses
3, 44, 62, 67, 83, 123, 136

Nursing Interventions
Monitoring
1. Monitor vital signs; treat for shock if child becomes hypotensive.

Supportive Care
1. Provide emergency care for bleeding.
    a. Apply pressure and cold on the area for 10 to 15 minutes to allow clot formation. This should be done especially after any venipuncture or injection.
    b. Place fibrin foam or absorbable gelatin foam in the wound.
    c. Suturing and cauterization should be avoided.
2. Immobilize the affected part and elevate above the level of the heart.
3. Avoid rapid administration of coagulation factors to minimize the possibility of transfusion reaction; usually 2 or 3 mL per minute; consult package inserts. Stop the transfusion if hives, headaches, tingling, chills, flushing, or fever occur.
4. Apply fibrinolytic agents to wound for oral bleeding.
5. Keep child quiet during treatment to decrease pulse and rate of bleeding.
6. Provide protection against bleeding.
    a. Avoid taking rectal temperatures.

H

    b. Avoid injections; give medications orally whenever possible.

    c. If injection is necessary, use subcutaneous rather than intramuscular route. Apply pressure to injection site for 10 to 15 minutes, then apply pressure dressing with self-adhesive gauze.

 EMERGENCY ALERT Patients with hemophilia should not receive aspirin or compounds containing aspirin because this medication affects platelet function and prolongs bleeding time.

7. Maintain a safe environment and teach parents safety measures (eg, padding crib or bed rails, inspecting toys for sharp or rough edges, and so forth).

8. Be aware that increased pain usually means that there is continuing bleeding, and further replacement therapy may be needed.

9. Provide supportive care for hemarthrosis, immobilize in slight flexion, elevate and ice for initial treatment. If not severe, after 48 hours, begin passive range-of-motion exercises. Refer patient for a physical therapy consultation if needed.

10. Assess pain level and manage through analgesics and non-pharmacologic measures, such as hypnosis, biofeedback, relaxation techniques, and transcutaneous electrical nerve stimulation.

11. Provide emotional support to the child and family. Encourage the parents to allow the child to participate in as many normal activities as possible within the realm of safety.

Education and Health Maintenance

1. Encourage parents to educate teachers, baby-sitters, and others involved in child's care so they can respond in an emergency.

2. Advise that patient wear a medical alert bracelet.

3. Remind parents not to administer aspirin to the child.

4. Teach emergency treatment for hemorrhage.

5. Encourage regular medical and dental supervision.

    a. Preventive dental care is important. Soft-bristled or sponge-tipped toothbrushes should be used to prevent bleeding. Factor replacement therapy is necessary for extensive dental work and extractions.

b. Hepatitis B vaccine is necessary to protect against hepatitis from blood transfusions.

6. Teach healthy diet to avoid overweight, which places additional strain on the child's weight-bearing joints and predisposes to hemarthroses. Also, teach child to avoid sharp utensils, hard candy, suckers, and other foods and straws with sharp edges that may cause mucosal lacerations.

7. Assist the parents in teaching the child to understand the exact nature of the illness as early as possible. Special attention should be given to the signs of hemorrhage, and the child should be told of the need to report even the slightest bleeding to an adult immediately.

8. Provide teaching and referrals to initiate a home care program for infusion therapy at home when hemorrhage begins.

COMMUNITY CARE CONSIDERATIONS

Perform or encourage parents to perform a home-safety survey to identify potential hazards to the hemophiliac child, such as cluttered furniture the child may bump into, sharp edges on furniture or other objects, loose rugs that promote falls, slippery tub or floor surfaces, rocks or holes in backyard, or concrete play areas.

9. Advise family that genetic counseling and family planning are available for parents and adolescent patients.

10. Educate regarding hepatitis B and C and HIV disease, and risks of treatment.

11. For additional information and support, refer to National Hemophilia Foundation, *www.hemophilia.org.*

HEMORRHOIDS AND OTHER ANORECTAL CONDITIONS

Hemorrhoids are vascular masses that protrude into the lumen of the lower rectum or perianal area. They result when increased intra-abdominal pressure causes engorgement in the vascular tissue lining the anal canal. Loosening of vessels from surrounding connective tissue occurs with protrusion or prolapse into the anal canal. There are two main types of hemorrhoids: external hemorrhoids appear outside the external sphincter, and internal hemorrhoids appear above the internal sphincter. When blood within the hemorrhoids becomes clotted because of obstruction, the hemorrhoids are referred to as being *thrombosed*.

Predisposing factors include pregnancy, prolonged sitting or standing, straining at stool, chronic constipation or diarrhea, anal infection, rectal surgery or episiotomy, genetic predisposition, alcoholism, portal hypertension (cirrhosis), coughing, sneezing, or vomiting, loss of muscle tone attributable to old age, and anal intercourse. Complications include hemorrhage, anemia, incontinence of stool, and strangulation.

Hemorrhoids are the most common of a variety of anorectal disorders.

Assessment
1. Pain (more so with external hemorrhoids), sensation of incomplete fecal evacuation, constipation, and anal itching. Sudden rectal pain may occur if external hemorrhoids are thrombosed.
2. Bleeding may occur during defecation; bright red blood on stool caused by injury of mucosa covering hemorrhoid.
3. Visible and palpable masses at anal area.

Diagnostic Evaluation
1. External examination with anoscope or proctoscope shows single or multiple hemorrhoids.
2. Barium enema or colonoscopy rules out more serious colonic lesions causing rectal bleeding such as polyps.

Collaborative Management
Therapeutic Interventions
1. High-fiber diet to keep stools soft
2. Warm sitz baths to ease pain and combat swelling
3. Reduction of prolapsed external hemorrhoid manually

Pharmacologic Interventions

1. Stool softeners to keep stools soft and relieve symptoms.
2. Topical creams, suppositories or other preparations such as Anusol, Preparation H, and witch-hazel compresses to reduce itching and provide comfort.
3. Oral analgesics may be needed.

Surgical Interventions

1. Injection of sclerosing solutions to produce scar tissue and decrease prolapse is an office procedure.
2. Cryodestruction (freezing) of hemorrhoids is an office procedure.
3. Surgery may be indicated in presence of prolonged bleeding, disabling pain, intolerable itching, and general unrelieved discomfort.
    a. Anoscopy with ligation with a rubber band is treatment of choice. Internal hemorrhoid is encircled at the base. After a period, the hemorrhoid sloughs away.
    b. Dilatation of the anal canal and lower rectum may be performed under general anesthesia. This procedure is not advocated for patients whose main complaints are prolapse or incontinence. It is also not recommended for aging patients with weak sphincters.
    c. An acutely thrombosed hemorrhoid may be incised to remove clot.
    d. Hemorrhoidectomy may be used to remove internal and external hemorrhoids.

Nursing Diagnoses

2, 16, 24

H

Nursing Interventions

Supportive Care

1. After thrombosis or surgery, assist with frequent repositioning using pillow support for comfort.
2. Provide analgesics, warm sitz baths, or warm compresses to reduce pain and inflammation.
3. Apply witch-hazel dressing to perianal area or anal creams or suppositories, if ordered, to relieve discomfort.

4. Observe anal area postoperatively for drainage and bleeding; report if excessive.
5. Administer stool softener or laxative to assist with bowel movements soon after surgery, to reduce risk of stricture.

Education and Health Maintenance

1. Teach anal hygiene and measures to control moisture to prevent itching.
2. Encourage the patient to exercise regularly, follow a high-fiber diet, and have an adequate fluid intake (8 to 10 glasses per day) to avoid straining and constipation, which predisposes to hemorrhoid formation.
3. Discourage regular use of laxatives; firm, soft stools dilate the anal canal and decrease stricture formation after surgery.
4. Tell patient to expect a foul-smelling discharge for 7 to 10 days after cryodestruction.
5. Determine the patient's normal bowel habits and identify predisposing factors to educate patient about preventing recurrence of symptoms.

HEPATITIS, VIRAL

Hepatitis is a viral infection of the liver associated with a broad spectrum of clinical manifestations from asymptomatic infection through icteric hepatitis to hepatic necrosis. Currently, five forms of viral hepatitis have been identified, as follows:

Type A hepatitis (HAV) is caused by an RNA virus of the enterovirus family. It spreads primarily by the fecal–oral route, usually through the ingestion of infected food or liquids. It may also be spread by person-to-person contact and, rarely, by blood transfusion. Type A hepatitis occurs worldwide, especially in areas with overcrowding and poor sanitation.

Type B hepatitis (HBV) is caused by a double-shelled virus containing DNA. Type B hepatitis spreads primarily through blood (percutaneous and permucosal route). It can also spread by way of saliva, breast-feeding, or sexual activity (blood, semen, saliva, or vaginal secretions). Male homosexuals are at high risk for infection. After acute infection, 10% of patients progress on to carrier status or develop chronic hepatitis. Worldwide, HBV is the main cause of cirrhosis and hepatocellular carcinoma.

Type C hepatitis (HCV), formerly called non-A, non-B hepatitis, usually spreads through blood or blood product transfusion, usually from asymptomatic blood donors. It may also be transmitted through unsterile piercing or tattooing tools or dyes. It commonly affects I.V. drug users and renal dialysis patients and personnel. HCV is the most common form of posttransfusion hepatitis. Approximately 50% of cases develop chronic liver disease, and at least 20% progress to cirrhosis.

Type D hepatitis (HDV), or delta hepatitis, is caused by a defective RNA virus that requires the presence of hepatitis B—specifically, hepatitis B surface antigen (HBsAg)—to replicate. Hence, HDV occurs along with HBV or may superinfect a chronic HBV carrier, and cannot outlast a hepatitis B infection. HDV cases in the United States occur primarily in I.V. drug abusers or those who have had multiple blood transfusions, but the highest incidence is in the Mediterranean, Middle East, and South America. HDV causes approximately 50% of cases of fulminant hepatitis, which has an extremely high mortality rate.

Type E hepatitis (HEV) is caused by a nonenveloped, single-strand RNA virus. It is transmitted by the fecal—oral route but is hard to detect because it is inconsistently shed in the feces. Its occurrence is primarily in India, Africa, Asia, or Central America. Not much is known about HEV.

Fulminant hepatitis is a rare but severe complication of hepatitis, which may require liver transplantation.

H

Assessment

1. Type A hepatitis (incubation period, 3 to 5 weeks)
   a. Prodromal symptoms: fatigue, anorexia, malaise, headache, low-grade fever, nausea, vomiting. Highly contagious at this time, usually 2 weeks before onset of jaundice.
   b. Icteric phase: jaundice, tea-colored urine, clay-colored stools, right upper quadrant pain and tenderness.
   c. Symptoms often milder in children.

2. Type B hepatitis (incubation period, 2 to 5 months)
   a. Prodromal symptoms (insidious onset): fatigue, anorexia, transient fever, abdominal discomfort, nausea, vomiting, headache.
   b. May also have myalgias, photophobia, arthritis, angioedema, urticaria, maculopapular rash, vasculitis.
   c. Icteric phase occurs 1 week to 2 months after onset of symptoms.
3. Type C hepatitis (incubation period, 6 weeks to several months)
   a. Similar to HBV but less severe.
4. Type D hepatitis (unclear incubation period)
   a. Similar to HBV but more severe.
5. Obtain a patient history. Ask about I.V. drug use, blood transfusions, contact with infected persons (including sexual activity), travel to endemic areas, and ingestion of possible contaminated food or water to help determine cause of hepatitis.

Diagnostic Evaluation

1. All forms of hepatitis: elevated serum transferase levels (aspartate aminotransferase, alanine aminotransferase); may have abnormal clotting tests.
2. HAV: radioimmunoassay detects immunoglobulin M (IgM) antibodies to hepatitis A virus in the acute phase.
3. HBV: radioimmunoassays detect hepatitis B surface antigen (HBsAg), antibody to hepatitis B core antigen (anti-HBc), anti-HBsAg in various stages of hepatitis B infection. (See *Figure H-2*.)
4. HCV: hepatitis C antibody may not be detected for 3 to 6 months after onset of illness (used for screening); polymerase chain reaction testing evaluates viral activity.
5. HDV: anti-delta antibodies in the presence of HBsAg, or detection of IgM in acute disease and IgG in chronic disease.
6. Hepatitis E antigen (with HCV ruled out).
7. If indicated, prepare the patient for liver biopsy to detect chronic active disease, track progression, and evaluate response to therapy.

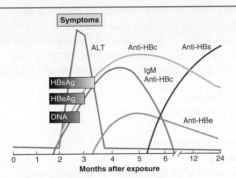

FIGURE H-2 Time course for clinical, laboratory, and virologic features of acute hepatitis B infection. ALT: alanine aminotransferase; anti-HBc: antibody to hepatitis B core antigen; anti-HBe: antibody to hepatitis Be antigen; anti-HBs: antibody to hepatitis B surface antigen; HBeAg: hepatitis Be antigen; HBsAg: hepatitis B surface antigen.

Collaborative Management

Therapeutic Interventions

1. Provide adequate rest according to the patient's level of fatigue.
2. Hospitalization for protracted nausea and vomiting or life-threatening complications. Universal and enteric precautions are maintained.
3. Provide small, frequent feeding of a high-calorie, low-fat diet. Proteins are restricted when the liver cannot metabolize protein by-products, as demonstrated by symptoms.
4. After jaundice has cleared, encourage gradual increase in physical activity. This may require many months.

Pharmacologic Interventions

1. Vitamin K injected subcutaneously (S.C.) if prothrombin time is prolonged.
2. I.V. fluid and electrolyte replacements as indicated.
3. Antiemetic for nausea.

H

4. Long-term interferon therapy in combination with oral ribavirin may produce remission in HCV patients. Peginterferon alfa-2b is a long-acting preparation given S.C. once per week, and ribavirin is taken twice daily.
5. Antiviral treatment is being investigated for HBV.

Nursing Diagnoses
1, 24, 35, 51, 92, 93, 123, 136

Nursing Interventions
Monitoring
1. Monitor hydration through intake and output.
2. Monitor prothrombin time and for signs of bleeding.
3. In severe infection, monitor for signs of encephalopathy — lethargy, confusion, excitability, and asterixis (irregular flapping of forcibly dorsiflexed outstretched hands).

Supportive Care
1. Encourage the patient to eat meals in a sitting position to reduce pressure on the liver.
2. Encourage pleasing meals in an environment with minimal noxious stimuli (odors, noise, interruptions).
3. Administer or teach self-administration of antiemetics as prescribed. Avoid phenothiazines such as chlorpromazine, which have a cholestatic effect and may cause or worsen jaundice.
4. Encourage frequent oral fluids or administer I.V. fluids, as indicated.
5. Encourage rest during symptomatic phase, according to level of fatigue.
6. Encourage diversional activities when recovery and convalescence are prolonged.
7. Encourage gradual resumption of activities and mild exercise during convalescent period.
8. Stress importance of proper public and home sanitation and proper preparation and dispensation of foods.
9. Encourage specific protection for close contacts.
   a. Immune globulin as soon as possible to household contacts of HAV patients

b. Hepatitis B immune globulin as soon as possible to blood or body fluid contacts of HBV patients, followed by HBV vaccine series

10. Explain precautions about transmission and prevention of transmission to others to the patient and family.
    a. Good hand washing and hygiene after using bathroom
    b. Avoidance of sexual activity (especially for HBV) until free of HBsAg
    c. Avoidance of sharing needles, eating utensils, and toothbrushes to prevent blood or body fluid contact (especially for HBV)

11. Report all cases of hepatitis to public health officials.

12. Warn the patient to avoid trauma that may cause bruising; limit invasive procedures, if possible, and maintain adequate pressure on needle-stick sites.

Education and Health Maintenance

1. Identify individuals or groups at high risk, such as I.V. drug abusers or their sexual contacts, and those living in crowded conditions with potentially poor hygiene or sanitation, and teach them proper hygiene, waste disposal, food preparation, use of condoms, not sharing needles, and other preventive measures.

2. Encourage vaccination for HBV with series of three shots (at 0, 1, and 6 months) for high-risk adults, such as health care workers or institutionalized patients, and for all children at birth or during adolescence.

3. Instruct all patients who have received a blood transfusion to avoid donating blood for 6 months (the incubation period of HBV). After hepatitis infection, blood should not be given if the patient is a hepatitis B carrier or was infected with hepatitis C.

4. Stress the need to follow precautions with blood and secretions until the patient is deemed free of HBsAg.

5. Explain to HBV carriers that their blood and secretions will remain infectious.

6. Emphasize that most hepatitis is self-limiting, but follow-up is needed for liver function tests.

HERNIA, ABDOMINAL

A *hernia* is a protrusion of an organ, tissue, or structure through the wall of the cavity in which it is normally contained. It is often called a "rupture." *Abdominal hernias* are likely to occur with congenital or acquired structural weakness or trauma to the abdominal wall, which yields to increased intra-abdominal pressure from heavy lifting, obesity, pregnancy, straining, coughing, or proximity to a tumor. Many types of abdominal hernias occur, classified by site.

In an *inguinal hernia* (most common), viscera protrudes into the inguinal canal at the point where the spermatic cord emerges in the male, and the round ligament in the female. Through this opening, an indirect inguinal hernia extends down the inguinal canal and even into the scrotum or the labia. A direct inguinal hernia protrudes through the posterior inguinal wall.

A *femoral hernia* occurs where the femoral artery passes into the femoral canal, and appears below the inguinal ligament below the groin.

An *umbilical hernia* results from failure of the umbilical orifice to close. It occurs most often in obese women, in children, and in patients with increased intra-abdominal pressure from cirrhosis and ascites.

A *ventral* or *incisional hernia* occurs through the abdominal wall because of weakness, possibly because of a poorly healed surgical incision.

A *parastomal hernia* may protrude through the fascial defect around a stoma and into the subcutaneous tissue.

Hernias may be reducible, where the protruding mass can be placed back into the abdominal cavity; irreducible, where the mass cannot be replaced; incarcerated, where intestinal flow is completely obstructed; or strangulated, where blood flow and intestinal flow are completely obstructed. Complications of hernias are bowel obstruction and recurrence of hernia.

PEDIATRIC ALERT Umbilical hernias are more common in black infants and in those with Down syndrome and hypothyroidism. Because spontaneous closure is common, surgery is deferred until the child is age 3 or 4 or if the opening is greater than 2 inches (5 cm).

Inguinal hernias are more common in premature male infants due to the delayed closing of the processus vaginalis, the route by which the testicles descend.

Assessment
1. Hernia bulges when the patient stands or strains (Valsalva maneuver) and disappears when supine
2. Discomfort or pulling sensation
3. Strangulation — severe pain, vomiting, swelling of hernial sac, rebound tenderness, fever

Diagnostic Evaluation
1. Abdominal X-ray shows abnormally high level of gas in the bowel or bowel obstruction.
2. Complete blood count and serum electrolytes may show hemoconcentration (increased hematocrit), increased white blood cells, and electrolyte imbalance, if strangulation occurs.

Collaborative Management
Therapeutic Interventions
1. If hernia is reducible and patient is a poor surgical candidate, a truss (pad and belt) may be positioned snugly over the area to prevent viscera from entering the hernial sac. A similar appliance is available for a reducible parastomal hernia.

Surgical Interventions
1. Surgery is recommended to correct the defect and prevent strangulation. Procedures include:
   a. Herniorrhaphy — removal of hernial sac; contents replaced into the abdomen; layers of muscle and fascia sutured; may be done by way of laparoscopy as outpatient
   b. Hernioplasty — involves reinforcement of suturing (often with mesh), for extensive hernia repair
   c. Bowel resection for ischemic bowel along with hernia repair in strangulated hernia

H

Nursing Diagnoses
3, 24, 122, 135

Nursing Interventions
Also see *Gastrointestinal or Abdominal Surgery,* page 381.

Monitoring
1. Monitor for signs of bowel obstruction or strangulation: abdominal distention, change in bowel sounds (increased, short, high-pitched sounds, then silent abdomen), pain, fever, nausea, and vomiting.
2. Monitor postoperative patient for signs of infection: fever, chills, malaise, and diaphoresis.

Supportive Care
1. If ordered, fit the patient with truss or belt when hernia is reduced. Advise the patient to wear truss under clothing, and to apply it before getting out of bed in the morning, when hernia is reduced.
2. Position the patient for comfort to reduce pressure on hernia such as semi-Fowler's position.
3. Immediately report signs of hernial incarceration or strangulation. Keep patient on NPO and insert nasogastric tube as directed to reduce intra-abdominal pressure above the obstruction and relieve pressure on herniated sac.
4. Postoperatively, have the patient splint the incision site with hand or pillow when coughing to lessen pain and protect site from increased intra-abdominal pressure.
5. Administer analgesics, as ordered.
6. Check scrotum or labia for swelling after inguinal hernia repair, and apply ice and other comfort measures.
7. Encourage ambulation as soon as permitted.
8. Advise patient that difficulty in urinating is common after surgery; encourage fluids to promote elimination. Catheterize patient, if necessary.
9. Check dressing for drainage and incision for redness and swelling; report signs of infection.
10. Administer antibiotics, as directed.

Education and Health Maintenance

1. Using bed rest, intermittent ice packs, and scrotal elevation, teach the patient to reduce scrotal edema expected for 24 to 48 hours after repair of an inguinal hernia.
2. Teach the patient to monitor and report continued difficulty in voiding or signs of infection: pain, drainage from incision, and temperature elevation.
3. Advise patient to avoid heavy lifting for 4 to 6 weeks. Athletics and extremes of exertion should be avoided for 8 to 12 weeks postoperatively, per health care provider instructions.

HERNIA, HIATAL

A *hiatal hernia* is a protrusion of part of the stomach through the hiatus of the diaphragm and into the thoracic cavity. There are two types of hiatal hernias (see Figure H-3). In a *sliding hernia*, the upper stomach and gastroesophageal junction move upward into the chest and slide in and out of the thorax (most common); in a *paraesophageal hernia* (rolling hernia), part of the greater curvature of the stomach rolls through the diaphragmatic defect next to the gastroesophageal junction. Hiatal hernia results from muscle weakening caused by aging or other conditions, such as esophageal carcinoma, trauma, or after certain surgical procedures. Treatment can prevent incarceration of the involved portion of the stomach in the thorax, which constricts gastric blood supply.

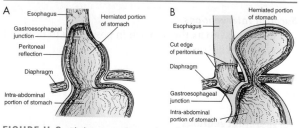

FIGURE H-3 Sliding esophageal and paraesophageal hernias. (**A**) Sliding esophageal hernia. (**B**) Paraesophageal hernia.

Assessment

1. May be asymptomatic.
2. Patient may report feeling of fullness or chest pain resembling angina.
3. Sliding hernia may cause dysphagia, heartburn (with or without regurgitation of gastric contents into the mouth), or retrosternal or substernal chest pain from gastric reflux.
4. Severe pain or shock may result from incarceration of stomach in thoracic cavity with paraesophageal hernia.

Diagnostic Evaluation

1. Upper GI series with barium contrast shows outline of hernia in esophagus.
2. Endoscopy visualizes defect and rules out other disorders, such as tumors or esophagitis.

Collaborative Management

Therapeutic Interventions

1. Elevate head of bed 6 to 8 inches (15 to 20 cm) to reduce nighttime reflux.

Pharmacologic Interventions

1. Antacids neutralize gastric acid and reduce pain.
2. If patient has esophagitis, give histamine-2 receptor antagonist (such as cimetidine or ranitidine) or proton pump inhibitor (such as omeprazole) to decrease acid secretion.

Surgical Interventions

1. Gastropexy to fix the stomach in position is indicated if symptoms are severe.

Nursing Diagnoses

13, 24, 92

Nursing Interventions

Also see *Gastrointestinal or Abdominal Surgery*, page 381.

Supportive Care and Education

1. Advise the patient about preventing reflux of gastric contents into esophagus by:
   a. Eating smaller meals to reduce stomach bulk
   b. Avoiding stimulation of gastric secretions by omitting caffeine and alcohol, which may intensify symptoms
   c. Refraining from smoking, which stimulates gastric acid secretion
   d. Avoiding fatty foods, which promote reflux and delay gastric emptying
   e. Refraining from lying down for at least 1 hour after meals
   f. Losing weight, if obese
   g. Avoiding bending from the waist or wearing tight-fitting clothes
2. Advise the patient to report to health care facility immediately at onset of acute chest pain — may indicate incarceration of paraesophageal hernia.
3. Reassure patient that he or she is not having a heart attack, but all instances of chest pain should be taken seriously and reported to the patient's health care provider.

HERNIATED INTERVERTEBRAL DISC (RUPTURED DISC)

A *herniated intervertebral disc* results from protrusion of the nucleus of the disc into the annulus (fibrous ring around the disc), with subsequent compression of nerve roots. Herniation may result from trauma, degeneration attributable to aging, and congenital malformations. It may take from months to years to develop, producing acute and chronic symptoms. Most herniations occur in the lumbar and lumbosacral region, but they can occur in any portion of the vertebral column (see *Figure H-4*, page 460). If untreated, the disorder may cause permanent neurologic dysfunction (weakness, numbness).

Assessment

1. Cervical herniation
   a. Pain and stiffness in the head, neck, top of shoulders, scapular region, and upper extremities

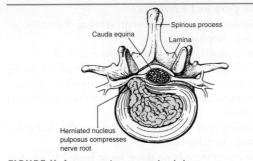

Spinous process

Cauda equina

Lamina

Herniated nucleus
pulposus compresses
nerve root

FIGURE H-4 Ruptured intervertebral disc.

  b. Paresthesia, numbness, and weakness of upper extremities
  2. Lumbar and lumbosacral herniation
    a. Low back pain with radiation into buttocks and down leg.
    b. Positive straight leg raising test—radiation of pain below the knee when the leg is elevated at 45 degrees from supine position (indicates lumbosacral nerve root involvement). Pain at a lesser elevation may indicate a worsening condition.
    c. Varying degrees of sensory and motor dysfunction (weakness and asymmetric reflexes).
    d. Postural deformity of the lumbar spine may also be evident.

EMERGENCY ALERT Cauda equina syndrome is an emergency caused by compression of the cauda equina (a group of spinal nerves extending just below the end of the spinal cord proper). Symptoms include bowel, bladder, or sexual dysfunction, or saddle area numbness. It must be recognized early, and compression must be relieved to prevent permanent loss of these functions.

Diagnostic Evaluation
  1. CT scan or MRI identifies herniated disc.
  2. Myelography determines the level of disc herniation.
  3. Electromyography localizes spinal nerve involvement.

Collaborative Management
Therapeutic and Pharmacologic Interventions
1. Conservative therapy for 4 to 6 weeks, if no progressive neurologic deficit
   a. Anti-inflammatory drugs, such as ibuprofen or prednisone.
   b. Opioids may be necessary during acute phase.
   c. Muscle relaxants to relieve associated spasm.
   d. Bed rest on a firm mattress for first 2 days followed by physical therapy.
   e. Heat or ice application to affected area.
2. Complimentary and alternative therapies, such as acupuncture, manipulative therapy, and homeopathic remedies.

ALTERNATIVE INTERVENTION

Acupuncture, chiropractic manipulation, homeopathic remedies, and other complementary therapies may be used with some success for herniated disc symptoms; however, the patient should notify the health care provider of worsening neurologic deficit.

Surgical Interventions
1. Surgery is indicated if there is progression of neurologic deficit or failure to improve with conservative management. Procedures include discectomy, laminectomy, spinal fusion, microdiskectomy, or percutaneous discectomy; hemilaminectomy with excision of the involved disc is the procedure of choice for lumbar disc disease.
2. Chemonucleolysis for lumbar disc herniation is a possible alternative to surgery. It involves injection of chymopapain to dissolve the nucleus pulposus and relieve pressure on the nerve root. May cause severe complications, including transverse myelitis, allergic reactions, and persistent muscle spasm.

H

Nursing Diagnoses
3, 24, 62, 136

Nursing Interventions

Also see *Orthopedic Surgery*, page 680.

Monitoring

1. Assess the patient's response to conservative pain control regimen.
2. Inspect the skin several times per day while patient is on bed rest for redness and evidence of pressure ulcer development.
3. Monitor for progression of motor, sensory, or reflex deficits.
4. If the patient has had surgery, monitor and report any sudden reappearance of radicular pain (may indicate nerve root compression from slipping of bone graft or collapsing of disc space) or burning back pain radiating to buttocks (may indicate arachnoiditis).
5. Monitor vital signs and surgical dressings frequently because hemorrhage is a possible complication.

Supportive Care

1. Be sure to administer or teach self-administration of anti-inflammatory drugs with food or antacid to prevent GI upset.
2. Use bed boards under mattress and maintain bed rest except for short trips to bathroom; maintain the patient in supine or low Fowler's position or in side-lying position with slight knee flexion and a pillow between the knees.
3. Apply heat or ice massage to affected area of back as desired.
4. Encourage relaxation techniques, such as imagery and progressive muscle relaxation.
5. Properly fit and use a cervical collar or traction (if ordered) to maintain alignment.
6. Provide massage and good skin care to pressure-prone areas.
7. Encourage range-of-motion exercises while in bed.
8. Encourage compliance with physical therapy treatments to prevent contractures and maintain rehabilitation potential.
9. If the patient is undergoing surgery:

a. Document baseline neurologic assessment to compare after surgery.

b. Provide routine postoperative care, including frequent assessment of vital signs and neurologic function, frequent turning, coughing and deep breathing, pain control, and ambulation on the first postoperative day.

c. Reinforce surgical dressing and maintain patency of blood drainage system, if in place.

d. Assess movement and sensation of extremities and report any new deficits.

e. Administer analgesics and corticosteroid medications to control pain from surgical incision and resultant swelling around nerve roots and spinal cord.

f. Maintain cervical collar if ordered.

g. Position for comfort with small pillow under head (but avoid extreme neck flexion) and pillow under knees to take pressure off lower back. Logroll patient for position changes.

h. If the patient has had cervical surgery, assess for hoarseness, indicating recurrent laryngeal nerve injury; may cause ineffective cough. Watch for dysphagia caused by edema of the esophagus, and provide blenderized diet.

i. Provide fluids as soon as gag reflex and bowel sounds are noted.

j. Make sure that the patient voids after surgery; report urinary retention.

k. Encourage ambulation as soon as possible by having the patient lie on side close to edge of bed and push up with arms while swinging legs toward floor in one motion; alternate walking with bed rest, discourage sitting.

Education and Health Maintenance

1. Teach the patient the importance of complying with bed rest, use of cervical collar, and other conservative measures to reduce inflammation and heal disc herniation.

H

2. Tell the patient who has had a cervical disc herniation to avoid extreme flexion, extension, or rotation of the neck and to keep the head in a neutral position during sleep.

3. Encourage the patient to do stretching and strengthening exercises of extremities and abdomen after acute symptoms have subsided and start an aerobic program such as walking.

4. Teach the patient about proper body mechanics to prevent recurrence. Leg and abdominal muscles should always be used rather than the back. Knees should be bent on lifting, and load should be carried close to midtrunk.

5. Encourage follow-up with physical therapy as indicated for reconditioning and work hardening.

6. Instruct the patient to report any changes in neurologic function or recurrence of radicular pain.

7. Encourage good nutrition, avoidance of obesity, smoking cessation, and proper rest to reduce risk of recurrence.

HERPES ZOSTER

Herpes zoster (shingles) is an inflammatory skin condition in which the varicella zoster virus produces a painful vesicular eruption along the nerve tracks leading from one or more dorsal root ganglia. After a primary chickenpox infection, the virus persists in a dormant state in the dorsal ganglia. The virus may become active again in later years, either spontaneously or in association with immunosuppression, to cause the eruptions.

Herpes zoster may progress to chronic pain syndrome (postherpetic neuralgia), characterized by constant aching and burning pain or intermittent lancinating pain or hyperesthesia of affected skin after healing. Ophthalmic complications include involvement of the ophthalmic branch of the trigeminal nerve with keratitis, uveitis, corneal ulceration and, possibly, blindness. Facial and auditory nerves may become involved, with hearing deficits, vertigo, and facial weakness. If the virus spreads to the viscera, it may cause pneumonitis, esophagitis, enterocolitis, myocarditis, or pancreatitis.

Assessment

1. Eruption may be accompanied or preceded by fever, malaise, headache, and pain. Pain may be burning, lancinating, stabbing, or aching.
2. Inflammation is usually unilateral, involving the cranial, cervical, thoracic, lumbar, or sacral nerves in a bandlike configuration.
3. After 3 or 4 days, patches of grouped vesicles appear on erythematous, edematous skin.
4. Early vesicles contain serum; these later rupture and form crusts. Scarring usually does not occur unless the vesicles are deep and involve the dermis.
5. Patient may have a painful eye if ophthalmic branch of the facial nerve is involved.
6. Lesions usually resolve in 2 or 3 weeks.

EMERGENCY ALERT A susceptible person can acquire chickenpox if he or she comes in contact with the infective vesicular fluid of a zoster patient. A person with a previous history of chickenpox is immune and, thus, not at risk from infection after exposure to zoster patients. Varicella zoster virus may be a life-threatening condition to the patient who is immunosuppressed, is receiving cytotoxic chemotherapy, or is a bone marrow transplant recipient.

Diagnostic Evaluation

1. Culture of varicella zoster virus from lesions or detection by fluorescent antibody techniques, including monoclonal antibodies (MicroTrak).

Collaborative Management
Pharmacologic Interventions

1. Antivirals, such as acyclovir or valacyclovir, interfere with viral replication; may be used orally in all cases but especially for treatment of immunosuppressed or debilitated patients (I.V. route). Antivirals are most effective if started within 48 hours of onset of symptoms.
2. Corticosteroids *early* in illness for severe herpes zoster if symptomatic measures fail; given for anti-inflammatory effect and relief of pain (controversial).

H

3. Aspirin, acetaminophen, nonsteroidal anti-inflammatory drugs, or opioids to manage pain during the acute stage; good pain control may reduce the incidence of postherpetic neuralgia.

Nursing Diagnoses
3, 13, 63, 135

Nursing Interventions
Supportive Care
1. Assess the patient's level of discomfort and medicate as prescribed.
2. Teach the patient to apply wet dressings and calamine lotion for soothing and cooling effect on inflamed tissue.
3. Encourage diversional activities.
4. Teach relaxation techniques, such as deep breathing, progressive muscle relaxation, and imagery, to help control pain.
5. Apply antibacterial ointments (after acute stage) as prescribed to soften and separate adherent crusts and prevent secondary infection.

Education and Health Maintenance
1. Teach the patient to use proper hand-washing techniques to avoid spreading herpes zoster virus.
2. Advise the patient not to open the blisters to avoid secondary infection and scarring.
3. Reassure the patient that shingles is a viral infection of the nerves; "nervousness" does not cause shingles.
4. A caregiver may be required to assist with dressings and meals. In older persons, the pain is more pronounced and incapacitating. Dysesthesia and skin hypersensitivity are distressing.

HIGH BLOOD PRESSURE
See *Hypertension.*

HIP ARTHROPLASTY
See *Arthroplasty and Total Joint Replacement.*

HIP DYSPLASIA, DEVELOPMENTAL

Developmental dysplasia of the hip (formerly known as *congenital hip dysplasia* or *congenital dislocation of the hip*) refers to conditions involving abnormalities of the developing hip, including subluxation, dislocation, and dysplasia of the hip joint. With dysplasia, the acetabulum is shallow or sloping instead of cup shaped; with dislocation, there is no contact between the femoral head and the acetabulum; with subluxation, the femoral head maintains contact, but is not fully within the hip joint.

The cause of hip dysplasia is unknown. Risk factors include twin births, firstborns, ligamentous laxity of fetal joints, breech presentation, family history, in utero restrictions to fetal movement, and postnatal swaddling in which the hips are adducted and extended. Dysplasia may be unilateral or bilateral (20% of patients); unstable dysplasia occurs in 10 per 100 live births, whereas complete dislocation is rarer, occurring in 1 per 100 live births. Females are eight times more commonly affected than males.

Unless treated early, hip dysplasia may lead to lost range of motion, early osteoarthritis, and recurrent dislocation or unstable hip. Avascular necrosis may occur after hip reduction.

Assessment
1. Asymmetry of thigh folds or gluteal folds
2. Limitation in abduction of the hip
3. Leg length inequality
4. Ortolani's sign and positive Barlow's test (see *Figure H-5*, page 468)
5. Abnormal gait pattern: Trendelenburg's sign — downward tilt of the pelvis on the affected side
6. Pain in the older child

Diagnostic Evaluation
1. X-rays of the cartilaginous femoral head; it is difficult to visualize in the neonate. As the child ages, the ossification center can be better viewed, and the efficacy of this

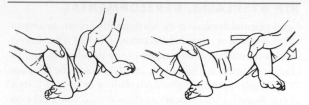

FIGURE H-5 Adduction and depression of the femur dislocates hip (Barlow's test), and a "click" is felt when dislocated hip is abducted and relocated (Ortolani's sign).

examination increases. It can be useful in ruling out other pelvic, spinal, and femoral anomalies.
2. Ultrasound examination by a skilled technician is highly accurate in diagnosis in children younger than age 6 months.

Collaborative Management
Therapeutic Interventions
1. Use of Pavlik harness in children age 6 to 9 months.
2. Once standing, change to abduction brace until hip joint is normal.
3. If successful, closed reduction and traction.
4. Follow-up until skeletal maturity.

Surgical Interventions
1. Closed reduction under general anesthesia and placement of the child in a hip-spica cast is the preferred treatment for dislocation (age 18 to 36 months).
2. Open reduction and osteotomy with hip-spica cast and abduction bracing may be necessary.
3. Surgery is also necessary for older children with subluxation and dysplasia.

Nursing Diagnoses
22, 62, 133, 134, 136

Nursing Interventions
Monitoring
1. Assess the skin around the edges of the cast or brace daily for signs of skin irritation.
2. Assess neurovascular status frequently after application of cast or brace, then daily to detect compromise. Watch for discoloration or cyanosis, impaired movement, loss of sensation, edema, absent pulses, and pain disproportionate to injury or not relieved by analgesics.

Supportive Care
1. Encourage parents to avoid swaddling the infant, and to hold the child with hips abducted.
2. Reassure parents that effective outcome depends on early intervention and compliance.
3. Prepare the child for casting or immobilization procedure by showing materials to be used and describing procedure in age-appropriate terms.
4. Assess the need for pain medication, sedation, distraction techniques, or restraint, and administer as ordered.
5. Assist with application of the immobilization device as indicated.
6. If a cast or plaster splint was applied, help facilitate drying in proper position.
   a. Keep the child or affected part still until thoroughly dry.
   b. Support the curves of the cast with pillows.
   c. Avoid excessive handling of the cast, and use palms of hands when handling it.
7. Try to prevent skin breakdown by padding edges of device and telling child to avoid placing anything inside the device.
8. If child is in a hip-spica cast, prevent skin breakdown from frequent soiling around perineum.
   a. Line cast edges around perineum with a plastic covering to prevent soiling of cast.
   b. Use a fracture bedpan or urinal to facilitate toileting.

H

c. If child is not toilet trained, use a small diaper or perineal pad tucked under the edges of the cast, covered by a larger diaper, and change diapers as soon as soiled.

d. Wash the perineum frequently and dry thoroughly.

e. If the cast is synthetic and becomes soiled, clean it with a damp cloth and small amount of detergent.

9. Stimulate child with games and activities to exercise upper body and feet as able.

10. Turn the child frequently and encourage ambulation as able. Support the head and legs to reposition.

11. Encourage deep-breathing exercises at intervals to prevent atelectasis and hypostatic pneumonia. For example, children can blow whistles, party favors, soap bubbles, and cotton balls across the table as appropriate.

12. Encourage fluids and high-fiber diet to prevent constipation.

13. Prepare the child for cast removal by describing the sensation (warmth, vibration) and demonstrating the cast cutter by touching it lightly to your palm.

14. Provide and teach care of skin after cast, brace, or splint removal.

a. Wash with warm, soapy water.

b. Soak the area daily with warm water to facilitate removal of desquamated skin and secretions.

c. Advise child to avoid scratching; instead, apply lotion or oil to relieve itching.

d. Encourage exercise as prescribed to regain strength and function.

Education and Health Maintenance

1. If the child will be treated with an abduction splint, explain its purpose and demonstrate its application and removal to the parents.

a. Instruct the parents regarding if and when the device can be removed.

b. Instruct the parents to check fit of abduction splint at every diaper change.

c. Allow the parents to demonstrate their ability to properly place the device on the child.

    d. Follow with written instructions whenever possible.
2. Teach child or parents to look for and report redness, skin breakdown, localized pain, or foul odor that may indicate open wounds under device.
3. Encourage regular follow-up evaluations and regular health maintenance visits.

HIRSCHSPRUNG'S DISEASE

Hirschsprung's disease (congenital aganglionic megacolon) is the congenital absence of or arrested development of parasympathetic ganglion cells in the intestinal wall, usually in the distal colon. Symptoms are related to chronic intestinal obstruction and usually appear shortly after birth but may not be recognized until later in childhood or (rarely) in adulthood.

In this disorder, the lack of colorectal innervation inhibits peristalsis, and the affected portion of intestine becomes spastic and contracted. The internal rectal sphincter fails to relax, which prevents evacuation of fecal material and gas and causes severe abdominal distention and constipation. The most common site affected is the rectosigmoid colon (short segment disease). Less commonly, the upper descending colon and possibly the transverse colon are affected (long segment disease).

Other congenital disorders are common with Hirschsprung's disease. Complications of untreated disease include enterocolitis (a major cause of death); hydroureter or hydronephrosis; and cecal perforation.

Assessment

1. In the neonate:
   a. No meconium passed
   b. Vomiting—bile-stained or fecal
   c. Abdominal distention
   d. Constipation—occurs in all patients
   e. Overflow-type diarrhea
   f. Anorexia, poor feeding
   g. Temporary relief of symptoms with enema

H

PEDIATRIC ALERT Suspect Hirschsprung's disease in any infant who fails to pass meconium within the first 24 hours and requires repeated rectal stimulation to induce bowel movements.

2. Older child (symptoms not prominent at birth):
    a. History of obstipation at birth
    b. Distention of abdomen — progressive enlarging
    c. Thin abdominal wall with observable peristaltic activity
    d. Constipation — no fecal soiling; relieved temporarily with enema
    e. Stool appears ribbonlike, fluidlike, or in pellet form
    f. Failure to grow — loss of subcutaneous fat; appears malnourished; perhaps has stunted growth
    g. Anemia

Diagnostic Evaluation

1. Rectal examination demonstrates absence of fecal material in long segment disease; in short segment disease, rectal impaction may be present and, when the finger is removed, it may cause a rush of stool as the obstruction is temporarily relieved.
2. X-rays show severe gaseous distention of the bowel, with absence of gas in the rectum.
3. Radiopaque markers, when ingested, measure intestinal transit time. Children with short segment disease retain the markers in the rectum for long periods.
4. Barium enema shows narrowed intestine proximal to anus and dilated intestine proximal to narrow segment.
5. Rectal biopsy may be done to demonstrate absent or reduced number of ganglion nerve cells, and confirm diagnosis.
6. Anorectal manometry may be done to record the reflex response of anal sphincter; requires cooperation of the child.
7. Ultrasonogram may be done to demonstrate dilated colon.

Collaborative Management
Therapeutic Interventions
1. Enemas or colonic irrigation with physiologic saline solution.
2. Older child whose symptoms are chronic but not severe may be treated with isotonic enemas, stool softeners, and a low-residue diet.

Pharmacologic Interventions
1. Treatment of enterocolitis with I.V. or oral antibiotics, and colonic irrigation, followed by surgical decompression.

Surgical Interventions
1. Initially, a colostomy or ileostomy is performed to decompress intestine, divert fecal stream, and rest the normal bowel.
2. Definitive surgery is done to remove the nonfunctioning bowel segment with various pull-through procedures (abdominoperineal, endorectal, or rectorectal).

> **EMERGENCY ALERT** Enterocolitis is a potentially life-threatening event. Notify health care provider immediately if change in abdominal distention occurs (whether preoperatively or postoperatively) especially if accompanied by feces, diarrhea, vomiting, and lethargy.

3. Surgery may be delayed until child is age 9 to 12 months or until child weighs 15 to 20 lb (6.5 to 9 kg).

Nursing Diagnoses
3, 16, 51, 75, 104, 135, 136

Nursing Interventions
Monitoring
Preoperative
1. Monitor for respiratory difficulty that may result from abdominal distention; watch for rapid shallow respirations, cyanosis, and sternal retractions.
2. Monitor abdominal girths, for the presence of fluid waves, for increasing distention after enemas, and discrepancy

H

in output from enemas, which may indicate intestinal obstruction.

3. Monitor hydration and nutritional status through intake and output, weights, and skin turgor.
4. Monitor characteristics of stool in older children being treated medically.

Postoperative

1. Monitor vital signs and respiratory status closely. To avoid injuring rectal mucosa, take axillary or external ear temperature.
2. Monitor for proper functioning of colostomy, if present.
   a. Note drainage from colostomy — characteristics, frequency, fecal material, or liquid drainage.
   b. Note abdominal distention.
   c. Measure fluid loss from colostomy to help guide fluid replacement.
3. Monitor and report signs of obstruction (may be due to peritonitis, paralytic ileus, handling of bowel, or swelling): no output from colostomy, abdominal tenderness, irritability, vomiting, and increased temperature.
4. Monitor for respiratory distress, infection, hemorrhage, and shock.

Supportive Care
Preoperative

1. Assist in emptying the bowel by giving repeated enemas and colonic irrigations.
   a. Procedure for enema in an infant is similar to that in an adult, except that less fluid and pressure are used.
   b. Warm physiologic saline solution should be used for irrigations. Tap water may result in water intoxication.
   c. Record all intake and output of irrigant and drainage. Report marked discrepancies in retention or loss of fluid.
2. If abdominal distention is not relieved by enemas, discomfort is significant, and rectal tube insertion fails to give relief, consult doctor for a nasogastric (NG) tube.

a. Note drainage from NG tube, and chart characteristics.
b. Check for patency; saline irrigations may be requested. Carefully record input and output.
c. Give frequent mouth care.
d. Alternate nares when changing NG tube every 24 hours, and use minimal amount of tape to prevent skin irritation.

3. Offer pacifier for infant to suck if on parenteral fluids.
4. Encourage parents to hold and rock infant.
5. Maintain position of comfort with head elevated. Offer soothing stimulation (eg, music, touch, play therapy).
6. Offer small, frequent feedings. Low-residue diet will aid in keeping stools soft.
7. Administer parenteral nutrition if feeding causes additional discomfort because of distention and nausea.
8. For older child, provide demonstration and written and verbal instructions to family for saline enema administration and use of stool softeners.

Postoperative

1. Change wound dressing using sterile technique.
2. Prevent wound contamination from diaper.
3. Prevent perianal and anal excoriation by thorough cleaning and use of ointments after the infant soils (postoperative stools can number 7 to 10 per day).
4. Use careful hand-washing technique.
5. Report any wound redness, swelling or drainage, evisceration, or dehiscence immediately.
6. Suction oral secretions frequently to prevent infection of the tracheobronchial tree and lungs.
7. In older child, encourage frequent coughing and deep breathing to maintain respiratory status.
8. Allow the infant to cry for short periods to prevent atelectasis.
9. Change position of infant frequently to increase circulation and allow for aeration of all lung areas.
10. Maintain patency of NG tube immediately postoperatively.

H

a. Watch for increasing abdominal distention; measure abdominal girth.
b. Measure fluid loss because amount will affect fluid replacement.
11. Maintain NPO status until bowel sounds return and the bowel is ready for feedings as determined by health care provider.
12. Provide frequent oral hygiene while on NPO status.
13. Administer fluids to maintain hydration and replace lost electrolytes. Begin oral feedings as ordered.
14. Support the parents when teaching them to care for their child's colostomy. Reassure parents that colostomy will not cause delay in the child's normal development.
15. Initiate community nurse referral to help the parents care for the child at home, and obtain necessary equipment.

Education and Health Maintenance

1. Involve the entire family in teaching colostomy care to enhance acceptance of body change of the child.
   a. An older child should become totally responsible for his or her own colostomy care.
   b. Procedures need to be thoroughly understood and practiced, including preparation of skin, application of collecting appliance, care of appliance, and control of odor.
2. Teach parents to recognize and report signs of stomal complications: ribbonlike stool, diarrhea, failure of evacuation of stool or flatus, and bleeding.
3. Prepare parents and older child for colostomy closure as appropriate.
4. Review gastrostomy feeding techniques as well as procedures for care and dilation of anus as indicated.
5. Allow the parents to learn and practice these procedures long before the infant is to be discharged.
6. Emphasize the importance of treating the child as normally as possible to prevent behavior problems later.
7. Teach about good nutrition — diet needs to be understood by parents before discharge. Involve the dietitian as necessary.

8. Encourage close medical follow-up for Hirschsprung's disease, as well as general growth and development and immunizations.
9. Refer parents to helping agencies such as United Ostomy Association, Inc., *www.uoa.org*.

H.I.V. DISEASE AND A.I.D.S.

Acquired immunodeficiency syndrome (AIDS) is defined as the most severe form of a continuum of illnesses associated with infection by the *human immunodeficiency virus* (HIV). AIDS causes a slow degeneration of humoral and cell-mediated immune functions, eventually — if untreated — opening the way to the opportunistic infections and malignancies that characterize this disease.

HIV disease refers to the entire course of HIV infection from asymptomatic infection and early symptoms to fully developed AIDS.

HIV is transmitted by injection of blood or blood components, sexual contact (vaginal, anal, and oral intercourse), and perinatally from an infected mother to the child. High-risk groups for HIV transmission include homosexual or bisexual men, I.V. drug users, transfusion and blood product recipients (before 1985), heterosexual contacts of HIV-positive individuals, and neonates of HIV-positive mothers.

Most persons infected with HIV show no immediate signs of illness. However, some experience a brief flulike illness referred to as primary HIV infection, in which the immune system is compromised by a sudden decrease in CD4 T-helper lymphocytes for a brief period. Three to six months after initial infection, the body develops enough antibodies to HIV to produce a positive serologic test (seroconversion). Staging of HIV disease is based on the medical findings and the CD4 count (see *Figure H-6*, page 478). AIDS-related diseases develop years after HIV exposure without treatment.

Assessment

1. Persistent cough with and without sputum production, shortness of breath, chest pain, fever resulting from *Pneumocystis carinii* pneumonia (most common), bacterial pneu-

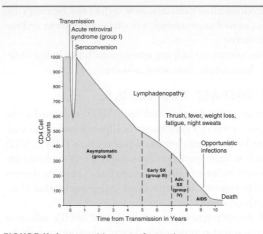

FIGURE H-6 Natural history of HIV disease.

monia, *Mycobacterium tuberculosis*, disseminated *Mycobacterium avium* complex, cytomegalovirus (CMV), *Histoplasma*, Kaposi's sarcoma, *Cryptococcus*, *Legionella*, and other pathogens.

2. Diarrhea, weight loss, anorexia, abdominal cramping, rectal urgency (tenesmus) result from enteric pathogens including *Salmonella*, *Shigella*, *Campylobacter*, *Entamoeba histolytica*, *Clostridium difficile*, CMV, M. *avium* complex, and others.

3. Oral manifestations include:

   a. Appearance of oral lesions, white plaques on oral mucosa and angular cheilitis from *Candida albicans* of mouth and esophagus.

   b. Vesicles with ulceration from herpes simplex virus.

   c. White thickened lesions on lateral margins of tongue from hairy leukoplakia.

   d. Oral warts attributable to human papillomavirus and associated gingivitis.

   e. Periodontitis progressing to gingival necrosis.

   f. Aphthous ulcers of unclear etiology.

4. Cognitive, motor, and behavioral symptoms (AIDS dementia complex or HIV encephalopathy) are demonstrated by mental slowing, impaired memory and concentration, loss of balance, lower extremity weakness, ataxia, apathy, and social withdrawal; may result from central nervous system (CNS) toxoplasmosis, cryptococcal meningitis, herpes virus infections, CMV (causing retinopathy and blindness), and CNS lymphoma.

5. Malignancies include:
   a. Kaposi's sarcoma (aggressive tumor involving skin, lymph nodes, GI tract, and lungs).
   b. Non-Hodgkin's lymphoma (see page 598).
   c. Cervical cancer (see page 120).

Diagnostic Evaluation

1. Enzyme-linked immunosorbent assay (ELISA) detects antibody to HIV; Western blot test — confirms a positive result on ELISA test
   a. Once infected with HIV, it can take the body up to 12 weeks to develop enough antibody to HIV for the ELISA result to be positive (seroconversion). Risk of false-negative test if evaluated early.
   b. Occasionally, a sample that shows reactivity by ELISA may give an indeterminate result by Western blot. The cause of an indeterminate result may be early HIV seroconversion or false-positive in a low-risk person. The test should be repeated every 2 or 3 months until Western blot becomes positive or infection with HIV is no longer suspected.
   c. There is a variety of rapid HIV screening tests using blood samples with results available in about 20 minutes. There is also a urine screening test and a test using saliva (sample is sent back to company and result is available in about 3 days). Positive results from any of these tests need to be confirmed by ELISA.

2. Lymphocyte panel shows decreased CD4 count. Normal CD4 count is 800 to 1,000/mm^3.

3. A complete blood count (CBC) may show anemia and a low white blood cell count.

4. Diagnostic procedures, such as biopsies, imaging studies, and cultures to confirm presence of indicator disease (eg, *Pneumocystis carinii* pneumonia, candidiasis of esophagus, Kaposi's sarcoma).

5. Viral load testing (quantitative HIV RNA) greater than 750,000 indicates greater viremia; undetectable viral load indicates less than 50 copies/mL of the virus in the blood, which is the goal of antiviral therapy.

Collaborative Management
Therapeutic Interventions
1. Treatment of reversible illnesses
2. Nutritional support
3. Palliation of pain
4. Dental management
5. Evaluation and management of psychological and social aspects of AIDS
6. Treatment to relieve symptoms (cough, diarrhea)
7. Treatment of depression

Pharmacologic Interventions
1. Antiviral therapy using combination of three drugs from at least two classes known as highly active antiretroviral therapy to try to decrease viral load to undetectable level (see *Table H-2*).
2. Therapy started if acute retroviral syndrome or known seroconversion within past 6 months; signs and symptoms of indicator diseases, such as oral thrush; or CD4 count of 200 to 350/mm^3 or less or viral load greater than 55,000 copies/mL

 DRUG ALERT If a patient on antiretroviral therapy develops abdominal pain or vomiting, notify the health care provider. A serious adverse effect, such as lactic acidosis, hypersensitivity, or pancreatitis, must be ruled out.

3. *P. carinii* pneumonia prophylaxis: trimethoprim-sulfamethoxazole (SM/TMP), dapsone, atovaquone, aerosolized pentamidine
   a. Therapy is started at a CD4 cell count of 200/mm^3 or less.

| **TABLE H-2** | **Highly Active Antiretroviral Therapy (HAART)** |

DRUG	**ADVERSE REACTIONS**

Nucleoside reverse transcriptase inhibitors (NRTIs)

• Zidovudine (AZT, Retrovir) • Didanosine (ddI, Videx) • Zalcitabine (ddC, Hivid) • Abacavir (Ziagen) • Stavudine (d4T, Zerit) • Lamivudine (3TC, Epivir) • Tenofovir (Viread) • Emtricitabine (Fmtriva)	• All NRTIs: Nausea, fatigue (initial month on drug), anemia, myalgias, leukopenia, granulocytopenia • Peripheral neuropathy may occur with didanosine and stavudine. Pancreatitis may occur with didanosine and zalcitabine. Hypersensitivity reaction occurs in 5% of patients treated with abacavir. Adverse reactions are rare with lamivudine, tenofovir, and emtricitabine. • Tenofovir should be used cautiously in patients with renal compromise.

Nonnucleoside reverse transcriptase inhibitors (NNRTIs)

• Nevirapine (Viramune) • Efavirenz (Sustiva) • Delavirdine (Rescriptor)	• All NNRTIs: Nausea, diarrhea, headache, dizziness, asthenia, rash, liver dysfunction. Efavirenz may cause strange dreams in the first 2 weeks.

Protease inhibitors (PIs)

• Indinavir (Crixivan) • Saquinavir (Fortovase; also as Invirase, hard capsules) • Nelfinavir (Viracept) • Ritonavir (Norvir) • Lopinavir with ritonavir (Kaletra) • Amprenavir (Agenerase) • Atazanavir (Reyataz)	• All PIs: Nausea, vomiting, diarrhea, inflammation at injection site. • All PIs may also cause long-term adverse effects in varying degrees, including drug-induced hepatitis, hyperlipidemia, insulin resistance.

Entry inhibitors

• Enfuvirtide (T-20, Fuzeon)	• Nausea, fatigue, diarrhea, inflammation at injection site; rarely peripheral neuropathy, pancreatitis, hypersensitivity, liver abnormality.

H

b. Decreases frequency, morbidity, and mortality of *P. carinii* infection.

4. Toxoplasmosis prophylaxis with SM/TMP when CD4 cell count is less than $100/mm^3$.

5. Tuberculosis screening yearly and immunization for pneumococcal pneumonia (every 5 years) and influenza (yearly) if CD4 cell count is greater than $100/mm^3$.

6. Vaccine studies are in progress.

Nursing Diagnoses
4, 5, 27, 28, 35, 43, 48, 51, 60, 69, 75, 86, 135

Nursing Interventions
Monitoring

1. Monitor nutritional status by weighing patient periodically; recording calorie count; taking anthropometric measurements; and evaluating serum albumin and prealbumin, blood urea nitrogen, protein, and transferrin levels.

2. Monitor CBC every 4 weeks for 3 months, then every 2 or 3 months if stable for severe anemia caused by zidovudine therapy.

3. Monitor CBC, liver function tests, and amylase monthly for 3 months; then bimonthly, if stable, for complications of didanosine (ddI) therapy.

4. Monitor for sore throat, which progresses to dysphagia or odynophagia (pain on swallowing) or persistent heartburn — suggestive of esophageal candidiasis.

5. Tell the patient to monitor stools for blood and try to determine if bleeding is before, with, or after bowel movement to help determine source of bleeding.

6. Monitor intake and output; assess skin and mucous membranes for poor turgor and dryness, indicating dehydration.

7. Assess for depressive or suicidal symptoms — AIDS represents a significant risk for suicide.

8. Assess mental status daily; monitor for changes in behavior, memory, concentration ability, and motor system dysfunction — the patient may become vegetative and

unable to ambulate. Onset of dementia is usually insidious but may be abrupt, precipitated by acute infection.

9. Frequently assess for chills, fever, tachycardia, and tachypnea and watch for sudden change in respiratory function — the patient may be developing a secondary infection.

Supportive Care

1. Never assume the family or loved ones know that the patient is HIV positive.

2. Always ask the patient who knows of the HIV status. Confidentiality must be maintained. However, encourage the patient to share the diagnosis to decrease isolation. Offer to be with the patient when sharing the diagnosis; role-playing before you meet with family or loved ones can be helpful.

3. Offer counseling services, especially when AIDS is initially diagnosed and as the patient enters terminal phase of illness.

4. Obtain social service referral for available resources and services, such as housekeeping, food shopping, support groups, cancer counseling agencies, hospice, and Social Security Administration.

COMMUNITY CARE CONSIDERATIONS

If the patient is homebound, there are many agencies that are HIV specific and that provide home visits for services, such as legal counseling, hospice care, respite care, housekeeping, food preparation, care for pets, and companionship. Assist the patient or significant other to locate these agencies in the community.

H

5. Encourage the patient to arrange personal business. Anticipate necessity of advance directives, guardianship, durable power of attorney for health care, informed consent, and so forth, because cognitive deterioration may make it impossible for the patient to act on his or her own behalf at later date.

6. Assure the patient of palliative care, pain control, and help with anxiety and depression as disease progresses.

7. Follow universal precautions for all patients; use strict enteric precautions for diarrhea.

8. Administer and teach meticulous skin care, especially to the perianal area if having diarrhea.

9. Employ aseptic techniques when performing invasive procedures.

10. Consult with dietitian to develop strategies for nutritional therapy. Be aware that antiviral therapy and other drugs cause nausea and anorexia.
   a. Administer or teach the patient to administer prescribed antiemetic 30 minutes before meals.
   b. Encourage small, frequent meals because these may make best use of limited absorptive capacity.

11. For the patient with oral or esophageal pain from *Candida* esophagitis, herpetic esophagitis, or endotracheal Kaposi's sarcoma:
   a. Avoid highly seasoned or acidic foods.
   b. Offer fluids and blenderized foods to minimize chewing and ease swallowing.
   c. Suggest nutrition—dense supplements, such as instant breakfast drinks or protein-fortified drinks—for home care.

12. Discourage excessive alcohol intake—has immunosuppressive effect.

13. Prepare the patient for enteral or parenteral feedings when necessary.

14. Administer or teach the patient to administer prescribed antifungal mouth rinses or lozenges for oral candidiasis or acyclovir (oral or I.V.) for herpes simplex.

15. Perform or encourage oral care two to three times per day.

16. Advise the patient to eliminate caffeine, alcohol, dairy products, foods high in fats, fresh juices, and acidic juices if diarrhea occurs. Drink liquids at room temperature.

17. Advise the patient to report increased weakness, dizziness, and continuing weight loss.

18. Reorient the patient to time and place frequently if dementia occurs; use structured care plan.

19. Provide for patient safety: bed rails up; call signal available; and things within the patient's reach.
20. Provide supplemental oxygen as indicated for pneumonia.
21. Encourage smoking cessation to enhance pulmonary ciliary defense.
22. Administer saline nebulization to induce sputum collection for culture and sensitivity.
    a. Wear mask and gloves during sputum collection.
    b. Instruct the patient to brush tongue, buccal surfaces, teeth, and palate with water before sputum induction — to decrease contamination of specimen.
    c. Instruct the patient to gargle and rinse mouth with tap water.

ALTERNATIVE INTERVENTION

St. John's wort is used by many people for depression; however, it interacts with indinavir, so it should not be used by AIDS patients on this drug. Grapefruit juice should also be avoided by people on protease inhibitors.

Education and Health Maintenance

1. Indicate that the patient is a source of infection to others and should take actions to prevent transmission (no exchange of blood or body fluids). Casual contact, such as holding hands and hugging, will not cause transmission, however.
2. Encourage the patient to disclose HIV status to sex and needle-sharing partners.
3. Emphasize to HIV-positive woman that children should be tested for HIV.
4. Discuss family planning with HIV-positive woman; the rate of transmission from mother to neonate is approximately 30%. If she does not want more children, discuss birth control options.
5. Establish a primary care provider for the patient and encourage the need for regular follow-up care; should in-

H

clude yearly Pap smears for women and routine dental and eye examinations.

6. Teach the patient to recognize and report important symptoms:
   a. Change in pattern or magnitude of temperature elevation
   b. Development of a new focal complaint: skin spots, sore mouth, or diarrhea

DRUG ALERT If the patient decides to stop antiretroviral therapy, he or she must stop all medications at once to prevent resistance, which could compromise treatment options for the future.

7. Emphasize to injection drug users that continued use may expose them to additional infection and such infections may activate viral replication.
8. Encourage the patient to modify sexual behaviors for safer sex:
   a. Use latex male condoms.
   b. If the man will not use a condom, the woman should use a female condom.
   c. Refrain from oral and anal sex.
   d. Consult various AIDS action groups for additional safe-sex techniques.
9. If the patient is a substance abuser:
   a. Enroll in a treatment program.
   b. Do not share needles ("works").
   c. If no access to unused needles, clean needles before using with a bleach and water solution.
10. Teach the patient to optimize immune system function by sound dietary practices, exercise, and regular periods of sleep.
11. Refer the patient to resources such as National AIDS Hotline, *www.ashastd.org/nah*.

H.I.V. DISEASE AND A.I.D.S. IN CHILDREN

Infection with the human immunodeficiency virus (HIV) in infants, children, and adolescents is represented by a continuum of immunologic and clinical manifestations ranging from no to severe suppression of the immune system and associated symptomatology. HIV is transmitted through sexual contact, contaminated blood products, perinatally, or through breast milk. Perinatal transmission has greatly decreased in the United States due to drug treatment for the woman and neonate. Progressive destruction of the immune system leads to increased incidence of serious bacterial infections; opportunistic infections; *Pneumocystis carinii* pneumonia (PCP), esophageal candidiasis, and *Mycobacterium avium* infection; aggressive viral infections; cancers; and wasting syndromes.

🔲 **PEDIATRIC ALERT** Because of the potential to transmit HIV through breast milk, bottle-feeding is recommended for all infants born to HIV-infected mothers.

Assessment

1. Generalized lymphadenopathy, especially in less common sites, such as epitrochlear and axillary nodes
2. Persistent or recurrent oral candidiasis
3. Failure to thrive
4. Developmental delays or loss of previously acquired milestones
5. Hepatomegaly and splenomegaly
6. Persistent diarrhea
7. Parotitis (enlarged parotid glands)
8. Unexplained anemia, thrombocytopenia
9. Unexplained cardiac and kidney disease
10. Recurrent serious bacterial infections

Diagnostic Evaluation

1. Infants younger than age 18 months:
   a. Two separate HIV tests by culture, polymerase chain reaction (PCR) or p24 antigen are positive, or
   b. The child is HIV antibody-positive and meets criteria for diagnosis of acquired immunodeficiency syndrome (AIDS)
2. In infants who have been born to HIV-positive mothers, testing should be done during the first 48 hours of life, at 1 or 2 months, and again at 3 to 6 months.
   a. Umbilical cord blood should not be used.

H

   b. HIV infection is never diagnosed based on a single laboratory result; it must be confirmed on a second specimen.
3. Children older than age 18 months:
   a. Repeated HIV antibody tests by reactive enzyme immunoassay and confirmatory tests are positive, or
   b. Same as 1a
4. A child is considered HIV negative when two or more negative PCR or HIV culture test results were obtained after age 1 month and again when the child was older than age 4 months.

Collaborative Management
Therapeutic Interventions
1. Nutritional support
2. Evaluation and treatment of developmental delays
3. Support for child and family in the areas of disclosure issues, parental guilt, and long-term care (including caretakers for child in the event of maternal death)

Pharmacologic Interventions
1. Initiation of PCP prophylaxis when indicated by low CD4 counts based on age with trimethoprim-sulfamethoxazole (first choice), pentamidine, atovaquone, or dapsone.
2. Antiretroviral therapy for all infants younger than age 1 year who have HIV infection, regardless of clinical manifestations, immune parameters, or viral load. For children older than age 1 year, antiretroviral therapy for those with clinical symptoms or evidence of immune suppression or HIV PCR level (viral load). Combination therapy is recommended with nucleoside reverse transcriptase inhibitors, non-nucleoside reverse transcriptase inhibitors, protease inhibitors, and fusion inhibitors.
3. Use of I.V. immune globulin in infected children who have had two or more serious bacterial infections within 1 year or for the treatment of HIV-related thrombocytopenia.
4. Antifungal drugs, such as nystatin or fluconazole, for oral candidiasis.

5. Use of antivirals such as acyclovir or ganciclovir for recurrent viral infections.
6. Prompt treatment of additional infections.

Nursing Diagnoses
10, 14, 27, 28, 43, 44, 48, 49, 51, 60, 79, 92, 97, 107, 111, 132, 135, 152

Nursing Interventions
Monitoring
1. Monitor absolute neutrophil counts, which may drop with antiretroviral therapy and predispose to infection.
2. Monitor hydration status if diarrhea is present (see *Assessment of degree of dehydration*, page 297).
3. Monitor for fever and report any core temperature over 101° F (38.3° C).
4. Monitor growth parameters and developmental milestones.

Supportive Care
1. Prevent secondary infections by maintaining a clean environment, employing aseptic technique for invasive procedures, providing good skin care, and encouraging proper food preparation.
2. Encourage high-calorie, nutritious diet in small, frequent feedings.
3. Provide fluids and blenderized foods and avoid highly seasoned or acidic foods if oral candidiasis is present.
4. If diarrhea is present, provide careful skin care of anal area, including application of barrier cream. Use strict enteric precautions.
5. While child is febrile, institute comfort measures, such as sponge baths, dry linens, and antipyretics, as ordered.
6. Assess the family's coping skills and provide emotional and situational support. Refer to social services and community resources.
7. Allow the family to use denial as a protective mechanism, if needed, but help them move toward setting realistic goals and expectations for the child.

H

8. Accept that some families may not be able to disclose the nature of the disease to their child, even after much support and guidance. Answer the child's questions as honestly as possible within parental constraints.

9. Assess the child for pain and administer analgesics as indicated. Allay fear by explaining all procedures in age-appropriate terms and providing distraction techniques.

Education and Health Maintenance

1. Teach standard precautions. Gloves are recommended when handling any potentially contaminated body fluids but are not considered necessary for routine diaper changes unless bloody diarrhea or hematuria exists.

2. Offer guidance as to how to initiate discussion of the child's HIV status with school and day-care settings. It is not currently required that schools and day-care settings be advised, but it is advantageous in that this alerts the school to notify parents in the event of a breakout of infectious disease (such as varicella) that could pose a threat to the HIV-infected child.

3. Advise reporting fever over 101° F (38.3° C) and other signs of illness.

4. Encourage all recommended immunizations according to pediatric schedule including the new pneumococcal conjugate vaccine and yearly influenza (after age 6 months). Live virus vaccines should not be administered; the only exception is the measles, mumps, rubella vaccine, which is recommended if the child is not severely immunocompromised.

5. For more information, refer to National AIDS Hotline, *www.ashastd.org/nah*.

HODGKIN'S DISEASE

Hodgkin's disease is a malignant lymphoma of the reticuloendothelial system that results in an accumulation of dysfunctional, immature lymphoid-derived cells. The disease generally spreads by lymphatic channels, involving lymph nodes, spleen, and ultimately (through the bloodstream) to extralymphatic sites, such as GI tract, bone marrow, skin, upper air passages, and other organs. Hodgkin's disease is most common in patients ages 20 to 40 and in those older than age 60. Its cause is unknown.

Hodgkin's disease is more readily cured than other lymphomas. More than one treatment strategy is available, and combinations of radiation and chemotherapy are commonly used. Depending on location and extent of malignancy, complications may include splenomegaly, hepatomegaly, thromboembolism, and spinal cord compression.

Assessment

1. Fatigue, fever, chills, night sweats, painless swelling of lymph nodes (generally unilateral), pruritus, weight loss
2. Wide variety of symptoms may occur if there is pulmonary involvement, superior vena cava obstruction, hepatic or bone involvement, and involvement of other structures

Diagnostic Evaluation

Tests are used to determine extent of disease involvement before treatment and repeated periodically to assess response to treatment.

1. Lymph node biopsy detects characteristic Reed-Sternberg giant cell, helping to confirm diagnosis.
2. Complete blood count and bone marrow aspiration and biopsy determine whether there is bone marrow involvement.
3. X-rays, CT scan, and MRI detect deep nodal involvement.
4. Lymphangiogram detects size and location of deep nodes involved, including abdominal nodes, which may not be readily seen by CT scan.
5. Liver function tests and liver biopsy determine hepatic involvement.
6. Gallium-67 scan detects areas of active disease; determines aggressiveness of disease.
7. Surgical staging (laparotomy with splenectomy, liver biopsy, multiple lymph node biopsies) may be done in selected patients.

H

Collaborative Management
Therapeutic Interventions
1. Radiation therapy is treatment of choice for localized disease.
   a. Areas of body where lymph node chains are located can generally tolerate high radiation doses.
   b. Vital organs are protected during radiation treatments with lead shielding.

Pharmacologic Interventions
1. Chemotherapy may be used in combination with radiation.
   a. Initial treatment often begins with a specific four-drug regimen known as MOPP (Mustargen, Oncovin, procarbazine, and prednisone).
   b. Three or four drugs may be given in intermittent or cyclical courses, with periods of treatment to allow recovery from toxicities.

Surgical Interventions
1. Autologous or allogeneic bone marrow or stem cell transplantation

Nursing Diagnoses
27, 43, 44, 60, 67, 135

Nursing Interventions
Supportive Care
1. To protect the skin receiving radiation, avoid rubbing, powders, deodorants, lotions, or ointments (unless prescribed) or application of heat or cold.
2. Encourage patient to keep clean and dry, and to bathe the area affected by radiation gently with tepid water and mild soap.
3. Encourage wearing loose-fitting clothes and to protect skin from exposure to sun, chlorine, and temperature extremes.

4. To protect oral and GI tract mucous membranes, encourage frequent, small meals, using bland and soft diet at mild temperatures.

5. Teach patient to avoid irritants, such as alcohol, tobacco, spices, and extremely hot or cold foods.

6. Administer or teach self-administration of pain medication or antiemetic before eating or drinking, if needed.

7. Encourage mouth care at least twice per day and after meals using a soft toothbrush or toothette and mild mouth rinse.

8. Assess for ulcers, plaques, or discharge that may be indicative of superimposed infection.

9. For diarrhea, switch to low-residue diet and administer antidiarrheals as ordered.

10. Provide support throughout the diagnostic and treatment process.

Education and Health Maintenance

1. Teach patient about risk of infection. Advise patient to monitor temperature and report any fever or other sign of infection promptly; to avoid crowds; and to use condoms and other safer-sex practices.

2. Teach patient how to take medications as ordered; advise patient about possible adverse effects and their management.

3. Explain to patient that radiation therapy may cause sterility: male patients should be given opportunity for sperm banking before treatment; female patients may develop ovarian failure and require hormone replacement therapy.

4. Refer patient to support group if appropriate.

5. Reassure the patient that fatigue will decrease after treatment is completed; encourage frequent naps and rest periods.

HUMAN IMMUNODEFICIENCY VIRUS

See *HIV Disease and AIDS*.

HYDROCEPHALUS

Hydrocephalus is characterized by an abnormal increase in cerebrospinal fluid (CSF) volume within the intracranial cavity and by enlargement of the head in infancy. Pressure from increased fluid volume can damage brain tissue.

Hydrocephalus results from two major causes: obstruction of CSF flow (noncommunicating hydrocephalus) or faulty CSF absorption or overproduction of CSF (communicating hydrocephalus). In the noncommunicating type, obstruction may result from congenital defects, infections, trauma, spontaneous intracranial bleeding, and neoplasms. In the communicating type, faulty CSF absorption may result from meningeal adhesions or excessive production of CSF fluid caused by a tumor or from unknown causes. Complications of hydrocephalus include seizures, spontaneous arrest due to natural compensatory mechanisms, persistent increased intracranial pressure (ICP), brain herniation, and developmental delays.

Assessment

Infants

1. Excessive head growth (may be seen up to age 3)
2. Alteration of muscle tone of the extremities
3. Delayed closure of the anterior fontanelle
4. Fontanelle tense and elevated above the surface of the skull
5. Signs of increased ICP — vomiting, restlessness and irritability, high-pitched and shrill cry, alteration in vital signs (increased systolic blood pressure, decreased pulse), pupillary changes, lethargy, and seizures
6. Late physical findings include:
   a. Forehead becomes prominent ("bossing").
   b. Scalp appears shiny, with prominent scalp veins.
   c. Infant has difficulty holding head up.
   d. Eyebrows and eyelids may be drawn upward, exposing the sclera above the iris.
   e. Infant cannot gaze upward, causing "sunset eyes."
   f. Strabismus, nystagmus, and optic atrophy may occur.

Older children — present with signs of increased ICP

1. Headache, especially on awakening
2. Vomiting
3. Lethargy, fatigue, apathy
4. Personality changes
5. Separation of cranial sutures (may be seen up to age 10)
6. Double vision, constricted peripheral vision, sudden appearance of internal strabismus, and pupillary changes
7. Alteration in vital signs similar to those seen in infants
8. Difficulty with gait
9. Stupor, coma
10. Papilledema

Diagnostic Evaluation

1. CT scan is the diagnostic tool of choice; it helps differentiate between hydrocephalus and other intracranial lesions.
2. Skull radiographs show widening of the fontanelle and sutures and erosion of intracranial bone.

Collaborative Management

Surgical Interventions

1. Surgical procedures include:
   a. Extracranial shunt (most common), diverts fluid from the ventricular system to an extracranial compartment, frequently the peritoneum or right atrium.
   b. Intracranial shunt may be used in selected cases of noncommunicating hydrocephalus, to divert fluid from the obstructed segment of the ventricular system to the subarachnoid space.
   c. Direct operation on the lesion causing the obstruction such as a tumor.
2. Most shunts have the following components:
   a. Ventricular tubing
   b. A one-way or unidirectional pressure-sensitive flow valve
   c. A pumping chamber
   d. Distal tubing
3. Shunt complications

H

a. Need for shunt revision frequently occurs because of occlusion, infection, or malfunction.

b. Shunt revision may be necessary because of growth of the child. Newer models, however, include coiled tubing to allow the shunt to grow with the child.

c. Shunt dependency frequently occurs. The child rapidly manifests symptoms of increased ICP if the shunt does not function optimally.

d. Children with ventriculoatrial shunts may experience endocardial contusions and clotting, leading to bacterial endocarditis, bacteremia, and ventriculitis, or thromboembolism and cor pulmonale.

Nursing Diagnoses
6, 51, 88, 104, 123, 135, 135

Nursing Interventions
Monitoring

1. Observe for evidence of increased ICP and report immediately.

EMERGENCY ALERT Brain stem herniation can occur with increased ICP and is manifested by opisthotonic positioning (flexion of head and feet backward). This is a grave sign and may be followed by respiratory arrest. Obtain help and prepare ventricular tap. Have emergency equipment on hand for resuscitation.

2. After surgery, monitor the child's temperature, pulse, respiration, blood pressure, and pupillary size and reaction every 15 minutes until stable; then monitor every 1 or 2 hours.

3. Monitor patient postoperatively for excessive drainage of CSF.
   a. Sunken fontanelle, agitation, restlessness (infant)
   b. Decreased level of consciousness (LOC) (older child)

4. Monitor patient postoperatively for increased ICP, indicating shunt malfunction.
   a. Note especially change in LOC, change in vital signs, vomiting, and pupillary changes.
   b. Report these changes immediately to prevent cerebral hypoxia and possible brain herniation.

5. Accurately measure and record total fluid intake and output.

6. When oral feeding is begun after surgery, observe for and report any decrease in urine output, increased urine specific gravity, diminished skin turgor, dryness of mucous membranes, or lethargy, indicating dehydration.

7. After surgery, assess for fever (temperature normally fluctuates during the first 24 hours after surgery), purulent drainage from the incision, or swelling, redness, and tenderness along the shunt tract.

Supportive Care

1. For diagnostic studies to be accurate, a sedative may be prescribed. Give 30 minutes before the procedure to ensure its effectiveness.

   DRUG ALERT Sedatives are contraindicated in many cases because increased ICP predisposes the child to hypoventilation or respiratory arrest. If sedatives are administered, observe the child very closely for evidence of respiratory depression.

2. Offer patient small, frequent feedings.
   a. Be aware that feeding is often a problem because the child may be listless, anorectic, and prone to vomiting.
   b. Complete nursing care and treatments before feeding so the child will not be disturbed after feeding.
   c. Hold the infant in a semi-sitting position with head well supported during feeding. Allow ample time for burping.
   d. Place the child on side with head elevated after feeding to prevent aspiration.

3. Because pressure sores of the head are a frequent problem, prevent sores by placing the child on a sponge rubber or lamb's-wool pad or an alternating-pressure or convoluted foam mattress to keep weight evenly distributed. Keep the scalp clean and dry.

4. Provide meticulous skin care to all parts of the body and observe skin for the effects of pressure.

5. Turn the child's head frequently; change position at least every 2 hours.

H

a. When turning the child, rotate head and body together to avoid straining the neck.

b. A firm pillow may be placed under the head and shoulders for further support when lifting the child.

6. Perform passive range-of-motion exercises with the extremities, especially the legs.

7. Keep the eyes moistened with artificial tears if the child is unable to close eyelids normally. This prevents corneal ulcerations and infections.

8. Prepare the parents for their child's surgery by answering questions, describing what nursing care will take place postoperatively, and explaining how the shunt will work.

9. Prepare the child for surgery by using dolls or other form of play to describe what interventions will occur.

10. After surgery, take precautions to prevent hypothermia or hyperthermia.

11. Aspirate mucus from the nose and throat as necessary to prevent respiratory difficulty.

12. Turn the child frequently.

13. Promote optimal drainage of CSF through a surgical shunt by pumping the shunt and positioning the child as directed.

a. Report difficulties in pumping the shunt.

b. Gradually elevate the head of child's bed to 30 to 45 degrees as ordered. (Initially, the child is positioned flat to prevent excessive CSF drainage.)

14. Avoid placing excessive pressure on skin overlying shunt.

15. Administer I.V. fluids as prescribed; carefully monitor infusion rate to prevent fluid overload.

16. Use a nasogastric (NG) tube if necessary for abdominal distention.

a. Most frequently used when a ventriculoperitoneal shunt has been performed.

b. Measure the drainage and record amount and color.

c. Monitor for return of bowel sounds after NG suction has been disconnected for at least 30 minutes.

17. Give frequent mouth care while the child is NPO.

18. Begin oral feedings once the child is fully recovered from the anesthetic and displays interest.

19. Encourage the parents to treat the child as normally as possible, providing appropriate toys and love.
20. Help the parents to assist siblings to understand hydrocephalus and the child's special needs. Encourage parents to spend individual time with siblings and not neglect their needs as well. Suggest family counseling if needed.

Education and Health Maintenance

1. Stress the importance of recognizing symptoms of increased ICP and reporting them immediately.
2. Advise parents to report shunt malfunction or infection immediately to prevent increased ICP.
3. Teach parents that illnesses that cause vomiting and diarrhea or that prevent an adequate fluid intake are a great threat to the child who has had a shunt procedure. Advise parents to consult with the child's health care provider about immediate treatment of fever, control of vomiting and diarrhea, and replacement of fluids.
4. Tell the parents that few restrictions are required for children with shunts and to consult with the health care provider about specific concerns.
5. Help parents locate additional resources, such as a social worker, discharge planner, visiting or home health nurse or aide, parent group or community agencies, and special programs at school.
6. For additional information, refer to Hydrocephalus Association, *www.hydroassoc.org*.

HYPEROSMOLAR HYPERGLYCEMIC NONKETOTIC SYNDROME

H

Hyperosmolar hyperglycemic nonketotic syndrome (HHNS), also called *hyperosmolar coma*, is an acute complication of diabetes mellitus (particularly type 2) characterized by hyperglycemia, dehydration, and hyperosmolarity, but little or no ketosis. The disorder is caused by inadequate levels of endogenous or exogenous insulin to control hyperglycemia, but enough to prevent ketosis. Precipitating factors include cardiac failure, burns, or chronic illness that increases need for insulin; use of agents, such as corticosteroids or immunosuppressants that increase blood glucose levels; and procedures that cause stress and increase blood glucose levels, such as hyperosmolar hyperalimentation or peritoneal dialysis.

HHNS is a medical emergency that can cause coma and death if not treated properly.

Assessment
1. Early symptoms include fatigue, malaise, polyuria, signs of dehydration, nausea, and vomiting.
2. Later signs are muscle weakness, hypothermia, seizures, stupor, and coma.

Diagnostic Evaluation
1. Serum glucose and osmolality greatly elevated.
2. Serum and urine ketone bodies are minimal or absent.
3. Serum sodium and potassium may be elevated, depending on degree of dehydration, despite total body losses.
4. Serum blood urea nitrogen and creatinine may be elevated because of dehydration.
5. Urine specific gravity is elevated because of dehydration.

Collaborative Management
Therapeutic Interventions
1. Correct fluid and electrolyte imbalances with I.V. fluids.
2. Evaluate complications, such as stupor, seizures, and shock; treat appropriately.
3. Identification and treatment of underlying illnesses or events that precipitated HHNS.

Pharmacologic Interventions
1. I.V. regular insulin drip to counteract hyperglycemia

Nursing Diagnoses
23, 86, 119

Nursing Interventions
Monitoring
1. Assess for signs of dehydration, such as poor turgor, reduced urine output, thirst, and dry mucous membranes.

2. Monitor glucose and electrolyte levels during I.V. therapy.
3. Monitor hourly intake and output and urine specific gravity for hydration status.
4. Monitor for shock: rapid, thready pulse, cool extremities, and hypotension.
5. Monitor respiratory rate and breath sounds for signs of aspiration pneumonia.

Supportive Care

1. Institute fluid replacement therapy as ordered (usually normal or half-strength saline initially), maintaining patent I.V. line.
2. Assess patient for signs and symptoms of fluid overload and cerebral edema as I.V. therapy progresses.

> **EMERGENCY ALERT** Too-rapid infusion of I.V. fluids can cause cerebral edema and death.

3. Administer regular insulin I.V. as ordered, and add dextrose to I.V. infusion as blood glucose falls below 300 mg/dL, to prevent hypoglycemia.
4. Be aware that patient is at risk for aspiration; assess patient's level of consciousness and ability to handle oral secretions (cough and gag reflex, ability to swallow).
5. Properly position patient to reduce possibility of aspiration.
   a. Elevate head of bed unless contraindicated.
   b. If nausea is present, use side-lying position.
6. Suction as often as needed to maintain patent airway.
7. Withhold oral intake until patient is no longer in danger of aspiration.
8. If patient is comatose, insert nasogastric tube to prevent aspiration.
9. Provide mouth care to maintain adequate mucosal hydration.

Education and Health Maintenance

1. Advise the patient and family that it may take 3 to 5 days for symptoms to resolve.

2. Instruct patient and family about signs and symptoms of hyperglycemia and use of sick day guidelines.
3. Explain possible causes of HHNS.
4. Review any changes in medication, activity, meal plan, or glucose monitoring for home care. It may not be necessary to continue insulin therapy after HHNS; many patients can be treated with diet and oral agents alone.

HYPERLIPIDEMIA

Hyperlipidemia is a group of metabolic abnormalities resulting in combinations of elevated serum total cholesterol (hypercholesterolemia), elevated low-density lipoprotein (LDL), elevated triglycerides, and decreased high-density lipoprotein (HDL). Primary hyperlipidemias are relatively rare, due to genetic abnormalities, and run in families. Secondary hyperlipidemias occur in up to 50% of Americans and are multifactorial, related to obesity, other metabolic disorders such as diabetes and hypothyroidism, poor dietary habits, and use of certain medication such as beta-adrenergic blockers. Hyperlipidemia leads to accelerated atherosclerotic plaque formation in blood vessels, possible thromboembolism formation, and subsequent cardiovascular, cerebrovascular, and peripheral vascular disease.

Assessment

1. Usually asymptomatic until target organ damage is done.
   a. Chest pain and signs of myocardial infarction
   b. Transient ischemic attacks, stroke
   c. Intermittent claudication and signs of arterial occlusion
2. Metabolic signs may be present, particularly in primary hyperlipidemias: corneal arcus (opaque fatty ring around the cornea), xanthoma (fatty deposit in the skin or internal organs), xanthelasma (fatty deposit of the eyelid), and abdominal pain with pancreatitis.

Diagnostic Evaluation

1. A fasting lipid profile is recommended for all adults (age 20 and older) every 5 years, including cholesterol, LDL, HDL, and triglycerides.
   a. Cholesterol below 200 mg/dL is normal.
   b. LDL below 100 mg/dL is considered optimal.
   c. HDL greater than 40 mg/dL is considered optimal.
   d. Triglyceride level below 150 mg/dL is normal.
2. Additional testing may include thyroid function tests, fasting glucose, liver function tests, renal function tests, and others to rule out chronic diseases, which may affect lipid metabolism.
3. Lipoprotein electrophoresis may be done if primary (familial) hyperlipidemia is suspected.
4. Advanced testing for coronary risk factors associated with hyperlipidemia include homocysteine level, apolipoprotein B, lipoprotein a, and C-reactive protein.

Collaborative Management

Therapeutic Interventions

1. Therapeutic lifestyle changes are indicated as primary prevention for cardiovascular disease and adjunct therapy for established disease.
   a. Decrease saturated fat (below 7% of calories) and total cholesterol in diet.
   b. Increase soluble fiber in diet.
   c. Add plant sterol or stanol esters (dietary spread that lowers LDL).
   d. Lose weight if overweight or obese.
   e. Regular physical activity.

Pharmacologic Interventions

1. Initiation of drug treatment for hyperlipidemia is primarily based on LDL results and presence of other risk factors (smoking, diabetes, family history of premature coronary artery disease, hypertension, low HDL, high cholesterol); drug therapy is considered for the following:

H

a. LDL 100 to 129 mg/dL and patient has established coronary artery disease or is at high risk for it (possible drug therapy)

b. LDL greater than 130 mg/dL and patient has established coronary artery disease or is at moderate to high risk for it (definite drug therapy)

c. LDL greater than 160 mg/dL and patient is at moderate risk for coronary artery disease (two or more risk factors; definite therapy)

d. LDL 160 to 189 mg/dL and patient at low risk for coronary artery disease (zero to one risk factor; optional therapy)

e. LDL greater than 190 mg/dL (definite therapy even with no other risk factors)

2. Drug of choice for lowering LDL is a HMG CoA reductase inhibitor ("statin"), such as pravastatin or atorvastatin.

a. Most expensive agents

b. May cause serum transaminase elevations; monitor liver function tests at baseline, after 12 weeks, and periodically

c. May also cause myopathy, especially if used in combination with a fibrate

3. Fibrates (fibrinic acid derivatives) are most effective in lowering triglycerides, and may also raise HDL; include gemfibrozil, fenofibrate, and clofibrate.

a. Monitor liver function periodically; use cautiously in patients with renal impairment.

b. If patient complaints of muscle pain, check creatine kinase (CK) level and investigate for rhabdomyolysis.

c. Potentiate anticoagulants.

4. Bile acid sequestrants are effective in reducing LDL, especially in combination with statins; include cholestyramine and colestipol.

a. May cause constipation, bloating, and flatus

b. Inhibit absorption of many other drugs; give other drugs 1 to 2 hours before or 4 to 6 hours after bile acid sequestrant

5. Nicotinic acid is most effective in raising HDL, but also lowers LDL and triglycerides.
   a. Major adverse effect is severe flushing; taking aspirin 325 mg 1 hour before dose may help.
   b. Monitor liver function tests every 6 to 12 weeks for 1 year, then periodically; monitor for hyperglycemia and hyperuricemia.
   c. May potentiate antihypertensives and interfere with antidiabetic agents.
6. Cholesterol absorption inhibitors is a newer class of drugs that contains ezetimibe to lower LDL, triglycerides, and apoprotein B.
   a. If used as monotherapy, no need for monitoring of liver function.
   b. GI adverse effects are very mild.

DRUG ALERT Anticoagulant doses may need to be reduced by 50% if a fibrate is added because of an increased risk of bleeding.

Nursing Diagnoses
24, 52

Nursing Interventions
Monitoring
1. Monitor lipid profile 6 weeks after initiating therapy and every 3 to 6 months thereafter to determine effectiveness of therapy.
2. Monitor liver function tests, renal function tests, and CK levels as indicated by drug therapy.
3. Monitor for complaints of muscle aches and weakness, which may indicate acute rhabdomyolysis; withhold drug therapy and notify health care provider.
4. Monitor for signs of developing vascular disease such as carotid or femoral bruits, chest pain, intermittent claudication, and transient ischemic attacks.

H

Supportive Care
1. Provide education about hyperlipidemia and its association with coronary artery disease, cerebrovascular disease,

and peripheral vascular disease. Reassure the patient that therapy can be effective to reduce risks.

2. Teach diet basics and obtain a nutritional consult.
   a. If patient is overweight, diet should be designed to stimulate 1- to 2-lb (0.5- to 1-kg) weight loss per week.
   b. Total fat content should be 25% to 35% of total calories with saturated fat less than 7%.
   c. Plant sterol or stanol spreads, such as Take Control, are available over the counter in grocery and health food stores and can lower cholesterol by 10%.
3. Encourage patient to engage in 30 minutes of moderate exercise per day such as walking, bicycling, and housecleaning.
4. Encourage patient to quit smoking.

Education and Health Maintenance

1. Encourage follow-up for laboratory work and checkups, even if patient is feeling well.
2. Teach about medication adverse effects and dosage schedule; statins are usually taken at bedtime.
3. Advise patient that a fat-soluble vitamin supplement (A, D, E, K) is sometimes recommended with long-term bile acid sequestrant therapy.
4. Urge patients to report unexplained muscle pain or weakness, dark-colored urine, light-colored stools, unusual bleeding, or jaundice immediately.
5. Refer for more information to American Heart Association, *www.americanheart.org*.

HYPERPARATHYROIDISM

Hyperparathyroidism results from hypersecretion of parathyroid hormone (PTH), which causes calcium resorption by bone and increased calcium absorption by the kidneys and gut, among other effects. The disorder occurs in primary and secondary forms. Primary hyperparathyroidism most commonly results from a single parathyroid adenoma (approximately 80% of cases), and primarily affects women older than age 50. Secondary hyperparathyroidism is usually caused by kidney failure, which stimulates excessive compensatory production of PTH.

Early diagnosis is difficult. Complications include renal stones and kidney disease, GI ulceration, demineralization of bones causing fractures, and hypoparathyroidism after surgery.

Assessment

1. Depression of neuromuscular function: the patient may trip, drop objects, or show general fatigue, loss of memory for recent events, emotional instability, and changes in level of consciousness with stupor and coma
2. Cardiac arrhythmias, hypertension, and possible cardiac standstill
3. Skeletal pain, backache, pain on weight bearing, and pathologic fractures

Diagnostic Evaluation

1. Persistently elevated serum calcium (11 mg/100 mL); test is performed on at least two occasions to determine consistency of results. Other causes of hypercalcemia must be ruled out: malignancy (usually bone or breast cancer), vitamin D excess, multiple myeloma, sarcoidosis, milk-alkali syndrome, Cushing's disease, hyperthyroidism, or effects of drugs such as thiazides.
2. PTH levels are increased.
3. Alkaline phosphatase levels are elevated, and serum phosphorus levels are decreased.
4. X-rays show skeletal changes such as deformities and bony cysts.
5. Cine CT scan shows parathyroid tumors more readily than radiography.

Collaborative Management
Therapeutic Interventions

1. Restrict dietary calcium, and discontinue all drugs that might cause hypercalcemia (thiazides, vitamin D) as directed.
2. Dialysis may be necessary in patients with resistant hypercalcemia or who have renal failure.

H

Pharmacologic Interventions

1. Hydration with I.V. saline solution and diuretics to increase urinary excretion of calcium in patients not in renal failure.
2. Oral phosphate may be used as an antihypercalcemic agent.
3. Pamidronate, calcitonin, and etidronate disodium inhibit bone resorption of calcium.

> **EMERGENCY ALERT** If a patient is taking digoxin, reduce dosage because a patient with hypercalcemia is more sensitive to drug's toxic effects.

Surgical Interventions

1. Primary hyperparathyroidism is treated surgically to remove parathyroid lesion.
2. Treatment risks hypoparathyroidism if too much of the gland tissue is removed.

Nursing Diagnoses
1, 13, 23, 24, 136

Nursing Interventions
Monitoring

1. Closely monitor the patient's fluid intake and output and dietary calcium intake.
2. Monitor serum blood urea nitrogen, creatinine, potassium, magnesium, and calcium.
3. Observe for signs of urinary tract infection, hematuria, and renal colic. Strain all urine.
4. Monitor electrocardiogram to detect changes secondary to hypocalcemia: Shortened QT interval; with extreme hypercalcemia, widening of the T wave is seen.
5. After surgery, monitor serum calcium level and evaluate for signs and symptoms of hypocalcemia (paresthesias of extremities and around mouth) and onset of tetany.

Supportive Care

1. Prevent or promptly treat dehydration by reporting vomiting or other sources of fluid loss.

2. Increase fluid intake to 3,000 mL per day to maintain hydration and prevent precipitation of calcium and formation of stones.
3. Assist the patient in hygiene and activities if bone pain is severe or if the patient experiences musculoskeletal weakness.
4. Protect the patient from falls or injury.
5. Turn the patient cautiously, and handle extremities gently to avoid fractures.
6. Encourage the patient to participate in mild exercise gradually as symptoms subside.
7. Instruct and demonstrate correct body mechanics to reduce strain, backache, and injury.
8. Administer analgesia as prescribed; assess pain level and patient's response to analgesia.
9. Reassure the patient about skeletal recovery: bone pain diminishes fairly quickly, and fractures can be treated by orthopedic procedures.

Education and Health Maintenance
1. Instruct the patient about administration and adverse effects of calcium-reducing medications.
   a. Teach subcutaneous administration of calcitonin.
   b. Avoid calcium-containing foods within 2 hours of etidronate.
   c. Administer pamidronate over 24 hours mixed with I.V. saline or dextrose solutions; do not mix with Ringer's solution and keep other I.V. drugs separate.
2. Instruct the patient to avoid dietary sources of calcium, such as dairy products, broccoli, and calcium-containing antacids.
3. Teach the patient to recognize and report signs and symptoms of hypocalcemic tetany (apprehensiveness, numbness and tingling in extremities or around the mouth).

HYPERTENSION

Hypertension (high blood pressure) is a disease of vascular regulation resulting from malfunction of arterial pressure control mechanisms (central nervous system, renin-angiotensin-

BOX H-1   Accelerated Hypertension

Accelerated hypertension (malignant hypertension) is severely elevated and sustained diastolic blood pressure that puts strain on the arterial walls, possibly leading to cerebral, myocardial, and renal ischemia. The blood pressure must be reduced promptly but not too rapidly because the patient's usual range may not be tolerated. The patient may manifest headaches, vision problems, confusion, disorientation, irritability, lethargy, and nausea and vomiting. Be alert for signs of seizure activity and pulmonary edema. If diastolic blood pressure exceeds 115 to 130 mm Hg, the condition is assessed very carefully. Hospitalization in an intensive care unit is recommended for seizures, pulmonary edema, severe occipital headache, and neurologic abnormalities. Antihypertensive treatment includes vasodilators such as nitroprusside or hydralazine; adrenergic inhibitors, such as labetalol and methyldopa; and possibly diuretics, all given I.V. Vasopressor agents should be available if the blood pressure responds too vigorously to antihypertensive agents.

Nursing responsibilities include continuous monitoring of blood pressure and electrocardiogram; monitoring urine output; monitoring for adverse effects of medications such as tachycardia and orthostatic hypotension; maintaining seizure precautions; providing a restful, quiet environment; maintaining cardiac monitoring; and reporting signs of central nervous system or cardiac complications.

aldosterone system, extracellular fluid volume). The cause is unknown, and there is no cure. The basic explanation is that blood pressure is elevated when there is increased cardiac output plus increased peripheral vascular resistance.

The two major types of hypertension are *primary (essential) hypertension*, in which diastolic pressure is 90 mm Hg or higher and systolic pressure is 140 mm Hg or higher in absence of other causes of hypertension (approximately 95% of patients); and *secondary hypertension*, which results primarily from renal disease, endocrine disorders, and coarctation of the aorta. Either of these conditions may give rise to *accelerated hypertension — a medical emergency —* in which blood pressure elevates very rapidly to threaten one or more of the target organs: the brain, kidney, or heart (see *Box H-1*).

Hypertension is one of the most prevalent chronic diseases for which treatment is available; however, most patients with hypertension are unaware, untreated, or inadequately treated. Risk factors for hypertension are age between 30 and 70; black; overweight; sleep apnea; family history; cigarette smoking; sedentary lifestyle; and diabetes mellitus. Because hypertension presents no overt symptoms, it is termed the "silent killer." The untreated disease may progress to retinopathy, renal failure, coronary artery disease, heart failure, and stroke.

Hypertension in children is defined as the average systolic or diastolic blood pressure greater than or equal to the 95th percentile for age and sex with measurement on at least three occasions (charts available from *www.nhlbi.nih.gov/health/ public/heart/nbp/dash*). The incidence of hypertension in children is low, but it is increasingly being recognized in adolescents; and it may occur in neonates, infants, and young children with secondary causes.

Assessment

1. Elevated blood pressure above 140/90 mm Hg in adults on at least two occasions (see *Table H-3*); varies in children based on age and sex-related norms

TABLE H-3	Classification of Blood Pressure for Adults Ages 18 and Older		
CATEGORY	**BLOOD PRESSURE (MM HG)**		
	Systolic		**Diastolic**
Normal	< 120	and	< 80
Prehypertension	120-139	or	80-89
Stage 1 hypertension	140-159	or	90-99
Stage 2 hypertension	≥160	or	≥100

From Joint National Committee on Prevention, Detection, Evaluation, and Treatment of High Blood Pressure. (2003). Available at *www.nhlbi.nih.gov/guidelines/hypertension/jncintro.htm*.

H

a. Measure blood pressure under the same conditions each time, and avoid taking blood pressure readings immediately after stressful or taxing situations.

b. Use correct size blood pressure cuff; width should be 20% greater than width of measured extremity, and length should be sufficient to encircle measured extremity.

c. Be aware that falsely elevated blood pressures may be obtained with a cuff that is too narrow; falsely low readings may be obtained with a cuff that is too wide.

d. Auscultate and record precisely the systolic and diastolic pressures based on Korotkoff sounds.

e. The finding of an isolated elevated blood pressure does not necessarily indicate hypertension. However, the patient should be regarded as at risk for high blood pressure until further assessment through history taking, physical examination, and repeated blood pressure measurement confirms or denies the diagnosis.

2. Associated findings:

a. Shift of the point of maximal impulse to the left, which occurs in heart enlargement caused by chronic strain

b. Bruits over peripheral arteries indicating the presence of atherosclerosis, which may be manifested as obstructed blood flow

c. Possible vascular changes on funduscopic examination of the eyes: edema, spasm, and hemorrhage of the eye vessels

3. Headache, dizziness, and blurred vision — indicate greatly elevated blood pressure and possibly development of accelerated hypertension

Diagnostic Evaluation

1. 12-lead electrocardiogram evaluates effects of hypertension on the heart (left ventricular hypertrophy, ischemia) and detects underlying heart disease

2. Chest X-ray detects possible cardiomegaly

3. Blood samples for chemistry evaluation

a. Elevated serum blood urea nitrogen and creatinine indicate kidney disease as a cause or effect of hypertension

b. Decreased serum potassium indicates primary hyperaldosteronism; increased potassium indicates Cushing's syndrome — both conditions cause secondary hypertension

4. Checking first morning spot urine for microalbumin or random spot urine for microalbumin creatinine ratio are screening tests for renal involvement; 24-hour urine samples for protein and creatinine clearance evaluate extent of renal disease

5. Collection of 24-hour urine for increased catecholamines, indicating pheochromocytoma

6. Renal scan, CT scan, and other special tests detect causes of secondary hypertension

Collaborative Management
Therapeutic Interventions

1. Lifestyle modifications as initial therapy:
   a. Lose weight, if more than 10% above ideal weight.
   b. Limit alcohol (no more than 1 oz [30 mL] of ethanol per day).
   c. Get regular aerobic exercise three times per week.
   d. Cut sodium intake to less than 2.4 g (2,400 mg) per day.
   e. Include recommended daily allowances of potassium, calcium, and magnesium in diet. This can be accomplished through the Dietary Approaches to Stop Hypertension diet, which is rich in fruits and vegetables, low-fat dairy products, and fiber; and low in saturated and total fat (see *www.dash.bwh.harvard.edu*).
   f. Stop smoking.
   g. Reduce caffeine intake.

H

ALTERNATIVE INTERVENTION

Licorice is used by some people to treat GI upset and peptic ulcer disease; however, it may worsen hypertension, and can worsen hypokalemia in patients on diuretics.

Pharmacologic Interventions

1. Antihypertensive medications, if, despite lifestyle changes, the blood pressure remains at or above 140/90 mm Hg over 3 to 6 months. Depending on the patient's condition, possible drugs include diuretics, beta-adrenergic blockers, alpha-receptor blockers, angiotensin-converting enzyme inhibitors, calcium antagonists (calcium channel blockers), and angiotensin II receptor blockers (see *Table H-4*).

   PEDIATRIC ALERT First-line drug therapy for hypertension in children includes thiazide diuretics and beta-adrenergic blockers.

2. If hypertension is not controlled with the first drug within 1 to 3 months, three options can be considered:
   a. If the patient has faithfully taken the drug and not developed any adverse effects, the dose of the drug may be increased.
   b. If the patient has had adverse effects, another class of drugs can be substituted.
   c. A second drug from another class could be added. If adding the second drug lowers the pressure, the first drug may be slowly withdrawn.

3. A third drug (particularly a diuretic if not already prescribed) may be added if the desired blood pressure is still not achieved after adding a second drug. Medications may include centrally acting alpha-agonists, peripheral adrenergic antagonists, or direct vasodilators.

Nursing Diagnoses
24, 108, 109

TABLE H-4	Select Adverse Reactions of Antihypertensives

DRUG CLASS AND DRUGS	ADVERSE REACTIONS
Thiazide diuretics hydrochlorothiazide, chlorthalidone	Increased glucose, cholesterol, and uric acid; decreased potassium, sodium, and magnesium
Beta-adrenergic blockers atenolol, metoprolol, propranolol	Bronchospasm, bradycardia, heart failure, may mask insulin-induced hypoglycemia, fatigue, hypertriglyceridemia
Calcium antagonists diltiazem, verapamil, amlodipine	Conduction defects, gingival hyperplasia, nausea and headache with diltiazem, constipation with verapamil, ankle edema with amlodipine
Angiotensin-converting enzyme inhibitors enalapril, captopril, lisinopril, ramipril	Cough, angioedema, hyperkalemia, rash, loss of taste, leukopenia
Alpha-adrenergic blockers doxazosin, prazosin, terazosin	Headache, fatigue, dizziness, postural hypotension
Angiotensin II receptor blockers losartan, valsartan, irbesartan	Dizziness, hyperkalemia, rare angioedema

H

Nursing Interventions
Monitoring

1. Monitor the patient's blood pressure at regular intervals, based on condition.
2. Monitor patient's response to drug therapy. Check for orthostatic changes caused by medication.
3. Monitor patient's weight and diet.

4. Monitor laboratory results for changes in kidney function and electrolyte levels due to hypertension and to drug therapy.
5. Monitor for signs of target organ disease.

Supportive Care and Education

1. Educate the patient about the disease, its treatment, and control. The goals of treatment are to control blood pressure, reduce risk of complications, and use the minimum number of drugs with lowest dosage necessary to accomplish control.
2. Warn that, unless blood pressure is greatly elevated, the patient cannot tell by the way he or she feels whether blood pressure is normal or elevated.
3. Stress that hypertension is chronic and requires persistent therapy and mandatory follow-up health care visits.
4. Explain the pharmacologic control of hypertension. Discuss possible adverse effects of drugs.

GERONTOLOGIC ALERT The multiple drugs required to control blood pressure may be difficult for the elderly patient to comprehend. The names of drugs are frequently difficult for the patient to pronounce. Color-coding of medication bottles with an accompanying color-coded time of administration chart is one way to help the patient remember when to take medications. Elderly patients are also more sensitive to therapeutic levels of drugs and may demonstrate adverse effects while on an otherwise average dosage. They may be more sensitive to postural hypotension and should be cautioned to change positions with great care.

5. Educate the patient about situations that may potentiate antihypertensive drugs and report if lightheadedness (if severe) or fainting occurs.
   a. Remember that certain circumstances produce vasodilation — a hot bath, hot weather, febrile illness, or consumption of alcohol (which may potentiate antihypertensives).
   b. Be aware that blood pressure is decreased when circulating blood volume is reduced — eg, during dehydration, diarrhea, or hemorrhage. Fluid volume replacement is essential.

6. Advise patient to follow a low-sodium diet and enlist his or her cooperation in redirecting lifestyle in keeping with therapy guidelines.

COMMUNITY CARE CONSIDERATIONS

Teach the patient how to take blood pressure readings at home and at work, as directed by the health care provider. Tell the patient which readings should be reported. Have patient bring home blood pressure monitor to health care facility to check accuracy against sphygmomanometer.

HYPERTHYROIDISM

Hyperthyroidism is an overproduction of thyroid hormone, which creates far-reaching metabolic effects. Hypertrophy and hyperplasia of the thyroid gland occur with increased vascularity. Most of the clinical manifestations result from increased metabolic rate, excessive heat production, increased neuromuscular and cardiovascular activity, and hyperactivity of the sympathetic nervous system. The condition is more common in women than in men and occurs in several forms.

Graves' disease, diffuse thyroid hyperfunctioning associated with ophthalmopathy, is the most prevalent form in adults and children. It has been linked to an autoimmune reaction. It may also occur after an emotional shock, stress, or infection. The disorder can be mild, characterized by remissions and exacerbations, or it may progress to emaciation, extreme nervousness, delirium, disorientation, thyroid storm, and death.

In toxic nodular goiter, one or more thyroid nodules become hyperproductive. It is more common in older women with preexisting goiter.

Autoimmune thyroiditis (Hashimoto's disease) may cause initial hyperthyroidism before developing into hypothyroidism.

Factitious hyperthyroidism results from ingestion of excessive amounts of thyroid hormone medication.

Thyroid storm (thyrotoxicosis, thyroid crisis) can be precipitated by stress (surgery, infection, and so forth) or inadequate surgical preparation of a patient with known hyperthy-

H

roidism. It requires emergency treatment. Other complications include infiltrative ophthalmopathy in 50% of patients with Graves' disease, development of goiter (hyperplasia of thyroid) from overstimulation, and hypothyroidism caused by overtreatment.

Assessment

1. Nervousness, emotional lability, irritability, apprehension, insomnia
2. Fine tremor of hands
3. Profuse perspiration; flushed skin (eg, hands may be warm, soft, moist); heat intolerance
4. Increased appetite but progressive weight loss
5. Change in bowel habits; diarrhea or frequent stools
6. Muscle fatigability and weakness
7. Amenorrhea
8. Children may be tall and underweight for age
9. Rapid pulse at rest as well as on exertion (ranges between 90 and 160 beats per minute)
10. Palpitations, possible atrial fibrillation
11. Infiltrative ophthalmopathy with Graves' disease
    a. Exophthalmos (bulging eyes) creates a startled expression
    b. Weakness of extraocular muscles, lid edema, lid lag
12. Possible enlarged thyroid gland (goiter); a bruit may be auscultated over gland

EMERGENCY ALERT Thyroid storm is characterized by hyperpyrexia, diarrhea, dehydration, tachycardia, arrhythmias, extreme irritation, and delirium. Coma, shock, and death result if not adequately treated.

Diagnostic Evaluation

1. Elevated triiodothyronine (T_3) and thyroxine (T_4), elevated serum T_3 resin uptake; possibly suppressed thyroid-stimulating hormone.
2. Microsomal antibodies elevated in initial stage of autoimmune thyroiditis.
3. Thyroid scan shows increased uptake of radioactive iodine (^{131}I). (Results may also be below normal, depend-

ing on the underlying cause of the disorder.) Also needed to rule out cold nodules that may indicate thyroid cancer.

Collaborative Management
Therapeutic Interventions

1. Treatment aims to restore the patient's basal metabolic rate to normal as soon as possible, and then to maintain it. The specific approach depends on the cause, age of the patient, severity of disease, and complications.
2. Radioactive iodine therapy limits thyroid hormone secretion by destroying thyroid tissue. Dosage is controlled to avoid provoking hypothyroidism.
   a. Chief advantage over drug therapy is that a lasting remission can be achieved; chief disadvantage is that permanent hypothyroidism can be caused by overtreatment.
   b. Radiation thyroiditis (a transient exacerbation of hyperthyroidism) may result from leakage of thyroid hormone into the circulation from damaged follicles.
3. Emergency management of thyroid storm includes treatment of hyperthermia with cooling blanket and acetaminophen; reversal of dehydration with I.V. fluids and electrolytes. The precipitating event must also be identified and treated, if possible.

Pharmacologic Interventions

1. Thyroid hormone antagonists — thionamide drugs such as propylthiouracil and methimazole — inhibit thyroid hormone formation.
   a. Duration of treatment depends on reduction of thyroid gland, and normalization of T_4 and T_3 uptake. Treatment continues until patient becomes clinically euthyroid (from 3 months to 1 or 2 years).
   b. Drug is withdrawn gradually to prevent exacerbation.
   c. If euthyroidism cannot be maintained without therapy, then radiation or surgery is recommended.

 DRUG ALERT Observe the patient for evidence of iodine toxicity when taking a thionamide: swelling of buccal mucosa, excessive

H

salivation, coryza, and skin eruptions. Discontinue thionamides and notify the health care provider.

2. Beta-adrenergic blocker propranolol may be given to abolish tachycardia, tremor, excess sweating, and nervousness until antithyroid drugs or radioiodine can take effect; it also inhibits peripheral conversion of T_4 to T_3.

3. Glucocorticoids may be given to suppress peripheral conversion of T_4 to T_3, a more potent thyroid hormone.

4. Lugol's iodine solution may be used to inhibit hormone release in thyroid storm.

5. Diuretics may be used for ophthalmopathy, along with lubricating eyedrops; in severe cases, corticosteroids or orbital radiation may be necessary.

Surgical Interventions

1. Used for patients with very large goiters or for those who cannot be treated with thionamides or radioiodines. Surgery or radioiodine is preferred for nodular toxic goiter and thyroid carcinoma.

2. Subtotal thyroidectomy involves removal of most of the thyroid gland. Entire thyroid gland is not removed to spare parathyroid function.

Nursing Diagnoses
6, 24, 34, 51, 134, 135, 136

Nursing Interventions
Also see *Thyroidectomy*, page 927.

Monitoring

1. Monitor for signs of acute agranulocytosis due to drug therapy (fever, sore throat, low white blood cell count), thrombocytopenia (unusual bleeding, low platelet count), and aplastic anemia (fatigue, shortness of breath, low hemoglobin and other values on complete blood count [CBC]). Report these and signs of allergic reaction (rash, urticaria) immediately.

2. Monitor temperature for impending thyroid storm.

3. Monitor the patient's fluid and nutritional status: weigh the patient daily, accurately record daily intake and output, and monitor vital signs and skin turgor.
4. Monitor thyroid function tests for return of euthyroid state.

Supportive Care

1. To provide adequate nutrition, give high-calorie foods and fluids consistent with the patient's requirements.
2. Provide a quiet, calm environment; reduce environmental stressors (light, television and radio, visitors) as necessary.
3. Restrict stimulants (tea, coffee, chocolate) and alcohol; explain rationale to patient.
4. Assess for fatigue and prevent overactivity.
5. Promote sleep and relaxation through use of prescribed medications, massage, relaxation exercises, and clustering nursing care activities.

PEDIATRIC ALERT Disrupted sleep pattern is an important issue for children with hyperthyroidism as well as their parents. Acknowledge their lack of sleep and encourage parents to rest whenever possible.

6. Employ safety measures to reduce risk of trauma or falls if patient is agitated.
7. Bathe the patient frequently with cool to warm (not hot) water (avoid soap to prevent drying skin) to counteract diaphoresis; change linens when damp. Use lubricant skin lotions to protect pressure points.
8. Clear up treatment misconceptions, especially about radioactive iodine.
   a. Radioactive iodine pill will cause destruction of thyroid tissue only.
   b. Small levels of radiation will be eliminated through urine and feces, which should be disposed of promptly.

Education and Health Maintenance

1. Emphasize to the patient and family the importance of following the prescribed medication regimen.

2. Advise the patient to have periodic blood evaluations to monitor CBC and thyroid hormone levels.
3. Teach patient about signs of hypothyroidism (lethargy, weight gain, feeling cold, constipation, bradycardia, short attention span, edema, and menorrhagia) due to overtreatment; instruct patient to report them.
4. Teach the patient and family to recognize and immediately report signs and symptoms of thyroid storm (tachycardia, hyperpyrexia, extreme irritation) and alert them to predisposing factors (infection, surgery, stress, abrupt withdrawal of antithyroid medications and adrenergic blockers).
5. Encourage well-child visits for evaluation of growth and development.

HYPOPARATHYROIDISM

Hypoparathyroidism results from a deficiency of parathyroid hormone (PTH) caused by accidental surgical removal or destruction, malignancy, idiopathic (may be familial or autoimmune), or resistance to PTH action. With inadequate PTH secretion, less calcium is resorbed by the kidneys and bones, and less calcium is absorbed by the GI tract, causing serum calcium levels to fall. Neuromuscular irritability and possible tetany result.

Acute complications related to hypocalcemia include seizures, tetany (which may cause airway obstruction), and mental disorders, all of which can be reversed with calcium therapy. Long-term complications include subcapsular cataracts, calcification of the basal ganglia, and papilledema, caused by precipitation of calcium out of serum and deposition in tissues; and shortening of the fingers and toes, and bowing of the long bones, caused by inadequate PTH and additional genetic abnormalities. Of these complications, only papilledema is reversible.

Assessment

1. Tetany — general muscular hypertonia and attempts at voluntary movement result in tremors and spasmodic or uncoordinated movements.

a. Positive Chvostek and Trousseau's signs (see page 929)
b. If onset is acute, may cause laryngeal spasm.
2. Severe anxiety and apprehension
3. Renal colic is often present if the patient has history of stones; preexisting stones loosen and migrate into the ureter — also cause hematuria and signs of infection.

Diagnostic Evaluation

1. Serum phosphorus is elevated; serum calcium is decreased to low level (7.5 mg/100 mL or less).
2. PTH is decreased in most cases; may be normal or elevated in pseudohypoparathyroidism.
3. Periodic 24-hour urine for calcium determines hypercalciuria and risk for kidney stones.

Collaborative Management
Therapeutic and Pharmacologic Interventions

1. I.V. calcium solution is used to treat hypocalcemic tetany.
   a. A syringe and ampule of a calcium solution (calcium chloride, calcium gluceptate, calcium gluconate) is kept at the bedside at all times.
   b. Most rapidly effective calcium solution is ionized calcium chloride (10% solution).
   c. For rapid relief of severe tetany, calcium solution is given every 10 minutes.
   d. When tetany is controlled, I.M. or oral calcium is given.
   e. Later, add vitamin D to calcium intake to increase calcium absorption and raise serum calcium levels.
   f. Thiazide diuretic may also be added because of its calcium-retaining effect on the kidney; doses of calcium and vitamin D may then be lowered.
2. Treatment of kidney stones and possible hypercalciuria.

Nursing Diagnoses
24, 136

H

Nursing Interventions
Monitoring
1. Monitor respiratory and neuromuscular status closely for impending tetany and laryngeal spasm.
2. Closely monitor patient's intake and output and serum calcium and phosphorus levels.

Supportive Care
1. Make sure that dosage of calcium is correct based on preparation used:
   a. Calcium chloride 10% 500 mg to 1 g (5 to 10 mL)
   b. Calcium gluconate 10% 500 mg to 2 g (5 to 20 mL); children 0.5 to 0.7 mEq/kg
   c. Calcium glucceptate 1 or 2 g (5 to 10 mL)

DRUG ALERT Administer all I.V. calcium preparations slowly, at rates of approximately 0.5 to 1 mL per minute, to avoid severe irritation, thrombosis, flushing, and possible cardiac arrest. Use small needle in large vein. Stop infusion if any discomfort occurs, and resume when symptoms disappear.

2. Promote high-calcium diet if prescribed — dairy products, green leafy vegetables, and calcium-enhanced foods, such as cereals and juices.
3. Use caution in administering other drugs to the patient with hypocalcemia.
   a. The hypocalcemic patient is sensitive to digoxin; as hypocalcemia is reversed, the patient may rapidly develop digoxin toxicity.
   b. Cimetidine interferes with normal parathyroid function, especially in the patient with renal failure, which increases the risk of hypocalcemia.

Education and Health Maintenance
1. Explain to the patient and family the function of PTH and the role of vitamin D and calcium in maintaining good health.
2. Discuss the importance of complying with the medication regimen. Warn the patient not to substitute any over-the-counter drugs without prior advice and consent of the health care provider.

3. Instruct the patient about signs and symptoms of hypocalcemia (anxiety, hypertonia, spasms) and hypercalcemia (fatigue, weakness, clumsiness, emotional instability, arrhythmias) that should be reported.
4. Advise the patient to wear a medical alert tag.
5. Stress the rationale and importance of lifelong periodic follow-up examinations.

HYPOSPADIAS

Hypospadias is a congenital malposition of the urethral opening. It is the most common congenital anomaly involving the penis and is more common in boys. It may result partly from decreased testosterone production in early gestation. In males, the urethra opens on the ventral aspect of the penis. In severe cases, the urethra may open on the shaft of the penis and deflect the penis downward. Hypospadias is rare in females, in which the urethra opens into the vagina. In about 10% of the cases, an associated unilateral or bilateral cryptorchidism is present. Subsequent male siblings are at increased risk of hypospadias. Severe forms may interfere with the ability to procreate.

Assessment
1. Inspection of the genitalia shows abnormal placement of urethra.
2. The male infant or child cannot void with the penis in the normal elevated position.
3. In females, urine dribbles from the vagina.

Diagnostic Evaluation
1. Usually not difficult to diagnose because of visual anomaly.
2. Severe cases require genotypic or phenotypic sex determination, chromosomal, and hormonal studies.
3. Renal ultrasound, I.V. pyelography, or voiding cystourethrography may be done to determine associated defects.

H

Collaborative Management
Surgical Interventions
1. Surgical reconstruction may be required beginning before age 1.
2. Two-stage procedure is needed for extensive defects.

PEDIATRIC ALERT Circumcision should not be performed on an infant with hypospadias, however mild. All the tissue is needed for surgical repair at a future date.

Nursing Diagnoses
3, 6, 24, 30, 44, 67, 69, 123, 135

Nursing Interventions
Monitoring
1. Postoperatively, monitor daily weights and intake and output.
2. Monitor vital signs for hypotension or tachycardia.
3. Assess patient's skin turgor and mucous membranes for signs of dehydration.
4. Observe and record characteristics of urinary drainage, occurrence of bladder spasms, and appearance of dressing and the incision. Promptly report if urine or bloody drainage from the incision occurs.

Supportive Care
1. Explain all diagnostic tests before their occurrence, and prepare the parents and child for surgery.
2. Emphasize that the parents or child are not to blame for the illness.
3. Postoperatively, maintain patency of suprapubic catheter and perineal dressing. Restrain child as necessary to prevent inadvertent removal.
4. Maintain child in bed in a supine position for 2 or 3 days and with limited activity in bed for several more days to prevent disruption of surgical site. Use bed cradle as necessary to prevent pressure of bedclothes on surgical site.
5. Administer analgesics as needed and anticholinergics for sharp painful bladder spasms.

6. Encourage fluids and high-fiber diet to prevent constipation associated with bed rest.
7. Provide diversional activity and reassurance while on bed rest.

Education and Health Maintenance

1. Teach prompt diaper changes and cleaning of skin after bowel movements to prevent irritation of skin and contamination of healing wound.
2. Encourage long-term follow-up to ensure healing and acceptable cosmetic appearance.
3. Advise parents to report curvature of the penis, decreased force of urinary stream, or any change in voiding that may indicate complication requiring dilation or other surgical intervention.

HYPOTHERMIA

Hypothermia is a condition in which the core temperature of the body falls below 95° F (35° C) because of exposure to cold. In response to a decreased core temperature, the body will attempt to produce or conserve more heat through three mechanisms: by shivering, which produces heat through muscular activity; by peripheral vasoconstriction, which decreases heat loss; and by raising the basal metabolic rate. Treatment of this life-threatening condition requires immediate resuscitation, careful monitoring, and gradual rewarming of the body without precipitating cardiac arrhythmias.

Assessment

1. Progressive neurologic deterioration marked by apathy, poor judgment, ataxia, dysarthria, drowsiness, and eventually, coma.
2. Speech is slow and may be slurred.
3. Shivering may be suppressed below a temperature of 90° F (32.2° C).
4. Initial tachypnea followed by slow and shallow respirations; possibly 2 or 3 breaths per minute in severe hypothermia.

H

5. Breath may have fruity or acetone odor, indicating metabolism of fat because of decreased insulin levels.

6. If the body temperature falls below 86° F (30° C; severe hypothermia), heart sounds may not be audible even if the heart is still beating. Tissues conduct sound poorly at low temperatures.

7. Blood pressure readings may be extremely difficult to hear.

8. Pupil reflexes may be blocked by a decrease in cerebral blood flow, so the pupils may appear fixed and dilated.

EMERGENCY ALERT A severely hypothermic patient may present like a patient in cardiac arrest, with fixed dilated pupils, no pulse, and no blood pressure.

9. A variety of cardiac arrhythmias may be seen. A hypothermic heart is extremely susceptible to ventricular fibrillation. Very cold hearts do not respond to drugs or defibrillation.

Diagnostic Evaluation

1. Electrocardiogram (ECG) and continuous cardiac monitoring determine heart rate and rhythm.

2. Arterial blood gas (ABG) analysis detects acidosis.

3. Serum electrolytes and kidney function tests monitor condition.

Therapeutic Interventions

1. Assist breathing and oxygenation with supplemental oxygen at 100%, or bag-valve-mask device.

EMERGENCY ALERT If intubation is necessary, extreme caution should be used because ventricular fibrillation may be precipitated.

2. If pulse and respirations are absent, provide cardiopulmonary resuscitation (CPR) until the patient is adequately rewarmed and further evaluation through ECG and hemodynamic monitoring can be done.

3. Start I.V. therapy with normal saline. Ringer's lactate is not recommended, because a cold liver may not be able to metabolize the lactate.

4. Initiate rewarming. The type of rewarming (passive or active external rewarming; active core rewarming) depends

on the degree of hypothermia. Rewarming should continue until the core body temperature is 93.2° F (34° C). If the patient is in cardiac arrest, rewarming should continue until a temperature of 89.6° F (32° C) has been reached. Death in hypothermia is defined as a failure to revive after rewarming.

Nursing Diagnoses
19, 35, 50, 75, 87, 88

Nursing Interventions
Monitoring
1. Continuously monitor core temperatures with a low-reading rectal thermometer.
2. Continuously monitor ECG. Because pulse may be unobtainable due to hypothermia, rely on the cardiac monitor to determine the need for CPR.
3. Monitor the patient's condition through vital signs, central venous pressure and other hemodynamic methods, urinary output, and ABG values.
   a. Maintain an arterial line for recording blood pressure and to facilitate blood sampling. This allows rapid detection of acid–base disturbances and assessment of adequacy of ventilation and oxygenation.
   b. Urine output may show increase in response to peripheral vasoconstriction, "cold diuresis."

Supportive Care
1. Handle the patient *carefully and gently* to avoid triggering ventricular fibrillation.

> **EMERGENCY ALERT** Extreme caution should be used in moving or transporting patients because the heart is near fibrillation threshold in hypothermia.

2. Provide passive external rewarming for patients with temperature above 90° F (32.2° C).
   a. Remove all the wet or cold clothing and replace with warm clothing.
   b. Provide insulation by wrapping the patient in several blankets.

H

    c. Provide warmed fluids to drink.
3. Provide active external rewarming for patients with temperature above 82° F (27.7° C), as directed.
    a. Apply external heat, for example, warm hot water bottles to the axilla, neck, or groin (do not apply hot water bottles directly to the skin), or warm water immersion.
    b. May cause peripheral vasodilation, returning cool blood to the core, causing an initial lowering of the core temperature.
    c. May cause acidosis because of the "washing out" of lactic acid from the peripheral tissues.
    d. May cause an increase in the metabolic demands before the heart is warmed to meet these needs.
4. Assist with active core rewarming for patient with temperature less than 82° F, as directed.
    a. Inhalation of warmed, humidified oxygen by mask or ventilator
    b. Warmed I.V. fluids
    c. Warmed gastric lavage
    d. Peritoneal dialysis with warmed standard dialysis solution
    e. Mediastinal irrigation through open thoracotomy has been used successfully but has serious complications.
    f. Cardiopulmonary bypass

Education and Health Maintenance

1. Ensure adequate follow-up to enhance full recovery.
2. Review safety measures to prevent hypothermia, such as wearing adequate warm, dry clothing when exposed to cool, wet, windy weather conditions.
3. Discourage the use of alcohol while engaging in sports and recreation outdoors in cool weather because alcohol increases the risk of hypothermia.

 GERONTOLOGIC ALERT Elderly patients are at increased risk of hypothermia due to altered compensatory mechanisms.

HYPOTHYROIDISM

Hypothyroidism (also known as *myxedema* if symptomatic) refers to a low level of thyroid hormone in the bloodstream. This condition is caused by thyroid dysfunction, which may result from autoimmune disease (Hashimoto's thyroiditis); treatment for hyperthyroidism with surgery, radioactive iodine, or antithyroid drugs; iodine deficiency; subacute thyroiditis; or lithium toxicity. Hypothyroidism may also be congenital (1 in 4,000 live births). Secondary hypothyroidism refers to inadequate levels of thyroid-stimulating hormone (TSH), caused by disease of the pituitary gland.

Inadequate secretion of thyroid hormone leads to a general slowing of all physical and mental processes. General depression of most cellular enzyme systems and oxidative processes is represented by decreased metabolic activity and decreased production of body heat. The signs and symptoms of the disorder range from vague, nonspecific complaints that make diagnosis difficult, to severe symptoms that may be life-threatening if unrecognized and untreated. Complications include mental retardation in the young child who is untreated from birth; short stature and delayed physical development in the older child; and myxedema coma in all ages, which has a high mortality.

Assessment

1. The neonate may have very subtle signs, if any: markedly open posterior fontanelle, prolonged physiologic jaundice, feeding difficulties, cool and mottled skin, hypotonia, and umbilical hernia.
2. After age 6 months, signs may include growth failure, large and protruding tongue, coarse facial features, poor feeding, and constipation.
3. Older children with acquired hypothyroidism may exhibit slow growth rate, lethargy, obedient and nonaggressive behavior, cold intolerance, and poor school performance.
4. Signs and symptoms in adults include:
   a. Fatigue, lethargy, reduced attention span.
   b. Weight gain.

H

c. Complaints of cold hands and feet.

d. Decreased libido.

e. Menorrhagia or amenorrhea; difficulty conceiving or spontaneous abortion.

f. Subnormal temperature and pulse rates.

g. Thick, puffy skin; subcutaneous swelling in hands, feet, and eyelids (myxedema); thinning hair, with loss of the lateral one-third of each eyebrow.

h. Polyneuropathy, ataxia, muscle aches or weakness, clumsiness, prolonged deep tendon reflexes (especially ankle jerk).

i. Constipation, decreased peristalsis.

5. Myxedema is evidenced by hypotension, bradycardia, hyponatremia, (possibly) seizures, hypothermia, cerebral hypoxia, and coma.

DRUG ALERT Patients with hypothyroidism have increased response to hypnotic, sedative, and anesthetic agents.

Diagnostic Evaluation

1. Thyroid function tests show low triiodothyronine (T_3) and thyroxine (T_4) levels and elevated TSH level.

2. Thyroid microsomal antibodies may be elevated in autoimmune thyroiditis.

3. Elevated cholesterol.

4. Possible enlarged heart on chest X-ray.

5. Children may have delayed bone age on X-ray.

6. Electrocardiogram may show sinus bradycardia, low voltage of QRS complexes, and flat or inverted T waves.

Collaborative Management
Therapeutic Interventions

1. In severe hypothyroidism with myxedema coma, vital functions must be supported.

2. I.V. fluids are given cautiously if hyponatremia is present to prevent water intoxication.

3. Rapid rewarming techniques are avoided in myxedema to prevent increased oxygen requirements and possible cardiovascular collapse.

Pharmacologic Interventions

1. To restore normal metabolic state (euthyroid) in severe hypothyroidism:
   a. Because T_3 acts more quickly than T_4, this is given by nasogastric tube if patient is unconscious.
   b. Levothyroxine (T_4) can be administered parenterally until consciousness is restored to restore thyroxine level.
   c. Later, the patient is continued on oral thyroid hormone therapy.
   d. With rapid administration of thyroid hormone, plasma thyroxine levels may initiate adrenal insufficiency; hence, steroid therapy may be initiated.
2. Mild symptoms in the alert patient or asymptomatic cases (with abnormal laboratory work only) require only low-dose thyroid hormones, such as levothyroxine, to be given orally.

GERONTOLOGIC ALERT Care must be taken with elderly patients and those with coronary artery disease when starting thyroid hormone replacement, to avoid coronary ischemia caused by increased oxygen demands of heart. Preferably, start with low doses and increase gradually, taking 1 to 2 months to reach full replacement doses.

Nursing Diagnoses

1, 16, 19, 24, 43

Nursing Interventions

Monitoring

1. Monitor the patient to anticipate successful response to treatments:
   a. Diuresis, decreased puffiness
   b. Improved reflexes and muscle tone
   c. Accelerated pulse rate
   d. A slightly higher T_4 level and decreased TSH
   e. All signs of hypothyroidism should disappear over a 3- to 12-week period
2. As thyroid hormone levels gradually return to normal, monitor for arrhythmias, chest pain, and signs of heart failure.

H

3. Monitor a child's behavior, including sleep, eating pattern, bowel habits, level of alertness, and school performance.
4. Assess a child's growth pattern, weight gain, and head circumference.

Supportive Care

1. Prevent chilling to avoid increasing metabolic rate, which, in turn, places strain on the heart. Provide bed socks, bed jacket, and a warm environment.
2. Administer all prescribed drugs with caution before and after thyroid replacement begins. After thyroid replacement is initiated, the thyroid hormones may increase the effects of digoxin (monitor pulse) and anticoagulants (watch for signs of bleeding).
3. Report occurrence of angina.
4. Teach energy conservation techniques and need to increase activity gradually.

Education and Health Maintenance

1. Stress that thyroid hormone replacement therapy is a lifelong treatment.
2. Teach patients to take medications every day.

PEDIATRIC ALERT Advise parents not to mix thyroid medication in a bottle because feeding may not be finished; instead mix with small amount of fluid and give with dropper or syringe. If thyroid hormone pill is being chewed rather than swallowed, have child avoid brushing teeth immediately after to avoid washing away some of dose.

3. Teach about signs and symptoms of insufficient and excessive medication.
   a. Underdosage — fatigue, slow pulse, constipation
   b. Overdosage — feeling jittery, insomnia, increased pulse, palpitations
4. Reinforce the necessity of having blood evaluations periodically to determine thyroid levels.
5. Encourage adequate fluid intake and use of fiber to prevent constipation.
6. Advise controlling dietary intake to limit calories and reduce weight.

7. Advise obtaining further information through American Thyroid Association, *www.thyroid.org*.

HYSTERECTOMY

Hysterectomy is the surgical removal of the uterus primarily to treat cancer, benign tumors, bleeding disorders of the uterus, uterine prolapse, chronic pelvic pain, and endometriosis. Sixty-five percent of these procedures occur during the reproductive years. Hysterectomy is classified as subtotal (cervical stump remains); total (the entire uterus, including cervix, is removed); or total hysterectomy with bilateral salpingo-oophorectomy (BSO). Sometimes, the uterus is removed through a vaginal rather than an abdominal approach, with the cervical stump remaining. Laparoscopically assisted vaginal hysterectomy and laparoscopic supracervical hysterectomy may also be performed.

Potential Complications
1. Incisional or pelvic infection
2. Hemorrhage, thrombolic complications
3. Urinary tract injury
4. Bowel obstruction

Nursing Diagnoses
3, 30, 69, 135, 156

Collaborative Management and Interventions
Preoperative Care
1. Determine if the patient knows reason for hysterectomy, what the procedure involves, and what to expect postoperatively.
2. Keep the patient NPO from midnight the night before surgery and have the patient void before surgery.
3. Administer an enema before surgery to evacuate the bowel and prevent contamination and trauma during surgery.
4. Perform vaginal irrigation before surgery to cleanse the area and ensure that a skin preparation is done if ordered.
5. Administer preoperative medication to help the patient relax.

H

Postoperative Care

1. Provide adequate pain control.
2. Encourage the patient to splint incision when moving.
3. Encourage the patient to ambulate as soon as possible to decrease flatus and abdominal distention.
4. Institute sitz baths or ice packs as prescribed to alleviate perineal discomfort.

EMERGENCY ALERT Be alert for calf tenderness or leg swelling (which may indicate deep vein thrombosis) or sudden onset of shortness of breath and tachycardia (which could indicate pulmonary embolism).

5. Monitor intake and output, bladder distention, and for signs and symptoms of bladder infection.
6. Make sure that patient voids after surgery. Catheterize the patient intermittently if uncomfortable or has not voided in 8 hours. Maintain patency of indwelling catheter if one is in place.
7. Catheterize for residual urine after the patient voids, if ordered; should be less than 3 oz (100 mL). Continue to check if more than 3 oz voided to prevent bladder infection.
8. Encourage the patient to empty bladder around the clock, not only when feeling the urge because of loss of sensation of bladder fullness.
9. Ensure adequate hydration to decrease risk of urinary infection.
10. Assess vaginal drainage for amount, color, and odor. Assess incision site and vital signs for signs of infection.
11. Administer antibiotics as prescribed.
12. Assist with use of incentive spirometer, coughing and deep breathing, and ambulation to decrease risk of pulmonary infection.
13. Discuss changes about sexual functioning such as shortened vagina and possible dyspareunia due to dryness.
14. Offer suggestions to improve sexual functioning.
    a. Use of water-soluble lubricants
    b. Change position—female dominant offers more control of depth of penetration.

Education and Health Maintenance

1. Advise the patient that a total hysterectomy with BSO produces a surgical menopause. The patient may experience hot flashes, vaginal dryness, and mood swings unless hormonal replacement therapy is instituted.

2. Advise the patient not to sit too long at one time, as in driving long distances, because of risk of pooling of blood in the lower extremities or pelvis, causing thromboembolism.

3. Advise that the patient follow the surgeon's instructions to delay driving a car because even pressing the brake pedal puts stress on the lower abdomen.

4. Tell the patient to expect a tired feeling for the first few days at home and, therefore, not to plan too many activities for the first week. She will be able to perform most of her usual daily activities within 1 month, and feel herself again within 2 months.

5. Tell the patient not to feel discouraged if at times during convalescence she experiences depression, feels like crying, and seems unusually nervous. This is common but will not last.

6. Remind the patient to ask her surgeon about any strenuous or lifting activities, which are usually delayed for 4 to 6 weeks.

7. Reinforce instructions given by the surgeon on intercourse, douching, and use of tampons, which are usually discouraged for 4 to 6 weeks. Sexual intercourse should be resumed cautiously to prevent injury and discomfort.

8. Showers are permitted, but tub baths are deferred until healing is complete.

9. Instruct the patient to report fever greater than 100° F (37.8° C), heavy vaginal bleeding, drainage, and foul odor of discharge.

10. Emphasize the importance of follow-up and routine physical and gynecologic examinations.

H

IJ

IMPERFORATE ANUS AND OTHER ANORECTAL MALFORMATIONS

An arrest in embryonic development at the eighth week may result in a variety of lower rectal, anal, and genitourinary abnormalities. These abnormalities include imperforate anal membrane, rectoperineal fistula, anal atresia and stenosis, anal agenesis, anorectal malformation with rectourinary fistula (males), anorectal malformation with fistula and cloaca (embryonic nondifferentiation of lower GI, reproductive, and urinary tracts), and cloacal exstrophy (abnormal lower GI, urinary, and reproductive organs open to the outside). Complications include permanent bowel and bladder incontinence, intestinal obstruction, infection, and reproductive problems. Other congenital abnormalities, such as Down syndrome, congenital heart disease, spinal malformations, and esophageal atresia, may be present.

Assessment

Condition is usually evident at birth or within several hours.

1. Absent or abnormally placed anal opening
2. Meconium stool is absent; stool may be passed through fistula
3. Thermometer or rectal tube cannot be inserted into rectum
4. Abdominal distention progresses

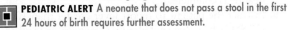 **PEDIATRIC ALERT** A neonate that does not pass a stool in the first 24 hours of birth requires further assessment.

Diagnostic Evaluation

1. Urine examination may show meconium and epithelial debris, indicating fistula.
2. Voiding cystourethrogram shows abnormality.
3. Cross-table lateral abdominal X-ray with infant in prone position with pelvis elevated may show blind rectum.

4. Sonogram may be done to locate rectal pouch.
5. MRI may be done.

Collaborative Management
Surgical Interventions

Surgical procedure depends on the location and type of abnormality.

1. Imperforate anal membrane and agenesis, and anal stenosis may be repaired through relatively minor procedure at birth.
2. More complex and higher level lesions require more extensive surgery in two or three steps.

Nursing Diagnoses
69, 104, 123, 132, 134, 136

Nursing Interventions
Monitoring

1. Observe the infant carefully for any signs of distress, abdominal distention, and vomiting. Monitor abdominal girth and intake and output.
2. Check vital signs frequently.
3. Monitor nasogastric (NG) decompression before and after surgery for amount and character of drainage.
4. Observe postoperatively for abdominal distention, bleeding from perineum, and respiratory difficulty. Especially note vomiting or stooling.
5. Monitor for return of peristalsis through auscultation after clamping of NG tube.
6. Monitor parenteral fluids and discontinue when oral intake is sustained.

Supportive Care
Preoperative Care

1. Withhold feedings. Note color and amount of vomiting.
2. Maintain NG tube passed to decompress the stomach.
3. Use an Isolette or radiant warmer to maintain stable temperature.
4. Keep fistula area clean.

IJ

5. Comfort the infant to prevent crying to minimize expenditure of energy.
6. Minimize handling of the infant between procedures to encourage rest and sleep.

Postoperative Care

1. Prevent infection of suture line.
   a. Do not put anything in rectum after anoplasty.
   b. Expose perineum to air and apply antibiotic ointment as directed.
   c. Position the infant for easy access to perineum for cleansing and minimal irritation of site.
2. Observe for redness, drainage, and poor healing.
3. Prevent skin breakdown around colostomy site with appropriate appliances and skin barrier. Consult an enterostomal therapist.
4. Administer I.V. antibiotics as directed.
5. Start oral feedings when bowel sounds are present and NG decompression is stopped (usually within hours after an anoplasty, longer with colostomy or pull-through).
6. Monitor for vomiting and record characteristics of stool.
7. Maintain patency of the urinary catheter.
8. Encourage parents to participate in care and provide emotional security for the child.
9. Initiate referral to community nurse, especially if the parents are particularly anxious about caring for the child at home.

Education and Health Maintenance

1. Review special care and procedures to be continued at home (colostomy, anal dilation). Involve parents and other caregivers in teaching.
2. Explain problems that may be encountered as the child grows:
   a. Fecal impaction because of lack of sensation to defecate.
   b. Future surgery if primary repair was not done.
   c. Toilet training may be delayed, especially after a pull-through procedure.

     d. Inability to control fecal seepage from rectum.
3. Provide some practical guidelines to help parents cope:
     a. Fecal control may not be achieved until age 10.
     b. Encourage bowel habit training or patterning of defecation (eg, after breakfast) early.
     c. Promote diet modifications; teach about foods that have a laxative effect (plums, prunes, chocolate, nuts, corn) and foods that have a binding effect (peanut butter, bananas, cheese).
     d. Stool softeners or antidiarrheal medications may be effective.
     e. Rectal inertia may cause fecal impaction in rectosigmoid colon with soiling from fluid overflow. Bisacodyl suppository or cleansing enema provides assistance in management.
4. Encourage mutual support from other families who have a child with an anorectal malformation. For additional information, refer to the National Organization for Rare Disorders, Inc., *www.rarediseases.org*.

INFECTIVE ENDOCARDITIS

See *Endocarditis, Infective*.

INTESTINAL OBSTRUCTION

Intestinal obstruction is an interruption in the normal flow of intestinal contents along the intestinal tract. The block may occur in the small (most common) or large intestine, may be complete or incomplete, may be mechanical or functional (paralytic), and may or may not compromise the vascular supply. Obstruction most frequently occurs in the very young and the very old.

    Mechanical obstruction is a physical blockage to the passage of intestinal contents. It may result from postsurgical adhesions, hernia (most common nonsurgical cause), volvulus, hematoma, tumor, intussusception (telescoping of intestinal wall into itself), stricture, stenosis, foreign body, fecal or barium impaction, or polyp.

    Functional obstruction (paralytic ileus), in contrast, involves no physical obstruction. Peristalsis is ineffective, blood sup-

IJ

ply is not interrupted, and the condition usually disappears spontaneously after 2 to 3 days. Causes of functional obstruction include spinal cord injuries, vertebral fractures, peritonitis, pneumonia, GI or abdominal surgery, and wound dehiscence (opening).

Severity depends on the degree of obstruction, the area affected, and the degree to which circulation in the bowel wall is disrupted.

Untreated, intraluminal pressure increases due to accumulating secretions and gas. Bacteria and toxins pass across the intestinal wall, leading to peritonitis. Eventually, intestinal wall ischemia and necrosis may occur, leading to shock and death.

Assessment

1. Crampy abdominal pain that may occur in waves (colic).

■ **PEDIATRIC ALERT** Episodes of severe abdominal pain combined with vomiting in the infant suggest intussusception.

2. No bowel movements; however, blood or mucus may be passed.
3. Vomiting, first of stomach contents, then bilious, finally containing fecal matter (if obstruction of ileum or distal).
4. Abdominal distention.
5. Signs of dehydration — malaise, thirst, dry mucus membranes, oliguria.
6. Signs and symptoms of large bowel obstruction develop more slowly with constipation being prominent.
7. Signs of shock — pallor, hypertension, tachycardia, reduced level of consciousness.

■ **GERONTOLOGIC ALERT** Watch for air-fluid lock syndrome in elderly patients, who often remain in the recumbent position for extended periods. In this syndrome, fluid collects in dependent bowel loops, and peristalsis is too weak to push fluid "uphill." The obstruction primarily occurs in the large bowel. Turn the patient every 10 minutes until enough flatus is passed to decompress the abdomen. A rectal tube may help.

Diagnostic Evaluation

1. Abdominal X-rays show intestinal gas or fluid.

2. Barium enema shows a distended, air-filled colon or a closed sigmoid loop.
3. Decreased serum sodium, potassium, and chloride levels because of vomiting; elevated white blood cell counts with necrosis, strangulation, or peritonitis; and increased serum amylase levels from irritation of the pancreas by the bowel loop.
4. Arterial blood gas analysis may indicate metabolic acidosis or alkalosis.
5. Flexible sigmoidoscopy or colonoscopy may be done to identify cause.

Collaborative Management
Therapeutic Interventions
1. Correct fluid and electrolyte imbalances:
   a. Na^+, K^+, blood component therapy
   b. Normal saline or Ringer's lactate to correct interstitial fluid deficit
2. Nasogastric (NG) decompression of GI tract to reduce gastric secretions; nasointestinal tubes, such as the Cantor or Miller Abbott, may also be used.
3. Treatment for shock and peritonitis with I.V. fluids, vasopressors, or antibiotics.
4. Hyperalimentation to correct protein deficiency from chronic obstruction, paralytic ileus, or infection.
5. Ambulation to try to induce peristalsis in a patient with a paralytic ileus.

Surgical Interventions
1. Bowel resection with end-to-end anastomosis
2. Closed bowel procedure such as lysis of adhesions or reduction of volvulus
3. Double-barrel ostomy if end-to-end anastomosis too risky
4. Loop colostomy to divert fecal stream and decompress bowel, with bowel resection to be done as second procedure

IJ

Nursing Diagnoses
3, 6, 16, 23, 75, 135, 136

Nursing Interventions

Also see *Gastrointestinal or Abdominal Surgery*, page 381.

Monitoring

1. Frequently check the patient's level of responsiveness; decreasing responsiveness may indicate impending shock or increasing electrolyte imbalance.
2. Monitor vital signs closely for tachycardia or drop in blood pressure, indicating hypovolemia and impending shock.
3. Monitor intake and output, including vomitus and NG drainage, to guide fluid replacement.

> **EMERGENCY ALERT** Be alert for signs of worsening obstruction that may require surgery — worsening pain, increasing distention, and increasing NG output — and report them promptly.

Supportive Care

1. Recognize the patient's concerns and provide care confidently and calmly to ensure cooperation and allay fears.
2. Evaluate effectiveness of pain relief regimen.
3. Maintain NG suction and monitor drainage.
4. Record intake and output, taking into account I.V. fluids, hyperalimentation, blood products, NG drainage, urine, and other output.
5. After ostomy procedure, empty drainage bag frequently or connect tubing to drainage bottle at side of bed; expect considerable amount of fecal drainage during the first 12 to 15 hours (17 to 34 oz [500 to 1,000 mL]).
   a. Observe drainage equipment frequently for patency.
   b. If there is difficulty with drainage, it may be necessary to inject 0.5 oz (15 mL) of warm saline solution into the enterostomy tube every 2 to 4 hours, with approval of health care provider.
   c. Protect skin around ostomy with a skin barrier such as a karaya preparation.
6. Record amount and consistency of stools, and test for occult blood.
7. Keep the patient in Fowler's position to promote ventilation and relief from abdominal distention.

8. Remove NG tube (when drainage has ceased, bowel sounds have returned, and patient is passing flatus), as directed.
   a. Keep tube clamped with suction off for period of time before removal, and monitor for return of bowel sounds.
   b. When ready for removal, remove tape and instruct the patient to take a deep breath and hold it.
   c. Withdraw the tube slowly and evenly, covering it with a towel as it emerges; pull quickly when tube reaches nasopharynx.
   d. Allow the patient to clear nose and mouth of secretions and provide mouth care supplies.

Education and Health Maintenance

1. Teach care after bowel resection or temporary colostomy.
2. Teach proper diet, fluid intake, and activity to prevent constipation and recurrence of partial obstruction.
3. Advise prompt recognition and reporting of recurrent symptoms.

INTRACRANIAL ANEURYSM

See *Aneurysm, Intracranial.*

INTUSSUSCEPTION

Intussusception is the invagination or telescoping of a portion of the intestine into an adjacent, more distal section of the intestine causing mechanical obstruction. The cause may be idiopathic (unknown but following a viral infection); lead point (change in the mucosa from another condition such as cystic fibrosis, Meckel's diverticulum, or hematoma); or post-operative.

Intussusception occurs in children younger than age 3, most commonly ages 5 to 10 months. Without prompt treatment, necrosis of the involved segment leads to shock, perforation, and peritonitis.

IJ

Assessment

1. Paroxysmal abdominal pain; legs drawn up, child is inconsolable; may be comfortable between episodes

2. Blood in stool, or later "currant-jelly" stools containing sloughed mucosa, blood, and mucus
3. Vomiting
4. Increasing absence of stools
5. Abdominal distention, bowel sounds diminished, absent or high pitched
6. Sausagelike mass palpable in abdomen (Dance's sign)
7. Unusual-looking anus; may look like rectal prolapse
8. Dehydration and fever
9. Shocklike state with rapid pulse, pallor, marked sweating

 PEDIATRIC ALERT Incarcerated hernia and testicular torsion are the differential diagnosis; these can be palpated.

Diagnostic Evaluation

1. X-ray of abdomen may show absence of gas or mass in right upper quadrant.
2. Barium enema is done if there is no appearance of peritonitis; shows a concave filling defect (will help reduce the invagination).
3. Ultrasonogram may be done to locate area of telescoped bowel.
4. Color Doppler sonography determines whether reducible. Absence of blood flow indicates ischemia and, therefore, enema reduction should be avoided.

Collaborative Management
Therapeutic Interventions

1. Hydrostatic reduction of telescoped bowel with air or barium enema used during first 24 hours after onset may reduce intussusception in 70% to 90% of patients. However, recurrence and perforation may occur.

EMERGENCY ALERT Clinical findings of peritonitis, shock, or signs of perforation indicate that enemas are contraindicated.

Surgical Interventions

1. Intussusception can be surgically reduced; resection may be necessary if bowel is nonviable.

Nursing Diagnoses
3, 44, 75, 123, 135, 136

Nursing Interventions
Also see *Gastrointestinal or Abdominal Surgery*, page 381.

Monitoring
1. Monitor I.V. fluids and intake and output to guide fluid balance.
2. Be alert for respiratory distress due to abdominal distention. Watch for grunting or shallow, rapid respirations if patient is in shocklike state.
3. Monitor vital signs, urine output, pain, distention, and general behavior preoperatively and postoperatively.

Supportive Care
1. Observe infant's behavior as indicator of pain; may be irritable and very sensitive to handling or lethargic or unresponsive. Handle the infant gently.
2. Explain cause of pain to parents, and reassure them about purpose of diagnostic tests and treatments.
3. Administer analgesics as prescribed.
4. Maintain NPO status as ordered.
   a. Wet lips and give mouth care.
   b. Give infant pacifier to suck.
5. Restrain infant as necessary for I.V. therapy.
6. Insert nasogastric tube if ordered to decompress stomach.
   a. Irrigate at frequent intervals.
   b. Note drainage and return from irrigation.
7. Continually reassess condition because increased pain and bloody stools may indicate perforation.

PEDIATRIC ALERT Passage of one normal brown stool may occur, clearing the colon distal to the intussusception. Passage of more than one normal brown stool may indicate that the intussusception has reduced itself. Report any stools immediately to the health care provider.

8. After reduction by hydrostatic enema, monitor vital signs and general condition — especially abdominal tenderness, bowel sounds, lethargy, and tolerance to fluids — to watch for recurrence.

IJ

9. Prepare the patient for surgery if in shocklike state or febrile.

Education and Health Maintenance

1. Explain that recurrence is 5% to 7% and usually occurs within 36 hours after reduction. Review signs and symptoms of recurrence with parents.
2. Review activity restrictions with parents (eg, positioning on back or side, quiet play, and avoidance of water sports until wound heals).
3. Encourage follow-up care.
4. Provide anticipatory guidance for developmental age of child.

IRON DEFICIENCY ANEMIA

See *Anemia, Iron Deficiency.*

KAWASAKI DISEASE

Kawasaki disease (mucocutaneous lymph node syndrome) is a form of vasculitis identified by an acute febrile illness with multiple systems affected. The cause is unknown, but autoimmunity, infection, and genetic predisposition are believed to be involved. It affects mostly children between ages 3 months and 8 years; 80% are younger than age 5. It occurs more commonly in Japanese children or those of Japanese decent. It has seasonal epidemics, usually in late winter and early spring.

Although Kawasaki disease is a multisystem disease, the cardiovascular system appears to be the primary site with coronary artery vasculitis, aneurysm development, thrombosis, and myocardial thrombosis progressing over days to weeks. Approximately 15% to 25% of patients develop cardiac complications (coronary thrombosis or rupture, myocardial infarction, heart failure, vasculitis of the aorta or peripheral arteries); however, mortality is low.

Assessment
Stage I — Acute Febrile Phase (First 10 days)
1. The child appears severely ill and irritable.
2. Major diagnostic criteria established by the Centers for Disease Control and Prevention (CDC) are as follows:
   a. High, spiking fever for 5 or more days
   b. Bilateral conjunctival injection
   c. Oropharyngeal erythema, "strawberry" tongue, or red and dry lips
   d. Erythema and edema of hands and feet, periungual desquamation
   e. Erythematous generalized rash
   f. Cervical lymphadenopathy greater than 0.6 inch (1.5 cm)
3. Pericarditis, myocarditis, cardiomegaly, heart failure, and pleural effusion.

K

549

4. Other associated findings include meningitis, arthritis, sterile pyuria, vomiting, and diarrhea.

Stage II — Subacute Phase (Days 11 to 25)
1. Acute symptoms of stage I subside as temperature returns to normal. The child remains irritable and anorectic.
2. Dry, cracked lips with fissures.
3. Desquamation of toes and fingers.
4. Coronary thrombosis, aneurysm, myocardial infarction, and heart failure.
5. Thrombocytosis peaks at 2 weeks.

Stage III — Convalescent Phase (Until sedimentation rate and platelet count normalize)
1. The child appears well.
2. Transverse grooves of fingers and toenails (Beau's lines).
3. Coronary thrombosis, aneurysms may occur.

Diagnostic Evaluation
1. Diagnosis is based on criteria developed by the CDC — during stage I, fever and four of six other criteria must be present.
2. Complete blood count shows leukocytosis during stage I.
3. Erythrocyte sedimentation rate (ESR) is elevated.
4. Erythrocytes and hemoglobin are slightly decreased.
5. C-reactive protein is positive.
6. Platelet count is increased during second to fourth weeks of illness.
7. Urinalysis detects proteinuria and leukocytes.
8. Liver enzymes are elevated.
9. Chest X-ray, electrocardiogram, and echocardiogram are done to detect cardiovascular effects.

Collaborative Management
Therapeutic Interventions
1. Treatment aims to ameliorate symptoms and prevent coronary thrombosis, coronary aneurysm, and death.
2. Supportive measures:

    a. Maintain fluid and electrolyte balance; give nutritional support.

    b. Provide comfort.

3. Cardiac follow-up by pediatric cardiologist with serial two-dimensional echocardiograms, angiography, and cardiac isoenzyme studies. Rarely, coronary bypass surgery is required.

Pharmacologic Interventions

1. Immune globulin (gamma globulin) I.V. therapy—IVGG (2 g/kg/day) is initiated during stage I in one 8- to 10-hour infusion to reduce the incidence of coronary artery abnormalities.

EMERGENCY ALERT Infusion of IVGG sometimes causes blood pressure to drop sharply, which may mimic anaphylaxis. This effect may be related to the infusion rate. Monitor blood pressure and heart rate at the start of infusion, after 15 and 30 minutes, and then hourly until infusion is complete. Slow the infusion and have the patient evaluated for any drop in blood pressure. Premedicate the child as directed and have diphenhydramine and epinephrine available to treat anaphylactic reaction.

2. Aspirin therapy:

    a. Anti-inflammatory dose (80 to 100 mg/kg/day) divided qid during stage I.

    b. Antiplatelet dose (3 to 10 mg/kg/day) given after fever is controlled, then continued for 2 to 3 months after illness (when the echocardiogram is normal), or until ESR and platelet count are normal, to reduce risk of spontaneous coronary thrombosis. Aspirin may be continued indefinitely if there are coronary abnormalities.

3. Thrombolytic therapy may be required during stages I, II, or III. Dipyridamole or pentoxifylline may be given as a platelet aggregation inhibitor if aneurysms are present.

Nursing Diagnoses

3, 15, 19, 23, 60, 63

K

Nursing Interventions
Monitoring

1. Monitor pain level and child's response to analgesics.
2. Institute continual cardiac monitoring and assessment for complications; report arrhythmias.
   a. Take vital signs as directed by condition; report abnormalities.
   b. Assess for signs of myocarditis (tachycardia, gallop rhythm, chest pain).
   c. Monitor for heart failure (dyspnea, nasal flaring, grunting, retractions, cyanosis, orthopnea, crackles, moist respirations, distended jugular veins, edema).
3. Closely monitor intake and output, and administer oral and I.V. fluids as ordered.
4. Monitor hydration status by checking skin turgor, weight, urinary output, specific gravity, and presence of tears.
5. Observe mouth and skin frequently for signs of infection.

Supportive Care

1. Allow the child periods of uninterrupted rest. Offer pain medication routinely rather than as needed during stage I; avoid nonsteroidal anti-inflammatory drugs if the child is on aspirin therapy.
2. Perform comfort measures related to the eyes:
   a. Conjunctivitis can cause photosensitivity, so darken the room, offer sunglasses.
   b. Apply cool compresses.
   c. Discourage rubbing eyes.
   d. Instill artificial tears to soothe conjunctiva.
3. Monitor temperature every 4 to 8 hours, every 2 hours if elevated. Give tub or sponge baths for temperature over 101° F (38.3° C), or use a cooling blanket for higher temperatures unresponsive to antipyretics.
4. Perform comfort measures related to joint pain and tender lymph nodes.
   a. Use passive range-of-motion exercises every 4 hours while the child is awake because movement may be restricted.

b. Encourage the child to move about freely under supervision; provide soft toys and quiet play and encourage use of hands and fingers.

5. Provide quiet, peaceful environment with diversional activities.

6. Provide care measures for oral mucous membranes.

a. Offer cool liquids (ice chips and ice pops); progress to soft, bland foods.

b. Give mouth care every 1 to 4 hours with special mouth swabs; use soft toothbrush only after healing has occurred.

c. Apply petroleum jelly to dried, cracked lips.

7. Provide care measures to improve skin integrity.

a. Avoid use of soap because it tends to dry skin and make it more likely to break down.

b. Elevate edematous extremities.

c. Use sheepskin, egg-crate mattress, and smooth sheets.

d. If clothes are used, encourage use of soft flannel or terry cloth garments that fit loosely.

e. Apply emollients to skin, as ordered.

f. Protect peeling skin; observe for signs of infection.

8. Offer clear liquids every hour when child is awake.

9. Encourage the child to eat meals and snacks with adequate protein to prevent hypoalbuminemia.

10. Infuse I.V. fluids through a volume control device if dehydration is present, and check the site and amount hourly.

11. Explain all procedures to the child and family.

12. Provide respite for parents during irritable stage of illness when child may be inconsolable.

13. Encourage the parents and child to verbalize their concerns, fears, and questions.

14. Practice relaxation techniques with child, such as relaxation breathing, guided imagery, and distraction.

15. Prepare the child for cardiac surgery or thrombolytic therapy if complications develop.

16. Keep the family informed about progress and reinforce stages and prognosis.

K

Education and Health Maintenance

1. Make sure that the family understands the medications, follow-up tests, and physical activity levels that have been prescribed for the child based on the extent of cardiac involvement.

2. Teach parents that long-term care after discharge is critical because complications may occur months after illness.

3. Provide written instructions about cardiac complications and stress the need to report the development of symptoms.

4. Teach family members cardiopulmonary resuscitation.

5. Teach parents to recognize and report signs of possible salicylate toxicity—tinnitus, nausea, vomiting, GI distress, blood in stool, and increased respirations.

COMMUNITY CARE CONSIDERATIONS

Risk of Reye's syndrome increases with children who are taking aspirin and develop varicella or influenza. Parents need to notify their health care provider immediately if the child has been exposed. Aspirin therapy may be temporarily discontinued.

6. Encourage parents not to overprotect the child. Discuss with parents the grief and mourning process of denial, anger, bargaining, depression, and acceptance that they may be going through because of the chronic illness.

7. Advise parents to allow child to be as active as desired unless coronary ischemia is present or the child is on anticoagulants. Try to protect the child from injury if on anticoagulants (no sharp toys, no contact sports) and develop a plan with the child's school for safety.

8. Discuss regression that might occur as a result of hospitalization or the disease process and suggest ways to deal with these changes.

PEDIATRIC ALERT The effectiveness of live virus vaccines, such as measles-mumps-rubella, may be reduced after receiving gamma globulin. Therefore, if the child is due for a live virus vaccine, it should be delayed until 5 months after receiving gamma globulin.

9. For additional information, refer to such agencies as the American Heart Association, *www.americanheart.org*.

KIDNEY SURGERY AND URINARY DIVERSION

Kidney surgery may include *nephrectomy*, *kidney transplantation*, procedures to remove obstruction such as stones or tumors, procedures to insert drainage tubes for *nephrostomy* or *ureterostomy*, or procedures to insert stents (ureteral stent) to bypass obstruction. Incisional approaches vary but may involve the flank, thoracic, and abdominal regions. Nephrectomy is usually performed for malignant tumors of the kidney but may also be indicated for trauma and kidneys that no longer function because of obstructive disorders and other renal disease. Loss of one kidney does not impair renal function when the remaining kidney is normal. Nephrectomy and other procedures are now being done laparoscopically to decrease pain, blood loss, and length of stay.

Kidney transplantation is done for end-stage renal failure, as an alternative to hemodialysis. *Urinary diversion* refers to providing an alternate pathway for urinary excretion other than through the bladder and urethra. Urinary diversion may be necessary due to trauma, genitourinary cancer, congenital malformation, or in severe urinary tract infections that threaten the kidneys. A number of operative procedures are performed to achieve this (see *Box K-1*, pages 556 to 558).

Potential Complications

1. Hemorrhage and shock
2. Pulmonary complications (atelectasis, pneumonia, pneumothorax)
3. Thromboembolism (thrombophlebitis and pulmonary embolism)
4. Paralytic ileus
5. Urinary infection
6. Obstruction of urinary drainage
7. Rejection of transplant

(*Text continues on page 558.*)

K

BOX K-1 Methods of Urinary Diversion

ILEAL CONDUIT (BRICKER'S LOOP)

Most common; ureters are transplanted into an isolated section of the terminal ileum; one end is brought through the abdominal wall to create a stoma. Urine flows from the kidney through the ileal conduit and exits through the stoma. The ureters may also be transplanted into the transverse colon (colon conduit).

CONTINENT URINARY RESERVOIR (KOCK POUCH, INDIANA POUCH, MAINZ POUCH, AND OTHERS)

Transplants the ureters into a pouch created from small bowel or large and small bowel. The existing ileocecal valve or a surgically created intussuscepted nipple valve provides the continence mechanism. The patient does not have to wear an external appliance, but the procedure does require intermittent self-catheterization of the pouch.

ORTHOTOPIC BLADDER REPLACEMENT (HEMI-KOCK POUCH, NEOBLADDER, AND OTHERS)

Pouch created from small or large and small bowel is anastomosed to urethral stump in men; voiding is through the urethra. The patient usually has nocturnal incontinence. Not all patients are candidates for this procedure.

NURSING CONSIDERATIONS

1. An enterostomal therapist or surgeon will mark stoma site preoperatively in good anatomic location where patient can see it. Site may also be marked for orthotopic bladder replacement in case intraoperative findings prevent such a procedure.
2. Postoperatively monitor drains—sudden increase in drainage suggests a urine leak; send specimen of drainage for blood urea nitrogen (BUN) and creatinine, if ordered. (Presence of measurable BUN and creatinine in drainage indicates urine in drainage, confirming a urine leak.)
3. Maintain protection of ureteral stents used to protect ureterointestinal anastomoses (with ileal or colon conduit); stents will emerge from stoma or through separate wound and are removed in approximately 3 weeks.
4. Maintain transparent urostomy pouch over stoma postoperatively to allow easy assessment. Observe for normal urine (but not fecal) drainage at all times.

Methods of Urinary Diversion (continued)

5. Inspect stoma for color; size; whether it is flush, nippled, or retracted; and the condition of peristomal skin. Document baseline information.
6. With continent urinary diversions, maintain patency of drainage catheters placed into internal urinary pouch during surgery; irrigate with 1 oz (30 mL) saline every 2 to 4 hours to prevent obstruction from mucus accumulation.
7. Teach patient how to change pouch. Emphasize that peristomal skin must be clean and dry or appliance will not adhere.
   a. Tell patient that frequency of pouch changes depends on type of pouch used—generally, pouches should be changed every 3 days (for one-piece pouches) to every 4 to 7 days (for two-piece pouches).
   b. Advise emptying the pouch when it is one-third to one-half full to prevent weight of urine from loosening adhesive seal. Open drain valve for periodic emptying.

COMMUNITY CARE CONSIDERATIONS

Advise changing pouch in morning before fluids are taken or before bedtime when urine output is lowest. Have the patient insert a small piece of gauze into the stoma or over the stoma to prevent drainage while changing appliance.

   c. Advise using a belt to keep the pouch in place during the day and using a bedside urinary drainage bag at night if desired.
8. Teach patient with continent urinary reservoir how to catheterize stoma every 2 hours at first and gradually lengthen time until reservoir is holding 13.5 to 17 oz (400 to 500 mL) of urine and patient is catheterizing four to five times per day.
9. For patients with orthotopic bladder replacement, after removal of catheter, teach patient to void by straining abdominal muscles. Initially voiding must be done every 2 hours during day and every 3 hours at night. Gradually, intervals are lengthened.
   a. Teach pelvic floor–strengthening exercises to minimize incontinence.
   b. Patience with exercise and voiding schedule will optimize results.

(continued)

K

> **Methods of Urinary Diversion** (continued)
>
> 10. Advise the patient to report problems with peristomal skin or with leakage from pouch or development of fever, chills, pain, change in color of urine (cloudy, bloody), or diminishing urine output.
> 11. For additional information and support refer to United Ostomy Association, Inc., *www.uoa.org.*

8. Postinfarction syndrome (if renal artery embolization was done)

Nursing Diagnoses
3, 6, 24, 30, 69, 123, 135

Collaborative Management and Interventions
Preoperative Care

1. Prepare the patient for surgery with information about operating room routine and postoperative care; administer preoperative antibiotics and bowel-cleansing regimen.
2. Assess for risk factors for thromboembolism (smoking, hormonal contraceptive use, varicosities of lower extremities), and apply antiembolism stockings if ordered. Review leg exercises with the patient, and describe pneumatic compression device that will be used postoperatively.
3. Assess pulmonary status (presence of dyspnea, productive cough, other related cardiac symptoms), and teach deep-breathing exercises, effective coughing, and use of an incentive spirometer.
4. If embolization of the renal artery is being done preoperatively for patients with renal cell carcinoma, monitor for and treat symptoms of postinfarction syndrome (flank pain, fever, leukocytosis, and hypertension), which may last for up to 3 days.

Postoperative Care

1. Closely monitor intake and output, especially after kidney transplantation.
   a. Expect normal urine output to be 30 to 100 mL/hour.
   b. Report oliguria with less than 30 mL/hour, or polyuria of 100 to 500 mL/hour.
2. Monitor serum electrolyte results and electrocardiogram for changes caused by electrolyte imbalance. Report arrhythmias or other cardiac symptoms immediately.
3. Monitor blood pressure and heart rate, central venous pressure, and pulmonary artery pressure (if indicated) to anticipate adjustment of fluid replacement.

EMERGENCY ALERT Frequently monitor blood pressure, pulse, and respirations to recognize signs of hemorrhage (and shock), the chief dangers after renal surgery. Watch for pain, blood in wound drainage, or an expanding flank mass. Prepare for rapid blood and fluid replacement and reoperation.

4. Avoid using the same extremity being used for dialysis access when inserting I.V. or intra-arterial lines. Prepare for hemodialysis in postoperative period if kidney transplant was done, until transplanted kidney is functioning well. Monitor patency of vascular access.
5. Assess pain location, intensity, and characteristics.
   a. Transient renal coliclike pain may be caused by passage of blood clots down the ureter; report increased or persistent pain that may indicate hemorrhage or obstruction of urinary drainage.
   b. Assess bowel sounds, abdominal distention, and pain that may indicate paralytic ileus and need for nasogastric decompression.
6. Administer pain medications; evaluate effectiveness of patient-controlled analgesia.
7. Assist the patient with use of incentive spirometer, coughing and deep breathing, and ambulation to decrease risk of pulmonary infection. Provide meticulous chest tube care. Encourage splinting of incision when turning or coughing.
8. Maintain patency of urinary drainage tubes or catheters as indicated. Prevent kinking or pulling.

K

9. Use frequent hand washing and asepsis when providing care and handling of urinary drainage system (especially important for the patient taking immunosuppressants).

10. Make sure indwelling catheter is dependent and draining.
    a. Report decrease in output or excessive clots.
    b. Be alert for signs of urinary infection, such as cloudy urine, fever, and aching pain in bladder or flank.

11. Administer antibiotics as prescribed.

12. Change dressings promptly if drainage is present.

13. Provide regular skin care and assist with hygiene.

14. Obtain specimens for bacteriologic testing of urine, wound drainage, sputum, and discontinued catheters, drains, and I.V. lines as indicated.

15. For kidney transplantation patients, administer immunosuppressant drugs, and monitor for early signs of rejection:
    a. Temperature greater than 100.4° F (38° C)
    b. Decreased urine output
    c. Weight gain of 3 or more pounds (1.4 kg) overnight
    d. Pain or tenderness over the graft site
    e. Hypertension
    f. Increased serum creatinine level

16. For kidney transplantation patients, give oral antifungal agent to prevent mucosal candidiasis, which commonly occurs due to immunosuppression.

Education and Health Maintenance

1. Provide information about postoperative recovery measures: regular exercise, refraining from heavy lifting or strenuous activities, and resuming normal dietary intake.

2. Advise the patient to wear a medical alert bracelet and to inform all health care providers of single-kidney status.

3. Reinforce the need for close follow-up, and urge the patient to seek immediate medical attention for signs of urinary infection or urinary tract disease involving the remaining kidney.

4. After stent placement, such as a Double-J stent for ureteral obstruction, advise the patient to report any of the following symptoms that last longer than 3 days: fever, flank pain, frequency, dysuria, or hematuria. These could indicate infection or stent migration. Also remind patient that stent needs to be replaced in 3 to 9 months as directed.

5. After kidney transplantation:

   a. Explain and reinforce symptoms of rejection — fever, chills, sweating, lassitude, hypertension, weight gain, peripheral edema, and decrease in urine output. Reassure the patient that acute rejection, although common, is usually reversible. It commonly occurs during the first 2 months after transplantation.

   b. Prepare the patient for possible need for maintenance dialysis when rejection occurs. If the transplanted kidney is rejected, it may be removed in the initial postoperative period. In chronic rejection, the kidney is not usually removed.

   c. Explain need for continued protection of vascular access graft — which may still be enlarged and tender — that is associated with edema of overlying tissue.

   d. Encourage compliance with laboratory tests (serum and urine chemistry, hematology, bacteriology) to monitor immune status and detect early signs of rejection.

   e. Instruct the patient and family about prescribed immunosuppressants and possible complications of therapy (infection or incomplete control of rejection). Review other medications, such as antacids, to prevent stress ulcers, vitamins, and iron replacement.

   f. Review in detail postoperative self-care regimen (may be inpatient or outpatient), including adequate fluid intake, daily weight, measurement of urine, stool test for occult blood, prevention of infection, and exercise.

   g. Advise the patient to avoid contact sports for life to prevent trauma to the transplanted kidney.

   h. Stress that follow-up care after transplantation is a lifelong necessity.

K

6. For additional support and information, refer to the American Association of Kidney Patients, *www.aakp.org*.

KNEE ARTHROPLASTY

See *Arthroplasty and Total Joint Replacement.*

KNEE INJURIES

Knee injuries result from rapid position changes involving flexing and twisting of the joint. Severe stresses are applied to knee ligaments and cartilage during many sport activities. The knee ligaments provide stability to the knee joint. These ligaments promote rotational stability (anterior and posterior cruciate ligaments) and prevent varus and valgus instability (medial and lateral collateral ligaments). Pieces of cartilage that stabilize the knee internally are known as the medial and lateral menisci. Anterior cruciate ligament (ACL) injuries and medial meniscus tears are common because of sports injuries.

Assessment

1. Torn cartilage (meniscus)
   a. Pain, tenderness, joint effusion
   b. Clicking sensations
   c. Decreased range of motion
2. Torn ligaments
   a. Pain on ambulation, swelling
   b. Joint instability
   c. Possible rupture of patellar tendon causing anterior bulge

Diagnostic Evaluation

1. Special assessment techniques are done to detect injury to the ACL:
   a. *Anterior drawer test:* patient is placed supine with knee in 90 degrees of flexion with foot flat on table. Proximal tibia is pulled forward by examiner using two hands. Forward subluxation of tibia on femur indicates ACL injury.

   b. *Lachman test:* patient is placed supine with knee in 15 to 20 degrees of flexion. Distal femur is grasped by examiner with one hand while other hand grasps proximal tibia and applies forward pressure. Forward subluxation of tibia on femur indicates ACL injury.

   c. *Pivot shift test (evaluates anterolateral rotational stability):* patient is placed supine with knee slightly flexed. Examiner grasps patient's ankle in one hand and places palm of other hand over lateral aspect of knee distal to the joint. Lower leg is extended and internally rotated, applying a valgus (lateral) stress to knee. Tibia subluxes and reduces itself ("pivots and shifts"), indicating ACL injury.

2. MRI shows extent of soft tissue injury.

Collaborative Management
Therapeutic Interventions
1. Some injuries may be immobilized (splint, brace, or cast) and treated with physical therapy.

Surgical Interventions
1. ACL reconstruction frequently indicated.
   a. Arthroscopic surgery preferred using synthetic ligaments where ligaments failed. Graft rejection is a complication.
   b. Postoperative continuous passive motion used.
   c. ACL rehabilitation program includes progressive range of motion, bracing (not done with synthetic ligaments).
   d. Long-term bracing during sports is controversial.
2. Meniscal injury—damaged cartilage removed:
   a. Arthroscopic or open meniscectomy.
   b. Rehabilitation includes progressive range of motion and quadriceps strengthening.

Nursing Diagnoses
3, 62, 135

Nursing Interventions
Also see *Orthopedic Surgery*, page 680.

K

Supportive Care

1. After arthroscopic surgery, ensure proper use of crutches and encourage pain control through medications as prescribed and rest, ice, compression, and elevation.
2. For open joint surgery, evaluate incision for drainage and signs of infection. Maintain immobility as ordered.
3. Encourage exercises prescribed by physical therapy.

Education and Health Maintenance

1. Teach the patient strengthening exercises for affected extremity.
2. Teach the patient to prevent fatigue through rest periods and conservation of energy.
3. Advise the patient to prevent injuries by using proper equipment and wearing proper footwear for sports.

L

LARYNGEAL CANCER
See *Cancer, Laryngeal.*

LEAD POISONING

Lead poisoning is a chronic disorder resulting from consumption of lead from hand-to-mouth activities that introduce lead into children's mouths from dust, soil, and nonfood sources such as paint chips. Lead-painted earthenware may also transfer lead to food and liquids.

Lead is absorbed from the GI tract, is stored in the soft tissue, and primarily affects the central nervous system (CNS), bone marrow, and kidneys. CNS effects include learning disabilities, mental retardation, encephalopathy, paralysis, blindness, and seizures. Lead in bone marrow impairs production of hemoglobin and red blood cells, resulting in anemia and respiratory distress. In the kidneys, lead damages proximal tubules, causing increased excretion of amino acids, protein, glucose, and phosphate. Although lead poisoning primarily occurs in young children, it may develop at any age.

Assessment
1. GI: anorexia, sporadic vomiting, intermittent abdominal pain, constipation
2. CNS: hyperirritability; decreased activity; personality changes; loss of recently acquired developmental skills; falling, clumsiness, loss of coordination (ataxia); local paralysis; peripheral nerve palsies
3. Hematologic: anemia, pallor
4. Cardiovascular: hypertension, bradycardia

PEDIATRIC ALERT Assess all children for pica (eating nonfood substances such as paint chips or dirt) and initiate screening for lead poisoning. Pica is usually associated with a more severe degree of poisoning than picking up lead dust in the hands.

Diagnostic Evaluation

1. Elevated serum lead levels; a repeat level is done at a time based on initial level:
   a. If greater than 70 mcg/dL, repeat immediately.
   b. If 60 to 69 mcg/dL, repeat in 24 hours.
   c. If 45 to 59 mcg/dL, repeat in 48 hours.
   d. If 20 to 44 mcg/dL, repeat in 1 to 4 weeks.
   e. If 10 to 19 mcg/dL, repeat in 3 months.
2. Complete blood count indicates iron deficiency anemia.
3. Erythrocyte protoporphyrin (EP) level is not sensitive enough to identify lead levels below approximately 25 mg/dL. It can be used to follow blood lead levels after medical and environmental interventions for poisoned children. A progressive decline in EP levels indicates that management is successful.
4. A 24-hour urine specimen is more accurate than a single voided specimen in determining elevated urine components that correspond with elevated blood lead levels.
5. Edetate calcium disodium (CaEDTA) provocation chelation test is used only in selected medical centers treating large numbers of lead-poisoned children. It demonstrates increased lead levels in urine over an 8-hour period after injection of CaEDTA.
6. Flat plate of abdomen may show radiopaque material if lead has been ingested during the preceding 24 to 36 hours.
7. Radiologic examination of long bones is unreliable for diagnosis of acute lead poisoning, although it may provide some indication of past lead poisoning or length of time poisoning has occurred.

Collaborative Management
Therapeutic Interventions

1. Removal of leaded paint or paint chips or lead-containing objects from the child's environment. Child should be away from environment during paint-stripping process.
2. High-iron diet and iron supplements to treat associated anemia.
3. Low-fat diet and small, frequent feedings will reduce the GI absorption of lead.

4. Foods high in vitamin C and calcium are encouraged.

Pharmacologic Interventions

1. Chelation therapy if blood lead level is between 45 and 70 mcg/dL. If greater than 70 mcg/dL, hospitalization is required.

2. Ethylenediaminetetraacetic acid (EDTA), British anti-Lewisite (BAL), and succimer (Chemet) bind with lead in the blood to form nontoxic compounds that are excreted by bowel and kidney.

3. Effectiveness of therapy depends on degree and duration of lead poisoning.

4. BAL is given first to decrease the chance of seizures.
   a. Used alone in patients with encephalopathy.
   b. Do not give with iron supplements, and avoid in patients with plant allergies.
   c. Avoid in patients with glucose-6-phosphate dehydrogenase deficiency caused by hemolysis.
   d. Administered deep I.M., results in pain and tissue necrosis at the injection site.

5. EDTA may be toxic to the kidneys.
   a. Monitor urinary output as well as kidney and liver function studies.
   b. Administer I.V.

6. Chemet was approved for use in 1991.
   a. Do not give to patients with encephalopathy, those receiving iron, or those who are continually exposed to lead.
   b. Administer orally.
   c. Monitor hematologic parameters.
   d. Dosage depends on individual drug, the child's weight, severity of poisoning, history, and whether other chelating agents are being used simultaneously.

7. Chelating drugs are usually given every 4 hours for 5 days. A second course of therapy may be needed if there is a rebound in the blood lead level.

8. Increased oral and I.V. fluids are given to enhance excretion, except if increased intracranial pressure (ICP) is present.

9. D-penicillamine, a third-line agent with a high incidence of adverse effects that chelates heavy metals, may be given for long-term chelation only if current exposure to lead is definitely excluded. If this drug is used, it should be given on an empty stomach, 2 hours before breakfast.

10. Supplemental calcium, phosphorus, and vitamin D are given to help lead move from the blood (where it is toxic) to the bones (where it is nontoxic).

11. For the child with encephalopathy, corticosteroids are given, and intensive care management is maintained until acute stage is resolved.

Nursing Diagnoses
3, 15, 25, 136

Nursing Interventions
Monitoring

1. In a child with encephalopathy, observe for signs of increased ICP:
   a. Rising blood pressure
   b. Papilledema
   c. Slow pulse
   d. Seizures
   e. Unconsciousness

2. In chelation therapy, monitor intake and output and blood studies such as electrolytes, and liver and kidney function tests as directed.

3. When working with children, look for these high-risk groups for lead: those who live in homes built before 1950; those with iron deficiency anemia; those who are exposed to contaminated dust or soil; those with developmental delays; those who have been abused or neglected; or those with a family history of lead poisoning.

Supportive Care

1. Be aware that encephalopathy may occur 4 to 6 weeks after first symptoms (sudden onset of vomiting, ataxia, altered consciousness, coma, seizures).

2. Maintain seizure precautions for a child with encephalopathy.
   a. Elevate and pad crib or bed rails.
   b. Have tongue blade and suction equipment at bedside.
3. Provide supportive care to maintain vital functions.
4. In chelation therapy, plan appropriate play activities to prepare the child for injections and as an outlet for pain and anger child feels.
5. Implement measures to decrease pain at injection site.
   a. Rotate injection sites.
   b. Apply warm packs to site to decrease pain.
   c. Move painful areas slowly.
6. Provide and encourage activities that will help the child to learn and progress from current developmental state to meet next appropriate milestone.
7. Initiate appropriate referrals for assessment of developmental delays or learning difficulties.
8. Share the results of developmental testing with the parents, and discuss ways to provide stimulation for the child at home.
9. Use sensitivity in interviewing and teaching to avoid causing or increasing guilt feelings about the poisoning and to establish a positive, trusting relationship between the family and the health care facility.

Education and Health Maintenance
1. Explain to the parents why long-term follow-up is important. Inform them that residual lead is liberated gradually after treatment and may result in renewal of symptoms, increase serum lead to a dangerous level, and cause additional CNS damage, which may not become apparent for several months.
2. Stress that acute infections must be recognized and treated promptly because these may reactivate the disease.
3. Inform that iron supplementation may be continued to treat anemia. Advise on administration and adverse effects and periodic complete blood count monitoring.

4. Advise parents that the most important factor in managing childhood lead poisoning is reducing the child's re-exposure to lead.

COMMUNITY CARE CONSIDERATIONS

Children should not be discharged from the hospital until their home environment is lead-free.

5. Initiate referrals to community outreach workers so environmental case management is conducted. Lead abatement must be conducted by experts, not untrained parents, property owners, or contractors.
6. Suggest periodic, focused household cleaning to remove the lead dust; use a wet mop.
7. Encourage hand washing before meals and at bedtime to eliminate lead consumption from normal hand-to-mouth activity.
8. Make certain that the family can closely supervise the child, or assist them to make necessary arrangements.
9. Provide either targeted or universal screening of blood lead levels based on local and state health official recommendations.
10. Initiate and support educational campaigns through schools, day-care centers, and news media to alert parents and children to hazards and symptoms of lead poisoning.
11. For additional information, contact the state or local health department or the Centers for Disease Control and Prevention at *www.cdc.gov*.

LEARNING DISABILITIES

See *Attention Deficit Disorder and Learning Disabilities*.

LEGG-CALVÉ-PERTHES DISEASE

Legg-Calvé-Perthes disease is a self-limiting condition of the proximal femur, in which avascular necrosis of the femoral head leads to its eventual deformation. Four stages are recognized. In stage I (avascularity), the blood supply to the upper femoral epiphysis is halted spontaneously and bone growth is halted (lasts a few weeks). In stage II (revascularization), new blood vessels arise to supply the necrotic area, and bone resorption and deposition take place (lasts several months to 1 year). However, the new bone lacks strength and pathologic fractures may occur; the weakened epiphysis may be progressively deformed. In stage III (reossification), the head of the femur gradually reforms as dead bone is replaced with new bone, which gradually spreads to heal the lesion (lasts 2 to 4 years). Finally (without treatment), in stage IV (postrecovery), the femoral head becomes permanently distorted, with resultant joint misalignment.

Legg-Calvé-Perthes disease occurs primarily in boys ages 4 to 8. Etiology is unclear but may be due to genetics, hormonal changes, trauma, infection, or metabolic abnormalities. Without treatment, early degenerative joint disease and loss of hip function may result in later life. With timely treatment, the femoral head can be reformed to preserve joint function and mobility.

Assessment

1. Synovitis causing limp (may be intermittent initially or last for several months)
2. Pain to hip, knee, inner thigh, or groin with activity
3. Limited abduction and internal rotation of the hip
4. Mild to moderate muscle spasm on rotation of the hip
5. Limited internal rotation, flexion, and abduction
6. Trendelenburg gait — tilt on one side when weight bearing

Diagnostic Evaluation

1. Hip X-ray with anterior-posterior and frog leg lateral views can determine extent of epiphyseal involvement and stage. Early findings may be normal.
2. MRI has been useful in demonstrating the pathologic process, but not in showing stage.
3. Bone scans can detect early disease.
4. Arthrograms may be useful to evaluate sphericity of femoral head.

Collaborative Management
Therapeutic and Pharmacologic Interventions
1. Limitation of activities, bed rest with or without skin traction.
2. Salicylates or anti-inflammatory agents are given to relieve synovitis, muscle spasm, and pain in the joint and help restore motion.

Surgical Interventions
1. Inominate osteotomy; varus osteotomy; osteotomy of the proximal femur, acetabulum (Salter innominate), or a combination of these may be required.

Nursing Diagnoses
3, 8, 62, 86

Nursing Interventions
Also see *Orthopedic Surgery,* page 680.

Monitoring
1. Monitor and assess pain level using age-appropriate pain measurement tool.
2. Assess for gait, spasm, or presence of contractures.

Supportive Care and Education
1. Instruct child and parents to maintain activities that promote range of motion, such as swimming and bicycling, but to avoid contact sports and high-impact running.
2. Provide equipment to assist with mobility (eg, wheelchair, walker) if needed.
3. Teach parents and siblings to assist only as needed.
4. Allow child to care for self and participate as able.
5. Reinforce to child that he or she is only temporarily restricted. Stress positive aspects of activity.
6. Encourage follow-up.

LEUKEMIA, ACUTE LYMPHOCYTIC AND ACUTE MYELOGENOUS

Leukemias are malignant neoplasms of the cells derived from either the myeloid or lymphoid line of the hematopoietic stem cells in the bone marrow (see *Figure L-1*). Proliferating abnormal and immature cells (blasts) spill out into the blood and infiltrate the spleen, lymph nodes, and other tissue. Acute leukemias are characterized by rapid progression of symptoms. High numbers (greater than 50,000/mm^3) of circulating blasts weaken blood vessel walls, with high risk for rupture and bleeding, including intracranial hemorrhage.

Lymphocytic leukemias involve immature lymphocytes and their progenitors. They arise in the bone marrow but infiltrate the spleen, lymph nodes, central nervous system (CNS), and other tissues. Myelogenous leukemias involve the pluripotent myeloid stem cells and, thus, interfere with the maturation of granulocytes, erythrocytes, and thrombocytes. Acute

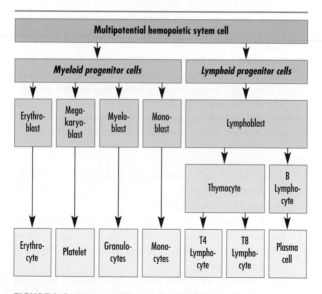

FIGURE L-1 Steps in differentiation of blood cells.

myelogenous leukemia (AML) and acute lymphocytic leukemia (ALL) have similar presentations and courses. Approximately half of new leukemias are acute. Approximately 85% of acute leukemias in adults are AML, and incidence of AML increases with age. ALL is the most common cancer in children, with peak incidence between ages 2 and 9.

Although the cause of leukemias is unknown, predisposing factors include genetic susceptibility, exposure to ionizing radiation or certain chemicals and toxins, some genetic disorders (Down syndrome, Fanconi's anemia), and human T-cell leukemia-lymphoma virus. Complications include infection, leukostasis leading to hemorrhage, renal failure, tumor lysis syndrome, and disseminated intravascular coagulation.

Assessment

1. Weight loss, fever, frequent infections (with ALL), weakness, progressively increasing fatigability, abnormal bleeding and bruising, and lymphadenopathy (ALL).
2. Bone and joint pain, headache, splenomegaly, hepatomegaly, and neurologic dysfunction may also be present.

PEDIATRIC ALERT The most common presenting signs and symptoms (in order of incidence) in children with ALL are hepatosplenomegaly, fever, pallor, lymphadenopathy, petechiae or purpura, bone or joint pain, and anorexia. In AML the most common presenting signs and symptoms are hepatosplenomegaly, respiratory symptoms, fever, bleeding, pallor, anorexia, bone or joint pain, and lymphadenopathy.

Diagnostic Evaluation

1. White blood cell count varies widely from 1,000 to 100,000/mm^3. Peripheral smear shows large number of abnormal immature cells (blasts).
2. Anemia may be profound (decreased hemoglobin and hematocrit); platelet count may be low, and coagulopathies (abnormal prothrombin time and partial thromboplastin time) may exist.
3. Bone marrow aspiration and biopsy classifies leukemia and checks for chromosomal abnormalities and immunologic markers.

4. Lymph node biopsy detects disease spread.
5. Lumbar puncture detects leukemic cells (especially in ALL) with CNS spread.

Collaborative Management

Therapeutic Interventions

1. Radiation therapy, particularly of CNS, in ALL; indicated for patients with CNS disease at the time of diagnosis.
2. Autologous or allogenic bone marrow or stem cell transplantation for failure to respond to conventional therapy.
3. Leukapheresis, or exchange transfusions in infants, may be used when abnormally high numbers of white cells are present to reduce the risk of leukostasis and tumor burden before chemotherapy.

Pharmacologic Interventions

1. High-dose chemotherapy given as an induction course to obtain a remission (elimination of abnormal cells from bone marrow and blood) and then in cycles as consolidation or maintenance therapy to prevent disease recurrence.
2. Granulocyte colony-stimulating factor to stimulate neutrophil production and prevent serious infection while undergoing chemotherapy.
3. Antibiotics to treat infection.
4. Analgesics and antiemetics.
5. Allopurinol is used to prevent tumor lysis syndrome (rapid destruction of large numbers of malignant cells leads to hyperuricemia, hyperkalemia, hyperphosphatemia, and hypocalcemia).

Nursing Diagnoses

1, 3, 44, 51, 135, 136

Nursing Interventions
Monitoring

1. Monitor vital signs every 4 hours to assess for changes indicating infection or bleeding.
2. Monitor for other signs of infection including sore throat, earache, cough, dysuria, skin warmth and redness.

> **EMERGENCY ALERT** Fever may not develop with infection if the patient is immunosuppressed because of chemotherapy. A fever of 101° F (38.3° C) may indicate overwhelming infection and impending septic shock.

3. Assess respiratory function every 4 hours while symptoms are present; otherwise, every 8 hours.
4. Assess for changes in mental status every 8 hours.
5. Monitor platelet counts daily.
6. Monitor granulocyte counts; concentrations under 500/mm^3 indicate serious risk of infection.
7. Monitor for signs of minor bleeding, such as petechiae, ecchymosis, conjunctival injection, epistaxis, bleeding gums, oozing at puncture sites, vaginal spotting, and heavy menses (initiate pad count).

> **EMERGENCY ALERT** Be alert for and report signs of serious bleeding, such as headache with change in responsiveness, blurred vision, hemoptysis, hematemesis, melena, hypotension, tachycardia, and dizziness.

8. Monitor urine, stool, and emesis for gross and occult blood.

Supportive Care

1. Use meticulous hand washing; observe reverse isolation precautions or use laminar airflow room, as directed.
2. Avoid invasive procedures and trauma to skin or mucous membrane to prevent entry of microorganisms.
3. Use the following rectal precautions to prevent infection:
   a. Avoid diarrhea and constipation, which can irritate the rectal mucosa.
   b. Avoid rectal thermometers.
   c. Keep perianal skin clean and well lubricated to prevent breakdown.
4. Encourage and assist the patient with personal hygiene, bathing, and oral care.

5. Keep the patient on bed rest during bleeding episodes.

6. Report the following, which may indicate an infection: fever; significant changes in vital signs such as tachycardia, tachypnea, and hypotension; chills; and mental status changes.

7. Administer pain medication as directed, but avoid aspirin and anti-inflammatory agents in the thrombocytopenic patient because they may interfere with platelet function.

8. Be aware of potential adverse effects of chemotherapeutic agents being used, including bone marrow suppression, nausea, vomiting, mucositis, pulmonary toxicity, cardiac toxicity, hepatotoxicity, cerebellar toxicity, dermatitis, keratoconjunctivitis, alopecia, and vesicant properties.

9. Provide family support with frequent discussions about diagnostic process, treatment options, and prognosis. Provide resources for the entire family — patient, parents, siblings, and others. Provide referral to other professionals as needed, such as social workers, psychologists, and clergy.

Education and Health Maintenance

1. Teach the use of good hand washing and avoidance of sources of infection, such as crowds, unnecessary hospital visits, undercooked food, and standing water.

2. Teach recognition and reporting of signs and symptoms of infection.

3. Advise parents to report exposure to chickenpox if child has not had the disease or the vaccine.

 PEDIATRIC ALERT Immunosuppressed children are at risk for developing disseminated varicella if they are exposed to chickenpox and they may be treated prophylactically with varicella immune globulin.

4. Encourage adequate nutrition to prevent emaciation from chemotherapy.

5. Encourage regular dental visits to detect and treat dental infections and disease.

6. Inform how constipation can be avoided with increased fluid and fiber intake and good perianal care.

7. Teach bleeding precautions, such as use of electric razor, avoidance of aspirin or nonsteroidal anti-inflammatory drugs, avoidance of sharp objects, avoidance of straining at stool, or forceful nose blowing.
8. After discharge from the hospital, encourage and support a return to as normal a life as possible. Communicate with school, home health agencies, and primary care providers to help reentry into normal routines.
9. For information and support, refer to The Leukemia & Lymphoma Society, *www.leukemia-lymphoma.org*.

LEUKEMIA, CHRONIC LYMPHOCYTIC

Chronic lymphocytic leukemia (CLL) involves more mature cells than acute leukemia and is characterized by proliferation of abnormal lymphocytes. Five forms are recognized according to cell origin: B cell, T cell, lymphosarcoma, prolymphocytic leukemia, and hairy cell leukemia. B cell lymphocytic leukemia is the most common type (95% of cases) and is also the most common leukemia in the United States and Europe. It occurs in twice as many men as women; most patients are older than age 50.

Usually insidious in onset, CLL may be discovered during a routine physical examination. The specific cause is unknown, although hereditary and hormonal factors may play a role. The disease may be indolent for years with gradual malignant transformation with eventual infection, bleeding, and thrombophlebitis due to venous or lymphatic obstruction.

Assessment

1. Early signs and symptoms include frequent skin or respiratory infections, symmetric lymphadenopathy, and mild splenomegaly.
2. Advanced symptoms include pallor, fatigue, activity intolerance, easy bruising and bleeding, skin lesions, bone tenderness, and abdominal discomfort.

Diagnostic Evaluation

1. Increased lymphocytes (10,000 to 150,000/mm³); decreased hemoglobin and hematocrit; decreased platelets on complete blood count.
2. Decreased serum immunoglobulins may be evident.
3. Bone marrow aspiration and biopsy detect lymphocytic infiltration.
4. Lymph node biopsy detects spread of disease.

Collaborative Management
Therapeutic and Surgical Interventions

1. Close observation until patient becomes symptomatic.
2. Splenic irradiation or splenectomy for painful splenomegaly, platelet sequestration, or hemolytic anemia.
3. Irradiation of painful enlarged lymph nodes.
4. Supportive treatment includes transfusion therapy to replace platelets and red blood cells.
5. Bone marrow transplantation with combination chemotherapy may be used.

Pharmacologic Interventions

1. Chemotherapy (chlorambucil, cyclophosphamide, prednisone) to control lymphocyte proliferation.
2. The B-cell type may be treated with fludarabine.
3. Monoclonal antibodies, such as alemtuzumab and rituximab, may be used.
4. Hairy cell leukemia is a specific type of B cell CLL that can be treated with cladribine, pentostatin, or alpha interferon.
5. I.V. immunoglobulins or gamma globulin to treat hypogammaglobulinemia.
6. Antibiotics, antivirals, and antifungals to treat infection.

Nursing Diagnoses
1, 3, 43, 135, 136

Nursing Interventions
Monitoring

1. Monitor for signs of infection, especially pneumonia.

2. Monitor for signs of thrombophlebitis—swollen, painful extremity with tenderness and red streaking.
3. Monitor platelet count and for signs of bleeding.

Supportive Care

1. Administer or teach the patient to administer analgesics on regular schedule, as prescribed.
2. Teach the use of relaxation techniques, such as relaxation breathing, progressive muscle relaxation, distraction, and imagery to control pain.
3. Encourage frequent rest periods alternating with ambulation and light activity as tolerated.
4. Assist with hygiene and physical care as necessary.
5. Encourage balanced diet or nutritional supplements as tolerated.
6. Teach the patient to use energy conservation techniques while performing activities of daily living such as sitting while bathing.

Education and Health Maintenance

1. Teach the patient to minimize risk of infection: immediately clean any abrasion or wound of mucous membranes or skin; monitor temperature and report fever or other sign of infection promptly; and use condoms and other safe sex practices.
2. Teach the patient use of medications as ordered, and possible adverse effects and their management; also to avoid aspirin and nonsteroidal anti-inflammatory drugs, which may interfere with platelet function.
3. For information and support, refer to The Leukemia & Lymphoma Society, *www.leukemia-lymphoma.org*.

LEUKEMIA, CHRONIC MYELOGENOUS

Chronic myelogenous leukemia (CML), also known as *chronic granulocytic* or *chronic myelocytic leukemia*, results from malignant transformation of the pluripotent myeloid stem cells. This leads to proliferation of the myeloid cell line of granulocytes, monocytes, platelets, and occasionally red cells. The specific cause is unknown but associated with the Philadelphia (Ph) chromosome. This disorder accounts for 25% of adult leukemias, generally in people ages 25 to 60, with peak incidence in the mid-40s. It causes fewer than 5% of childhood leukemias.

In its terminal phase, CML resembles an acute leukemia, with an accelerated phase and, possibly, a blast crisis. With the exception of possible cures using bone marrow transplant, CML is usually fatal, with an average survival time of 3 years. Complications include leukostasis from overproduction of cell types, infection, bleeding, and organ damage.

Assessment

1. Insidious onset; may be discovered on routine physical examination by laboratory changes or splenomegaly.
2. Common symptoms include fatigue, pallor, weight loss, night sweats, and activity intolerance.

Diagnostic Evaluation

1. Complete blood count shows increased granulocytes (typically more than 100,000/mm^3); later thrombocytopenia may occur.
2. Bone marrow aspiration and biopsy show hypercellular marrow and usually demonstrate presence of Ph chromosome.

Collaborative Management
Therapeutic and Pharmacologic Interventions

1. Imatinib mesylate is a relatively new agent that provides highly effective treatment orally for chronic or accelerated cases.
   a. As a protein-tyrosine kinase inhibitor, it inhibits proliferation of abnormal cells, causing cell death.
   b. Adverse effects include edema, GI irritation, hematologic toxicity and, rarely, hepatotoxicity.
2. Alfa interferon is used in patients who cannot tolerate imatinib mesylate to eliminate blasts; adverse effects may be severe and include fever and fatigue.
3. Allogenic bone marrow transplantation (related or unrelated donor) is potentially curative.

4. Treatment during accelerated phase or blast crisis aims to restore chronic phase through use of high-dose chemotherapy and leukopheresis, as used in acute myelogenous leukemia.
5. Additional treatment during chronic phase is usually palliative to control symptoms; may include chemotherapy (busulfan, hydroxyurea), irradiation, or splenectomy.

Nursing Diagnoses
1, 43, 44, 135, 136

Nursing Interventions
Also see *Acute Leukemia*, page 573.

Monitoring
1. Monitor for signs of infection.
2. Monitor for signs of bleeding.
3. Monitor for signs of thrombophlebitis caused by leukostasis.

Supportive Care
1. Encourage the patient to verbalize feelings and concerns.
2. Prevent infection by using good hand-washing technique, encouraging good hygiene, and preventing exposure to pathogens.
3. Provide good skin care, handle the patient gently, and prevent falls that may lead to bleeding.
4. Encourage fluids and ambulation to counteract leukostasis.
5. Assist the patient in identifying resources and support (eg, family and friends, spiritual support, community or national organizations, support groups).

Education and Health Maintenance
1. Teach the patient to take medications as prescribed and monitor for adverse effects.
2. Teach interferon injection technique.
3. For information and support, refer to The Leukemia & Lymphoma Society, *www.leukemia-lymphoma.org*.

LIVER CANCER

See *Cancer, Liver*.

LIVER FAILURE, FULMINANT

Fulminant liver failure (FLF), also called *fulminant hepatitis*, is acute, massive necrosis of liver tissue in the absence of pre-existing chronic liver disease, resulting in collapse of liver function. This rare syndrome is usually a complication of hepatitis B or D, or of drug toxicity (see *Box L-1*), but may also be caused by hepatic vein obstruction, autoimmune disease, Budd-Chiari syndrome, and fatty liver of pregnancy. It progresses rapidly to hepatic encephalopathy within 8 weeks of onset. Acute respiratory failure, infections and sepsis, cardiac dysfunction, kidney failure, brain stem herniation, respiratory arrest, and hemorrhage may also occur. Mortality is high (60% to 85%) despite intensive treatment.

Assessment

1. Malaise, anorexia, nausea, vomiting, fatigue

BOX L-1	Potential Causes of Liver Failure

FDA-APPROVED DRUGS
- acetaminophen (Tylenol)
- tetracycline (Tetracyn)
- isoniazid (INH)
- halogenated anesthetics
- monamine oxidase inhibitors
- valproate (Depakene)
- amiodarone (Cordarone)
- methyldopa (Aldomet)

HERBAL AGENTS
- Amanita mushrooms
- Comfrey (*Symphytum officinale*)
- Borage oil (*Borago officinalis*)
- Chaparral (*Larrea tridentate* or *L. divaricata*)
- Kava-kava (*Piper methysticum*)
- Mistletoe (*Viscum album, V. abietis, V. austriacum*)

2. Jaundice of skin and sclera; tea-colored, frothy urine; pruritus
3. Steatorrhea and diarrhea caused by decreased fat absorption
4. Ascites and edema caused by hypoproteinemia
5. Easy bruising, petechiae, overt bleeding caused by clotting deficiency
6. Fetor hepaticus: acetone breath odor
7. Altered levels of consciousness, ranging from irritability and confusion to stupor, somnolence, and coma
8. Asterixis tremor of hands; change in deep tendon reflexes — initially hyperactive, become flaccid

Diagnostic Evaluation
1. Prolonged prothrombin time, decreased platelet count
2. Elevated ammonia, amino acid, and mercaptan levels
3. Hypoglycemia or hyperglycemia
4. Dilutional hyponatremia or hypernatremia, hypokalemia, hypocalcemia, and hypomagnesemia

Collaborative Management
Therapeutic Interventions
1. Restrict dietary protein and sodium while maintaining adequate caloric intake with prescribed diet or hypertonic dextrose solutions.
2. Hemodialysis, hemofiltration, hemoperfusion, or plasmapheresis may be indicated.

Pharmacologic Interventions
1. Administration of lactulose orally or rectally to minimize formation of ammonia and other nitrogenous by-products in the bowel.
2. Administration of neomycin rectally to suppress urea-splitting enteric bacteria in the bowel and decrease ammonia formation.
3. Administration of low-molecular-weight dextran or albumin followed by a potassium-sparing diuretic (spironolactone) to enhance fluid shift from interstitial back to intravascular spaces.

4. Administration of pancreatic enzymes, if diarrhea and steatorrhea are present, to permit better tolerance of diet.
5. Supplemental vitamins (A, B complex, C, and K) and folate.
6. Mannitol I.V. to manage cerebral edema, if present.
7. Administration of cholestyramine to promote fecal excretion of bile salts and reduce itching.
8. Administration of antacids and histamine-2 antagonists to reduce the risk of bleeding from stress ulcers.
9. Infusion of fresh frozen plasma to maintain prothrombin time; cryoprecipitate as needed for bleeding.

Surgical Interventions
1. Liver transplantation is the preferred treatment.

Nursing Diagnoses
23, 30, 35, 48, 51, 75, 134, 135, 136

Nursing Interventions
Monitoring
1. Monitor vital signs frequently.
2. Weigh patient daily and keep an accurate intake and output record; record frequency and characteristics of stool.
3. Measure and record abdominal girth daily.
4. Monitor respiratory rate, depth, use of accessory muscles, nasal flaring, and breath sounds.
5. Evaluate results of arterial blood gas analysis and hemoglobin and hematocrit evaluations.
6. Be alert for signs of infection such as fever, cloudy urine, and abnormal breath sounds.
7. Observe for subtle changes in behavior, worsening of sample of handwriting, and change in sleeping pattern to detect worsening hepatic encephalopathy.

Supportive Care
1. Elevate the head of the bed to lower diaphragm and decrease respiratory effort.
2. Turn the patient frequently to prevent pressure ulcers and pooling of respiratory secretions.

3. Administer oxygen therapy as needed.

4. Provide small, frequent meals or dietary supplements to conserve the patient's energy.

5. Encourage the patient to eat in a sitting position to decrease abdominal tenderness and feeling of fullness.

6. Provide frequent mouth care if the patient has bleeding gums or fetor hepaticus.

7. Provide enteral and parenteral feedings as needed.

8. Bathe the patient without soap and apply soothing lotions.

9. Keep the patient's fingernails short to prevent scratching from pruritus. Administer antipruritics as prescribed.

10. Assess for signs of bleeding from broken areas on the skin.

11. Use good hand-washing and aseptic technique when caring for breaks in the skin or mucous membranes.

12. Restrict visits with anyone who may have an infection.

13. Maintain close observation, side rails, and nurse call system.

14. Assist with ambulation, as needed, and avoid obstructions to prevent falls.

15. Keep room well lit, and reorient the patient frequently.

16. Support the patient and family to help accept the poor prognosis and make the patient comfortable; provide clergy or counselor as indicated.

Education and Health Maintenance

1. Teach the patient and family to notify health care provider of increased abdominal discomfort, bleeding, increased edema or ascites, hallucinations, or lapses in consciousness.

2. Instruct the patient to avoid activities that increase the risk of bleeding, such as scratching, falling, forceful nose blowing, aggressive tooth brushing, and use of straight-edge razor.

3. Advise the patient to limit activities when fatigued and to rest frequently.

4. Maintain close follow-up for laboratory testing and evaluation.

LOU GEHRIG DISEASE

See *Amyotrophic Lateral Sclerosis*.

LOW BACK PAIN

See *Back Pain, Low*.

LUNG CANCER

See *Cancer, Lung*.

LUPUS ERYTHEMATOSUS, SYSTEMIC

Systemic lupus erythematosus (SLE) is a chronic, multisystem disease involving connective tissue that appears to result from production of autoantibodies. Immune complexes and other immune system constituents combine to form complement that is deposited in organs, causing inflammation and tissue necrosis. The disease may be mistaken for rheumatoid arthritis, especially early in the course of the disease. Course of the disease is highly variable, but complications of SLE include infection, renal failure, permanent neurologic impairment, and death. The disease is more common in women than men, usually women of childbearing age, but can affect children ages 5 to 15.

Discoid lupus is a variant that affects primarily the skin. Other variants include *subacute cutaneous lupus* (skin and mild systemic manifestations), *drug-induced lupus* (resolves when drug is withdrawn), and neonatal lupus.

PEDIATRIC ALERT The neonatal variant of SLE involves transient skin lesions, heart block, and hematologic abnormalities.

Assessment

1. Skin-related manifestations:
   a. "Butterfly" rash of the molar region of the face characterized by erythema and edema
   b. Alopecia
   c. Discoid lesions are scarring ringed-shaped lesions involving the shoulders, arms, and upper back; they may result in erythematous, scaly plaques on the face, scalp, and external ear

2. Arthritis:
   a. Generally bilateral and symmetric, involving the hands and wrists as well as other joints.
   b. May resemble rheumatoid arthritis, but is nonerosive (no joint destruction is seen on radiograph).
   c. Tendon involvement is common and may lead to deformities or tendon rupture.
3. Cardiac manifestations:
   a. Pericarditis
   b. Pleural effusion
   c. Myocarditis
   d. Endocarditis
   e. Coronary arteritis — less common
4. Pulmonary manifestations:
   a. Pleuritis
   b. Pleural effusion
   c. Lupus pneumonitis
   d. Pulmonary hemorrhage
   e. Pulmonary embolism
5. GI manifestations:
   a. Oral ulcers
   b. Acute or subacute abdominal pain
   c. Pancreatitis
   d. Spontaneous bacterial peritonitis
   e. Bowel infarction
6. Renal manifestations: occur in 50% of patients, more common and severe in children, with up to 15% developing renal failure
   a. Nephritis (several forms) — may develop within 2 years
   b. Renal vein thrombosis (rare)
7. Central nervous system manifestations:
   a. Neuropsychiatric disorders: depression, psychosis
   b. Transient ischemic attacks, stroke
   c. Epilepsy
   d. Migraine headache
   e. Myelopathy
   f. Guillain-Barré syndrome
   g. Chorea, other movement disorders
8. Hematologic manifestations:

a. Hemolytic anemia
b. Leukopenia
c. Thrombocytopenia
9. Constitutional manifestations:
   a. Fever, fatigue
   b. Weight loss
   c. Raynaud's phenomenon
   d. Lymphadenopathy
   e. Hepatomegaly and splenomegaly

PEDIATRIC ALERT Neonates born to mothers with SLE will have positive antinuclear antibodies transmitted transplacentally. There may be clinical evidence of SLE, but all manifestations are expected to resolve in 3 to 4 months. There is a slight increased risk of developing SLE at some time in the child's life.

Diagnostic Evaluation

1. Complete blood count: leukopenia, anemia (may be hemolytic), thrombocytopenia.
2. Antinuclear antibodies: positive in more than 90% of patients with SLE (Predominant pattern is homogeneous. Additional antibodies such as anti-dsDNA, anti-ssDNA, anti-nRNP, anti-Ro, and anti-La may be done if diagnosis is unclear or to identify clinical variant.)
3. Erythrocyte sedimentation rate is generally elevated.
4. Complement levels are generally decreased in active disease.
5. Hematuria, proteinuria, and "active sediment" (red cell casts) on urinalysis.
6. 24-hour urine for protein may be elevated, and creatinine clearance may be decreased in kidney disease.
7. Serum chemistry determines renal function and other system involvement.
8. Serologic test for syphilis will be false-positive due to antibody cross-sensitivity.
9. Hand and wrist X-rays may show nondestructive arthritis.
10. CT scan or MRI of the brain defines any neurologic manifestations; of the abdomen, rules out other abdominal processes in a patient with abdominal pain.

11. Cerebral arteriography may be done to detect cerebral vasculitis.

Collaborative Management
Therapeutic Interventions

1. Prevention of exacerbation through avoidance of bright sunlight, rest, and adequate nutrition.
2. Joint protection and energy conservation.
3. Application of heat or cold to affected areas.
4. Dialysis and kidney transplant may become necessary for renal involvement.

Pharmacologic Interventions

1. Anti-inflammatories, such as corticosteroids and non-steroidal anti-inflammatory drugs to control joint pain, fever, and inflammation.
2. Oral corticosteroids are indicated for renal or neurologic involvement, or hemolytic anemia; I.V. corticosteroids are used in severe SLE, but have little long-term effect.
3. Antimalarials, such as hydroxychloroquine, to relieve joint symptoms and rash.
4. Immunosuppressants to suppress autoantibody production.
5. Topical corticosteroids may suppress skin lesions.
6. Antihypertensives and diuretics may be necessary.

Nursing Diagnoses
1, 3, 6, 13, 43, 60, 134, 135

Nursing Interventions
Monitoring

1. Monitor degree of renal involvement:
   a. Intake and output, urine specific gravity.
   b. Measure urine protein, microalbumin, or obtain 24-hour creatinine clearance, as ordered.
   c. Check serum blood urea nitrogen and creatinine.
2. Monitor control of joint pain.
3. Monitor temperature every 4 hours.

4. Monitor for signs of dehydration due to fever, such as decreased urine output, dry mucous membranes, poor skin turgor, and thirst.
5. Monitor for adverse effects of corticosteroids, such as hyperglycemia, weight gain, edema, and hypertension.

DRUG ALERT When administering I.V. corticosteroid therapy, monitor pulse and blood pressure every 15 minutes for 1 hour, then every 30 minutes for 1 hour. Slow the rate of infusion and notify the health care provider if there are significant changes.

Supportive Care

1. Administer analgesics as directed and suggest the use of hot or cold applications, relaxation techniques, and nonstrenuous exercise to enhance pain relief.
2. Encourage oral fluids or provide I.V. fluids as directed to make up for fluid lost through fever.
3. Administer antipyretics as directed, and apply sponge baths as needed.
4. Encourage good nutrition, sleep habits, exercise, rest, and relaxation to improve general health and help prevent infection.
5. Suggest alternate hairstyles or wearing of scarves or wigs to cover significant areas of alopecia.
6. Encourage good oral hygiene and inspect mouth for oral ulcers.
7. Advise the patient that fatigue level will fluctuate with disease activity. Encourage the patient to modify schedule to include several rest periods during the day; use energy conservation techniques in daily activities.
8. Teach relaxation techniques, such as deep breathing, progressive muscle relaxation, and imagery to reduce emotional stress that causes fatigue.
9. Make sure that child has appropriate diversional activities. Use play therapy to dispel misconceptions and relieve fears.

Education and Health Maintenance

1. Stress that close follow-up is mandatory, even in times of remission, to detect early progression of organ involve-

ment and to alter drug therapy. Laboratory tests may be needed to monitor medication effects.

2. Avoid direct exposure to sunlight to reduce the chance of exacerbation.
   a. Use sunscreens with a sun protection factor 15 or higher on all sun-exposed areas.
   b. Wear protective clothing (hats, long-sleeved shirts, lightweight)
3. Advise frequent ophthalmologic examinations with hydroxychloroquine therapy to detect corneal and retinal changes to prevent blindness.
4. Advise using special cosmetics to cover skin lesions.
5. Advise about reproduction:
   a. Avoid pregnancy during time of severe disease activity.
   b. Immunomodulators may have teratogenic effects.
   c. Use of some drugs for treatment of SLE can cause sterility.
6. Advise on need for all regular childhood immunizations as well as pneumococcal vaccine and yearly influenza vaccine.
7. For additional information and support, refer to the Lupus Foundation, *www.lupus.org*.

LYME DISEASE

Lyme disease is a chronic, inflammatory, multisystemic disorder caused by a spirochete, *Borrelia burgdorferi*. This organism is transmitted by small ticks, which inject the organism into the bloodstream as they feed (see *Figure L-2*). Originally found in Lyme, Connecticut, in 1975, the disease is endemic to the northeast, mid-Atlantic, the upper north-central regions, and several counties in northwest California.

Onset is commonly in the summer, among people visiting heavily wooded areas. Three to 32 days after initial infection, *Borrelia* spreads through the skin to form a characteristic circular rash, erythema chronicum migrans (ECM). It then migrates through the blood and lymphatics to large joints and meningeal sites, where it may eventually cause meningitis,

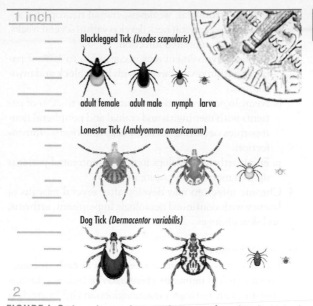

FIGURE L-2 Three human-biting tick species found in the United States. Only *Ixodes* ticks are known to transmit the Lyme disease bacterium to humans. Source: CDC Division of Vector-Borne Infectious Diseases. *www.cdc.gov/ncidod/dvbid/lyme/4ticks_cm.htm.*

arthritis, various neuropathies (chorea), or cardiac abnormalities (atrioventricular block).

Assessment
1. ECM is the initial manifestation of acute infection.
   a. Annular lesion appears at site of tick bite, expands over days or weeks to up to 6 inches (15 cm) in diameter, bright red with central clearing.
   b. Lesion is warm to touch but not painful.
   c. Frequently appear on axilla, thighs, and groin.
   d. Occurs in 60% of patients.
2. Flulike symptoms develop alone or along with ECM— malaise, fever, headache, myalgia, and lymphadenopathy. Some patients have no rash or flulike symptoms.

3. Migratory arthralgias, weakness, cranial neuropathy, severe headache, and stiff neck develop within several weeks, indicating disseminated infection.
   a. Cardiac involvement may occur in 5% to 10% of patients within several weeks, with heart block and myocarditis.
   b. Neurologic involvement occurs in 15% to 20% of patients with meningitis and cranial and peripheral neuropathies occurring several weeks to months after infection.
   c. Frank arthritis develops in 60% of untreated patients up to 6 months after acute infection.
4. Chronic infection may develop after several months of latency with continued neurologic impairment, arthritis, and skin changes.

Diagnostic Evaluation
1. Erythrocyte sedimentation rate is high in early disease.
2. Enzyme-linked immunosorbent assay or indirect fluorescent antibody testing for immunoglobulin (Ig) M and IgG antibodies — are very sensitive several weeks after infection and remain elevated indefinitely. These are confirmed with the more specific Western immunoblot test.

Collaborative Management
Pharmacologic Interventions
1. Oral antibiotics over a 21- to 28-day course for early Lyme disease: doxycycline, amoxicillin, cefuroxemine, or erythromycin is used.
2. For meningitis or cranial or peripheral neuropathies, I.V. penicillin or ceftriaxone, are usually used for 4 weeks. Treatment is usually repeated for recurrent symptoms.
3. Analgesics, antipyretics, and other symptomatic management

Nursing Diagnoses
3, 24, 49

Nursing Interventions
Supportive Care
1. Reassure the patient and family that Lyme disease cannot be transmitted person to person and, although treatment may be long, prognosis is good for most patients.
2. Administer pain medications and antipyretics as ordered.
3. Ask about drug allergies before giving prescribed antibiotics.
4. Monitor cardiac rhythm if heart block develops.
5. Administer I.V. fluids as directed.

Education and Health Maintenance
1. Teach avoidance of tick-infested areas, particularly in the spring and summer when nymphal ticks feed. Ticks are plentiful in a moist, shaded environment where there is leaf litter, low-lying vegetation, or overgrown grasses, and abundant deer and rodents.
2. Advise use of insect repellent containing DEET while outdoors.
3. Advise wearing light-colored clothing with long sleeves and high boots or pant legs tucked into socks.
4. Because transmission of *B. burgdorferi* is unlikely before 36 hours of tick attachment, encourage self tick checks daily followed by prompt removal.
5. Emphasize that ticks should be removed from skin with fine-tipped tweezers or forceps. There is no hazard if mouth parts remain in skin, but the area should be cleaned with an antiseptic.
6. For more information refer to the Centers for Disease Control and Prevention, *www.cdc.gov/ncidod/dvbid/lyme/index.htm*.

LYMPHEDEMA AND LYMPHANGITIS

Lymphedema is a swelling of the lymphatic tissues in the extremities (particularly in the dependent position), produced by obstructed lymph flow of the lymph nodes and lymphatic vessels. Lymphedema may be associated with radical mastectomy, varicose veins, chronic phlebitis, or a congenital condition.

Lymphangitis is an acute inflammation of lymphatic channels, which most commonly arises from a focus of infection in an extremity. Recurrent lymphangitis is commonly associated with lymphedema.

Complications include abscess formation, lymphedema praecox (firm, nonpitting lymphedema unresponsive to treatment), septicemia, or elephantiasis (chronic fibrosis of subcutaneous tissue).

Assessment

1. Edema may be massive and is usually firm in lymphedema.
2. Red streaks extend up the extremity in lymphadenitis, with local pain, tenderness, and swelling along involved lymph vessels. Lymph nodes may be enlarged, red, and tender.
3. Areas of necrotic, pus-producing abscesses indicate suppurative lymphadenitis (rare).
4. Fever and chills accompany lymphangitis.

Diagnostic Evaluation

1. Lymphangiography outlines the lymphatic system.
2. Lymphoscintigraphy, a reliable alternative to lymphangiography using a radioactive contrast medium, helps detect obstruction and inflammation.
3. CT scanning and MRI detect underlying cause.

Collaborative Management
Therapeutic Interventions

1. Bedrest with legs elevated
2. Active and passive exercises
3. External compression devices to treat lymphedema; elastic stockings when ambulatory
4. Application of moist heat for lymphangitis
5. Lymphedema therapy by a physical therapist

Pharmacologic Interventions

1. Diuretics in lymphedema to control excess fluid (controversial)

2. Antibiotics in lymphangitis because causative organisms are usually streptococci and staphylococci

Surgical Interventions

1. For lymphedema unresponsive to other approaches, procedures include replacement of affected subcutaneous tissue and fascia with skin grafts; or transfer of superficial lymphatics to the deep lymphatic system by means of a buried dermal flap.
2. In lymphangitis, incision and drainage may be necessary if necrosis and abscess formation take place.

Nursing Diagnoses
3, 24, 134, 135

Nursing Interventions
Monitoring

1. Assess extremity for response to therapy or worsening inflammation and edema.
2. Observe for signs of postoperative infection.
3. Watch for postoperative complications, such as flap necrosis, hematoma, abscess under flap, and cellulitis.

Supportive Care

1. Advise the patient to rest frequently with the affected extremity elevated, each joint higher than the preceding one. In lymphangitis, apply hot, moist dressings.
2. Apply elastic bandages or stocking (in lymphedema or after acute attack with lymphangitis); apply before getting out of bed.
3. To relieve postoperative pain:
   a. Encourage comfortable positioning and immobilization of affected area.
   b. Use a bed cradle to relieve pressure from bed covers.
   c. Administer, or teach patient to administer, analgesics as prescribed; monitor for adverse effects.
4. Recommend isometric exercises with extremity elevated.
5. Advise the patient to follow moderately restricted diet.

Education and Health Maintenance

1. Encourage patient to use elastic bandage or stocking when ambulatory. Advise patient that it may be needed for several months to prevent long-term edema.
2. Advise the patient to avoid trauma to extremity and to inspect daily for breaks in the skin.
3. Advise the patient to practice good hygiene to avoid superimposed infections.

LYMPHOMA, NON-HODGKIN'S

Non-Hodgkin's lymphomas are a group of malignancies of lymphoid tissue arising from T- or B-lymphocytes or their precursors. Malignant transformation arises in lymphocytes at some stage during hematopoiesis. The level of differentiation and type of lymphocyte affected influences the course of illness and prognosis. Although the cause is unknown, the disorder may be associated with defective or altered immune function. Incidence is higher in patients receiving immunosuppression for organ transplantation, in individuals infected with the human immunodeficiency virus, and in the presence of some viruses. Incidence rises steadily from approximately age 40. Unlike Hodgkin's disease, this disorder is more likely to be in an advanced stage at presentation. Complications of non-Hodgkin's lymphomas depend on the location and extent of malignancy and may include thromboembolism and spinal cord compression.

Assessment

1. Common symptoms include fatigue, fever, chills, night sweats, painless enlargement of lymph nodes (generally unilateral), and weight loss.
2. Examination findings include splenomegaly, hepatomegaly, and generalized lymphadenopathy.
3. Wide variety of manifestations may occur if there is pulmonary involvement, superior vena cava obstruction, or hepatic or bone involvement.

Diagnostic Evaluation

1. Lymph node biopsy determines the type of lymphoma.

2. Complete blood count (CBC) and bone marrow aspiration and biopsy determine whether there is bone marrow involvement.
3. X-rays, CT scanning, positron emission tomography, and MRI detect deep nodal involvement.
4. Lymphangiogram detects size and location of deep nodes involved, including abdominal nodes, which may not be readily seen by CT scan.
5. Liver function tests and liver scan detect liver involvement.
6. Lumbar puncture detects involvement of the central nervous system.
7. Surgical staging (laparotomy with splenectomy, liver biopsy, multiple lymph node biopsies) may be done in selected patients.

Collaborative Management
Therapeutic Interventions
1. Radiation therapy is palliative, not curative treatment.
2. Autologous or allogenic bone marrow or stem cell transplantation.

Pharmacologic Interventions
1. Chemotherapy regimens, including CHOP (cyclophosphamide, Adriamycin, Oncovin, and prednisone) or BACOP (bleomycin, Adriamycin, cyclophosphamide, Oncovin, and prednisone) regimen.
2. Monoclonal antibody therapy with rituximab and other agents may be given with combination chemotherapy.

Nursing Diagnoses
1, 24, 43, 48, 51, 135

Nursing Interventions
Monitoring
1. Monitor vital signs, breath sounds, level of consciousness, and skin and mucous membranes frequently for signs of infection.

2. Monitor for complications of radiation therapy (fatigue, rash, mucositis, cough, and shortness of breath) and chemotherapy (liver toxicity, cardiotoxicity, peripheral neuropathy, alopecia, nausea, vomiting, and vesicant effect).

Supportive Care

1. To minimize the risk of infection in a patient with altered immune response, provide care in protected environment with strict hand-washing technique.
2. If possible, avoid such invasive procedures as urinary catheterization.
3. Assess patient frequently for signs of infection, and notify health care provider if fever occurs or if the patient's condition changes.
4. If infection is suspected, obtain cultures of suspected infected sites or body fluids.

Education and Health Maintenance

1. Teach the patient infection precautions: avoid crowds and infected individuals; avoid raw or undercooked food; wash hands frequently; and use condoms and other safer sex practices.
2. Encourage frequent follow-up for monitoring of CBC and condition.

MALABSORPTION SYNDROME

Malabsorption syndrome is a group of symptoms and physical signs resulting from poor nutrient absorption in the small intestine, especially of fats and fat-soluble vitamins A, D, E, and K. Poor absorption of other nutrients, including carbohydrates, minerals, and proteins, may also occur. Malabsorption has multiple causes, including gallbladder or pancreatic disease, lymphatic obstruction, vascular impairment, or bowel resection. (See *Table M-1*, page 602.) Two common causes are lactase deficiency and celiac disease. In lactase deficiency, the lack of this enzyme prevents the digestion of lactose found in milk, causing osmosis of water into the lumen of the intestine when milk products are ingested.

Celiac disease, also called *gluten-sensitive enteropathy*, is a disease of the small intestine marked by atrophy of the villi and microvilli caused by an immune-mediated inflammatory response to gluten, a protein found in common grains such as wheat, rye, oats, and barley. The cause is unknown, but genetic, environmental, and immunologic elements may be involved. The disease is triggered by surgery, pregnancy, viral infection, or severe emotional distress. It is most common in young children ages 6 to 24 months but can occur at any age. Symptoms typically diminish or disappear in adolescence and reappear in early adulthood. Complications include impaired growth, inability to fight infection, electrolyte imbalance, clotting disturbance, and possible predisposition to malignant lymphoma of the small intestine. Celiac disease will be highlighted here, but other malabsorption syndromes present similar manifestations.

Assessment
Ages 3 to 9 Months
1. Acutely ill; severe diarrhea and vomiting
2. Irritability

TABLE M-1 Malabsorption Syndromes

MECHANISM	CAUSE
Reduced digestion	
Pancreatic exocrine deficiency	Cystic fibrosis, pancreatitis, Schwachman syndrome
Bile salt deficiency	Cholestasis, biliary atresia, hepatitis, cirrhosis, bacterial deconjugation
Enzyme defects	Lactase, sucrase, enterokinase, lipase deficiencies
Reduced absorption	
Primary absorption defects	Glucose–galactose malabsorption, abetalipoproteinemia, cystinuria, Hartnup disease
Decreased mucosal surface area	Crohn's disease, malnutrition, short bowel syndrome, antimetabolite chemotherapy, familial villous atrophy
Small intestinal disease	Celiac disease, tropical sprue, giardiasis, immune or allergic enteritis, Crohn's disease, lymphoma, acquired immunodeficiency syndrome
Lymphatic obstruction	Lymphangiectasia, Whipple disease, lymphoma, chylous ascites
Other	
Drugs	Antibiotics, antimetabolites, neomycin, laxatives
Collagen vascular	Scleroderma
Infestations	Hookworms, tapeworm, giardiasis, immune defects

3. Possible failure to thrive

Ages 9 to 18 Months
1. Slackening of weight followed by weight loss
2. Abnormal stools
   a. Pale, soft, bulky
   b. Offensive odor
   c. Greasy (steatorrhea)
   d. May increase in number
3. Abdominal distention
4. Anorexia, discoloration of teeth
5. Muscle wasting: most obvious in buttocks and proximal parts of extremities
6. Hypotonia, seizures
7. Mood changes: ill humor, irritability, temper tantrums, shyness
8. Mild clubbing of fingers
9. Vomiting: usually occurs in evening
10. Aphthous ulcers, dermatitis

Older Child and Adult
1. Signs and symptoms are commonly related to nutritional or secondary deficiencies resulting from disease
   a. Anemia, vitamin deficiency (A, D, E, K)
   b. Hypoproteinemia with edema
   c. Hypocalcemia, hypokalemia, hypomagnesemia
   d. Hypoprothrombinemia from vitamin K deficiency
   e. Disaccharide (sugar) intolerance
   f. Osteoporosis due to calcium deficiency
2. Anorexia, fatigue, weight loss
3. May have colicky abdominal pain, distention, flatulence, constipation, and steatorrhea (bulky, greasy, pale stools)

Diagnostic Evaluation
1. Small-bowel biopsy, which demonstrates characteristic abnormal mucosa.
   a. Severely damaged or flat, villous lesions
   b. Histologic recovery after gluten elimination

M

   c. Histologic recurrence of villous injury within 2 years of gluten reintroduction
2. Hemoglobin, folic acid, and vitamin K levels may be reduced.
3. Prothrombin time may be prolonged.
4. Elevated immunoglobulin (Ig) A endomysium antibodies and IgA anti-tissue transglutaminase antibodies.
5. Total protein and albumin may be decreased.
6. 72-hour stool collection for fecal fat is increased.
7. D-xylose absorption test—decreased blood and urine levels.
8. Sweat test and pancreatic function studies may be done to rule out cystic fibrosis in child.

Collaborative Management
Therapeutic Interventions
1. Dietary modifications include a lifelong gluten-free diet, avoiding all foods containing wheat, rye, barley and, possibly, oats.
   a. Biopsy reverts to normal with appropriate diet.
   b. Clinical signs of improvement should be seen 1 to 4 weeks after proper diet is initiated.
2. In some cases, fats may be reduced.
3. Lactose and sucrose may be eliminated from diet for 6 to 8 weeks, based on reduced disaccharidase activity.

Pharmacologic Interventions
1. Supplemental vitamins and minerals:
   a. Folic acid for 1 to 2 months
   b. Vitamins A and D because of decreased absorption
   c. Iron as needed for anemia
   d. Vitamin K if there is evidence of hypoprothrombinemia and bleeding
   e. Calcium if milk is restricted
2. Pancreatic enzymes are given for pancreatic insufficiency (cystic fibrosis, pancreatitis).

Nursing Diagnoses
3, 23, 51, 107, 134, 135

Nursing Interventions
Monitoring

1. Monitor dietary intake, fluid intake and output, weight, serum electrolytes, and hydration status.
2. Monitor growth parameters and milestones of development.
3. Monitor characteristics of stool, bowel sounds, abdominal distention, and pain.

Supportive Care

1. Make sure that diet is free of causative agent, but inclusive of essential nutrients, such as protein, fats, vitamins, and minerals.
2. Maintain NPO status during initial treatment of celiac crisis or during diagnostic testing; take special precautions to ensure proper restriction if the child is ambulatory.
3. Provide parenteral nutrition as directed.
4. Provide meticulous skin care after each loose stool and apply lubricant to prevent skin breakdown.
5. Encourage small frequent meals, but do not force eating if child has anorexia.
6. Be prepared to temporarily eliminate food items if symptoms increase.
7. Use meticulous hand-washing technique and other procedures to prevent transmission of infection.
8. Teach parents that child usually perspires freely and has a subnormal temperature with cold extremities; prevent dampness and chilling, and dress child appropriately.
9. Assess for fever, cough, irritability, or other signs of infection.
10. Teach the parents to develop an awareness of the child's condition and behavior; recognize changes and care for child accordingly.
11. Explain that the toddler may cling to infantile habits for security. Allow this behavior; it may disappear as physical condition improves.
12. Help the parents to understand that, after initial rapid weight gain, further improvement may be slow.

Education and Health Maintenance

1. Teach dietary therapy guidelines.
   a. Provide a specific list of restricted and acceptable foods; however, there is much variation among packaged foods, so it is best to check with the manufacturer.
   b. Teach how to read labels on foods to rule out those containing gluten.
   c. Provide information on substitutes for wheat, rye, barley, and oats, such as corn, rice, soybean flour, and gluten-free flour.
   d. Warn that advancing diet too rapidly may result in a setback. Total elimination of gluten is necessary to ensure proper growth.
2. Encourage regular medical follow-up.
3. Advise that prolonged fasting and use of anticholinergic drugs may precipitate celiac crisis.
4. Encourage good hygiene to prevent infection.
5. Explain that the emotional climate in the home and around the patient is vitally important in maintaining the patient's medical and physical stability.
6. Stress that the disorder is lifelong; however, changes in the mucosal lining of the intestine and in general clinical conditions are reversible when dietary gluten is avoided.
7. For additional information and support, refer to the Celiac Sprue Association, *www.csaceliacs.org*.

MANIC DEPRESSION

See *Bipolar Disorders*.

MASTECTOMY AND OTHER BREAST CANCER SURGERY

Surgery for breast cancer may involve breast and lymph node removal (mastectomy) or a breast-preserving procedure (lumpectomy and axillary dissection). Breast-preserving procedures aim to achieve a cosmetically acceptable breast while completely excising the tumor.

Simple mastectomy (removal of the breast with some nearby axillary nodes) is indicated for carefully selected patients who are at high risk for developing breast cancer, such as those with multifocal ductal carcinoma in situ. Modified radical mastectomy (removal of the entire breast with all axillary nodes) is indicated in advanced disease involving large or multifocal tumors, or in women with very small breasts that preclude local tumor excision, or who are ineligible for radiation therapy. Radical mastectomy itself (removal of the entire breast, pectoral muscles, and axillary nodes) is rarely performed except in advanced disease. If appropriate, breast reconstructive surgery may be performed after mastectomy. (See *Box M-1*, page 608.)

Research studies comparing breast conservation (lumpectomy) with mastectomy have demonstrated equivalent patient survival. The following discussion covers mastectomy and axillary node dissection.

Potential Complications
1. Infection
2. Hematoma, seroma
3. Lymphedema
4. Paresthesia, pain of axilla and arm
5. Impaired mobility of arm

Nursing Diagnoses
3, 6, 24, 30, 62, 88, 136, 156

Collaborative Management and Interventions
Preoperative Care
1. Explain the nature of the procedure and expected postoperative care, including care of surgical drains, location of the incision, and mobility of the involved arm.
2. Reinforce the health care provider's information about diagnosis and possibility of further therapy.
3. Recognize the extreme anxiety and fear that the patient, family, and significant others are experiencing.
   a. Discuss patient's concerns and usual coping mechanisms.
   b. Explore support systems with patient.
   c. Discuss concerns about body image changes.

| BOX M-1 | **Breast Reconstruction after Mastectomy** |

Breast reconstruction (mammoplasty) may be performed immediately or as long after surgery as desired. Benefits include improved psychological coping because of improved body image and self-esteem.

Implants are indicated for patients with inadequate breast tissue and skin of good quality. Prosthetic implants made of saline (and in the past, silicone) are placed in pocket under skin or pectoralis muscle. Tissue expansion with saline may be necessary before inserting implants. If opposite breast is ptotic (protruding downward), mastopexy may be necessary for symmetry. Complications include capsular contracture resulting in firmness, pain, and infection.

Nursing considerations for implants include:
1. Teach signs and symptoms of infection, hematoma, migration, and deflation.
2. Teach patient to massage breast to decrease capsule formation around implant.
3. Teach patient she may feel discomfort with the expansions, if used.

Flap grafts involve transfer of skin, muscle, and subcutaneous tissue from another part of the body to the mastectomy site. Latissimus dorsi flap graft tunnels skin, fat, and muscles of the back between shoulder blades under skin to front of chest. Transverse rectus abdominis myocutaneous (TRAM) flap tunnels muscle, fat, skin, and blood supply from abdomen to breast area. There is increased cost, hospitalization, time, and morbidity associated with this procedure. Complications include flap loss, hematoma, infection, seroma, and abdominal hernia.

Nursing considerations for TRAM flap grafts include:
1. Assess flap and donor site for color, temperature, and wound drainage.
2. Control pain.
3. Provide support with bra or abdominal binder to maintain position of prosthesis.
4. Teach patient to perform breast self-examination monthly and inform her that she may have some asymmetry.

Nipple-areolar reconstruction is usually done at a separate time from breast reconstruction. This procedure uses skin and fat from the reconstructed breast for the nipple, and upper thigh for the areola. Tanning or tatooing is done to obtain appropriate color.

4. Evaluate the patient's general medical condition by obtaining history of compliance with therapy for chronic illnesses, performing a systematic assessment as indicated, reviewing laboratory and diagnostic test results, and identifying major risk factors for perioperative morbidity and mortality, such as obesity, respiratory dysfunction, uncontrolled hypertension, and malnutrition.

GERONTOLOGIC ALERT Assessing the preoperative mental status of the older patient will help determine if cognitive changes occur postoperatively.

Postoperative Care

1. Assess dressing and wound after dressing is removed to note erythema, edema, tenderness, odor, and drainage.
   a. Initial dressing may consist of gauze held in place by elastic wrap; it is usually removed within 24 hours.
   b. Wound may be left open to the air or elastic wrap may be replaced if desired.
   c. Elastic wrap bandage should fit snugly but not so tightly that it hinders respiration. It should fit comfortably and support unaffected breast.
2. Assess drainage by way of suction drain for amount, color, and odor. Record amounts.
   a. May have 3½ to 7 oz (104 to 207 mL) serous to serosanguineous drainage in the first 24 hours.
   b. Report grossly bloody or excessive drainage.
3. Assess the involved arm for edema, erythema, and pain.
   a. Do not take blood pressure, draw blood, inject medications, or start I.V. in affected arm. Post sign over bed.
   b. Elevate affected arm on pillows, above level of heart, and position hand above elbow to promote gravity drainage of fluid.
   c. Teach the patient to massage the arm if prescribed, to increase circulation and decrease edema.
   d. Provide the patient with information about arm and hand care.
4. Assess mobility of affected arm and the patient's ability to perform self-care. At particular risk for lymphedema

are patients who undergo axillary node dissection in combination with radiation therapy to axilla.

   a. Initially, encourage wrist and elbow flexion and extension. Encourage use of arm for washing face, combing hair, applying lipstick, and brushing teeth. Encourage the patient to gradually increase use of the arm.
   b. Encourage the patient to avoid abduction initially to help prevent seroma formation. If prescribed, support arm in sling to prevent abduction of the arm.
   c. Instruct and provide patient with prescribed exercises to do when permitted.

5. Inspect wound and instruct patient to recognize and report signs of infection, hematoma, or seroma formation. Teach drain care, if appropriate.

GERONTOLOGIC ALERT Signs and symptoms of infection may not be obvious in older patients. Assess patients for mental status changes or urinary incontinence.

6. Teach patient to bathe the incision gently and blot carefully to dry, and later, with approval, massage the healed incision gently with cocoa butter to encourage circulation and increase skin elasticity.

7. Assess the mastectomy patient's knowledge of prosthesis and reconstruction options, and provide information as needed.

   a. Suggest clothing adjustments to camouflage loss of breast.
   b. Help the patient obtain a temporary prosthesis (may be provided by Reach to Recovery, an American Cancer Society program). Initial prosthesis should be light and soft to allow incision to heal. The patient may wear a heavier type, usually after 4 to 8 weeks, with the surgeon's approval.

8. Encourage the patient to allow herself to experience the grief process over the loss of her breast and to learn to cope with these feelings.

9. Discuss with the patient the effects of diagnosis and surgery on her view of herself as a woman.

   a. Encourage the patient to discuss these concerns with her partner.

b. Assist the patient and partner to look at the incision when ready.

COMMUNITY CARE CONSIDERATIONS

Home health nursing should provide the following after discharge: wound assessment and education about drainage tube and dressing; monitoring for complications; arm care and assessment for lymphedema; and help with the adjustment back to regular activities.

Education and Health Maintenance

1. Explain to the patient how the wound will gradually change and that the newly healed wound may have less sensation because of severed nerves.
2. Teach the patient how to care for arm to prevent lymphedema and infection after axillary node dissection. (See *Box M-2*, page 612.)
3. Teach importance of breast self-examination, mammograms, and regular follow-up visits.
4. Encourage discussion with health care provider about pregnancy after breast cancer, if indicated. Advise patient of premature menopause as adverse effect of chemotherapy.
5. Remind patient that stress related to breast cancer and mastectomy may persist for 1 year or more and to seek counseling as needed.
6. Encourage female relatives, especially sisters, daughters, and mother, to seek breast cancer surveillance.
7. Refer the patient to a postmastectomy support group as needed and desired. Community resources may be accessed through the telephone directory, the hospital information system, or the American Cancer Society, *www.cancer.org*.

> | **BOX M-2** | **Hand and Arm Care to Help Prevent Lymphedema and Infection** |
>
> After a mastectomy or axillary dissection, the arm may swell because of the excision of lymph nodes and their connecting vessels. Circulation of lymph fluid is slowed, making it more difficult for the body to combat infection. Special precautions should be taken to prevent lymphedema and infection.
> - Avoid burns while cooking or smoking.
> - Avoid sunburns.
> - Have all injections, vaccinations, blood samples, and blood pressure tests done on the other arm whenever possible.
> - Use an electric razor with a narrow head for underarm shaving to reduce the risk of nicks and scratches.
> - Carry heavy packages or handbags on the other arm.
> - Never cut cuticles; use hand cream or lotion instead.
> - Wear protective gloves when gardening and when using strong detergents, and so forth.
> - Use a thimble when sewing.
> - Avoid harsh chemicals and abrasive compounds.
> - Use insect repellent to avoid bites and stings.
> - Avoid elastic cuffs on blouses and nightgowns.
>
> From *Mastectomy: A Treatment for Breast Cancer.* NIH Pub No. 91-658.

MASTITIS, ACUTE

Acute mastitis is inflammation of the breast secondary to infection. The disorder usually occurs in first-time breast-feeding mothers. It may also occur later in chronic lactation mastitis and central duct abscesses. Milk stasis may lead to obstruction, followed by noninfectious inflammation, then infectious mastitis. If untreated, the disorder can progress to a breast abscess.

The infection may originate from hands of patient, personnel caring for patient, infant's nose or throat, or it may be bloodborne. Most common causative agents are *Staphylococcus aureus*, *Escherichia coli*, and *Streptococcus*.

Assessment
1. Redness, warmth, edema; breast may feel doughy and tough.
2. Patient may complain of dull pain in affected area and may have nipple discharge.
3. Fever may be present.
4. No diagnostic tests are necessary.

Collaborative Management
Therapeutic and Pharmacologic Interventions
1. Apply heat to resolve tissue reaction; however, may cause increased milk production and worsen symptoms.
2. May apply cold to decrease tissue metabolism and milk production.

Pharmacologic Interventions
1. Antibiotics for infection — usually a 10-day course of penicillinase-resistant agents, such as dicloxacillin, clindamycin, or a cephalosporin.
2. Antipyretics and nonopioid analgesics as needed.
3. If abscess develops, may need incision and drainage.

Nursing Diagnoses
3, 24, 89

Nursing Interventions
Monitoring
1. Monitor or teach the patient to monitor temperature and response to fever and pain control measures.
2. Inspect the breasts daily to note skin changes.
3. Observe for mammary abscess: increased fever, chills, malaise, purulent nipple discharge, and a palpable mass.

Supportive Care and Education
1. Have the patient wear firm breast support.
2. Encourage the breast-feeding patient to practice meticulous personal hygiene to prevent mastitis.

3. Discuss the issue of stopping or continuing breast-feeding with patient and health care provider; support the patient in her decision.

MÉNIÈRE'S DISEASE

Ménière's disease (endolymphatic hydrops) is a chronic disease of unknown cause that involves the inner ear. In this disorder, fluid distention of the endolymphatic spaces of the labyrinth destroys cochlear hair cells, which causes a triad of symptoms: vertigo, hearing loss, and tinnitus. If untreated, irreversible hearing loss results, with concomitant disability and social isolation. Ménière's disease occurs most commonly in patients ages 30 to 60. Other causes of vertigo are described in *Box M-3*.

Assessment

1. Sudden attacks of dizziness occur in which the patient feels the sensation of spinning (vertigo); attacks may last 10 minutes to several hours.
2. Tinnitus and reduced hearing occur on the involved side.
3. The patient reports headache, nausea, vomiting, and incoordination. Sudden head motion may precipitate vomiting.

Diagnostic Evaluation

1. Electronystagmography testing to help differentiate Ménière's disease from an intracranial lesion. This test battery evaluates the vestibuloocular reflex. One test (water or caloric) involves introducing water into the ear canal so that it hits the eardrum. Normal response is dizziness; lack of response may indicate an acoustic neuroma; and a severe attack of vertigo indicates Ménière's disease.
2. Audiometric tests to evaluate sensorineural hearing loss.
3. CT scanning and MRI may be used to rule out tumor.

Collaborative Management
Therapeutic Interventions

1. Keep a diary noting presence of aural symptoms (eg, tinnitus, distorted hearing) when episodes of vertigo occur,

BOX M-3 Vertigo

Vertigo is a type of dizziness characterized by the perception of spinning or movement. It is caused by vestibular dysfunction—either in the peripheral vestibular system (inner ear) or the central vestibular system (brain stem and cerebellum).

CAUSES
- Peripheral origin: Ménière's disease, labyrinthitis, acoustic neuroma, and benign paroxysmal positional vertigo (BPPV).
- Central origin: multiple sclerosis, basilar migraine, transient ischemic attack or stroke of the basilar artery, brain tumor, trauma, and cerebral hemorrhage.
- Other causes of dizziness: vaso-vagal syncope, hypovolemia, autonomic neuropathy of diabetes, severe anemia, aortic stenosis, hypoglycemia, hypoxia, hypocarbia, multiple sensory deficits, drug adverse effects, and emotional illness.

BPPV
BPPV is the most common cause of vertigo. Its onset is sudden, it can be severe in intensity, and it is always related to change in position of the head. It can be diagnosed by thorough history and physical examination including some provocative maneuvers such as the Dix-Hallpike maneuver. Diagnostic tests are only required to rule out central vestibular dysfunction and dizziness caused by other disorders. Patients with BPPV may be very concerned about their symptoms and at risk for injury due to imbalance.

NURSING CONSIDERATIONS
- Ensure safety by creating an uncluttered environment, using siderails and handrails as necessary, using proper footwear, and encouraging the patient to call for help.
- Teach patient to avoid sudden position changes, including simple head movements such as looking up or turning over in bed.
- Discourage use of alcohol and sedating drugs, which may further impair safe ambulation.
- Most episodes of BPPV last seconds to minutes and completely resolve within 3 months; however, if severe or prolonged, suggest referral to a physical therapist for vestibular rehabilitation if BPPV is prolonged.

to help determine which ear is involved and if surgery will be needed.

2. Lifestyle changes to decrease attacks: smoking cessation; avoidance of coffee, tea, alcohol, and stimulating drugs.

Pharmacologic Interventions

1. A vestibular suppressant, such as meclizine or diphenhydramine, may reduce symptoms.
2. Antiemetics, such as promethazine, may also be used to control symptoms.
3. Occasionally, a diuretic, such as acetazolamide, may be used.
4. In severe cases, transtympanic injection of gentamicin or I.M. streptomycin may be used to selectively destroy the vestibular apparatus to relieve vertigo.

Surgical Interventions

1. If drug therapy is ineffective, a conservative approach involves decompressing the endolymphatic sac or implanting an endolymphatic subarachnoid or mastoid shunt to relieve symptoms without destroying vestibular function.
2. Destructive procedures (labyrinthectomy or vestibular nerve neurectomy) may be required to provide relief. These cause total deafness of the affected ear.

Nursing Diagnoses
24, 33, 136, 159

Nursing Interventions
Supportive Care

1. Help the patient recognize aura symptoms to allow time to prepare for an attack. Also help the patient to identify specific trigger factors to control attacks.
   a. Move slowly because jerking or sudden movements may precipitate an attack.
   b. Avoid noises and glaring, bright lights, which may initiate an attack. Have patient close eyes if this lessens symptoms.

   c. Eliminate smoking and the intake of coffee, tea, alcohol, and stimulating drugs because of vasoconstriction effects.
   d. Control environmental factors and personal habits that may cause stress or fatigue.
   e. If there is a tendency toward allergic reactions to foods, eliminate those foods from the diet.
2. Encourage the patient to lie still in a safe place during the attack. Put side rails up on bed if in hospital.
3. Inform the patient that the dizziness may last for varying lengths of time. Maintain safety precautions until attack subsides.
4. Discuss feelings of isolation the patient may have due to hearing loss and debilitating symptoms.

Education and Health Maintenance
1. Teach the patient about medication regimen, including adverse effects of antihistamines, such as drowsiness and dry mouth.
2. Advise sodium restriction as adjunct to vestibular suppressant therapy.
3. Advise the patient to maintain a diary of attacks, triggers, and severity of symptoms.
4. Encourage follow-up hearing evaluations.
5. Teach patient to be aware of other sensory cues from the environment (visual, olfactory, tactile) if hearing is affected.
6. Teach the patient hearing-conservation methods, such as avoiding loud noise levels; wearing earplugs when necessary; avoiding smoking; and avoiding ototoxic drugs, such as aspirin, quinine, and some antibiotics.

MENINGITIS

Meningitis is an inflammation of the pia mater and arachnoid membranes that surround the brain and spinal cord. It is commonly preceded by an upper respiratory infection or, less commonly, may occur as a complication of other bacterial infections, such as sinusitis or otitis media, or through a wound, such as a lumbar puncture or puncture wound. Pathogenic bacteria cross the blood-brain barrier, invade the subarachnoid space, and cause an inflammatory response. Common causative organisms include *Neisseria meningitides* (meningococcal meningitis), *Haemophilus influenzae*, and *Streptococcus pneumoniae*. *Escherichia coli* and *Listeria monocytogenes* may also affect infants from birth to age 3 months. Fungal and parasitic meningitis may also occur, particularly of the immunocompromised. Onset is either insidious or fulminant, depending on causative organism.

If meningitis is caused by a virus, it is called *aseptic meningitis*. Aseptic meningitis may also result from a noninfectious cause such as blood in the subarachnoid space. Infants, children, college students (living in dorms) and elderly people are at highest risk for meningitis. Complications include seizures, increased intracranial pressure (ICP), brain stem herniation, syndrome of inappropriate antidiuretic hormone (SIADH), hearing loss, hydrocephalus, blindness, developmental delays, and learning disabilities.

Assessment

1. Headache, fever, neck stiffness, and photophobia
2. High fever and vomiting common in children
3. Altered mental status
4. Characteristic signs of meningeal irritation: nuchal rigidity, positive Brudzinski's and Kernig's signs (see *Figure M-1*)
5. Petechial or purpuric rash, which may indicate meningococcal or *Pseudomonas* meningitis

 PEDIATRIC ALERT Young children may display behavior changes, arching of the back, blank stare, refusal to feed, and seizures.

6. In children, the following may occur:
   a. Infants younger than age 2 months — irritability, lethargy, vomiting, poor feeding, seizures, high-pitched cry, fever, or hypothermia
   b. Infants ages 2 months to 2 years — above signs plus altered sleep pattern, tenseness of fontanelle, fever, or signs of meningeal irritation

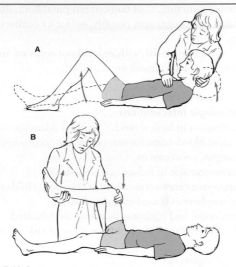

FIGURE M-1 Signs of meningeal irritation include nuchal rigidity and positive Brudzinski's and Kernig's signs. (**A**) To elicit Brudzinski's sign, place the patient supine and flex the head upward. Resulting flexion of both hips, knees, and ankles with neck flexion indicate meningeal irritation. (**B**) To test for the Kernig's sign, once again place the patient supine. Keeping one leg straight, flex the other hip and knee to a bent knee to form a 90-degree angle. Slowly extend the lower leg. This places a stretch on the meninges, resulting in pain and spasm of the hamstring muscle. Resistance to further extension can be felt.

    c. Children older than age 2—vomiting, headache, lethargy, confusion, photophobia, meningeal signs 12 to 24 hours after onset, progressive decline in responsiveness

Diagnostic Evaluation
1. Complete blood count with differential shows elevated white blood cells and neutrophils with shift to the left (immature neutrophils, called *bands*).
2. Blood, urine, and nasopharyngeal cultures help identify the causative organism.

3. Lumbar puncture, to obtain cerebrospinal fluid, show elevated cell counts and, possibly, isolate causative organism.
4. CT scanning or MRI, with and without contrast, rule out other neurologic disorders.

Collaborative Management
Pharmacologic Interventions

1. Antibiotics in large doses I.V. to allow adequate amount to cross blood-brain barrier: penicillins, cephalosporins, rifampin, vancomycin
2. Corticosteroids to reduce cerebral edema
3. Supportive care to critically ill or comatose child or adult
4. Plasmapheresis is used experimentally
5. Antifungal and antiparasitic agents as indicated
6. The meningococcal vaccine for those at risk

Nursing Diagnoses
3, 49, 51, 62, 88, 130

Nursing Interventions
Monitoring

1. Monitor level of consciousness (LOC), vital signs, and neurologic parameters frequently. Notify the health care provider of increasing temperature, decreasing alertness, onset of seizures, or periods of apnea, which signal deterioration.
2. Monitor for increased ICP (see page 86) or SIADH. SIADH causes inappropriate fluid retention and dilutional hyponatremia with signs and symptoms of anorexia, nausea, vomiting, edema, decreased urine output, lethargy, seizures, sluggish deep tendon reflexes, tachycardia, hyponatremia, and decreased serum osmolality.
3. Monitor central venous pressure and infusion of I.V. fluids to avoid fluid overload, which may worsen cerebral edema.
4. Monitor peak and trough blood levels of antibiotics to ensure adequate therapy.

Supportive Care

1. To reduce fever, administer antipyretics as ordered, and institute other cooling measures (eg, hypothermia blanket) as indicated. Administer I.V. fluids as ordered to avoid dehydration.
2. Administer analgesics as ordered; monitor for response and adverse reactions. Opioids should be avoided to prevent interference in assessment of LOC.
3. Maintain infection precautions for at least 24 hours after starting appropriate antibiotic therapy. Good hand washing and careful disposal of respiratory secretions are essential. Gowns and gloves may be considered.
4. Maintain quiet, calm environment and position of comfort with head of bed slightly elevated to prevent agitation, which may cause increased ICP.
5. Darken the room if photophobia is present.
6. Assist with positioning the patient for neck stiffness; be sure to turn the patient slowly and carefully with head and neck in alignment.
7. Be prepared to treat seizures.
8. Provide an opportunity for parents, spouse, or loved ones to ask questions and discuss concerns about the patient's progress.

Education and Health Maintenance

1. Advise the patient's close contacts that prophylactic treatment with rifampin may be indicated to protect against meningococcal meningitis; check with their health care providers or the local public health department.
2. Encourage following medication regimen as directed because infectious agent must be fully eradicated from body.
3. Advise on reporting recurrent fever, tense fontanelle in infant, or neurologic impairments such as decreased hearing after meningitis.
4. Encourage routine health evaluations for children to identify any developmental delays or other long-term complications.

COMMUNITY CARE CONSIDERATIONS

Encourage immunization practices that reduce the incidence of bacterial meningitis, including *Haemophilus influenzae* type b immunization in infants, *Neisseria meningitidis* immunization in high-risk groups such as college students, and *Streptococcus pneumoniae* immunization in patients age 65 and older and those with chronic disease.

MENOPAUSE

Menopause is described as the physiologic cessation of menses. It is caused by failing ovarian function and decreased estrogen production by the ovary. Menopause has occurred if menses have been absent for 1 year. Climacteric is the transition period (perimenopausal) during which the woman's reproductive function gradually diminishes and disappears. It usually occurs at approximately age 50. Artificial or surgical menopause may occur secondary to surgery or radiation involving the ovaries.

Assessment

1. Genitalia: atrophy of vulva, vagina, urethra results in dryness, bleeding, itching, burning, dysuria, thinning of pubic hair, loss of labia minora, and decreased lubrication.
2. Sexual function: dyspareunia, decreased intensity and duration of sexual response, but can still have active function.
3. Vasomotor: 60% to 70% of women experience "hot flashes," which may be preceded by an anxious feeling and accompanied by sweating.
4. Osteoporosis: decreased bone mass results in increased hip fractures, and spinal compression fractures.
5. Cardiovascular: increased coronary artery disease, cholesterol level, and palpitations.
6. Psychological: insomnia, irritability, anxiety, memory loss, fear, and depression may be experienced.

M

Diagnostic Evaluation
1. Luteinizing hormone and follicle-stimulating hormone levels are increased.
2. Estradiol fluctuates and eventually decreases.

Collaborative Management
Pharmacologic Interventions
1. Hormone replacement therapy — controversial
   a. Indicated to reduce symptoms, but long-term use slightly increases risk of breast cancer and cardiovascular disease.
   b. Topical preparations may be used for atrophic vaginitis.
   c. Progesterone preparation also given if uterus is intact to prevent endometrial hyperplasia and possible cancer.
   d. Should be prescribed for short-term therapy in the lowest effective dose.

ALTERNATIVE INTERVENTION

Estrogen and progesterone are available in synthetic, animal-based, and plant-source preparations. In addition to hormones, herbal products are available to take the place of estrogen in relieving menopausal symptoms, including soy products (isoflavones), ginseng, black cohosh, dong quai, and red clover. Encourage the patient to discuss the options with her health care provider and pharmacist.

2. Vaginal lubricants, such as Replens, to decrease vaginal dryness and dyspareunia
3. Vitamin E and B supplements to decrease hot flashes
4. Calcium supplements to prevent bone loss

Nursing Diagnoses
6, 24, 156

Nursing Interventions
Supportive Care

1. Provide patient with information related to estrogen replacement therapy, including dosage schedule, route, adverse effects, and what to expect of menstrual bleeding. Women who still have a uterus can expect a period at the end of every month if they are taking hormones cyclically. Alternatively, giving estrogen and lower-dose progesterone daily may cause some irregular spotting for 3 months to up to 1 year, after which most women experience no bleeding.
2. Explore with patient her feelings about menopause, clear up misconceptions about sexual functioning, and encourage her to discuss her feelings with her partner.
3. Instruct patient how to use water-based lubricant for intercourse to decrease dryness.

Education and Health Maintenance

1. Teach patient that sexual functioning does not decrease during menopause but may even increase because of loss of fear of pregnancy and increased time if children are grown.
2. Teach patient about foods that are high in calcium — dairy products, broccoli, and some fortified cereals — and to maintain weight-bearing activities to prevent osteoporosis.
3. Counsel patient on reducing risk factors for coronary artery disease.
4. Encourage patient to keep regular medical and gynecologic follow-up visits.
5. Advise patient that vulvovaginal infection and trauma are possible because of the dryness of the tissue, and to seek prompt evaluation if pain and discharge occur.

GERONTOLOGIC ALERT In the postmenopausal woman, if vaginal bleeding not associated with hormone replacement occurs, encourage the patient to see her health care provider immediately because cancer may be suspected.

MULTIPLE MYELOMA

Multiple myeloma is a malignant disorder of plasma cells. Neoplastic plasma cells are derived from a clone B lymphocyte and produce a homogeneous immunoglobulin (M protein or Bence-Jones protein) without any apparent antigenic stimulation. Abnormal immunoglobulin affects renal function and platelet function, lowers resistance to infection, and may cause hyperviscosity of blood. The abnormal plasma cells also produce osteoclast-activating factor, which causes extensive bone loss, severe pain, pathologic fractures, and, in some cases, spinal cord compression.

Multiple myeloma has no known cause. It generally affects elderly people (median age at diagnosis is 68) and is more common in blacks. Survival is generally 3 to 4 years. Complications include bacterial infections, renal failure or pyelonephritis, bleeding, and thromboembolism.

Assessment
1. Constant, often severe bone pain caused by bone lesions and pathologic fractures. Commonly affected sites include thoracic and lumbar vertebrae, ribs, skull, pelvis, and proximal long bones.
2. Fatigue and weakness related to anemia caused by crowding of marrow by plasma cells

Diagnostic Evaluation
1. Bone marrow aspiration and biopsy demonstrate increased number and abnormal form of plasma cells
2. Decreased hemoglobin and hematocrit related to anemia
3. Bence Jones protein found in urine and serum
4. Hypercalcemia (from bone destruction); increased uric acid; increased creatinine
5. Skeletal radiographs detect osteolytic bone lesions

Collaborative Management
Therapeutic Interventions
1. Plasmapheresis to treat hyperviscosity or bleeding
2. Radiation therapy for painful bone lesions

3. Hemodialysis to manage renal failure

Pharmacologic Interventions
1. Oral melphalan or cyclophosphamide as chemotherapeutic agents
2. Corticosteroids alone or in combination with chemotherapy and thalidomide, an antiangiogenesis agent
3. Alpha interferon as maintenance therapy
4. Bortezomib, a proteasome inhibitor to treat relapse
5. Allopurinol and fluids to treat hyperuricemia
6. Pamidronate, a potent bisphosphonate and calcium regulator, to inhibit bone resorption, treat hypercalcemia, and relieve bone pain

DRUG ALERT Pamidronate and other biphosphates may cause transient temperature elevation, hypophosphatemia, hypomagnesemia, hypocalcemia, and local reactions at the site of I.V. administration.

Surgical Interventions
1. Stabilization and fixation of fractures
2. Bone marrow or peripheral blood stem cell transplantation in selected cases (younger than age 50, no renal failure, few bone lesions, good organ function)

Nursing Diagnoses
3, 13, 24, 44, 62, 136

Nursing Interventions
Monitoring
1. Report sudden, severe pain, especially of back, which could indicate pathologic fracture.
2. Watch for nausea, drowsiness, confusion, or polyuria, which could indicate severe hypercalcemia caused by bony destruction and immobilization.
3. Monitor serum calcium levels.
4. Monitor serum blood urea nitrogen and creatinine to detect renal insufficiency.
5. Monitor intake and output to ensure adequate urine output, and weigh the patient daily.

Supportive Care

1. Administer analgesics as needed to control pain. Use adequate doses, regularly scheduled around the clock.
2. Administer biphosphonates I.V. over 4 hours or more, as directed, to prevent renal dysfunction.
3. Encourage the patient to wear back brace for lumbar lesion.
4. Recommend a consultation with a physical or occupational therapist.
5. Discourage bed rest to reduce hypercalcemia and prevent urolithiasis, but ensure safety of environment to prevent fractures.
6. Assist the patient with measures to prevent injury and decrease risk of fractures. Avoid lifting and straining; use walker and other assistive devices as appropriate.
7. Reassure the patient that you are available for support, to provide comfort measures, and to answer questions.
8. Encourage the patient to use own support network, such as church and community services and national agencies.

Education and Health Maintenance

1. Teach the patient about risk of infection caused by impaired antibody production; instruct the patient to monitor temperature and report any fever or other sign of infection promptly; also advise patient to use condoms and other safe sex practices.
2. Teach the patient to take medications as prescribed and monitor for possible adverse effects. Tell the patient to avoid aspirin and nonsteroidal anti-inflammatory drugs, unless prescribed, because these drugs may interfere with platelet function.
3. Teach the patient to minimize risk of fractures: use proper body mechanics and assistive devices as appropriate; avoid bed rest, remain ambulatory.
4. Advise patient to report new onset of pain, new location, or sudden increase in pain intensity immediately. Also, tell the patient to report new onset or worsening of neurologic symptoms (eg, changes in sensation) immediately.

5. Encourage the patient to maintain high fluid intake (2 to 3 qt [2 to 3 L]/day) to avoid dehydration and prevent renal insufficiency; also not to fast before diagnostic tests.

MULTIPLE SCLEROSIS

Multiple sclerosis (MS) is a relatively common, chronic central nervous system (CNS) disorder affecting young adults that is marked by demyelination of small areas of the white matter of the optic nerve, brain, and spinal cord. Demyelination results in disordered transmission of nerve impulses; concurrent inflammatory changes lead to scarring of the affected nerve fibers. The cause of MS is unknown but may be related to autoimmune dysfunction, genetic factors, or an infectious process. Although classed as a chronic disease, MS may flare up in acute exacerbations, after which the patient may go into remission. (See *Table M-3*.) Complications include respiratory dysfunction, infection or sepsis, and complications of immobility.

Assessment

1. Muscle weakness, fatigue, tremor, uncoordinated movements
2. Cranial nerve dysfunction, including vision disturbances (impaired and double vision, nystagmus) and impaired speech (slurring, dysarthria)
3. Absent or exaggerated deep tendon reflexes
4. Paresthesias, impaired deep sensation, impaired vibratory and position sense
5. Urinary dysfunction (hesitancy, frequency, urgency, retention, incontinence)
6. Symptoms are unpredictable, varying from person to person and from time to time in the same person.

Diagnostic Evaluation

1. Visual, auditory, and somatosensory evoked potential testing: slowed conduction is evidence of demyelination.
2. Lumbar puncture: electrophoresis shows abnormal immunoglobulin G antibody in cerebrospinal fluid.

TABLE M-3	Classification of Multiple Sclerosis

The National Multiple Sclerosis Advisory Committee recognizes four clinical forms of MS.

FORM	DESCRIPTION
Relapsing remitting (RR) 90% of cases at time of onset	Clearly defined acute attacks evolve over days to weeks. Partial recovery of function occurs over weeks to months. Average frequency of attacks is once every 2 years and neurologic stability remains between attacks without disease progression.
Secondary progressive (SP) (50% of those with RR will progress to SP within 10 years; 90% will progress within 25 years)	Always begins as RR but clinical course changes with declining attack rate with a steady deterioration in neurologic function unrelated to the original attack.
Primary progressive (PP) (10% of cases)	Characterized by steady progression of disability from onset without exacerbations and remissions. More preponderance among males and those with increased age at onset. Worst prognosis for neurologic disability.
Progressive relapsing (PR) (Rarest form)	Identical to PP except that patients experience acute exacerbations along with a steadily progressive course.

3. MRI: visualizes small plaques of demyelination scattered throughout white matter of CNS; magnetic resonance spectroscopy in development for use in monitoring plaques.

Collaborative Management
Therapeutic Interventions
1. Physical and occupational therapy to facilitate rehabilitation and maintenance of functional capacity
2. Nerve block for severe spasticity

3. Bowel and bladder programs to maintain control of elimination

Pharmacologic Interventions

1. Corticosteroids or adrenocorticotropic hormone to decrease inflammation and shorten duration of exacerbation of MS.
2. Immunosuppressive agents to help stabilize the course of the disease.
3. Interferon beta 1a and beta 1b are being used for treatment of rapid, progressing symptoms.
4. Glatiramer acetate is an immunomodulator, given daily subcutaneously, that has been shown to reduce relapse rate in relapsing-remitting MS.
5. Copolymer-1 has been effective in reducing relapse rates and disability in patients with relapsing-remitting MS.
6. Centrally acting muscle relaxants, such as baclofen or dantrolene, to control spasticity.
7. Amantadine and modafinil for fatigue; antidepressants
8. Anticholinergics such as oxybutynin for bladder control; prophylactic antibiotics may be used.
9. Stool softeners, bulk laxative, suppositories to control bowel function.
10. Carbamazepine to control dystonia and chronic pain.

Nursing Diagnoses
33, 43, 62, 69, 90, 156

Nursing Interventions
Monitoring

1. Observe for adverse reactions to drug therapy.
   a. Beta-interferon: flulike symptoms (fever, asthenia, chills, myalgias, sweating); local reaction at the injection site; liver function test elevation and neutropenia (Adverse effects may persist for up to 6 months of treatment before subsiding.)
   b. Glatiramer acetate: flulike symptoms; local reaction at injection site; nausea, diarrhea, GI distress; sweating, flushing, rash; palpitations, chest pain

c. Corticosteroids

d. Immunosuppressants: nausea, vomiting, leukopenia, thrombocytopenia, anemia, signs of serious infections

e. Muscle relaxants: drowsiness, dizziness, weakness, confusion, headache, hypotension, nausea, frequent urination

2. Monitor vital signs to detect changes.

3. Monitor for signs of respiratory or urinary infection, sepsis.

4. Monitor for signs of complications of immobility, such as pressure ulcers, contractures, constipation, pneumonia, and deep vein thrombosis.

Supportive Care

1. Perform muscle stretching and strengthening exercises daily or teach patient or family to perform; use stretch-hold-relax routine to minimize spasticity and prevent contractures.

2. Encourage ambulation and activities.

a. Teach use of braces, canes, walker, and so forth when necessary.

b. Advise the patient to avoid sudden changes in position and to use a wide-based gait to avoid injury from falls.

3. Encourage frequent position changes while immobilized to prevent contractures; advise that sleeping prone will minimize flexor spasm of hips and knees.

4. Explore ways to minimize fatigue.

a. Advise the patient to plan ahead and prioritize activities, and to take brief rest periods throughout the day.

b. Teach energy conservation techniques and avoidance of overheating or overexertion.

5. Advise the patient to avoid exposure to infectious agents.

6. Optimize sensory function.

a. Suggest use of an eye patch or frosted lens (alternate eyes) for patients with double vision.

b. If necessary, advise ophthalmologic consultation to maximize vision.

    c. Provide a safe environment for a patient with sensory alteration. Orient patient and make sure floors are free from obstacles or slippery areas.

7. Maintain urinary function.

    a. Ensure adequate fluid intake to help prevent infection and stone formation.

    b. Assess for urine retention; catheterize for residual urine as indicated.

    c. Initiate bladder-training program to reduce incontinence.

8. Promote the patient's sense of independence and well-being.

    a. Encourage verbal communication between patient and family members related to the disease and treatment.

    b. Explore adaptation of some roles so patient can still function in family unit; suggest dividing up household duties, and child care responsibilities to prevent strain on one person.

    c. Encourage counseling and use of church or community resources.

    d. If appropriate, encourage open communication between sexual partners; suggest consultation with sexual therapist to help promote sexual function.

Education and Health Maintenance

1. Encourage the patient to maintain previous activities although at a lower level of intensity.

2. Teach the patient to respect fatigue and to avoid physical overexertion, extremes in temperature, and emotional stress; remind patient that activity tolerance may vary from day to day.

3. Encourage the patient to follow a nutritious diet that is high in fiber to promote health and good bowel elimination.

4. Advise patient that some medications may accentuate weakness, such as some antibiotics, muscle relaxants, antiarrhythmics and antihypertensives, antipsychotics, hormonal contraceptives, and antihistamines; urge the pa-

tient to check with health care provider or pharmacist before taking new medications.

5. Include the whole family in teaching and explore ways each member can support the patient.

6. Instruct patient in self-injection technique for beta interferon and glatiramer acetate.

7. Refer the patient and family to such agencies as the National Multiple Sclerosis Society, *www.nmss.org*.

MUSCULAR DYSTROPHY

Muscular dystrophy is a group of hereditary disorders marked by progressive, symmetric weakness and wasting of skeletal muscles. The genetic defect may be X-linked, autosomal dominant or recessive. Common types include *Duchenne's muscular dystrophy*, *Becker's muscular dystrophy*, *myotonic dystrophy*, *facioscapulohumeral dystrophy*, and *limb-girdle dystrophy*. These disorders typically occur in childhood. Complications include infections and sepsis, cardiac arrhythmias, respiratory insufficiency, and depression.

Assessment

1. Progressive weakening and atrophy of muscles:
   a. *Duchenne's and Becker's:* involvement of iliopsoas, gluteal, and quadriceps muscles, pseudohypertrophy of calves, waddling gait, difficulty walking and climbing stairs; later, weakening of pretibial, pectoral girdle, and upper limbs (Becker's course is more benign.)
   b. *Myotonic:* levator palpebrae, facial, masseter, pharyngeal, laryngeal muscles affected (May have "swan neck" deformity from sternomastoid weakness.)
   c. *Facioscapulohumeral:* inability to raise arms over head; close eyes firmly or purse lips, scapular winging, "Popeye" effect of arms (large forearms, slim upper arms); atrophy of facial, shoulder, and arm muscles
   d. *Limb-girdle:* involvement of upper arm and pelvis, scapular winging (but absence of pseudohypertrophy of calves, sparing of facial muscles); lordosis; waddling gait

2. Hypotonia may result in delayed milestones or regression of milestones.

3. Heart muscle weakens and tachycardia develops.
4. Respiratory muscles weaken and ineffective cough leading to frequent infections.

Diagnostic Evaluation

1. Muscle biopsy shows deposits of fat and connective tissue (definitive diagnosis).
2. Nerve conduction test and electromyogram show weak bursts of electrical activity in affected muscles.
3. Serum creatine kinase level is usually elevated.

Collaborative Management
Therapeutic and Surgical Interventions

1. Physical and occupational therapy to preserve mobility and independence
2. Orthotic devices to promote spinal stability
3. Aids for ambulation
4. Respiratory therapy, such as chest percussion and inspirometry
5. Occasional surgical tendon release needed to treat contractures

Pharmacologic Interventions

1. Antiarrhythmics, bronchodilators, and corticosteroids are given to control manifestations.
2. Analgesics and antidepressants may be given to facilitate participation in activities.

Nursing Diagnoses
15, 19, 22, 62, 66, 75

Nursing Interventions
Monitoring

1. Monitor vital signs, respiratory effort, cardiac rhythm, and signs of heart failure, such as edema, adventitious breath sounds, and weight gain.
2. Monitor for signs of infections (pulmonary, urinary, systemic).

3. Monitor patient's emotional status; be alert for signs of depression.
4. Monitor muscle strength, atrophy, gait, and age-related motor development.

Supportive Care

1. When respiratory involvement occurs, encourage upright positioning to provide for maximum chest excursion.
2. Encourage coughing and deep breathing or perform chest physiotherapy as indicated, to strengthen respiratory muscles.
3. Suggest energy conservation techniques and avoidance of exertion.
4. Perform range-of-motion exercises to preserve mobility, prevent atrophy, and encourage stretching and strengthening exercises as taught by physical therapist.
5. Schedule activity with consideration of energy highs throughout the day.
6. Consult with occupational therapist for assistive devices to maintain independence.
7. Apply braces and splints, as directed, to prevent contractures.
8. Evaluate swallowing (gag reflex) and chewing.
9. Provide a diet that the patient can handle; blenderizing food may be necessary.
10. Encourage eating small, frequent meals and in upright position without talking.
11. Administer alternative enteral feeding if gag reflex is diminished.
12. Monitor intake and output and maintain I.V. or oral fluid intake as ordered.
13. Encourage diversional activities that prevent overexertion and frustration, but discourage long periods of bed rest and inactivity such as watching TV.
    a. If upper extremities are mostly affected, suggest walking or riding a stationary bike.
    b. If lower extremities are mostly affected, encourage use of a wheelchair to promote mobility, and performing simple crafts.

14. Help the patient investigate various methods of stress management to deal with frustration.

Education and Health Maintenance

1. Instruct the patient and family about range-of-motion exercises, pulmonary care, and methods of transfer and locomotion.
2. Stress the importance of maintaining fluid intake to decrease risk of urinary and pulmonary infections.
3. Advise patient or family to report signs of respiratory infection immediately to obtain treatment and prevent heart failure.
4. Encourage genetic counseling if indicated to determine options of family planning.
5. Help patient obtain services and devices that will promote maximal functioning, family functioning, and educational needs.
6. Refer the patient and family to The Muscular Dystrophy Association, *www.mdausa.org*.

MYASTHENIA GRAVIS

Myasthenia gravis is a chronic neuromuscular disorder affecting impulse transmission in the voluntary muscles of the body. The cause is unknown, but it is thought to result from impairment or destruction of acetylcholine (ACh) receptors at neuromuscular junctions by an autoimmune reaction. Reduced number of ACh receptors results in diminished amplitude of end-plate potentials and failed transmission of nerve impulses to skeletal muscles. Muscle contraction is impaired, leading to muscle weakness and fatigue.

A major complication is *myasthenic crisis*, which is severe weakness and respiratory distress caused by natural deterioration, emotional stress, upper respiratory infection, surgery, trauma, or as a result of adrenocorticotropic hormone therapy. A related emergency, *cholinergic crisis*, can result from overmedication with anticholinergic drugs, which release too much ACh at the neuromuscular junction. Presentation is similar to myasthenic crisis. *Brittle crisis* occurs when receptors at the neuromuscular junction become insensitive to anticholinergic medication.

Assessment

1. Cranial nerve dysfunction
   a. Vision disturbances: diplopia and ptosis from ocular weakness
   b. Masklike facial expression from involvement of facial muscles
   c. Dysarthria and dysphagia from weakness of laryngeal and pharyngeal muscles
2. Extreme muscular weakness and easy fatigability with repetitive activity and speech
3. Possible respiratory involvement with decreased vital capacity

Diagnostic Evaluation

1. Serum test for ACh receptor antibodies, which is positive in up to 90% of patients.
2. Tensilon test: I.V. injection temporarily improves motor response and relieves symptoms in myasthenic crisis; temporarily worsens symptoms in cholinergic crisis.
3. Electrophysiologic testing shows decremental response to repetitive nerve stimulation.
4. CT scan may show thymus hyperplasia, which is thought to initiate the autoimmune response.

Collaborative Management
Therapeutic and Surgical Interventions

1. In myasthenic or cholinergic crisis, airway maintenance, oxygen, and mechanical ventilation are indicated.
2. Plasmapheresis may be used to temporarily remove circulating ACh-receptor antibodies from the blood in crisis.
3. Thymectomy when thymoma or hyperplasia exists; may provide remission in some patients.

Pharmacologic Interventions

1. Anticholinergics such as neostigmine and pyridostigmine to enhance neuromuscular transmission. Neostigmine is given I.V. in myasthenic crisis.
2. Prednisone and/or azathioprine when weakness is not controlled by anticholinergics to suppress immune response.
3. Atropine is given I.V. in cholinergic crisis to reduce the effects of ACh.

Nursing Diagnoses
1, 33, 43, 44, 119, 159

Nursing Interventions
Monitoring

1. Monitor the patient's respiratory rate, use of accessory muscles, and oxygen saturation to watch for possible respiratory failure related to myasthenic or cholinergic crisis.
2. Be alert for signs of an impending crisis:
   a. Sudden respiratory distress
   b. Signs of dysphagia, dysarthria, ptosis, and diplopia
   c. Tachycardia, anxiety
   d. Rapidly increasing weakness of extremities and trunk
3. Monitor the patient's response to drug therapy.

DRUG ALERT Many drugs can accentuate the weakness experienced by the patient with myasthenia, including some antibiotics, antiarrhythmics, local and general anesthetics, muscle relaxants, and analgesics. Assess neurologic function after administering any new drug and report changes in the patient's condition.

Supportive Care

1. Administer medications so their peak effect coincides with meals or essential activities.
2. Help the patient develop a realistic activity schedule.
3. Allow for rest periods throughout the day to minimize fatigue.
4. Provide assistive devices to help patient perform activities of daily living despite weakness.

5. If the patient has diplopia, provide an eye patch to use on alternate eye to minimize risk of tripping and falling.
6. To avoid aspiration:
   a. Teach the patient to position the head in a slightly flexed position to protect the airway during eating.
   b. Have suction available that the patient can operate.
   c. If the patient is in crisis or has impaired swallowing, administer fluids I.V. and foods through nasogastric tube; elevate the head of bed after feeding.
   d. If the patient is on a mechanical ventilator, provide frequent suction, assess breath sounds, and check chest radiograph reports.
7. Show the patient how to cup chin in hands to support lower jaw to assist with speech.
8. If speech is severely affected, encourage the patient to use an alternative communication method, such as flash cards or a letter board.

Education and Health Maintenance

1. Instruct the patient and family about the symptoms of myasthenic crisis.
2. Teach the patient ways to prevent crisis and aggravation of symptoms.
   a. Avoid exposure to colds and other infections.
   b. Avoid excessive heat and cold.
   c. Tell the patient to inform the dentist of condition because use of procaine (Novocaine) is not well tolerated and may provoke crisis.
   d. Avoid emotional upset.
3. Teach the patient and family about the use of home suction.
4. Review the peak times of medications and how to schedule activity for best results.
5. Stress the importance of scheduled rest periods to avoid fatigue.
6. Encourage the patient to wear a medical alert bracelet.
7. Refer the patient and family to the Myasthenia Gravis Foundation, Inc., *www.myasthenia.org*.

MYOCARDIAL INFARCTION

Myocardial infarction (MI) refers to a dynamic process by which one or more regions of the heart muscle experience a severe and prolonged decrease in oxygen supply because of insufficient coronary blood flow. The affected muscle tissue subsequently becomes necrotic. Onset of an MI may be sudden or gradual, and the process takes 3 to 6 hours to run its course. MI is the most serious manifestation of acute coronary syndrome, a complication of coronary artery disease (CAD) (see page 233).

Approximately 90% of MIs are precipitated by acute coronary thrombosis (partial or total) secondary to severe CAD (greater than 70% narrowing of the artery). Other causative factors include coronary artery spasm, coronary artery embolism, infectious diseases causing arterial inflammation, hypoxia, anemia, and severe exertion or stress on the heart in the presence of significant coronary artery disease (eg, surgical procedures or shoveling snow).

In MI, the heart muscle experiences different degrees of damage, namely, necrosis, injury, and ischemia. In the *zone of necrosis,* death of the heart muscle has occurred; in the *zone of injury,* the muscle is inflamed and injured but can still be kept viable; and in the *zone of ischemia,* the tissue is at risk if the infarction spreads.

MIs are classified according to the layers of the heart muscle involved. In a transmural (Q-wave) infarction, necrosis occurs throughout the entire thickness of the heart muscle. In a subendocardial (nontransmural or non-Q-wave) infarction, the necrotic area is confined to the innermost layer of the myocardium lining the chambers.

EMERGENCY ALERT Patients with subendocardial infarctions should be considered as having an uncompleted MI; monitor carefully for signs and symptoms of spreading heart muscle damage.

MIs are also classified by the location of damaged heart muscle within the left ventricle (most common): anterior, inferior, lateral, and posterior wall. When an MI occurs in the right ventricle, it is commonly associated with damage to the inferior or posterior wall of the left ventricle. The region of the heart muscle that sustains damage is determined by the

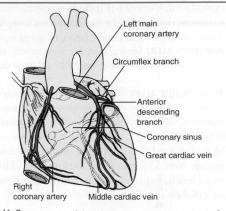

FIGURE M-2 Diagram of the coronary arteries arising from the aorta and encircling the heart. Some of the coronary veins are also shown.

Labels in figure:
Left main coronary artery
Circumflex branch
Anterior descending branch
Coronary sinus
Great cardiac vein
Right coronary artery
Middle cardiac vein

specific coronary artery that becomes obstructed (see *Figure M-2*).

Assessment

1. Chest pain
   a. *Character:* variable, but often diffuse, steady substernal chest pain. Other sensations include a crushing and squeezing feeling in the chest.
   b. *Severity:* pain may be severe; not relieved by rest or sublingual vasodilator therapy, requires opioids.
   c. *Location:* variable, but often pain resides behind upper or middle third of sternum.
   d. *Radiation:* pain may radiate to the arms (commonly the left), and to the shoulders, neck, back, or jaw.
   e. *Duration:* pain continues for more than 15 minutes.
2. Associated manifestations include anxiety, diaphoresis, cool clammy skin, facial pallor, hypertension or hypotension, bradycardia or tachycardia, premature ventricular or atrial beats, palpitations, dyspnea, disorientation, confusion, restlessness, fainting, marked weakness, nausea, vomiting, and hiccups.

3. Atypical symptoms of MI include epigastric or abdominal distress, dull aching or tingling sensations, shortness of breath, and extreme fatigue (more frequent in women).

EMERGENCY ALERT Some patients are asymptomatic, particularly patients with diabetes; these "silent MIs" still cause damage to the heart.

GERONTOLOGIC ALERT Elderly patients are more likely to experience silent MIs or have atypical symptoms: hypotension, low body temperature, vague complaints of discomfort, mild perspiration, strokelike symptoms, dizziness, and a change in sensorium.

4. Risk factors for MI include male gender, age over 45 for men, age over 55 for women, smoking, high blood cholesterol levels, hypertension, family history of premature CAD, diabetes, and obesity.

Diagnostic Evaluation

1. Serial 12-lead electrocardiograms (ECGs) detect changes that usually occur within 2 to 12 hours, but may take 72 to 96 hours.
   a. ST-segment depression and T-wave inversion indicate a pattern of ischemia; ST elevation indicates an injury pattern.
   b. Q waves indicate tissue necrosis and are permanent. (See *Figure M-3*.)

EMERGENCY ALERT A normal ECG does not rule out the possibility of infarction because ECG changes can be subtle and obscured by underlying conditions (bundle-branch blocks, electrolyte disturbances).

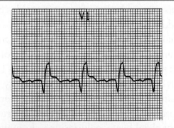

FIGURE M-3 Abnormal Q wave.

2. Nonspecific enzymes including aspartate transaminase, lactate dehydrogenase, and myoglobulin may be elevated.

3. More specific creatine phosphokinase isoenzyme CK-MB will be elevated.

4. Troponin T and I are myocardial proteins that increase in the serum about 3 to 4 hours after an MI, peak in 4 to 24 hours, and are detectable for up to 2 weeks; the test is easy to run, can help diagnose an MI up to 2 weeks earlier, and only unstable angina causes a false positive.

5. White blood cell count and sedimentation rate may be elevated.

6. Radionuclide imaging, positron emission tomography, and echocardiography may be done to evaluate heart muscle.

Collaborative Management
Therapeutic Interventions

1. Oxygen by way of nasal cannula to improve oxygenation of ischemic heart muscle

2. Bed rest to reduce myocardial oxygen demands

Pharmacologic Interventions

1. Pain control drugs to reduce catecholamine-induced oxygen demand to injured heart muscle.
   a. Opiate analgesics: morphine (to relieve pain, improve cardiac hemodynamics, and provide anxiety relief); meperidine (if allergic to morphine or sensitive to respiratory depression)
   b. Vasodilators: nitroglycerin (sublingual, I.V., paste; to promote venous [low-dose] and arterial [high-dose] relaxation as well as to relax coronary vessels and prevent coronary spasm; also to reduce myocardial oxygen demand with subsequent pain relief) (Persistent chest pain requires I.V. nitroglycerin.)
   c. Anxiolytics: benzodiazepines (used with analgesics when anxiety complicates chest pain and its relief)

2. Thrombolytic therapy by I.V. or intracoronary route, to dissolve thrombus formation and reduce the size of the infarction.

   a. Must be administered within 6 hours of the onset of chest pain to be effective, and they carry a risk of allergic reaction and bleeding.

   b. Reperfusion arrhythmias may follow successful therapy.

3. Anticoagulants or other antiplatelet medications as adjunct to thrombolytic therapy.

4. Beta-adrenergic blockers, to improve oxygen supply and demand, decrease sympathetic stimulation to the heart, promote blood flow in the small vessels of the heart, and provide antiarrhythmic effects.

5. Antiarrhythmics, such as lidocaine, decrease ventricular irritability commonly occurring after MI.

6. Calcium channel blockers, to improve oxygen supply and demand.

Surgical Interventions

1. Percutaneous transluminal intervention or coronary artery bypass graft surgery (see page 178) if revascularization of an evolving MI is deemed desirable.

Nursing Diagnoses
1, 3, 6, 19, 78, 88, 124, 136

Nursing Interventions
Monitoring

1. Monitor continuous ECG to watch for life-threatening arrhythmias (common within 24 hours after infarctions) and evolution of the MI (changes in ST segments and T waves). Be alert for any type of premature ventricular beats — these may herald ventricular fibrillation or ventricular tachycardia.

2. Monitor baseline vital signs before and 10 to 15 minutes after administering drugs; also monitor blood pressure continuously when giving nitroglycerin I.V.

3. Observe for signs of anxiety.

4. Monitor blood pressure every 1 or 2 hours or more frequently as indicated by condition.

5. Monitor respirations and auscultate lung fields every 2 to 4 hours or as indicated for crackles associated with left ventricular failure or pulmonary edema.

EMERGENCY ALERT Dyspnea, tachypnea, frothy pink sputum, and orthopnea may indicate left-sided heart failure, or pulmonary edema. Auscultation of clear lungs in the presence of cool, clammy skin, jugular vein distention, and hypotension may indicate right ventricular infarction.

M

6. Evaluate heart rate and heart sounds every 2 to 4 hours or as directed. Auscultate heart for the presence of a third heart sound (failing ventricle), fourth heart sound (stiffening ventricular muscle due to MI), friction rub (pericarditis), murmurs (valvular and papillary muscle dysfunction), or intraventricular septal rupture.

7. Evaluate major arterial pulses (weak pulse or presence of pulsus alternans indicates decreased cardiac output).

8. Monitor body temperature every 4 hours or as directed (most patients with MI develop increased temperature within 24 to 48 hours because of tissue necrosis).

9. Monitor skin color and temperature (cool, clammy skin and pallor — associated with vasoconstriction secondary to decreased cardiac output).

10. Observe for changes in mental status, such as confusion, restlessness, and disorientation.

11. Evaluate urine output (30 mL/hour) — decrease in volume reflects a decrease in renal blood flow.

12. Employ hemodynamic monitoring as indicated, including central venous pressure monitoring, pulmonary artery and pulmonary capillary wedge pressure monitoring, and arterial blood pressure monitoring.

Supportive Care

1. Handle the patient carefully while providing initial care, starting I.V. infusion, obtaining baseline vital signs, and attaching electrodes for continuous ECG monitoring. I.V. administration is the preferred route for analgesic medication because I.M. injections can cause elevations in serum enzymes, resulting in an incorrect diagnosis of an MI.

2. Reassure the patient that pain relief is a priority, and administer analgesics promptly. Place the patient in supine position during administration to minimize hypotension.

GERONTOLOGIC ALERT Elderly patients are extremely susceptible to respiratory depression in response to opioids. Substitute analgesic agents with less profound effects on the respiratory center. Anxiolytic agents should also be used with caution.

3. Emphasize importance of reporting any chest pain, discomfort, or epigastric distress without delay.

4. Explain equipment, procedures, and need for frequent assessment to the patient and significant others to reduce anxiety associated with facility environment.

5. Offer back massage to promote relaxation, decrease muscle tension, and improve skin integrity.

6. Promote rest with early gradual increase in mobilization to prevent deconditioning, which occurs with bed rest.
   a. Minimize environmental noise, provide a comfortable environmental temperature, and avoid unnecessary interruptions and procedures.
   b. Promote restful diversional activities for the patient (reading, listening to music, drawing, crossword puzzles, crafts).
   c. Encourage frequent position changes while in bed.
   d. Assist the patient to rise slowly from a supine position to minimize orthostatic hypotension caused by some drugs.
   e. Encourage passive and active range-of-motion exercises as directed while on bed rest.
   f. Elevate the patient's feet on chair when out of bed to promote venous return.

7. Take measures to prevent bleeding if patient is on thrombolytic therapy.
   a. Take vital signs every 15 minutes during infusion of thrombolytic agent and then hourly.
   b. Observe for presence of hematomas or skin breakdown, especially in potential pressure areas, such as the sacrum, back, elbows, and ankles.
   c. Be alert to the patient's complaints of back pain, which may indicate retroperitoneal bleeding.

d. Observe puncture sites every 15 minutes during infusion of thrombolytic therapy and then hourly for bleeding.

e. Apply manual pressure to venous or arterial sites if bleeding occurs. Use pressure dressings to cover access sites.

f. Observe for blood in stool, emesis, urine, and sputum.

g. Minimize venipunctures and arterial punctures; use heparin lock for blood sampling and medication administration.

h. Avoid I.M. injections.

i. Avoid use of automatic blood pressure device above puncture sites or hematoma. Use care in taking blood pressure; use arm not used for thrombolytic therapy.

j. Caution the patient about vigorous tooth brushing, hair combing, or shaving.

k. Monitor laboratory results: prothrombin time, partial thromboplastin time, hematocrit, and hemoglobin, and check for current blood type and crossmatch.

l. Administer antacids or histamine-2 blockers as directed to prevent stress ulcers.

8. Observe for persistence or recurrence of signs and symptoms of ischemia — chest pain, diaphoresis, and hypotension — may indicate extension of MI or reocclusion of coronary vessel. Report these manifestations immediately.

9. Be alert to signs and symptoms of sleep deprivation — irritability, disorientation, hallucinations, diminished pain tolerance, and aggressiveness.

10. Minimize possible adverse emotional response to transfer from the intensive care unit to the intermediate care unit. Introduce the admitting nurse from the intermediate care unit to the patient before transfer and inform the patient what to expect relative to physical layout of unit, nursing routines, and visiting hours.

Education and Health Maintenance

1. Explain basic cardiac anatomy and physiology; identify the difference between angina and MI; and describe how

the heart heals and that healing is not complete for 6 to 8 weeks after attack.

2. Emphasize the importance of rest and relaxation alternating with activity.

   a. Instruct the patient how to take pulse before and after starting activity, and to slow activity pace if sudden increase in heart rate occurs.

   b. Review signs and symptoms indicating a poor response to increased activity levels: chest pain, extreme fatigue, and shortness of breath.

3. Reinforce cardiac rehabilitation program with guidelines such as: 1) walk daily, gradually increasing distance and time as prescribed; 2) avoid activities that tense muscles, such as weight lifting, lifting heavy objects, isometric exercises, pushing or pulling heavy loads; 3) avoid working with arms overhead; 4) gradually return to work; 5) avoid extremes in temperature; and 6) do not rush; avoid tension.

4. Tell the patient that sexual relations may be resumed on advice of health care provider, usually after exercise tolerance is assessed. If the patient can walk briskly or climb two flights of stairs, sexual activity can usually be resumed with familiar partner. Advise the patient that sexual activity should be avoided after eating a heavy meal, after drinking alcohol, or when tired.

5. Advise the patient to get at least 7 hours of sleep each night and take 20- to 30-minute rest periods twice per day.

6. Advise the patient to eat three to four small meals per day rather than large heavy meals and to rest for 1 hour after meals.

7. Advise the patient to limit his or her caffeine and alcohol intake.

8. Tell the patient that driving a car must be cleared with health care provider at follow-up.

9. Teach the patient about medication regimen and adverse effects.

10. Instruct the patient to report the following symptoms: chest pressure or pain not relieved in 15 minutes by ni-

troglycerin or rest, shortness of breath, unusual fatigue, swelling of feet and ankles, fainting, dizziness, and very slow or rapid heartbeat.

11. Assist the patient to reduce risk of another MI by modifying risk factors (see *Coronary Artery Disease*, page 233).

12. For additional information and support, refer to the American Heart Association, *www.americanheart.org*.

M

MYOCARDITIS

Myocarditis is a focal or diffuse inflammation of the myocardium. It may be acute or chronic and can occur at any age. Myocarditis may be caused by viral infections (particularly Coxsackie group B viruses, as well as influenza A or B, and herpes simplex); infections by bacteria, fungi, parasites, protozoans, rickettsiae, and spirochetes; sarcoidosis and collagen vascular disorders; and chemotherapy (especially doxorubicin [Adriamycin]), or immunosuppressive therapy. Myocarditis may be self-limiting or may progress to heart failure or cardiomyopathy.

Assessment

1. Fatigue, fever, dyspnea, palpitations, and occasional chest pain. Be aware that disease severity depends on the type of infection, degree of myocardial damage, recuperative capacity of the myocardium, and host resistance. In some cases, symptoms may be minor and go unnoticed.

2. History of recent episodes of infection, chronic disease, and drugs that are myocardial toxins such as doxorubicin.

3. Displaced position of maximal impulse indicating heart enlargement; third heart sound; a systolic murmur in the apical area; and possibly a pericardial friction rub, if pericarditis is also present.

4. Signs of heart failure, such as pulsus alternans, dyspnea, and crackles.

> **EMERGENCY ALERT** Have equipment ready for resuscitation, cardiac defibrillation, and cardiac pacing if a life-threatening arrhythmia occurs.

Diagnostic Evaluation

1. 12-lead electrocardiogram (ECG) may show transient changes including flattened ST segment, T-wave inversion, conduction defects, extrasystoles, and supraventricular and ventricular ectopic beats.
2. Chest X-ray may show cardiomegaly and pulmonary congestion.
3. White blood cell count and sedimentation rate are elevated.
4. Throat or stool cultures isolate the offending agent.
5. Endomyocardial biopsy for definitive diagnosis.
6. Echocardiogram defines size, structure, and function of the myocardium.
7. MRI may be helpful to determine structural alterations.

Collaborative Management

Therapeutic and Pharmacologic Interventions

1. Strict bed rest to promote healing of damaged myocardium
2. Antipyretics to reduce fever
3. Antiarrhythmic therapy (usually quinidine or procainamide)
4. Antimicrobial therapy if causative bacteria are isolated
5. Diuretics and digoxin to treat symptoms of heart failure

DRUG ALERT Patients with myocarditis may be sensitive to digoxin. Assess for toxic signs and symptoms, such as anorexia, nausea, fatigue, weakness, yellow-green halos around visual images, and prolonged PR interval.

Nursing Diagnoses

1, 19, 22, 43, 49

Nursing Interventions

Monitoring

1. Monitor body temperature every 4 hours.
2. Record daily intake and output, daily weights, and check for edema to monitor for heart failure.
3. Maintain continuous ECG monitoring if arrhythmia develops.

4. Evaluate for clinical evidence that disease is subsiding by monitoring pulse, auscultating heart for improvement in murmur, auscultating lung fields, and monitoring respirations.

Supportive Care

1. Ensure strict bed rest to reduce heart rate, stroke volume, blood pressure, and heart contractility; bed rest also helps to decrease residual damage and complications of myocarditis, and promotes healing. Advise patient that bed rest may be prolonged until heart size is reduced and cardiac function improves.
2. Elevate the head of the bed, if necessary, to enhance respiration.
3. Allow the patient to use a bedside commode rather than a bedpan, to reduce cardiovascular workload.
4. Provide diversional activities for the patient.

Education and Health Maintenance

1. Because some residual heart enlargement is usually present, advise the patient that physical activity may be *slowly* increased. Discuss with the patient activities that can be continued after discharge to avoid fatigue. Tell the patient to begin with chair rest for increasing periods, followed by walking in the room, then outdoors for longer periods.
2. Tell the patient to immediately report any symptom in which the heart starts beating rapidly.
3. Advise the patient to avoid competitive sports, alcohol, and known myocardial toxins (such as doxorubicin).
4. Inform a female patient to avoid pregnancy if she has cardiomyopathy.
5. Advise the patient to get appropriate immunizations to avoid infectious diseases.

MYXEDEMA

See *Hypothyroidism*.

NECK DISSECTION, RADICAL

Radical neck dissection involves surgical removal of a tumor and all surrounding tissue from the ramus of the jaw down to the clavicle, from midline back to the angle of the jaw. In modified (functional) radical neck dissection, only the tumor and lymph nodes are removed. Part or all of the larynx may also be removed for some cancers. The procedure is commonly followed by radiation therapy. Surgical reconstruction may be performed with a rotational flap, skin graft, or free flap to promote healing and improve aesthetics.

This surgery is indicated for head and neck cancers (mostly squamous cell carcinomas), including tumors of the upper respiratory and digestive tracts. Specific sites include the ear, nasopharynx, nose and paranasal sinuses, palate, oral cavity, larynx, hypopharynx, and thyroid gland. Local extension to adjacent muscle, bone, and vital structures often occurs before detection, and metastasis to cervical lymph nodes is common.

Potential Complications
1. Salivary leakage, difficulty eating or swallowing
2. Malocclusion
3. Unintelligible speech
4. Unacceptable deformity

Nursing Diagnoses
3, 30, 51, 70, 75, 123, 135

Collaborative Management and Interventions
Preoperative Care
1. Improve nutritional status preoperatively through the use of nutritional supplements, parenteral nutrition, alcohol withdrawal, and counseling.

2. Assist with general health status evaluation and detection and treatment of underlying conditions, such as cirrhosis, obstructive pulmonary, and cardiovascular disease.

3. Assess level of understanding of disease process, treatment regimen, and follow-up care.

4. Provide intensive teaching and emotional preparation for major surgery, long rehabilitation, and change in body image.

Postoperative Care

1. Protect the airway and support respiration.
   a. After the patient has fully recovered from anesthesia, the endotracheal tube is removed (unless respiratory compromise occurs).
   b. Place the patient in Fowler's position.
   c. Observe for signs of respiratory difficulty, such as dyspnea, cyanosis, stridor, hoarseness, or dysphagia.
   d. Provide supplemental oxygen by facemask if necessary; if tracheostomy is present, provide oxygen by collar or T-piece to provide adequate humidification.
   e. Auscultate for decreased breath sounds, crackles, and wheezes; auscultate over the trachea in the immediate postoperative period to assess for stridor indicative of laryngeal edema.
   f. Encourage deep breathing and coughing.
   g. Assist the patient in assuming a sitting position to bring up secretions (support the patient's neck with the nurse's hands).
   h. Suction secretions orally or aseptically by tracheostomy if patient cannot cough them up.

2. Administer prophylactic antibiotics as directed to prevent infection caused by extensive incision, lymph node resection, and close proximity to oral secretions.

3. Assess vital signs for indication of infection (increased heart rate, elevation of temperature).

4. Closely monitor wound for hemorrhage, drainage, or tracheal constriction; reinforce dressings as needed.

5. Inspect incision for signs of infection (redness, warmth, swelling, and drainage). Ensure the incision site remains clean and dry; cleanse away secretions immediately.

6. If portable suction is used, expect approximately $2\frac{3}{4}$ to 4 oz (80 to 120 mL) serosanguineous secretions to be drawn off during the first postoperative day; this diminishes with each day. Aseptically cleanse skin area around drain exit, using saline or prescribed solution.

7. Provide I.V. fluids and parenteral nutrition, tube feedings by nasogastric tube or gastrostomy tube, or oral feedings of pureed food as soon as swallowing is established. Continue until oral intake is adequate and nutritional status is improved.

8. Provide mouth care before and after meals.

9. Watch for excessive or decreased salivation.

10. Make sure that emergency suctioning and airway equipment is available at the bedside during meals in the event of choking or aspiration.

11. Position patient in an upright position for feeding, supporting shoulders and neck with pillows if necessary.

12. If tracheostomy or laryngectomy has been performed, provide alternative methods of communication (letter board, chalk and slate, paper and pencil). Difficulty writing may result from denervation of the trapezius muscle.

13. Allow adequate time for patient to communicate. Recognize that patient may have difficulty nodding "yes" or "no" because of neck dissection.

14. Observe for lower facial paralysis because this may indicate facial nerve injury.

15. Watch for shoulder dysfunction, which may follow resection of spinal accessory nerves. Muscle exercises can improve range of motion.

16. Encourage the patient to verbalize concerns and feelings about body image and lifestyle changes in the areas of alcohol consumption and cigarette smoking.

Education and Health Maintenance

1. Advise the patient and family about exercises to prevent limited range of motion and discomfort.

a. Instruct the patient to perform exercises morning and evening. At first, exercises are done only once; then the number is increased by one each day until each exercise is done 10 times. The patient must relax after each exercise.

b. For neck, gently rotate head to each side as far as possible; tilt head to the right side as far as possible, then the left; drop chin to chest and then raise chin as high as possible.

c. For shoulder, place hand from unoperated side on chair for support and gradually swing arm on operated side up and back as far as tolerated. Each day, work toward finishing a complete circle.

2. Emphasize the need for frequent follow-up visits and completion of radiation therapy if prescribed.

3. If patient has a permanent tracheostomy or laryngectomy, instruct the patient and family about:

a. Need for humidification in the home.

b. Protective covering for stoma.

c. Activities to avoid that may cause aspiration.

d. Referral for a speech-language pathologist and social worker to meet ongoing communication needs.

NEPHROLITHIASIS AND UROLITHIASIS

Nephrolithiasis refers to the presence of stones, or calculi, in the renal pelvis, and *urolithiasis* refers to their presence in the urinary system. Stones are formed by crystallization of urinary solutes (calcium oxalate, uric acid, calcium phosphate, struvite, and cystine). They vary in size from granular ("sand or gravel") deposits to orange-sized bladder stones. In 80% of patients with urolithiasis, gravel stones pass spontaneously. Men are affected more frequently than women, and recurrences are possible.

Causes and predisposing factors include hypercalcemia and hypercalciuria caused by hyperparathyroidism; renal tubular acidosis; multiple myeloma; excessive intake of vitamin D, milk, and alkali; chronic dehydration, poor fluid intake, and prolonged immobility; abnormal purine metabolism (hyperuricemia and gout); genetic disorders (cystinuria); chronic infection with urea-splitting bacteria (*Proteus vulgaris*); chronic obstruction by foreign bodies in the urinary tract; and excessive oxalate absorption in inflammatory bowel disease, bowel resection, or ileostomy. Complications include obstruction, infection, and impaired renal function.

Assessment

1. Pain pattern (referred to as colic) depends on site of obstruction (see *Figure N-1*).
2. Chills, fever, dysuria, frequency, and hematuria may occur if infection is present secondary to obstruction.
3. Nausea, vomiting, diarrhea, and general abdominal discomfort may occur.

Diagnostic Evaluation

1. X-ray of kidneys, ureters, and bladder may show some stones.
2. Intravenous urography (IVU) locates stones and evaluates degree of obstruction.

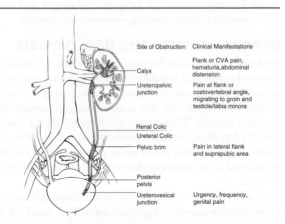

Site of Obstruction	Clinical Manifestations
Calyx	Flank or CVA pain, hematuria, abdominal distension
Ureteropelvic junction	Pain at flank or costovertebral angle, migrating to groin and testicle/labia minora
Renal Colic	
Ureteral Colic	
Pelvic brim	Pain in lateral flank and suprapubic area
Posterior pelvis	
Ureterovesical junction	Urgency, frequency, genital pain

FIGURE N-1 Areas where calculi may obstruct the urinary system. The ensuing clinical manifestations depend on the site of obstruction.

3. Ultrasonography may be sensitive for stone detection if technique is good.
4. Spiral CT technique identifies stone in ureter; faster than IVU and no preparation needed.
5. Laboratory analyses of passed or retrieved stone material identify type of stone.
6. Urinalysis may show hematuria and pyuria; culture and sensitivity studies identify infective organisms.
7. Serum renal function tests, electrolytes, calcium, phosphorous, uric acid, magnesium, and parathyroid hormone levels are evaluated.

Collaborative Management

Therapeutic and Pharmacologic Interventions

1. Conservative therapy for small stones (less than 0.2 inches [less than 5 mm]), which are usually passed spontaneously.
   a. Hydration to maintain high urinary volume
   b. Straining of urine and observation
   c. Pain management
   d. Hospitalization for intractable pain, persistent vomiting, high grade fever, obstruction with infection, and solitary kidney with signs of obstruction
2. *Extracorporeal shock wave lithotripsy* (ESWL), in which high-energy shock waves are directed at the kidney stone, disintegrating it into minute particles that pass in the urine.
   a. Treatment of choice for stones smaller than ¾ inch (2 cm) in diameter (80% of stones fall into this category), which are located in the ureter above the iliac crest.
   b. Eliminates need for surgery in most patients and can be repeated for recurrent stones with no apparent risk to kidney structure or function.
   c. Patient is placed on specially designed table and immersed in water or positioned over a cushion of water.

Surgical Interventions

1. *Percutaneous nephrolithotomy*, in which stones larger than 1 inch (2.5 cm) in the renal collecting system or proximal ureter are broken apart with hydraulic shock waves or a laser beam administered by nephroscope; fragments are removed using forceps, graspers, or basket.
   a. May be combined with ESWL
   b. Used for stones larger than 1 inch in diameter
2. *Percutaneous stone dissolution (chemolysis)*, in which a solvent is infused into the stone through a nephrostomy tube placed in the kidney. A second catheter may be used for drainage. Used to dissolve struvite, uric acid, and cystine stones.
   a. May be used in combination with other retrieval methods
   b. Irrigating solution introduced at a constant rate that patient can tolerate without flank pain
3. *Ureteroscopy*, in which stones are either removed by flexible or rigid ureteroscope with basket or grasper, or are fragmented with electrohydraulic, ultrasonic, or laser equipment.
   a. Used for distal ureteral calculi; may be used for midureteral calculi.
   b. Stent may be inserted to maintain patency of ureter.
4. Open surgical procedures are indicated for only 1% to 2% of all stones. Procedures include *pyelolithotomy*, *nephrolithotomy*, *nephrectomy*, *ureterolithotomy*, and *cystolithotomy*.

Nursing Diagnoses
3, 69, 135

Nursing Interventions
Monitoring
Also see *Kidney Surgery and Urinary Diversion*, page 555.
1. Monitor for complications of procedures for stone removal, including infection, hemorrhage, extravasation of urine, and obstruction from remaining stone fragments.

2. Monitor response to analgesics; because large doses of opioids are often necessary, monitor for respiratory depression and decrease in blood pressure.
3. Monitor urine output and patterns of voiding; report oliguria or anuria.
4. Monitor for fever, dysuria, frequency, and foul-smelling urine, which indicates infection.

Supportive Care

1. Encourage the patient to assume position of comfort.
2. Administer antiemetics (by I.M. or rectal suppository) as indicated for nausea.
3. Encourage oral fluid intake if able, or give I.V. if patient is vomiting to ensure adequate urine output.
4. Strain all urine through strainer or gauze to harvest the stone; uric acid stones may crumble. Crush clots and inspect sides of urinal or bedpan for clinging stones or fragments. Can discontinue straining 72 hours after symptoms resolve.

COMMUNITY CARE CONSIDERATIONS

Advise patient who is at home to strain urine through a coffee filter to catch stones, therefore documenting passage of stones. If these are recurrent stones, tell the patient to save them for analysis.

5. Assist the patient to walk, if possible, because ambulation may help move the stone through the urinary tract.

Education and Health Maintenance
To aid postoperative or postprocedure recovery

1. Encourage patient to drink fluids to accelerate passing of stone particles.
2. Teach patient about analgesics, which still may be necessary for colicky pain that may accompany passage of stone debris.
3. Warn patient that some blood may appear in urine for up to several weeks.

4. Encourage patient to walk frequently to assist in passage of stone fragments.

To prevent recurrent stone formation

1. Instruct patient about dietary requirements related to specific stone type: avoid excessive calcium and phosphorus for calcium oxalate stones; reduce purine intake (red meat, fish, and fowl) for uric acid stones.
2. Encourage patient to comply with prescribed drug therapy, such as thiazide diuretics to reduce urine calcium excretion, allopurinol to reduce uric acid concentration, D-penicillamine to lower cystine concentration, and sodium bicarbonate to alkalinize urine.
3. Teach patient with uric acid or cystine stones how to monitor urine pH with a test strip to maintain urine alkalinity.
4. Teach patient with struvite stones to recognize and quickly report signs and symptoms of urinary infection, and to seek prompt treatment.
5. Encourage patient to perform weight-bearing activity and avoid prolonged bed rest, which alters calcium metabolism.
6. Advise all patients with stone disease to drink enough fluids to achieve a urinary volume of 68 to 101 oz (2,011 mL to 2,990 mL) or more every 24 hours.

NEPHROTIC SYNDROME

Nephrotic syndrome is a clinical disorder of unknown cause characterized by proteinuria, hypoalbuminemia, edema, and hyperlipidemia. These conditions result from excessive leakage of plasma proteins into the urine because of impairment of the glomerular capillary membrane. Nephrotic syndrome is categorized as congenital, primary (idiopathic), and secondary. Most cases in children are minimal change nephrotic syndrome, a primary cause with minimal histologic change in the glomerular basement membrane. Upper respiratory infection and immunization are precipitating events. Secondary causes (more frequent in adults) are chronic glomerulonephritis, diabetes mellitus, renal amyloidosis, systemic lupus erythematosus, renal vein thrombosis, and malignancy. The loss of proteins, particularly albumin, reduces oncotic pressure and causes edema. The fluid shift out of the intravascular space stimulates the renin-angiotensin system to reabsorb water and sodium, which further contributes to edema. The mechanism of hyperlipidemia is not understood. Loss of immunoglobulins also predisposes the patient to infection. Other complications include thromboembolism, altered drug metabolism caused by decreased plasma proteins, and progression to end-stage renal disease.

N

Assessment

1. Insidious onset of pitting edema, including periorbital edema, dependent edema, and eventually ascites and pleural effusions
2. Decreased urine output; urine appears concentrated and frothy
3. Irritability, fatigue, anorexia, nausea, and vomiting
4. Profound weight gain (child may double weight)
5. Wasting of skeletal muscles

Diagnostic Evaluation

1. Urinalysis:
   a. Protein: 2+ or greater
   b. Casts: numerous
   c. Blood: absent or transient
2. Elevated 24-hour urine for protein; may be normal or decreased creatinine clearance
3. Urine protein electrophoresis characterizes protein
4. Serum chemistry
   a. Total protein and albumin reduced
   b. Cholesterol and triglycerides elevated
   c. May be normal or increased creatinine
5. Needle biopsy of kidney may be necessary to confirm diagnosis

Collaborative Management
Therapeutic Interventions

1. Treat causative glomerular disease

2. Restriction of sodium and fluids to control edema; liberal intake of potassium
3. Dietary protein supplements
4. Paracentesis for severe ascites
5. Low saturated fat diet

Pharmacologic Interventions

1. Corticosteroids and immunosuppressants to decrease proteinuria
   a. High-dose daily therapy for about 4 weeks.
   b. Taper and withdraw slowly to prevent adrenal insufficiency.
   c. If unresponsive to steroids or repeated relapse when steroids withdrawn, immunosuppressant agent may be used.
2. Diuretics and angiotensin-converting enzyme inhibitors to control edema if renal insufficiency is not severe
3. Infusion of salt-poor albumin to raise oncotic pressure and shift fluid from interstitial to intravascular space

Nursing Diagnoses
22, 24, 123, 134, 135

Nursing Interventions
Monitoring

1. Monitor edema, daily weights, urine specific gravity, and intake and output to gauge severity of condition; weigh diapers if indicated.
2. Monitor central venous pressure (if indicated), vital signs, orthostatic blood pressure, and heart rate measurements to detect hypovolemia.
3. Monitor serum blood urea nitrogen and creatinine to assess renal function.
4. Monitor for signs and symptoms of infection secondary to loss of immunoglobulins and therapy with immunosuppressants.

PEDIATRIC ALERT No immunizations should be given during active nephrosis or while child is receiving immunosuppressant therapy because response will be muted.

5. Monitor temperature and laboratory values for neutropenia due to immunosuppressant therapy.
6. Monitor for adverse effects of corticosteroid therapy: hyperglycemia, acne, striae, mood swings, increased appetite, and poor wound healing.
7. Monitor serum potassium during diuretic therapy.
8. Monitor the patient's response to other drug therapy; drug metabolism may be altered because of reduced plasma proteins.

Supportive Care

1. Encourage bed rest for a few days to help mobilize edema; however, some ambulation is necessary to reduce risk of thromboembolic complications.
2. Enforce mild to moderate sodium and fluid restriction if edema is severe; offer small amounts of fluid in appropriate-size cup at regular intervals.
3. Use aseptic technique for all invasive procedures and strict hand washing by the patient and all contacts; prevent patient contact with persons who may transmit infection.
4. Handle edematous extremities carefully, encourage change of position frequently, and inspect skin for breakdown caused by pressure of the edema.
5. Encourage high-protein, high-carbohydrate diet according to patient's interest.
6. Administer cyclophosphamide in the morning with fluid to reduce concentration of drug in the urine and increased susceptibility of cystitis.
7. Suggest quiet diversional activities during periods of bed rest.

Education and Health Maintenance

1. Teach the patient signs and symptoms of nephrotic syndrome; also review causes, purpose of prescribed treatments, and importance of long-term therapy to prevent end-stage renal disease.
2. Instruct patient and family of adverse effects of prescribed medications and methods of preventing infection if patient is taking immunosuppressants.

3. Carefully review with patient and family dietary and fluid restrictions; consult dietitian for assistance in meal planning.
4. Discuss the importance of maintaining exercise, decreasing cholesterol and fat intake, and changing other risk factors such as smoking, obesity, and stress to reduce risk of atherosclerosis and severe thromboembolic complications.
5. Encourage extended follow-up to ensure resolution of proteinuria and advise immediate reporting of edema and decreased urine output.

NEUROBLASTOMA

Neuroblastoma is a malignant tumor that arises from embryonic cells along the craniospinal axis of the sympathetic nervous system. Neuroblastoma is the most common extracranial solid tumor of childhood, occurring in approximately 1 in 7,000 children, mostly infants and young children. The tumor may spread to the liver, soft tissue, bones, and bone marrow, and nerve compression may cause neurologic deficits. In some cases, neuroblastoma may undergo spontaneous remission.

Assessment

1. Symptoms depend on the location of the tumor and the stage of the disease.
2. Most tumors are located within the abdomen and present as firm, nontender, irregular masses that cross the midline.
3. Other common signs include:
   a. Bowel or bladder dysfunction resulting from compression by a paraspinal or pelvic tumor
   b. Neurologic symptoms caused by compression by the tumor on nerve roots or because of tumor extension
   c. Supraorbital ecchymoses, periorbital edema, and exophthalmos resulting from metastases to the skull bones and retrobulbar soft tissue
   d. Lymphadenopathy, especially in the cervical area
   e. Bone pain and joint swelling with skeletal involvement

    f. Swelling of the neck or face, and cough with thoracic masses

    g. Anemic bleeding and infection secondary to bone marrow failure

    h. Pallor, anorexia, weight loss, and weakness with widespread metastasis

Diagnostic Evaluation

1. Workup done to document the extent of the disease throughout the body includes chest and skeletal X-rays, bone scan, bone marrow aspiration and possible biopsy, complete blood count, platelet count, ferritin level, 24-hour urine collection to detect elevated excretion of homovanillic acid and vanillylmandelic acid, and liver and kidney function tests.

2. Additional studies may include:
   a. CT scan of primary site and chest; MRI above the diaphragm
   b. Ultrasound examination
   c. Liver or spleen scan

3. N-*myc* oncogene blood screening and other forms of genetic testing — multiple copies associated with a poor prognosis

4. Tumors are staged primarily on the basis of the extent of disease.
   a. Evans staging system: stage I (tumor is confined to the organ or structure of origin) to stage IV (there is remote disease involving the skeleton, parenchymal organs, soft tissue, distant lymph nodes, or bone marrow)
   b. Stage IV-S refers to cases that would otherwise be stage I or II but have remote disease confined to one or more sites, such as the liver, skin, or bone marrow, without evidence of skeletal metastasis.

Collaborative Management
Pharmacologic Interventions

1. Stage II disease and greater generally requires combination therapy with chemotherapy, radiation, and surgery.

a. Chemotherapy drugs of choice include vincristine, dacarbazine, cyclophosphamide, doxorubicin, cisplatin, carboplatin, ifosfamide, and etoposide.

b. Factors that influence prognosis include stage of disease, age, site of primary tumor, pattern of metastasis, and genetic factors.

2. Newer chemotherapy agents, immunotherapy, and bone marrow or stem cell transplantation may improve survival.

Surgical Interventions

1. Surgery is both diagnostic and therapeutic — either primary (before chemotherapy or radiation) or delayed or secondary (after therapy).

2. When complete surgical resection of a stage I tumor is possible, this may be the only treatment required.

Nursing Diagnoses

1, 3, 6, 16, 30, 44, 69, 135

Nursing Interventions

Monitoring

1. Observe the surgical incision site for erythema, drainage, or separation of the incision. Report any of these changes.

2. Monitor and report an elevated temperature or sign of infection.

3. If the child is receiving chemotherapy or radiation, monitor for adverse effects, hydration status, and nutritional status.

EMERGENCY ALERT Monitor for increasing pain or development of pain in a new location, which might indicate progression of disease or pathologic fracture.

Supportive Care

1. Encourage the parents to ask questions and to understand fully the risks and benefits of surgery.

2. Prepare the child for surgery; explain procedures at the appropriate developmental level.

3. Continue supporting the parents during the postoperative period. They may be frightened and upset by the appearance of their child.
4. Explain why fatigue and shortness of breath may occur.
5. Plan frequent rest periods between daily activities.
6. Caution the child about physical overexertion; encourage rest frequently and warn child to expect a tired feeling.
7. Assess normal elimination patterns the child had before the illness began.
8. Keep careful intake and output records.
9. Assess for urinary overflow incontinence and loss of bowel function, depending on the age of the child.
10. Administer pain control medications as ordered in the immediate postoperative period.
11. Encourage the child to express feelings about the threat to body image resulting from chemotherapy.
12. Reassure the child that he or she will be able to wear a wig or a hat after recovery; hair will grow back from chemotherapy.
13. Assess need for other health professionals to help the child and family through this experience.

Education and Health Maintenance

1. Begin to develop a home care plan before discharge from the hospital to include school, peers, activities, follow-up appointments, and so forth.
2. Teach parents about the laboratory tests and radiographs needed at diagnosis and periodically throughout therapy.
3. Instruct parents about chemotherapy medications used and their potential adverse effects.
4. Inform parents about potential treatment methods, such as radiation therapy and bone marrow transplantation.
5. Advise parents to use good hand-washing practices and to prevent exposure to children with communicable diseases.
6. For further information, refer to the Candlelighters Childhood Cancer Foundation, *www.candlelighters.org*.

O

OBESITY

Obesity is an overabundance of body fat resulting in body weight 20% more than the average weight for the person's age, height, sex, and body frame. Body mass index (BMI) is now widely used to identify obesity (ratio of weight in kilograms to height in meters). The root cause is unknown, but a wide variety of predisposing factors have been identified. These include heredity, environment (availability of high-fat, high-calorie foods), psychological factors (eg, depression, anxiety), medications that increase appetite, age (puberty, old age), and, rarely, endocrine abnormalities (eg, Cushing's syndrome, hypothyroidism, hypogonadism, or hypothalamic lesions). Obesity is a risk factor for diabetes mellitus, cardiovascular disease, gallbladder disease, osteoarthritis, high blood pressure, and some cancers. There is shorter life expectancy of 13 to 20 years for persons with BMI greater than 45.

Assessment and Diagnostic Evaluation

1. Body weight exceeds 20% of acceptable weight for height and gender; or BMI 30 or greater (see *Table O-1*).
2. Nutritional assessment evaluates dietary habits and caloric intake.
3. Anthropometric assessment, including triceps skinfold measurement, and mid-upper arm circumference, evaluates body mass and fat; waist and hip measurements determine ratio, which may be an additional risk factor for cardiovascular disease.
4. Complete physical examination determines effect of obesity on body.
5. Selected hormonal studies (thyroid, adrenal) looks for underlying cause.

TABLE O-1	Body Mass Index (BMI)*					
WEIGHT			**HEIGHT**			
	5'	**5'3"**	**5'6"**	**5'9"**	**6'**	**6'3"**
140	27	25	23	21	19	18
150	29	27	24	22	20	19
160	31	28	26	24	22	20
170	33	30	28	25	23	21
180	35	32	29	27	25	23
190	37	34	31	28	26	24
200	39	36	32	30	27	25
210	41	37	34	31	29	26
220	43	39	36	33	30	28
230	45	41	37	34	31	29
240	47	43	39	36	33	30
250	49	44	40	37	34	31

*Body mass index = weight (kg)/height (m^2)

Collaborative Management

Therapeutic Interventions

1. Nutritional therapy is instituted to eliminate 1,000 calories per day to lose 2.2 lb (1 kg) of body weight per week.
   a. Diet should be individualized to create a calorie deficit that will be significant through reduced calorie intake and/or increased calorie expenditure.
   b. Elimination of an entire food group such as carbohydrates may present nutritional deficiencies and usually results in cravings for such foods.
   c. Vitamin and mineral deficiencies may result from a severely restricted diet. A very-low-calorie diet (800 to

1,000 calories per day) requires careful monitoring and use of vitamin and mineral supplements.
   d. The 2005 Dietary Guidelines for Americans from the U.S. Department of Agriculture outline healthy practices to attain ideal weight at *www.health.gov/ dietaryguidelines*.

ALTERNATIVE INTERVENTION

High-protein, high-fat, and low-carbohydrate diets have become popular; however, they have been associated with hyperlipidemia, uremia, rapid weight gain when discontinued, and other problems. Although reducing the carbohydrate ratio may be helpful (in some patients) to improve hyperglycemia and other metabolic problems, these diets are generally not recommended.

2. Daily exercise, such as walking or other aerobic activity, for approximately 180 minutes per week.
3. Behavior modification to reinforce diet program.
   a. Use food diary to identify and eliminate situations or cues leading to overeating or high-calorie foods.
   b. Provide positive reinforcement of proper diet habits.
   c. Stress-reduction techniques, such as visual imagery or progressive relaxation and peer support, may be helpful.

Pharmacologic Interventions

1. Pharmacologic therapy may be considered for some patients unable to achieve satisfactory weight loss with diet and exercise. Anorexiants of the amphetamine class and phentermine are not widely used because tolerance develops within 2 to 4 weeks and weight is usually regained when the drugs are discontinued.
2. Sibutramine (Meridia) is a mixed neurotransmitter uptake inhibitor that acts on the central nervous system to reduce appetite; long-term risks are unknown.
   a. Use cautiously with hypertension, coronary artery disease, heart failure, arrhythmia, renal and hepatic im-

pairment, narrow-angle glaucoma, and seizure disorders.

b. Many drug interactions include monoamine oxidase inhibitors, serotonin agents, 5-HT receptor agonists, lithium, dextromethorphan and, possibly, erythromycin and ketoconazole.

c. Adverse effects include dry mouth, constipation, dizziness, nervousness, and insomnia.

3. Orlistat (Xenical) is a GI lipase inhibitor, which blocks the breakdown and absorption of dietary fat in the intestines so that about 30% of fat is eliminated.

a. Long-term safety has not been established, but the addition of a fat-soluble vitamin is recommended 1 hour before or 2 hours after orlistat to prevent the theoretical deficiency of vitamins A, D, E, and K and beta-carotene.

b. Contraindicated in cases of malabsorption syndromes and cholestasis.

c. Adverse effects include oily stools, flatulence, and GI distress.

ALTERNATIVE INTERVENTION

There are no data to suggest that herbal products or liquid diet programs are effective for long-term weight loss; however, they are popular. Encourage patients to discuss products with their health care providers and to avoid any product containing ephedra (ma huang), which may cause hypertension, palpitations, tachycardia, stroke, seizures, and has led to death.

Surgical Interventions

1. Generally reserved for morbidly obese patients unable to lose weight through nonsurgical therapies (see *Figure O-1*, page 672)

a. Gastroplasty (gastric stapling) is vertical banding of the stomach to create a 30-mL pouch along the lesser gastric curvature with a small outlet.

b. Gastric bypass (Roux-en-Y gastroenterostomy) is the current procedure of choice. It creates distal and prox-

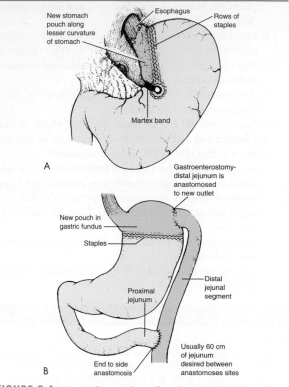

FIGURE O-1 Surgical procedures for obesity. **(A)** Gastroplasty with vertical banding. **(B)** Gastric bypass with Roux-en-Y anastomosis.

imal stomach pouches with horizontal stapling; the distal jejunum is attached to the proximal pouch, bypassing the distal stomach pouch. This procedure creates vitamin and mineral deficiency (malabsorption syndrome).

c. Gastric banding is the placement of a silicone band at the gastroesophageal junction, creating a small upper segment and a narrow passage into the larger remaining stomach.

Nursing Diagnoses
12, 52, 112, 135, 136

Nursing Interventions
Also see *Gastrointestinal or Abdominal Surgery,* page 381.

Monitoring
1. Monitor dietary intake for calorie count and essential nutrients.
2. Postoperatively, monitor vital signs, surgical incision, bowel sounds, and condition of the abdomen for signs of bleeding, obstruction, infection, or other complications.

Supportive Care
1. Assist the patient in assessing current dietary habits and identifying poor dietary habits.
2. Assist the patient in developing appropriate diet plan based on likes and dislikes, activity level, and lifestyle.
3. Suggest behavior modification strategies, such as using a smaller plate, shortening lunch break, preventing access to quick snacks, and eating only at mealtimes at the table.
4. Provide emotional support to the patient during weight-reduction efforts through positive reinforcement and creative problem solving.
5. Provide the patient with alternative coping mechanisms, including stress-reduction techniques, such as progressive relaxation and guided imagery.
6. Assess the patient's ability to tolerate exercise through measurement of vital signs before, during, and after exercise and asking about symptoms of shortness of breath and chest pain.
7. Provide postoperative care.
   a. Observe for and report increased pain and distention, which may indicate leakage at staple sites or obstruction.
   b. Provide I.V. fluids as directed, and, when bowel sounds return, give oral fluids to prevent dehydration.
   c. If fluids are tolerated, begin six small feedings for a total of 600 to 800 calories per day.

d. Watch for and report signs of dehydration (thirst, oliguria, dry mucous membranes) and hypokalemia (muscle weakness, anorexia, nausea, decreased bowel sounds, arrhythmias).

e. Warn patients that overeating will cause vomiting and painful esophageal distention.

COMMUNITY CARE CONSIDERATIONS

The 2005 Dietary Guidelines stress the following points:
- Personalized advice for diet and weight management
- Eat a variety of foods from every group in balance and moderation
- Pay attention to calorie consumption
- Achieve a balance between food intake and regular physical activity.

Education and Health Maintenance

1. Explain the purpose of a balanced diet based on the 2005 Dietary Guidelines for Americans.
2. Review the health hazards of obesity and the danger of regaining weight if good diet and exercise habits are not maintained.
3. Advise the patient of plateau period without weight loss for some time that may occur, but not to get discouraged.
4. Tell the patient to keep a food diary to show to nutritionist and to weigh self no more than once per week.
5. Refer patient to agencies such as American Dietetic Association, *www.eatright.org*.

OCCLUSIVE ARTERIAL DISEASE

See *Arterial Occlusive Disease*.

OCCUPATIONAL LUNG DISEASES

Occupational lung diseases result from long-term exposure to organic or inorganic (mineral) dusts and noxious gases. *Silicosis* is a chronic pulmonary fibrosis caused by inhaling silica dusts encountered in mining, ceramic, abrasive, and foundry industries. When silica particles are inhaled, nodular lesions are produced throughout the lungs, and the nodules undergo fibrosis, enlarge, and fuse. *Asbestosis* is a diffuse interstitial fibrosis caused by inhaling asbestos dust and particles from products encountered in numerous manufacturing and construction industries. Asbestos particles enter the alveoli and are obliterated by fibrous tissue. Fibrous pleural tissue produces restrictive lung disease, hypoxemia, and subsequent cor pulmonale. *Coal worker's pneumoconiosis* (CWP, "black lung") is a tissue reaction caused by inhaling coal dust (also kaolin, mica, or silica) from mining industries. When normal clearance mechanisms can no longer handle the dust load, the bronchioles and alveoli become clogged with coal dust, dying macrophages, and fibroblasts, leading to formation of the coal macule. Macules may enlarge, causing centrilobular emphysema.

Initial exposure to irritants may cause acute reaction of fever, chills, and cough in 4 to 12 hours; these recur with subsequent exposures. Chronic occupational lung diseases usually develop slowly, (over 20 to 30 years) and are asymptomatic in the early stages. Complications include respiratory failure and lung cancer. Asbestosis is strongly associated with bronchogenic cancer and with mesotheliomas of the pleura and peritoneal surfaces. Smoking increases the risk of lung cancer 50 to 100 times in patients with asbestosis.

Assessment
1. Characteristic symptoms include chronic cough (productive in silicosis and CWP); dyspnea on exertion (progressive and irreversible in asbestosis and CWP); and expectoration of varying amounts of black fluid in CWP. There is increased susceptibility to respiratory infections.
2. Auscultation reveals bibasilar crackles with asbestosis.

Diagnostic Evaluation
1. Chest radiograph may show nodules of upper lobes in silicosis and CWP and diffuse parenchymal fibrosis, especially of lower lobes, in asbestosis.
2. Pulmonary function tests primarily show a pattern of restrictive lung disease with possibly some obstructive component.

3. Bronchoscopy (with lavage) helps identify the specific exposure.
4. CT scanning, sputum examination, lung biopsy, and tuberculin testing may be done to rule out other disorders.

Collaborative Management
Therapeutic Interventions
1. There is no specific treatment; the exposure agent is eliminated, and the patient is treated symptomatically; smoking cessation is important to preserve remaining lung function and reduce the risk of lung cancer.
2. Home oxygen therapy may be required.

Pharmacologic Interventions
1. Isoniazid is given prophylactically to a patient with positive tuberculin test because silicosis is associated with high risk of tuberculosis.
2. Bronchodilators are given if any degree of airway obstruction is present.

Nursing Diagnoses
1, 24, 57, 73, 75

Nursing Interventions
Monitoring
1. Monitor for changes in baseline respiratory function.
2. Monitor changes in sputum quantity and quality.
3. If the patient has asbestosis, watch for signs and symptoms of lung cancer, such as changing cough, hemoptysis, and weight loss.

Supportive Care
1. Encourage smoking cessation, especially in patients who have been exposed to asbestos fibers, to decrease risk of lung cancer.
2. Encourage the patient to drink adequately and to perform breathing and coughing exercises to mobilize secretions.
3. Advise the patient to pace activities to prevent exertion.

Education and Health Maintenance

1. Teach the patient how to use bronchodilating inhalers or nebulizers.
2. Instruct the patient about methods of health maintenance, such as adequate nutrition and exercise, to avoid additional medical problems.
3. Advise the patient that compensation may be obtained for impairment related to occupational lung disease through the Workman's Compensation Act.
4. Provide information to healthy workers on preventing occupational lung disease, such as enclosing toxic substances to minimize their release into the air; using engineering controls to reduce exposure; monitoring air samples; ensuring adequate ventilation to reduce dust levels in the work atmosphere; and using protective devices, such as face masks, respirators, fume hoods, and so forth.

OCULAR SURGERY

Ocular surgery involves a variety of procedures on the eye and is usually done as outpatient surgery. Some common procedures include:

Extracapsular or intracapsular lens extraction: Cataract lens is removed by cryosurgery or phacoemulsification (use of ultrasonic needle), and an intraocular lens may be implanted if the capsule is left in place.

Iridectomy: Excision of a small portion of the iris whereby aqueous humor can bypass the pupil to treat acute glaucoma; iridotomy is done by laser to create multiple tiny incisions in the iris.

Trabeculectomy: Partial-thickness scleral resection with small part of trabecular meshwork removed along with an iridectomy, indicated for repeated acute glaucoma attacks.

Scleral buckling: Sclera is shortened to allow a buckling to occur, which forces the pigment epithelium closer to the retina.

Corneal transplantation: Transplantation of a donor cornea to repair a corneal scar, burn, deformity, or dystrophy.

Vitrectomy: Removal of the vitreous humor, the gelatin-like substance behind the lens, for hemorrhage due to diabetic retinopathy, intraocular foreign body, retinal tear, and other problems; saline is infused to replace the vitreous, and, at the end of the procedure, gas or oil is introduced to keep the retina in place.

Enucleation: Complete removal of the eyeball for trauma, infection, or tumor; a ball implant is inserted into the socket and the conjunctiva is closed, until an individualized prosthesis can be fitted 4 to 6 weeks later.

Refractive surgery: Involves reshaping the cornea to correct myopia; a variety of procedures using microsurgical instruments and lasers are used.

Laser photocoagulation, electrodiathermy, and *cryosurgery:* Additional procedures that may be done for various eye diseases.

Potential Complications
1. Hemorrhage
2. Infection
3. Postoperative glaucoma
4. Graft dislocation or rejection (corneal transplant)
5. Implant extrusion (enucleation)

Nursing Diagnoses
3, 24, 33, 44, 135, 136

Collaborative Management and Interventions
Preoperative Care
1. Assess the patient's general state of health and functional ability.
2. Assess for and try to minimize any other sensory deficits that may impact on patient's functional ability postoperatively.
3. Explain to the patient what to expect after surgery including pain, positioning, bandaging, and ability to see.
4. Instruct the patient to wash hair the evening before surgery and have hair away from face.

5. Make sure that the patient removes dentures, contact lenses, any metal fasteners or jewelry, and any prostheses before going to operating room.
6. Make sure that operative permit is signed and all questions are answered.
7. Wash the patient's face with antibacterial solution as directed.
8. Administer preoperative medications, including eyedrops, if ordered.

GERONTOLOGIC ALERT Be aware that many older adults have additional sensory or perceptual deficits, such as decreased hearing and position sense, which increases the risk of falls and feeling of isolation.

Postoperative Care

1. Immediately after surgery, position the patient as directed and maintain four side rails until the patient is completely alert and oriented.
2. Instruct the patient to ask for help rather than strain with activity and risk increasing intraocular pressure (IOP).
3. Arrange personal care articles nearby the patient and maintain a safe environment.
4. Encourage the patient to express fear and anxiety about loss of vision; comment on the positive aspects of recovery.
5. Provide diversional activities and occupational therapy consultation as appropriate.
6. Caution the patient against rubbing eyes or wiping them with soiled tissues.
7. If an eye patch is used, maintain its security and monitor for bleeding.
8. Check the patient's level of discomfort and administer analgesic as directed.
9. Assess the patient for signs of infection, which include eye drainage, increased pain or redness, warmth, and swelling.
10. Apply cold compresses as desired to reduce edema and discomfort.
11. Maintain a safe environment while vision is impaired.

PEDIATRIC ALERT Avoid overfeeding infant after ocular surgery to prevent regurgitation, which may increase IOP and place tension on sutures.

Education and Health Maintenance

1. Reinforce activity restriction, if any, and instruct the patient about the following:
   a. Initially, avoid straining at stool, lifting, bending over, coughing, and vomiting to prevent increase in IOP.
   b. May resume regular activities in 1 to 3 days with most procedures.
   c. Prolonged bed rest, possibly with face-down position to maintain placement of the retina, for patients who underwent a vitrectomy.
2. Advise the patient to report increased pain, swelling, drainage, and change in vision.
3. Teach the patient how to instill eyedrops and ointments.
4. Instruct the patient with corneal transplant to watch for signs of graft rejection in 10 to 14 days; these include decreased vision, ocular irritation, corneal edema, and red sclera.
5. Advise the patient that adjustment to vision change with many procedures is gradual, and to follow up as directed.

ORAL CANCER

See *Cancer, Oral.*

ORTHOPEDIC SURGERY

Orthopedic surgery includes a wide variety of procedures performed on bones, joints, and surrounding structures for trauma, musculoskeletal, and systemic disorders. Procedures include:

1. *Open reduction:* Reduction and alignment of the fracture through surgical incision
2. *Internal fixation:* Stabilization of the reduced fracture by use of metal screw, plates, nails, or pins
3. *Bone graft:* Placement of autologous or homologous bone tissue to replace, promote healing of, or stabilize diseased bone

4. *Arthroplasty:* Repair of a joint; may be done through arthroscope (arthroscopy) or open joint repair

5. *Joint replacement:* Type of arthroplasty that involves replacement of joint surfaces with metal, plastic, or ceramic materials

6. *Total joint replacement:* Replacement of both articulatory surfaces within a joint

7. *Meniscectomy:* Excision of damaged meniscus (fibrocartilage) of the knee

8. *Tendon transfer:* Movement of tendon insertion point to improve function

9. *Fasciotomy:* Cutting muscle fascia to relieve constriction or contracture

10. *Amputation:* Removal of a body part

O

Potential Complications

1. Compartment syndrome
2. Shock
3. Atelectasis and pneumonia
4. Osteomyelitis, wound infections
5. Thromboembolism
6. Fat embolus

Nursing Diagnoses

3, 24, 51, 62, 75, 123, 135, 136, 140, 141

Collaborative Management and Interventions
Preoperative Care

1. Assess nutritional status; hydration, protein and caloric intake. Maximize healing and reduce risk of complications by providing I.V. fluids, vitamins, and nutritional supplements as indicated.

GERONTOLOGIC ALERT Many elderly patients are at risk for poor healing because of undernutrition. Check the patient's serum albumin and prealbumin levels and suggest nutritional consult for decreased results.

2. Determine if the patient has had previous corticosteroid therapy—could contribute to current orthopedic condition (aseptic necrosis of the femoral head; osteoporosis),

as well as affect his or her response to anesthesia and the stress of surgery. The patient may need corticotropin postoperatively.

3. Determine if the patient has an infection (cold, dental, skin, urinary tract infection); it could contribute to development of osteomyelitis after surgery. Administer preoperative antibiotics as ordered.

4. Prepare patient for postoperative routines, which include coughing and deep breathing, frequent vital sign and wound checks, and repositioning.

5. Have patient practice voiding in bedpan or urinal in recumbent position before surgery. This helps reduce the need for postoperative catheterization.

6. Acquaint the patient with traction apparatus and the need for splint or cast, as indicated by the type of surgery.

Postoperative Care

1. Monitor for hemorrhage and shock, which may result from significant bleeding and poor hemostasis of muscles that occur with orthopedic surgery.
   a. Evaluate the blood pressure and pulse rates frequently — report rising pulse rate or slowly decreasing blood pressure.
   b. Watch for increased oozing of wounds.
   c. Measure suction drainage if used. Anticipate up to 7 to 17 oz (200 to 500 mL) drainage in the first 24 hours, decreasing to less than 1 oz (30 mL) per 8 hours within 48 hours, depending on surgical procedure.
   d. Report increased wound drainage or steady increase in pain of operative area.

2. Administer I.V. fluids or blood products as ordered.

3. Monitor neurovascular status.
   a. Watch circulation distal to the part where cast, bandage, or splint has been applied; check pulses, color, warmth, and capillary refill.
   b. Prevent constriction leading to interference with blood or nerve supply; check for swelling.
   c. Note movement, and ask about sensation of distal extremities.

EMERGENCY ALERT Assess neurovascular status frequently, and notify surgeon and loosen cast or dressing immediately if compromise is identified.

4. Elevate affected extremity and apply ice packs as directed to reduce swelling and bleeding into tissues.

5. Monitor pain level and response to analgesia; administer patient-controlled analgesia or other method of pain relief as directed; notify health care provider if not effective or if the patient cannot tolerate adverse effects.

6. Immobilize the affected area and limit activity to protect the operative site and stabilize musculoskeletal structures.

7. Give analgesics that may cause respiratory depression cautiously. Monitor respiration depth and rate frequently. Opioid analgesic effects may be cumulative.

8. Change position and encourage use of incentive spirometer and coughing and deep-breathing exercises every 2 hours to mobilize secretions and prevent atelectasis. Auscultate lungs frequently.

9. Monitor vital signs for fever, tachycardia, or increased respiratory rate, which may indicate infection.
   a. Examine incision for redness, increased temperature, swelling, and induration.
   b. Note character of drainage.

10. Maintain aseptic technique for dressing changes and wound care.

11. Encourage the patient to move joints that are not fixed by traction or appliance through their range of motion as fully as possible. Suggest muscle-setting exercises (quadriceps setting) if active motion is contraindicated.

12. Apply antiembolism stockings, sequential compression, or give prophylactic anticoagulants, if prescribed, to prevent thromboembolism.

13. Encourage early resumption of activity.

14. Monitor for anemia, especially after fracture of long bones.

15. Avoid giving calcium supplements or large amounts of dairy products to orthopedic patients on bed rest, and encourage other fluids to prevent urinary calculi.

Education and Health Maintenance

1. Instruct the patient in dietary considerations to facilitate healing and minimize development of constipation and renal calculi.
   a. Encourage high-iron diet.
   b. Ensure adequate protein and vitamin C.
   c. Ensure balanced diet with increased fluids and fiber.
2. Inform the patient of techniques that facilitate moving while minimizing associated discomforts (eg, supporting injured area and practicing smooth, gentle position changes).
3. Teach proper technique for use of crutches, transferring to wheelchair, and use of all ambulatory aids.
4. Encourage long-term follow-up and physical therapy exercises as directed to regain maximum functional potential.

OSTEOARTHRITIS

Osteoarthritis, or degenerative joint disease, is a chronic, non-inflammatory, progressive disorder that causes deterioration of articular cartilage. Progressive wear and tear on cartilage leads to thinning of joint surface and ulceration into bone. Increased blood supply to the joint leads to formation of abnormal bone spurs caused by hypertrophy of subchondral bone and secondary soft tissue changes around the joint. Osteoarthritis affects weight-bearing joints (hips and knees) as well as joints of the distal and proximal interphalangeal joints of the fingers. The cause is unknown, but aging and obesity are contributing factors; the disease generally affects adults ages 50 to 90, occurring equally in both sexes. Untreated disease leads to limited mobility and, in some cases, neurologic deficits associated with spinal involvement.

Assessment

1. Deep, aching joint pain; pronounced after weight bearing or exercise, usually relieved by rest
2. Joint swelling or deformity
3. Joint stiffness on awakening, usually lasting less than 30 minutes

4. Hard nodes on distal or proximal interphalangeal joints of the fingers; known as Heberden's nodes when present on distal interphalangeal joints and Bouchard's nodes when present on proximal interphalangeal joints

Diagnostic Evaluation
1. X-rays of affected joints show joint space narrowing, osteophytes (bone spurs), and sclerosis.
2. Radionuclide imaging (bone scan) may show increased uptake in affected bones.
3. Synovial fluid analysis will differentiate osteoarthritis from rheumatoid arthritis by low cell count.

Collaborative Management
Therapeutic Interventions
1. Conservative management includes physical therapy, isometric exercises, and graded exercises; diet to control weight if indicated; application of heat; and use of splints, traction, or other means of support as needed.
2. Patient education on joint conservation techniques to stop the progression of degeneration.

Pharmacologic Interventions
1. Analgesics, with acetaminophen as first-line therapy; other analgesics, such as nonsteroidal anti-inflammatory drugs (NSAIDs) and tramadol.
2. Occasionally, opioid analgesics are needed.
3. Injectable vesicosupplements include hyaluronate and hylan G-f 20; given intra-articularly once per week for several weeks to increase cartilage and reduce pain; contraindicated in patients allergic to avian products, including feathers.

ALTERNATIVE INTERVENTION

Glucosamine and chondroitin are herbal supplements that are being studied for their positive effect on cartilage and pain reduction in patients with arthritis. Advise patients to tell their health care provider if these are being taken as well as any other over-the-counter drug or supplement. Indian frankincense and devil's claw are additional remedies; however, little research has been done regarding these.

Surgical Interventions

1. Surgical intervention is considered when the pain becomes intolerable to the patient and mobility is severely compromised. Options include osteotomy, debridement, joint fusion, arthroscopy, and arthroplasty.

Nursing Diagnoses
13, 62

Nursing Interventions
Also see *Orthopedic Surgery*, page 680.

Monitoring

1. Monitor mobility and functional capacity to perform activities of daily living.
2. Monitor the patient's response to pain medications.
3. Monitor for adverse effects to NSAIDs, such as renal impairment and GI bleeding.

GERONTOLOGIC ALERT Elderly patients are at greater risk for GI bleeding and renal failure associated with NSAID use. Encourage administration of medication with meals, monitor stool for occult blood, and encourage use of medication as prescribed.

Supportive Care

1. Provide rest for involved joints. Excessive use aggravates the symptoms and accelerates degeneration.
   a. Use splints, braces, cervical collars, traction, or lumbosacral corsets as necessary.
   b. Have prescribed rest periods in recumbent position.
2. Advise the patient to avoid activities that precipitate pain.
3. Apply heat as directed to relieve muscle spasm and stiffness; avoid prolonged application of heat, which may cause increased swelling and flare symptoms.

4. Teach the patient correct posture and body mechanics. Postural alterations lead to chronic muscle tension and pain.

5. Advise the patient to sleep with a rolled terry cloth towel under the neck to relieve cervical pain.

6. Provide patient with crutches, braces, or a cane when indicated to reduce weight-bearing stress on hips and knees. Teach the patient how to use a cane in the hand on side opposite involved hip or knee.

7. Encourage patient to wear corrective shoes and metatarsal supports for foot disorders; also is helpful in treating arthritis of the knee and hip.

8. Encourage patient to lose weight to decrease stress on weight-bearing joints.

9. Support the patient undergoing orthopedic surgery for unremitting pain and disabling arthritis of joints.

10. Teach patient range-of-motion exercises to maintain joint mobility and muscle tone for joint support, to prevent capsular and tendon tightening, and to prevent deformities. Avoid flexion and adduction deformities by prolonged sitting.

11. Refer patient to physical and occupational therapy.

Education and Health Maintenance

1. Teach the patient isometric exercises and graded exercises to improve muscle strength around the involved joint.

2. Advise patient to put joints through range of motion after periods of inactivity (eg, automobile ride).

3. Suggest patient perform important activities in morning, after stiffness has abated and before fatigue and pain become a problem.

4. Advise patient on lifestyle modifications, such as wearing looser clothing without buttons, placing bench in tub or shower for bathing, and sitting at table or counter in kitchen to prepare meals.

5. Help patient with obtaining assistive devices, such as padded handles for utensils and grooming aids, to promote independence.

6. Suggest patient swims or performs water aerobics (eg, offered by the YMCA) as a form of nonstressful exercise to preserve mobility.
7. Encourage patient to have adequate diet and sleep to enhance general health.
8. Advise patient to avoid weight-bearing activities for 48 hours after intra-articular injection treatment, as directed.
9. Refer for additional information and support to local chapter of the Arthritis Foundation, *www.arthritis.org*.

OSTEOMYELITIS

Osteomyelitis is an infection of the bone. It results from hematogenous spread (through the bloodstream) of infection to an area of bone with lowered resistance, or by direct extension from a soft tissue infection or open wound. It may occur at any age. The most common causative organisms include *Staphylococcus aureus* (70% to 80%), *Escherichia coli*, *Pseudomonas*, *Klebsiella*, *Salmonella*, and *Proteus*. In acute osteomyelitis, the organisms grow and form pus within the bone, accompanied by edema, vascular congestion, thrombosis, and necrosis. The infection spreads into the medullary cavity and into adjacent soft tissue and joints. If an abscess forms, the area must be completely drained and excised for complete healing to take place. If treatment is unsuccessful, recurrent abscesses develop in chronic osteomyelitis. Other complications include pathologic fracture, joint destruction, skeletal deformities, and sepsis. Osteomyelitis may be life-threatening if unrecognized and untreated.

PEDIATRIC ALERT Osteomyelitis in children frequently affects the metaphyseal region of long bones. Bone deformity and limb-length discrepancy may develop without aggressive treatment.

Assessment

1. Localized pain, swelling, erythema, and fever; may be masked in early disease
2. Malaise, irritability
3. Limited range of motion; tenderness on palpation
4. May be signs of sepsis

GERONTOLOGIC ALERT Adults at risk for osteomyelitis include elderly people, obese people, poorly nourished people, people with diabetes, those with rheumatoid arthritis, and those on long-term corticosteroid therapy.

Diagnostic Evaluation

1. Blood cultures obtained before initiation of antibiotic therapy identify causative agent.
2. Needle aspiration of bone may be done if necessary to help identify causative agent. (Negative aspirate does not always rule out infection.)
3. Complete blood count shows marked leukocytosis, low hemoglobin.
4. Erythrocyte sedimentation rate is elevated.
5. X-rays may be negative in early stages.
   a. Rules out fracture
   b. Will eventually show periosteal elevation
6. Bone scan rules out multiple lesions.
7. MRI differentiates soft tissue from bone marrow involvement.

Collaborative Management
Pharmacologic Interventions

1. Broad-spectrum antibiotics until organism sensitivity obtained.
2. I.V. antibiotics for at least 3 to 4 weeks.
3. Additional 4 to 8 weeks of oral antibiotics at completion of I.V. therapy is recommended.

Surgical Interventions

1. Surgical incision and drainage if infection site is abscessed.
2. Chronic disease requires surgical removal of sequestra (dead bone).

Nursing Diagnoses
3, 13, 22, 24, 62

Nursing Interventions
Supportive Care
1. Maintain rest and immobilization of affected limb. Instruct patient about allowable activities: generally no weight bearing on affected limb and bed rest during acute phase.
2. Administer analgesics as indicated.
3. Increase fluid intake to prevent dehydration.
4. Monitor temperature and administer antipyretics as indicated.
5. Inspect and clean surgical wounds every 4 to 8 hours. Use strict aseptic technique.
6. Instruct patient and family in proper care of surgical wounds.
7. Teach proper I.V. catheter and site care.
8. Encourage use or exercise of unaffected limbs and joints.
9. Design diversional activities program that complies with activity restriction.
10. Initiate appropriate home care referrals for reinforcement and monitoring of I.V. therapy.

Education and Health Maintenance
1. Teach patient and family to recognize and report signs and symptoms of recurrent or chronic infection.
2. Stress the importance of compliance with treatment. Reinforce the need for maintaining serum levels of antibiotics after discharge even after signs and symptoms improve.
3. Encourage long-term follow-up to prevent recurrent abscesses.
4. Encourage early medical intervention of subsequent infections.

OSTEOPOROSIS

Osteoporosis is a condition in which the rate of bone resorption increases over the rate of bone formation, causing loss of calcium and phosphate salts and bone mass. Loss of bone mass and structure weakens the bones and makes them more susceptible to fractures. The diagnosis of osteoporosis is made when the bone mineral density is 2.5 standard deviations below the peak bone density for young adults (T score, –2.5). Decrease in bone density of 1.5 to 2.5 below that of a young adult is termed osteopenia (T score, –1.5 to –2.5). The disease occurs frequently in postmenopausal women, especially whites and Asians. Other risk factors include prolonged inactivity, chronic illness, medications such as corticosteroids, calcium and vitamin D deficiency, smoking, caffeine intake, small frame, and genetic predisposition.

Assessment

1. Asymptomatic until later stages; may then cause progressive kyphosis and chronic back pain.
2. Fracture after minor trauma may be first indication.
3. Most frequent fractures associated with osteoporosis include fractures of the distal radius, vertebral bodies, proximal humerus, pelvis, and proximal femur (eg, hip).
4. May have vague complaints related to aging process (eg, stiffness, pain, weakness).

Diagnostic Evaluation

1. X-rays show changes only after 30% to 60% bone loss.
2. Dual-energy X-ray absorptiometry shows reduced bone mineral density (T score, –2.5 or worse).
3. Serum bone GLA-protein (a marker for bone turnover) is elevated.
4. Bone biopsy shows thin, porous bone structure.

Collaborative Management
Therapeutic Interventions

1. Management is primarily preventive.
2. Fall prevention in elderly patients to prevent fractures.
3. Weight-bearing exercise (walking) throughout life.
4. Adequate intake of vitamin D through milk, exposure to sunlight, and dietary supplements to enhance absorption of calcium.
5. Intake of calcium (1 to 1.5 g/day) may be preventive.

GERONTOLOGIC ALERT With age there is decreased ability to absorb vitamin D through the skin. Therefore, replacement is usually necessary to obtain the recommended daily intake of 400 to 800 IU.

Pharmacologic Interventions
1. Calcium and vitamin D supplements.
2. Use of estrogen replacement therapy for postmenopausal women; however, there are a number of risks that may outweigh benefits in most cases.
3. Calcitonin administered by nasal spray preserves bone density; adverse effect is local irritation.
4. Alendronate and risedronate are bisphosphonates that increase bone density and reduce fracture risk.
5. An alternative to estrogen is an estrogen receptor agonist such as raloxifene, which shows some benefit in preserving bone density with no increase in breast cancer risk.

Nursing Diagnoses
13, 24, 128, 136

Nursing Interventions
Supportive Care
1. Administer analgesics as indicated for acute exacerbations of pain.

   GERONTOLOGIC ALERT Prolonged use of opioids in elderly patients is dangerous because opioids may impair mental status and may also contribute to falls and other accidents.

2. Assist patient with putting on back brace and ensure proper fit. Encourage use as much as possible, especially while ambulatory.
3. Administer bisphosphonates with food or fluid and have the patient remain upright for 30 minutes to prevent esophagitis.
4. Encourage compliance with physical therapy and practicing of exercises to increase muscle strength surrounding bones and to relieve pain.
5. Make sure safety measures are taken to prevent falls. (See *Box O-1.*)

BOX O-1   Prevention of Falls

- Familiarize patient with environment (ie, identify call light or bell to ring, label the bathroom, kitchen, closet).
- Have patient demonstrate ways to obtain help if needed.
- Place bed in low position with brakes locked if possible, or mattress on the floor.
- Make sure that footwear is fitted and nonslip, and is used properly.
- Determine appropriate use of side rails based on cognitive and functional status.
- Use nightlight.
- Keep floor surfaces clean and dry.
- Keep room uncluttered and make sure that furniture is in optimal condition.
- Make sure patient knows where personal possessions are and that he or she can safely access them.
- Make sure there are adequate handrails in bathroom (commode, shower, tub), bedroom, and hallway.
- Establish a care plan to maintain bowel and bladder function.
- Evaluate effects of medications that increase the patient's risk of falling.
- Encourage participation in functional activities and exercise at patient's highest possible level and refer to physical therapy as appropriate.
- Monitor patient regularly and encourage safe activities.

Education and Health Maintenance

1. Encourage exercise for all patients. Teach the value of walking daily throughout life to provide stress required for strong bone remodeling.
2. Explain that calcium can be obtained through milk and dairy products, some vegetables, fortified juices, and supplements. Advise that a patient with a history of urinary tract calculi should consult with health care provider before increasing his or her calcium intake.
3. Encourage young women at risk to maximize bone mass through nutrition and exercise.
4. Suggest that perimenopausal women confer with health care provider concerning need for calcium supplements and other therapy.

5. Teach strategies to prevent falls. Assess home for hazards (eg, throw rugs, slippery floors, extension cords, inadequate lighting). Encourage use of walking aids when balance is poor and muscle strength weakens.

6. For additional information, contact the National Osteoporosis Foundation, *www.nof.org*.

COMMUNITY CARE CONSIDERATIONS

Identify women at high risk for osteoporotic fractures in the community — frail, elderly, White or Asian women with poor dietary intake of dairy products and little exposure to sun — and provide education and safety measures to prevent falls and fractures. Encourage screening for all women older than age 65 or older than age 60 for those at risk.

OTITIS EXTERNA

Otitis externa (swimmer's ear) is an inflammation of the external ear canal that may occur 2 to 3 days after swimming and diving, especially in contaminated water. It may also be caused by trauma to the ear canal. Infection may be caused by bacteria, usually *Pseudomonas*, *Proteus vulgaris*, streptococci, and *Staphylococcus aureus*, or fungi, such as *Aspergillus Niger* or *Candida albicans*. Predisposing factors include seborrhea, psoriasis, stagnant water in the ear canal, and trauma to the canal from cleaning ears with blunt objects.

Assessment

1. Pain may be mild to severe, increased by jaw movement or manipulation of auricle or tragus, or may be pulsating ache.

2. Ear canal may be red and swollen and have foul-smelling, white, or purulent discharge. Fungal infection may produce blackish deposits.

3. Fever and periauricular lymphadenopathy may be present.

EMERGENCY ALERT Necrotizing malignant otitis externa is a serious infection into deeper tissue adjacent to the ear canal, which involves cellulitis and osteomyelitis. It is commonly caused by *Pseudomonas* and may be seen in people with diabetes, elderly people, and debilitated people.

Diagnostic Evaluation

1. Otoscopic evaluation may be difficult because of pain and swelling but shows characteristic swelling and exudate.
2. Culture and sensitivity tests may be done but usually are not necessary.

Collaborative Management

Therapeutic and Pharmacologic Interventions

1. Warm compresses and analgesics for pain.
2. Topical antibiotics or acetic acid (modifies pH) solution is used to treat infection.
3. Topical corticosteroids may be used to reduce inflammation and swelling.
4. If acute inflammation and closure of the ear canal prevent drops from saturating canal, a wick may need to be inserted so that drops will penetrate to walls of entire ear canal. Irrigation may be necessary to clear drainage when acute swelling subsides.
5. Burrow's solution (aluminum acetate solution) reduces drainage caused by eczema.
6. Alcohol may be used as a drying agent to prevent recurrences.
7. I.V. antibiotics are used for necrotizing malignant otitis externa.

Nursing Diagnoses

3, 24

Nursing Interventions

Supportive Care

1. Provide comfort measures, such as warm compresses and frequent cleaning of drainage from around ear canal, to relieve irritation.
2. Demonstrate proper application of eardrops:
   a. Lie or sit with head tilted to side and affected ear up.

    b. Pull auricle upward and outward (for adults) or downward and backward (for children) and instill four drops or amount prescribed.

    c. Maintain position for 5 minutes to ensure proper saturation.

    d. Do not put cotton in ear because cotton will absorb drops and impair contact with canal.

3. Advise the patient that otitis externa can be prevented or minimized by thoroughly drying the ear canal after coming into contact with water or moist environment.

Education and Health Maintenance

1. Tell the patient and family to use eardrops after swimming to help prevent swimmer's ear.

2. Advise the patient to use properly fitting earplugs for recurrent cases.

3. Teach the patient proper ear hygiene: clean auricle and outer canal with washcloth only, do not insert anything smaller than finger wrapped in washcloth in ear canal.

COMMUNITY CARE CONSIDERATIONS

Use of cotton-tipped applicators to dry the canal or remove earwax should be avoided because:

- Cerumen may be forced against the tympanic membrane.
- The canal lining may be abraded, making it more susceptible to infection.
- Cerumen that coats and protects the canal may be removed.

OTITIS MEDIA, ACUTE AND CHRONIC

Otitis media is an inflammation and infection of the middle ear caused by a dysfunctional eustachian tube. In acute otitis media (AOM), infection usually results from bacterial or viral infection. Most commonly found are *Streptococcus pneumoniae* (40% to 50%), viruses (30% to 40%), *Haemophilus influenzae* (20% to 30%), and *Moraxella catarrhalis* (10% to 15%). In otitis media with effusion (OME), no purulent infection occurs, but blockage of the eustachian tube causes negative pressure and transudation of fluid from blood vessels and development of effusion in the middle ear. This occurs frequently after resolution of an AOM. Chronic OME disease may lead to conductive hearing loss, mastoiditis (rare), and cholesteatoma.

AOM, with its rapid onset of signs and symptoms, is a major problem in children but may occur at any age. If not treated successfully, or if the causative organism is resistant to drugs, it can progress to recurrent and chronic otitis media. With the advent of antibiotics, the serious complications of AOM (eg, meningitis, brain abscess) have decreased to less than 3%.

Assessment

1. In AOM, pain is the most specific symptom. In young children, this may be indicated by pulling at ears, difficulty swallowing, or discomfort when lying down.
2. Associated symptoms of upper respiratory infection occur in 40% to 50%.
3. Fever may occur in 50%.
4. Purulent drainage (otorrhea) occurs if the tympanic membrane is perforated; may be odorless or foul smelling.

PEDIATRIC ALERT In infants and young children, irritability, difficult feeding or anorexia, nausea, vomiting, diarrhea, or cough may be the presenting symptoms of otitis media.

Diagnostic Evaluation

1. Pneumatic otoscopic examination shows a tympanic membrane that is full, bulging, and opaque with impaired mobility (or retracted with impaired mobility).
2. Specimens of ear discharge (from ruptured tympanic membrane) for cultures to help identify causative organism.
3. Tympanometry measures the compliance of the tympanic membrane; also can measure ear canal volume, which when increased may indicate a perforated tympanic membrane.
4. Tympanocentesis if severe otalgia or toxic appearance, poor response to antibiotics, neonates or immunosuppressed patients.

5. Audiometry may be ordered to evaluate conductive hearing loss in chronic disease.

Collaborative Management

Pharmacologic Interventions

1. In AOM, oral antibiotics are given. First-line antibiotic is amoxicillin or co-trimoxazole for initial treatment of AOM. If patient is symptomatic after 72 hours of treatment, has a recurrent AOM after complete course within 3 months, or lives in an area of known drug-resistant *Streptococcus pneumoniae*, second-line antibiotics should be used, such as amoxicillin clavulanate, azithromycin, cefprozil, or clarithromycin.

> **DRUG ALERT** Children younger than age 2 who attend day care or have been treated with antibiotics within the last 3 months are treated with high-dose amoxicillin 80 to 90 mg/kg/day (twice the usual dosage).

2. In recurrent disease (three AOM episodes in 6 months or four AOM episodes in 12 months), consider use of prophylactic antibiotics, particularly during winter months.
3. Nasal decongestants and antihistamines play a limited role to promote eustachian tube drainage.

Surgical Interventions

1. In AOM, myringotomy (incision in tympanic membrane to relieve pressure and drain pus from middle ear) may be done for antimicrobial failure; for severe, persistent pain; or for persistent conductive hearing loss.
2. In children with middle ear effusions lasting 4 months or longer, with conductive hearing loss, myringotomy with ventilating tube placement may be done.
3. In children with recurrent AOM who have breakthrough infections on prophylaxis or who are not good candidates for prophylaxis therapy, myringotomy with ventilating tube placement may be done.

Nursing Diagnoses
3, 33, 108

Nursing Interventions
Monitoring

1. Monitor the patient for headache, increasing irritability, fever, stiff neck, nausea, and vomiting, which indicate meningeal involvement.
2. Assess the patient's hearing regularly.
3. Check for speech and language delays in young children at regular intervals, caused by hearing impairment.

Supportive Care

1. Administer or teach self-administration of acetaminophen and other analgesics as directed. Sedation is usually avoided because it may interfere with early detection of central nervous system complications.
2. Encourage use of warm compresses to promote comfort and help resolve infectious process.
3. Perform and teach postoperative dressing changes because area is packed with gauze for drainage — this may be done daily or every other day; packing is removed on third or fourth day.

Education and Health Maintenance

1. Instruct the patient about activities to avoid after tympanic membrane rupture or surgery until healing takes place (swimming, shampooing hair, showering).
2. Advise the patient of hygienic practices that will prevent tympanic membrane injury (avoid ear-picking, inserting objects into ear).
3. Advise the patient to report symptoms that indicate recurrence (discomfort, pain, fever, dizziness).
4. Advise the patient to elevate head at night to promote drainage of middle ear into pharynx.
5. Postoperatively, teach patient to change dressing and comply with antibiotic therapy as ordered.
6. Stress the importance of follow-up hearing evaluations.
   a. If stapes has been removed or dislodged, then hearing is lost.

    b. If stapes or cochlea has not been removed or disturbed, then hearing will probably be regained; a hearing aid may be required.

7. Instruct parents on how to possibly prevent or decrease the frequency of AOM.

    a. Feed infants in upright position; do not prop bottles or give a bottle in bed.

    b. Breast-feeding for at least the first 3 months decreases risk of AOM.

    c. Exposure to smoke increases risk of AOM.

    d. Prolonged use of pacifiers increases risk of AOM.

    e. Enrollment in day care increases risk of AOM.

8. Advise parents of children with ventilating tubes that water should not enter ear canal. Eardrops should not be instilled in that ear, and tubes will come out spontaneously in 6 to 12 months.

OVARIAN CANCER

See *Cancer, Ovarian*.

OVARIAN CYSTS

Ovarian cysts are benign growths that arise from various ovarian tissues. They often arise from functional changes in the ovary, as from the Graafian follicle or from persistent corpus luteum; dermoid ovarian cysts may develop from abnormal embryonic epithelium. Incidence is highest during childbearing years. Masses found in women older than age 50 are more likely to become malignant. Ruptured cysts may cause peritoneal inflammation.

Assessment

1. Cysts may be asymptomatic or cause minor pelvic pain.
2. Menstrual irregularity may be noted.
3. Tender, palpable mass may be palpated.
4. Rupture causes acute pain and tenderness and may mimic appendicitis or ectopic pregnancy.

Diagnostic Evaluation
1. Pelvic sonogram to determine cyst size and characteristics.
2. Pregnancy test as directed to rule out ectopic pregnancy.
3. Suspicious cysts may be examined through biopsy at time of surgery.

Collaborative Management
Pharmacologic Interventions
1. Hormonal contraceptives for 1 to 3 months to suppress functional cysts smaller than 5 cm in diameter

Surgical Interventions
1. Laparoscopy or laparotomy to remove large or leaking cysts

Nursing Diagnoses
3, 123

Nursing Interventions
Also see *Gastrointestinal or Abdominal Surgery,* page 381.

Monitoring
1. Postoperatively, monitor the patient's vital signs frequently.
2. Assess patient frequently for abdominal distention caused by fluid and gas pooling in abdominal cavity.
3. Assess for effectiveness of pain management and return of bowel sounds.

Supportive Care
1. Encourage the use of analgesics as directed.
2. Teach patient the proper use of hormonal contraceptives if prescribed, along with adverse effects; encourage monthly follow-up to determine if cyst is resolving.
3. Tell the patient that heavy lifting, strenuous exercise, and sexual intercourse may increase pain.
4. Encourage patient to breathe deeply and cough postoperatively.

5. Administer antiemetics and insert a nasogastric tube, as ordered, to prevent vomiting.
6. Place the patient in semi-Fowler's position for greatest comfort, and encourage early ambulation after surgery to reduce distention. Help the patient arise slowly to prevent orthostatic hypotension.
7. As distention resolves and bowel sounds return, advance oral intake slowly.

Education and Health Maintenance

1. Reassure patient that, in most cases, ovarian function and fertility are preserved.
2. Reassure patient about low malignancy rate of cysts.
3. Encourage patient to report recurrent symptoms or worsening of pain if cyst is being treated medically.

PQ

PANCREATIC CANCER

See *Cancer, Pancreatic*.

PANCREATITIS

Acute pancreatitis refers to inflammation of the pancreas, which is most commonly caused by alcoholism and biliary tract diseases, such as cholelithiasis and cholecystitis. Other causes include infections, trauma, pancreatic tumors, and use of certain drugs (corticosteroids, thiazide diuretics, and hormonal contraceptives). Attacks may resolve with complete recovery, may recur without permanent damage, or may progress to chronic pancreatitis. Mortality is high (10%) because of shock, anoxia, hypotension, or fluid and electrolyte imbalances.

Chronic pancreatitis (see *Box P-1*, page 704) results in destruction of the secreting cells of the pancreas, causing maldigestion and malabsorption of protein and fat, and possibly diabetes mellitus if islet cells have been affected. As cells are replaced by fibrous tissue, the pancreatic and common bile ducts may be obstructed.

Assessment

1. Abdominal pain, usually constant in nature, midepigastric or periumbilical, radiating to the back or flank. Patient assumes a fetal position or leans forward while sitting (called *proning*) to relieve pressure of the inflamed pancreas on celiac plexus nerves.
2. Nausea and vomiting, diarrhea, and passage of stools containing fat.
3. Low-grade fever.
4. Involuntary abdominal guarding, epigastric tenderness to deep palpation, and reduced or absent bowel sounds.
5. Dry mucous membranes; hypotension; cold, clammy skin; cyanosis; and tachycardia, which may reflect mild to mod-

BOX P-1	Chronic Pancreatitis

In chronic pancreatitis, pain is similar to that of acute pancreatitis, but it is more constant and occurs at unpredictable intervals. As the disease progresses, recurring attacks of pain are more severe, more frequent, and of longer duration. As pancreatic cells are destroyed, malabsorption and steatorrhea occur, along with diabetes mellitus.

Treatment involves chronic pain management, pancreatic enzyme replacement, and insulin treatment for hyperglycemia. Surgery may be necessary to reduce pain, restore drainage of pancreatic secretions, correct structural abnormalities, and manage complications. Pancreaticojejunostomy is the side-to-side anastomosis of pancreatic duct to jejunum to drain pancreatic secretions into jejunum. Other procedures include revision of sphincter of ampulla of Vater, drainage of pancreatic cyst into stomach, resection or removal of pancreas (pancreatectomy), and autotransplantation of islet cells.

Nursing interventions involve assessing and assisting in pain management; assessing and assisting in nutritional management; teaching low concentrated carbohydrate diet and insulin therapy; and assessment of GI symptoms and characteristics of stool to guide pancreatic enzyme replacement. After surgery, provide meticulous care to prevent infection, promote wound healing, and prevent routine complications of surgery. Support total abstinence from alcohol to control symptoms and prevent progression.

EMERGENCY ALERT Warn the patient that a dangerous hypoglycemic reaction may result from use of insulin while still drinking alcohol and skipping meals.

erate dehydration from vomiting or capillary leak syndrome (third space loss).

6. Shock may be the presenting manifestation in severe episodes, along with respiratory distress and acute renal failure.

7. Purplish discoloration of the flanks (Grey Turner's sign) or of the periumbilical area (Cullen's sign) occurs in extensive hemorrhagic necrosis.

Diagnostic Evaluation

1. Serum amylase, lipase, glucose, bilirubin, alkaline phosphatase, serum transaminases, potassium, and cholesterol may be elevated.
2. Serum albumin, calcium, sodium, magnesium and, possibly, potassium levels may be low because of dehydration, vomiting, and the binding of calcium in areas of fat necrosis.
3. Abdominal X-rays show pancreatic calcification or peripancreatic gas pattern of a pancreatic abscess.
4. Chest X-ray detects infiltrate or pleural effusion as a complication.
5. CT scanning identifies pancreatic structural changes, such as calcifications, masses, ductal irregularities, enlargement, and cysts.

Collaborative Management
Therapeutic Interventions

PQ

1. Oxygen therapy to maintain adequate oxygenation, which is reduced by pain, anxiety, acidosis, abdominal pressure, or pleural effusions.
2. Withhold oral feedings to decrease pancreatic secretions.
3. Nasogastric (NG) intubation and suction to relieve gastric stasis, distention, and ileus.
4. I.V. crystalloid or colloid solutions or blood products to restore circulating blood volume.
5. Parenteral nutrition to treat malnutrition.

Pharmacologic Interventions

1. Opioid analgesics to alleviate pain and anxiety, which increases pancreatic secretions
2. Histamine-2 antagonists and antacids to suppress acid drive of pancreatic secretions and prevent stress ulcer complications of acute disease
3. Sodium bicarbonate to reverse metabolic acidosis
4. Regular insulin to treat hyperglycemia
5. Antibiotics to treat infection or sepsis

Surgical Interventions

1. Surgery is indicated if complications occur.
2. Incision and drainage of infection and pseudocysts.
3. Debridement or pancreatectomy to remove necrotic pancreatic tissue.
4. Cholecystectomy for gallstone pancreatitis.

Nursing Diagnoses

2, 13, 23, 51, 75, 78

Nursing Interventions

Also see *Gastrointestinal or Abdominal Surgery*, page 381.

Monitoring

1. When giving opioid analgesics, monitor patient for hypotension and respiratory depression.
2. Monitor and record vital signs, skin color, and temperature, and intake and output, including NG drainage.
3. Assess respiratory rate and rhythm, effort, oxygen saturation, and breath sounds frequently.
4. Monitor results of hemoglobin and hematocrit, albumin, and electrolytes.

GERONTOLOGIC ALERT The incidence of severe, systemic complications of pancreatitis increases with age. Monitor kidney function and respiratory status closely in elderly patients.

Supportive Care

1. Keep the patient NPO to decrease pancreatic enzyme secretion; administer adequate replacement I.V. fluids.
2. Provide frequent oral care.
3. Administer antacids followed by clamping of NG tube. Check pH of gastric aspirate periodically.
4. Report any increase in severity of pain, which may indicate pancreatic hemorrhage, rupture of a pseudocyst, or inadequate analgesic dosage.
5. Evaluate laboratory results for hemoglobin, hematocrit, albumin, calcium, potassium, sodium, and magnesium levels, and administer replacements as directed.

6. Position the patient in upright or semi-Fowler's position to enhance diaphragmatic excursion.
7. Administer oxygen supplementation as directed to maintain adequate oxygen levels.
8. Instruct the patient in coughing and deep breathing to improve respiratory function.

Education and Health Maintenance

1. Instruct the patient to gradually resume a low-fat diet.
2. Instruct the patient to increase activity gradually, providing for daily rest periods.
3. Reinforce information about the disease process and precipitating factors. Stress that subsequent bouts of acute pancreatitis destroy more and more of the pancreas and cause additional complications.
4. If the pancreatitis results from alcohol abuse, remind the patient of the importance of eliminating all alcohol; advise patient to join Alcoholics Anonymous or obtain other substance abuse counseling.

PQ

PARKINSON'S DISEASE

Parkinson's disease is a progressive neurologic disease affecting the brain centers responsible for control and regulation of movement. A deficiency of dopamine due to degenerative changes in the substantia nigra produces tremor, bradykinesia, rigidity, and autonomic dysfunction. The cause is not known. Complications of Parkinson's disease include dementia, aspiration, and injury from falls. The incidence of Parkinson's disease increases with age; approximately 1% of the population older than age 60 has this disorder.

Assessment

1. Characteristic resting tremor of the extremities (may be worse on one side), and possibly affecting the head and neck
2. Bradykinesia (slowness of movement)
3. Muscle rigidity in performing all movements, as well as at rest
4. Verbal fluency may be impaired

5. Signs of autonomic dysfunction (sleeplessness, salivation, sweating, orthostatic hypotension)
6. Depression, dementia
7. Masklike facies
8. Poor balance, gait disturbances, speech problems

Diagnostic Evaluation

1. Diagnosis is based on observation of clinical symptoms and consideration of patient's age and history; confirmed by favorable response to levodopa therapy.
2. CT scanning and MRI may be performed to rule out other disorders.

Collaborative Management
Pharmacologic Interventions

1. Various drugs can be used, often in combination to prolong effectiveness because tolerance develops. See *Table P-1.*
   a. Anticholinergics to reduce activation of cholinergic pathways, which are thought to be overactive in dopamine deficiency
   b. Amantadine, which may improve dopamine release in the brain
   c. Levodopa, a dopamine precursor, combined with carbidopa, a decarboxylase inhibitor, to inhibit destruction of L-dopa in the bloodstream, making more available to the brain
   d. Bromocriptine, a dopaminergic agonist that activates dopamine receptors in the brain
   e. Monoamine oxidase inhibitors as adjunct to levodopa therapy
   f. Catecholamine-O-methyltransferase (COMT) inhibitors, as adjunct therapy in combination with levodopa therapy; COMT is an enzyme that eliminates dopamine from the brain.

 GERONTOLOGIC ALERT Elderly patients may have reduced tolerance to antiparkinsonian drugs and may require smaller doses. Watch for and report psychiatric reactions, such as anxiety, confusion, and hallucinations; cardiac effects, such as orthostatic hypotension and

TABLE P-1 Parkinson's Disease Drugs

CLASS/DRUGS	NURSING CONSIDERATIONS
Anticholinergic • trihexyphenidyl (Artane) • benztropine (Cogentin) • procyclidine (Kemadrin)	• Most effective at controlling tremor but have significant adverse effects, such as dry mouth, constipation, blurred vision, drowsiness, confusion, and orthostatic hypotension. • Contraindicated in patients with urinary retention, prostatic hyperplasia, angle-closure glaucoma, and paralytic ileus.
Antiviral • amantadine (Symmetrel)	• Commonly used as early monotherapy but tolerance develops, so drug-free days may be introduced. • Adverse effects include light-headedness, drowsiness, and nausea.
Dopamine precursor • levodopa (Dopar) • levodopa with the enzyme inhibitor carbidopa (Sinemet)	• Must be used cautiously in a variety of chronic conditions. • Adverse effects similar to those of anticholinergics. • Pyridoxine may decrease effectiveness. • Eventually loses it effectiveness.
Dopaminergic agonist • bromocriptine (Parlodel) • pergolide (Permax) • ropinirole (Requip)	• Used alone or in combination with Simemet. • Adverse effects similar to those of anticholinergics. • Take with food if GI upset occurs.
Monoamine oxidase inhibitor • selegiline (Eldepryl)	• Used to boost the effect of Simemet when levodopa becomes less effective. • Contraindicated with use of opioids and other antidepressants. • Adverse effects similar to those of anticholinergics. • May cause severe hypertension if tyramine-containing foods are ingested.

(continued)

Parkinson's Disease Drugs *(continued)*	
CLASS/DRUGS	**NURSING CONSIDERATIONS**
Catecholamaine-O-methyltransferase inhibitor (COMT)	
▪ tolcapone (Tasmar) ▪ entacapone (Comtan)	▪ Used with levodopa to prolong the effect. ▪ Potentiates the effect of central nervous system depressants. ▪ Adverse effects similar to those of anti-cholinergics. ▪ May interact with other drugs, such as epinephrine, dopamine, dobutamine, methyldopa, erythromycin, ampicillin, and cholestyramine.

pulse irregularity; and blepharospasm (twitching of the eyelids), an early sign of toxicity.

Surgical Interventions

1. Medial pallidotomy to improve dyskinesia, rigidity, and tremor.
2. Chronic deep brain stimulation through electrodes implanted into the thalamus or globus pallidus to decrease tremor.
3. Brain tissue transplants through the use of stem cells and genetically engineered animal cells are a promising area of research.

Nursing Diagnoses
16, 43, 51, 62, 66, 70, 78

Nursing Interventions
Monitoring

1. Monitor drug treatment to note adverse reactions and allow for dosage adjustments. Monitor for liver function changes and anemia during drug therapy.
2. Monitor the patient's nutritional intake and check weight regularly.

3. Monitor the patient's ability to perform activities of daily living.

Supportive Care

1. To improve mobility, encourage the patient to participate in daily exercise, such as walking, riding a stationary bike, swimming, or gardening.
2. Advise the patient to perform stretching and postural exercises as outlined by a physical therapist.
3. Teach the patient walking techniques to offset parkinsonian shuffling gait and tendency to lean forward.
   a. Use wide-based gait.
   b. Swing arms at sides.
   c. Increase length of stride.
   d. Raise feet while walking.
4. Encourage the patient to take warm baths and massage muscles to help relax muscles.
5. Instruct the patient to rest often to avoid fatigue and frustration.

PQ

COMMUNITY CARE CONSIDERATIONS

Suggest various aids around the house to promote the patient's mobility and to help avoid injury from falls, such as grab rails on the tub or shower, raised toilet seat, handrails on both sides of stairway, a rope secured to the foot of the bed to help pull up to sitting position, and a straight-backed wooden chair with armrests.

6. To improve the patient's nutritional status, teach the patient to think through the sequence of swallowing.
   a. Chew deliberately and slowly, using both sides of mouth.
   b. Close lips with teeth together; lift tongue up with food on it; then move tongue back and swallow while tilting head forward.
7. Urge the patient to make a conscious effort to control accumulation of saliva (drooling) by holding head upright and swallowing periodically. Be alert for aspiration hazard.

8. Have the patient use secure, stabilized dishes and eating utensils.
9. Suggest the patient eat smaller meals and additional snacks.
10. To prevent constipation, encourage patient to consume foods containing moderate fiber content (whole grains, fruits, and vegetables), and to increase his or her water intake.
11. Obtain a raised toilet seat to help the patient sit and stand.
12. Encourage the patient to follow regular bowel routine.
13. Maintain the patient's communication ability.
    a. Encourage compliance with medication regimen to help preserve speech function.
    b. Suggest referral to a speech therapist.
    c. Teach the patient facial exercises and breathing methods to obtain appropriate pronunciation, volume, and intonation.
14. Strengthen the patient's coping ability.
    a. Help the patient establish realistic goals and outline ways to achieve those goals.
    b. Provide emotional support and encouragement.
    c. Encourage use of outside resources, such as therapists, primary care provider, social worker, and a social support network.
    d. Encourage open communication, discussion of feelings, and exchange of information about Parkinson's disease.
    e. Have the patient take an active role in activity planning and evaluating the treatment plan.
    f. Use soothing music to reduce anxiety, pain, and depression.

Education and Health Maintenance

1. Teach the patient about the medication regimen and adverse reactions.
2. Instruct the patient to avoid sedatives, unless specifically prescribed, which have additive effects with other medications.
3. Instruct the patient to avoid vitamin B preparations and vitamin-fortified foods that can reverse effects of medication.

4. Encourage follow-up visits and monitoring for diabetes, glaucoma, hepatotoxicity, and anemia while on drug therapy.
5. Teach the patient ambulation cues to avoid "freezing" in place.
   a. Raise head, raise toes, then rock from one foot to another while bending knees slightly.
   b. Or raise arms in a sudden short motion.
   c. Or take a small step backward, then start forward.
   d. Or step sideways, then start forward.
6. Instruct the family not to pull the patient during such "freezing" episodes, which may cause falling.
7. Refer the patient to agencies such as the National Parkinson Foundation, *www.parkinson.org*.

PELVIC INFLAMMATORY DISEASE

Pelvic inflammatory disease (PID) may involve the fallopian tubes, ovaries, uterus, or peritoneum. It is caused by infection with *Neisseria gonorrhoeae*, *Chlamydia trachomatis*, anaerobic bacteria, gram-negative bacteria, and streptococci. Predisposing factors include multiple sexual partners, early onset of sexual activity, use of intrauterine devices, and procedures such as therapeutic abortion, cesarean sections, and hysterosalpingograms. The disease has a high recurrence rate because of reinfections. Complications may include abscess rupture and sepsis, infertility caused by adhesions of fallopian tubes and ovaries, and ectopic pregnancy.

Assessment

1. Pelvic pain is the most common symptom; it is usually dull and bilateral.
2. Vaginal discharge, irregular bleeding, and urinary symptoms (dysuria and frequency) may be present.
3. On pelvic examination, mucopurulent cervical discharge and cervical motion tenderness may be present (especially with gonococcal infection).
4. Nausea and vomiting, abdominal tenderness, rebound, guarding, or presence of a mass may indicate abscess.

EMERGENCY ALERT Localized right or left lower quadrant tenderness with guarding, rebound, or palpable mass signifies tuboovarian abscess with peritoneal inflammation. Immediate evaluation and surgery are necessary to prevent rupture and widespread peritonitis.

5. Presentation with chlamydia may be mild.

Diagnostic Evaluation

1. Smears for endocervical culture or immunodiagnostic testing identify causative organisms.
2. Complete blood count may show elevated leukocytes.
3. Laparoscopy may be done to visualize the fallopian tubes.

Collaborative Management
Pharmacologic Interventions

1. Oral or parenteral antibiotics: combinations of doxycycline, aminoglycosides, quinolones, and cephalosporins depending on patient's condition
   a. Cefotetan 2 g I.V. every 12 hours plus doxycycline 100 mg every 12 hours I.V. (continue oral doxycycline for total of 14 days)
   b. Clindamycin 900 mg I.V. every 8 hours plus gentamicin 2 mg/kg I.V. or I.M. as loading dose, then 1.5 mg/kg every 8 hours (a single dose of gentamicin may be used)
   c. Ofloxacin 400 mg orally twice per day plus metronidazole 500 mg orally twice per day for 14 days
   d. Ceftriaxone 250 mg I.M. once plus doxycycline 100 mg orally twice per day for 14 days

COMMUNITY CARE CONSIDERATIONS

If patient with PID will be treated at home, stress the importance of follow-up, usually within 48 hours, to determine if oral antibiotic treatment is effective. Advise the patient to immediately report worsening of symptoms.

2. Inpatient treatment is required in uncertain diagnosis, abscess, pregnancy, severe infection, inability to take oral

fluids, if the patient is prepubertal, or if more aggressive antibiotic therapy is required to preserve fertility.

Surgical Interventions

1. Surgery may be needed to drain an abscess, or later to treat adhesions or tubal damage.

Nursing Diagnoses

3, 6, 24, 49, 101, 123

Nursing Interventions

Monitoring

1. Monitor the patient's vital signs and intake and output closely.
2. Monitor for abdominal rigidity and bowel sounds to detect development of peritoneal inflammation.
3. Monitor pain control.

PQ

Supportive Care

1. Administer or teach self-administration of analgesics as directed. Alert the patient to adverse effects or drowsiness.
2. Assist the patient to a position of pelvic dependence, with head and feet elevated slightly to relieve strain on pelvic structures.
3. Encourage the patient to apply a heating pad to lower abdomen or lower back.
4. Advise the patient to rest in bed for first 1 to 3 days.
5. Administer or teach self-administration of antibiotics as directed. Advise patient to keep strict dosage schedule and notify health care provider if a dose is lost through vomiting.
6. Administer antiemetics as indicated.
7. Maintain I.V. infusion of fluids until oral intake is adequate.
8. Restart oral intake with ice chips and sips of water after vomiting has ceased for 2 hours.
9. Provide clear fluids followed by soft bland diet as tolerated.

Education and Health Maintenance

1. Encourage patient to comply with antibiotic therapy for full length of prescription.
2. Stress the need for sexual abstinence until repeat cultures prove cure at follow-up, approximately 2 weeks after treatment.
3. Tell the patient to advise partners to seek treatment.
4. Teach the patient methods of preventing sexually transmitted diseases: abstinence, monogamy, and proper condom use.
5. Advise patient that gonorrhea is reported to the public health department, who will contact the patient for names of sexual partners to help prevent further spread.

PEPTIC ULCER DISEASE

A peptic ulcer is a lesion in the mucosa of the lower esophagus, stomach, pylorus, or duodenum (see *Figure P-1*). Causative factors include mucosal infection by the bacterium *Helicobacter pylori* (mechanism unclear); use of nonsteroidal anti-inflammatory drugs (NSAIDs), especially aspirin; Zollinger-Ellison syndrome (excessive secretion of gastrin); and genetic factors. Cigarette smoking, stress, and lower socioeconomic status may

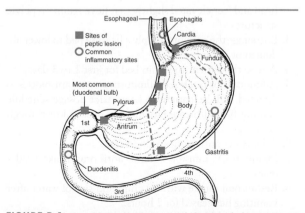

FIGURE P-1 Esophageal, gastric, and duodenal ulcer sites.

also play a role. Complications include GI hemorrhage, perforation, and gastric outlet obstruction.

Assessment

1. Abdominal pain
   a. Occurs in the epigastric area radiating to the back; described as dull, aching, and gnawing.
   b. Pain may increase when the stomach is empty, at night, or approximately 1 to 3 hours after eating. Pain is relieved by taking antacids (common with duodenal ulcers).
2. Nausea, anorexia, early satiety (common with gastric ulcers), belching.
3. Dizziness, syncope, hematemesis, melena with GI hemorrhage:
   a. Positive fecal occult blood
   b. Decreased hemoglobin and hematocrit, indicating anemia
   c. Orthostatic blood pressure and pulse changes

PQ

> ⚡ **EMERGENCY ALERT** Sudden, intense midepigastric pain radiating to the right shoulder may indicate ulcer perforation.

Diagnostic Evaluation

1. Upper GI series usually outlines ulcer or area of inflammation.
2. Endoscopy (esophagogastroduodenoscopy) visualizes duodenal mucosa and helps identify inflammatory changes, lesions, bleeding sites, and malignancy (through biopsy and cytology).
3. Gastric secretory studies (gastric acid secretion test, serum gastrin level test) are elevated in Zollinger-Ellison syndrome.
4. *H. pylori* antibody titer may be positive, especially in recurrent ulcers; however, there is a high rate of false-positive results; C-urea breath test or biopsy testing is more definitive test for *H. pylori*.

Collaborative Management
Therapeutic Interventions
1. Diet therapy includes well-balanced meals at regular intervals; avoid dietary irritants.
2. Eliminate cigarette smoking, which decreases rate of healing and increases rate of recurrence.
3. Eliminate NSAIDs from diet and reduce alcohol intake.

Pharmacologic Interventions
1. Histamine-2 (H_2) receptor antagonists such as ranitidine to reduce gastric acid secretion
2. Antisecretory or proton-pump inhibitor, such as omeprazole, to help ulcer heal quickly in 4 to 8 weeks
3. Cytoprotective drug sucralfate, which protects ulcer surface against acid, bile, and pepsin
4. Antacids to reduce acid concentration and help reduce symptoms
5. Antibiotics as part of a multidrug regimen to eliminate *H. pylori* to prevent reoccurrence
   a. Regimens generally include one or two antibiotics and an acid-controlling medication.
   b. Regimens are 4 to 14 days.
   c. Patient compliance may be an issue due to number of medications, length of time, and adverse reactions.

Surgical Interventions
Surgery is indicated for hemorrhage, perforation, obstruction, and when unresponsive to medical therapy. Procedures include:
1. Gastroduodenostomy (Billroth I) — partial gastrectomy with removal of antrum and pylorus; gastric stump is anastomosed to duodenum
2. Gastrojejunostomy (Billroth II) — partial gastrectomy with removal of antrum and pylorus; gastric stump is anastomosed to jejunum
3. Antrectomy — antrum (lower half of stomach), pylorus, and small cuff of duodenum are resected; stomach is anastomosed to jejunum and duodenal stump is closed

4. Total gastrectomy — removal of stomach with anastomosis of esophagus to jejunum or duodenum
5. Pyloroplasty — longitudinal incision is made in the pylorus, and closed transversely to permit the muscle to relax and establish an enlarged outlet; often performed with vagotomy
6. Vagotomy (severed vagus nerve) — may be selective (reduces acid secretion) or truncal (decreases acid secretion and gastric motility)

Nursing Diagnoses
3, 23, 24, 27, 51

Nursing Interventions
Also see *Gastrointestinal or Abdominal Surgery*, page 381, and *Gastrointestinal Bleeding*, page 377.

PQ

Monitoring
1. Monitor the patient for signs of bleeding through fecal occult blood, vomiting, persistent diarrhea, and change in vital signs.
2. Monitor intake and output.
3. Monitor the patient's hemoglobin, hematocrit, and electrolyte levels.

Supportive Care
1. Administer prescribed I.V. fluids and blood replacement, if acute bleeding is present.
2. Maintain nasogastric tube for acute bleeding, perforation, and postoperatively; monitor tube drainage for amount and color.
3. Perform saline lavage if ordered for acute bleeding.
4. Encourage bed rest to reduce stimulation that may enhance gastric secretion.
5. Provide small, frequent meals to prevent gastric distention if not actively bleeding.
   a. Decreases distention and release of gastrin.
   b. Neutralizes gastric secretions and dilutes stomach contents. However, small, frequent meals or snacks can

lead to acid rebound, which occurs 2 to 4 hours after eating.

6. Watch for diarrhea caused by antacids and other medications. Restrict foods and fluids that promote diarrhea and encourage good perianal care.

7. Advise patient to avoid extremely hot or cold food and fluids, to chew thoroughly, and to eat in a leisurely fashion to reduce pain.

8. Administer medications promptly and teach patient dose and duration of each medication.

Education and Health Maintenance

1. Advise patient to modify lifestyle to include health practices that will prevent recurrences of ulcer pain and bleeding.
   a. Plan for rest periods and avoid or learn to cope with stressful situations; avoid fatigue.
   b. Avoid specific foods known to cause gastric distress and pain.
   c. Avoid aspirin and NSAIDs, reduce consumption of alcohol and caffeine, and eliminate smoking.

2. Instruct patient to immediately report evidence of bleeding, tarry stools, or dizziness, which may indicate an acute bleeding episode.

3. Instruct patient about medications:
   a. Take antacids 1 hour after meals, at bedtime, and when needed. Be aware that antacids may cause changes in bowel habits.
   b. Do not take H_2-receptor antagonists at the same time as sucralfate. This reduces the therapeutic effect of H_2-blockers.
   c. Take medications for as long as prescribed (usually 8 weeks), even if symptoms subside.
   d. Avoid any alcohol intake while taking metronidazole because a severe reaction may occur.

4. Encourage follow-up to determine adequate healing.

PERICARDITIS

Pericarditis is an inflammation of the pericardium, the membranous sac enveloping the heart. It is commonly a manifestation of a more generalized disease. A pericardial effusion may occur in pericarditis, in which excess fluid accumulates in the pericardial cavity. In constrictive pericarditis, chronic inflammatory thickening of the pericardium compresses the heart so it cannot fill normally during diastole. Acute idiopathic pericarditis is the most common form; its cause is unknown.

Other causes of pericarditis include infection by viruses (influenza and Coxsackie virus), bacteria (staphylococcus, meningococcus, streptococcus, pneumococcus, gonococcus, and *Mycobacterium tuberculosis*), fungi, and parasites; connective tissue disorders such as systemic lupus erythematosus and periarteritis nodosa; myocardial infarction (MI) (early, 24 to 72 hours; or late, 1 week to 2 years, known as *Dressler's syndrome*); uremia; malignant disease such as lung or breast cancer; thoracic irradiation; chest trauma; heart surgery (including pacemaker implantation); or drug-induced reaction (as with procainamide or phenytoin).

PQ

Complications of pericarditis include cardiac tamponade, heart failure, and hemopericardium (especially in patients receiving anticoagulants after MI).

Assessment

1. Pain in anterior chest, which is aggravated by thoracic motion and relieved by sitting up and leaning forward
   a. May vary from mild to sharp and severe.
   b. Located in the precordial area (may be felt beneath clavicle, neck, scapular region).
   c. In post-MI patients, a dull, crushing pain may radiate to the neck, arm, and shoulders, mimicking an extension of infarction.
2. Dyspnea from compression of the heart and surrounding thoracic structures
3. Fever, sweating, and chills caused by inflammation of the pericardium

4. Arrhythmias
5. Pericardial friction rub: a scratchy, grating, or creaking sound occurring in the presence of pericardial inflammation

Diagnostic Evaluation

1. Chest X-ray to detect cardiac enlargement
2. Echocardiogram if pericardial effusion is suspected
3. 12-lead electrocardiogram (ECG) rules out acute MI
4. White blood cell count and differential to determine if infection is the cause
5. Chemistry panel including blood urea nitrogen to rule out uremia
6. Antinuclear antibodies rule out systemic lupus erythematosus (SLE); and antistreptolysin-O titers rule out rheumatic fever
7. Tuberculin testing rules out tuberculosis as a cause
8. Pericardiocentesis evaluates pericardial fluid and determines cause
   a. Position patient with head elevated 45 degrees and apply limb leads of ECG for cardiac monitoring.
   b. Have defibrillator and temporary pacemaker available.
   c. After pericardiocentesis, monitor for signs of cardiac tamponade.

EMERGENCY ALERT Because pericardiocentesis carries some risk of fatal complications, such as laceration of the myocardium or of a coronary artery, have emergency equipment ready at bedside.

Collaborative Management

Therapeutic Interventions

1. Dialysis and biochemical control of end-stage renal disease in uremic pericarditis
2. Radiation therapy for neoplastic pericarditis
3. Emergency pericardiocentesis if cardiac tamponade develops

Pharmacologic Interventions

1. Antimicrobial agents such as penicillin for bacterial pericarditis or amphotericin B for fungal pericarditis

2. Corticosteroids to treat rheumatic fever or SLE
3. Antituberculosis chemotherapy to treat tuberculosis
4. Intrapericardial chemotherapy to treat neoplastic pericarditis
5. Aspirin, nonsteroidal anti-inflammatory drugs, or corticosteroids in post-MI syndrome as well as other types of pericarditis to provide symptomatic relief of inflammation and pain

Surgical Interventions

1. Partial pericardiectomy (pericardial "window") or total pericardiectomy for recurrent constrictive pericarditis

Nursing Diagnoses

3, 19, 24

Nursing Interventions
Monitoring

1. Monitor heart rate, rhythm, blood pressure (BP), respirations, and hemodynamic parameters at least hourly in the acute phase.
2. Assess for signs of cardiac tamponade (increased heart rate, decreased BP, presence of paradoxical pulse, distended neck veins, restlessness, muffled heart sounds).

> ⚡ **EMERGENCY ALERT** The normal pericardial sac contains less than 0.8 to 1 oz (25 to 30 mL) fluid; pericardial fluid may accumulate slowly without noticeable symptoms. However, a rapidly developing effusion can produce serious hemodynamic alterations.

3. Assess patient for signs of heart failure (see page 424).
4. Institute continuous cardiac monitoring and monitor patient closely for the development of arrhythmias caused by compression of the heart.

Supportive Care

1. Give prescribed drugs on timely basis for pain and symptomatic relief.
2. Encourage patient to remain on bed rest when chest pain, fever, and friction rub occur.

3. Help the patient to a position of comfort, usually sitting upright.
4. Help relieve anxiety by explaining to the patient and family the difference between pain of pericarditis and pain of recurrent MI. (Patients may fear extension of myocardial tissue damage.) Explain that pericarditis does not indicate further heart damage.

Education and Health Maintenance

1. Instruct the patient about signs and symptoms of pericarditis and stress the need for long-term medication therapy to help relieve symptoms.
2. Review all medications with the patient, including their purpose, adverse effects, dosages, and special precautions.

PERITONITIS

Peritonitis is a generalized or localized inflammation of the peritoneum, the membrane that lines the abdominal cavity and covers visceral organs. This condition most often results from contamination by GI secretions and is a complication of appendicitis, diverticulitis, peptic ulceration, biliary tract disease, colitis, volvulus, strangulated obstruction, peritoneal dialysis, or abdominal neoplasms. It may also occur after abdominal trauma (gunshot or stab wounds, blunt trauma from motor vehicle accident) or GI surgery.

Primary peritonitis is relatively rare, occurring in patients with nephrosis or cirrhosis by *Escherichia coli;* or in young women because of infection introduced through fallopian tubes or through hematogenous spread.

Complications include intra-abdominal abscess, septicemia, and death.

Assessment

1. Localized abdominal pain becomes more diffuse, constant, and intense.
2. Fever, tachypnea, and tachycardia develop.
3. Anorexia, nausea, and vomiting develop as peristalsis decreases.

4. Abdominal distention and tenderness become prominent. Abdomen becomes rigid with rebound tenderness and absent bowel sounds. The patient lies very still, usually with legs drawn up.

5. Percussion shows resonance and tympany indicating paralytic ileus; loss of liver dullness may indicate free air in abdomen.

6. Signs of hypovolemia and shock may develop.

Diagnostic Evaluation

1. Complete blood count shows leukocytosis (increased white blood cells) or leukopenia if severe.

2. Abdominal radiograph detects gas and fluid accumulation in small and large intestines, generalized dilation.

3. CT scan of abdomen or sonography may show abscess formation.

4. Paracentesis may be done to demonstrate blood, pus, bile, bacteria, and amylase in the peritoneal cavity. Gram stain and culture can be done.

5. Arterial blood gas analysis may show metabolic acidosis with respiratory compensation.

6. Laparotomy may be necessary to identify the underlying cause.

Collaborative Management
Therapeutic and Pharmacologic Interventions

1. Treatment of inflammatory conditions preoperatively and postoperatively with antibiotics aims to prevent peritonitis.
   a. Initially, broad-spectrum antibiotics to cover aerobic and anaerobic organisms.
   b. Specific antibiotic therapy follows culture and sensitivity results.

2. Parenteral replacements of fluid and electrolytes.

3. Analgesics for pain; antiemetics for nausea and vomiting.

4. Nasogastric (NG) intubation to decompress the bowel; possibly rectal tube to facilitate passage of flatus.

5. Abdominal paracentesis to remove accumulating fluid.

Surgical Interventions

1. May be necessary to close perforations of abdominal organs, remove infection source (ie, inflamed organ, necrotic tissue), drain abscesses, and lavage peritoneal cavity.

Nursing Diagnoses
3, 19, 23, 51

Nursing Interventions
Monitoring

1. Monitor fluid status because large volumes of fluid can be shifted into peritoneal space.
   a. Weakness, pallor, diaphoresis, cold skin, dry mucous membranes, oliguria, postural hypotension, tachycardia, and diminished skin turgor reflect dehydration and hypovolemia.
   b. Shock (see page 865) and hypokalemia (see page 351) may result.
2. Monitor blood pressure and cardiac rhythm continuously in patients with shock.
3. Monitor central venous pressure and other hemodynamic parameters to guide fluid replacement.
4. Monitor intake and output, including amount of NG tube drainage and paracentesis fluid.

Supportive Care

1. Place the patient on bed rest in semi-Fowler's position to enable less painful breathing.
2. Maintain NPO status to reduce peristalsis; maintain NG decompression until gastric secretions have decreased.
3. Administer antiemetics as needed.
4. Administer antibiotics promptly as directed.
5. Infuse I.V. fluids, for initial fluid replacement and fluid maintenance needs; administer hyperalimentation, as ordered, to maintain positive nitrogen balance until patient can resume oral diet.
6. Reduce parenteral fluids and give oral food and fluids as directed, when the following occur:
   a. Temperature and pulse return to normal.

b. Abdomen becomes soft and bowel sounds return.

c. Flatus is passed and patient has bowel movement.

Education and Health Maintenance

1. Teach the patient and family how to care for open wounds and drain sites, if appropriate.

2. Assess the need for home care nursing to assist with wound care and assess healing; refer as necessary.

3. Teach the patient signs to report for recurrence of infection, namely fever, increasing abdominal pain, anorexia, nausea, vomiting, and abdominal distention.

PHEOCHROMOCYTOMA

Pheochromocytoma is a catecholamine-secreting tumor associated with hyperfunction of the adrenal medulla. It may occur as a component of multiple endocrine neoplasia II, an autosomal-dominant syndrome characterized by pheochromocytoma, thyroid carcinoma, hyperparathyroidism, and Cushing's syndrome. Pheochromocytomas located in the adrenal medulla produce both increased epinephrine and norepinephrine; those located outside the adrenal gland tend to produce epinephrine only. Excess catecholamine secretion produces hypertension, hypermetabolism, and hyperglycemia. Pheochromocytoma can occur at any age but is most common between ages 30 and 60. Most tumors are benign; 10% are malignant with metastasis.

Assessment

1. Hypermetabolic and hyperglycemic effects produce excessive perspiration, tremor, pallor or facial flushing, nervousness, elevated blood glucose levels, polyuria, nausea, vomiting, diarrhea, abdominal pain, and paresthesias.

2. Hypertension may be paroxysmal (intermittent) or persistent (chronic). The chronic form mimics essential hypertension but does not respond to antihypertensives. Headaches and vision disturbances are common.

3. Emotional changes, including psychotic behavior, may occur.

PQ

4. Predisposing factors that may trigger symptoms include physical exertion, emotional upset, and allergic reactions.

Diagnostic Evaluation

1. Elevated vanillylmandelic acid and metanephrine (metabolites of epinephrine and norepinephrine) on 24-hour urine.
2. Elevated epinephrine and norepinephrine in blood and urine while symptomatic.
3. Clonidine suppression shows no significant decrease in catecholamines in patients with pheochromocytoma.
4. CT scanning and MRI of the adrenal glands or entire abdomen identify tumor.

Collaborative Management
Pharmacologic Interventions

1. Preoperatively, an alpha-adrenergic blocker, such as phentolamine, is prescribed to inhibit the effects of catecholamines on blood pressure.
   a. Effective control of blood pressure may take 1 or 2 weeks.
   b. Blood volume needs to be expanded as blood vessels dilate with inhibition of catecholamines.
   c. Surgery is delayed until blood pressure is controlled and blood volume has been expanded.
2. Catecholamine synthesis inhibitors, such as metyrosine, preoperatively or for long-term management of inoperable tumors. Adverse effects include sedation and crystalluria leading to kidney stones.

Surgical Interventions

1. Surgery involves unilateral adrenalectomy or removal of nonadrenal tumor.
2. Bilateral adrenalectomy may be necessary if both adrenal glands are affected.
3. Manipulation of the tumor during surgery may cause release of stored catecholamines causing hypertension during and immediately after surgery.

Nursing Diagnoses
6, 88, 136

Nursing Interventions
Also see *Gastrointestinal or Abdominal Surgery*, page 381, and *Aldosteronism, primary*, page 7.

Monitoring
1. Monitor blood pressure frequently while patient is symptomatic.
2. Monitor patient for orthostatic hypotension after administration of phentolamine.
3. Monitor vital signs, cardiac rhythm, arterial blood pressure, neurologic status, and urine output closely because immediate postoperative hypertension, then hypotension, may occur.

Supportive Care

PQ

1. Remain with the patient during acute episodes of hypertension.
2. Ensure bed rest and elevate the head of bed 45 degrees during severe hypertension.
3. Instruct the patient about use of relaxation exercises.
4. Reduce environmental stressors by providing a calm and quiet environment. Restrict visitors.
5. Eliminate stimulants (coffee, tea, cola) from the diet.
6. Provide good skin care if symptomatic with diarrhea and diaphoresis.
7. Reduce events that precipitate episodes of severe hypertension, such as palpation of the tumor, physical exertion, and emotional upset.
8. Administer sedatives as directed to promote relaxation and rest.
9. Encourage oral fluids and maintain I.V. infusion preoperatively to ensure adequate volume expansion going into surgery.
10. Maintain adequate hydration with I.V. infusion postoperatively to prevent hypotension.

> ⚡ **EMERGENCY ALERT** Because reduction of catecholamines postoperatively causes vasodilation and enlargement of vascular space, hypotension may occur.

11. Provide routine wound care and prevention of postoperative complications.

Education and Health Maintenance

1. Instruct the patient how to take metyrosine if being treated medically.
   a. May cause sedation; need to avoid taking other central nervous system depressants and participating in activities that require alertness.
   b. Increase fluid intake to at least 2,000 mL per day to prevent kidney stones.
2. Inform patient regarding the need for continued follow-up for:
   a. Recurrence of pheochromocytoma.
   b. Assessment of any residual renal or cardiovascular injury related to preoperative hypertension.
   c. Documentation that catecholamine levels are normal 1 to 3 months postoperatively (by 24-hour urine).
3. Teach patient about corticosteroid replacement for rest of his or her life if bilateral adrenalectomy was performed; or for a few weeks if one adrenal gland was removed, until the stress of surgery is over and the remaining gland can compensate.

PITUITARY TUMORS

Pituitary tumors are usually adenomas of unknown origin that arise primarily in the anterior pituitary. Symptoms reflect tumor effects on target endocrine tissues or on local structures surrounding the pituitary gland. Tumors may be classified by size as microadenoma (smaller than 10 mm) or macroadenoma (larger than 10 mm), or by functional status as hormone secreting or nonsecreting.

Pituitary tumors respond well to early diagnosis and treatment and rarely metastasize. Without treatment, however, death or severe disability caused by stroke, blindness, or target endocrine disorders results.

Assessment

1. Effects of tumor on surrounding structures (mass effect)
   a. Headaches
   b. Possible nausea and vomiting
   c. Impairment of cranial nerves, such as visual field defects and diplopia, which may indicate pressure from tumor on the optic chiasm
2. Hormone imbalances caused by tumor hypersecretion or diminished secretion (see *Table P-2*, page 732)

Diagnostic Evaluation

1. Skull X-rays are usually normal but may show enlarged sella turcica.
2. MRI with attention to the sella turcica shows pituitary mass.
3. Serum hormone levels identify abnormalities suspected on clinical evaluation.
4. Provocative testing, such as glucose tolerance test and dexamethasone suppression test, detect abnormal hormone secretion.

PQ

Collaborative Management
Therapeutic Interventions

1. Ablation of tumor and much of gland by cryogenic destruction or stereotaxic radiofrequency coagulation
2. Radiation therapy

Pharmacologic Interventions

1. Drug therapy with bromocriptine (given daily) or cabergoline (twice weekly) for prolactinomas and, in some instances, growth hormone–secreting tumors.
2. Specific hormone replacement therapy is indicated for hypopituitarism after medical or surgical treatment.
   a. Hypothyroidism caused by lack of thyroid-stimulating hormone is treated with thyroxine-based medications.
   b. Adrenocortical insufficiency requires immediate hormone replacement with adrenocorticotropic hormone (ACTH) or hydrocortisone.

TABLE P-2	Clinical Manifestations Associated with Hormone Effects of Pituitary Tumors	
HORMONE	**HYPERPITUITARISM (INCREASED SECRETION)**	**HYPOPITUITARISM (DECREASED SECRETION)**
Growth hormone (GH)	• Gigantism (child) • Acromegaly (adult)	• Shortness of stature (child) • Silent (adult)
Prolactin	• Infertility and galactorrhea (female)	• Postpartum lactation failure (female)
Adrenocorticotropic hormone (ACTH)	• Cushing's disease	• Adrenocortical insufficiency
Thyroid-stimulating hormone (TSH)	• Hyperthyroidism	• Hypothyroidism
Luteinizing hormone (LH) and follicle-stimulating hormone (FSH)	• Gonadal dysfunction	• Hypogonadism

c. In women, menstruation ceases and infertility occurs almost always after total or near-total ablation; estrogen and progesterone may be indicated to prevent osteoporosis.

d. Transient or permanent diabetes insipidus may occur because of deficient antidiuretic hormone (ADH) secretion requiring desmopressin administration.

Surgical Interventions

1. Transsphenoidal hypophysectomy: direct approach through the sinus and nasal cavity to sella turcica.
2. Frontal craniotomy: Uncommon approach except where tumor occupies broad area (see page 238).
3. Manipulation of the posterior pituitary during surgery may cause transient syndrome of secretion of inappropriate antidiuretic hormone (SIADH) with excessive ADH secretion, requiring diuretics and fluid restriction.

Nursing Diagnoses

3, 44, 108, 135, 136

Nursing Interventions

Also see Craniotomy, page 238.

Monitoring

PQ

1. After transsphenoidal hypophysectomy, monitor vital signs, visual acuity, and neurologic status frequently for signs of cerebrospinal fluid (CSF) leak or infection.
2. Monitor for and report increased urine output and low urine specific gravity, indicating diabetes insipidus.
3. Monitor serum electrolytes (hyponatremia) and serum osmolality (low) for SIADH.

Supportive Care

1. Provide emotional support through the diagnostic process and answer questions about treatment options.
2. Prepare the patient for surgery or other treatment by describing nursing care thoroughly.
3. Stress likelihood of positive outcome with ablation therapy.
4. Assess for signs of sinus infection before transsphenoidal procedure, and administer antibiotics as directed.
5. Administer hydrocortisone preoperatively because the source of ACTH is being removed and surgery is a significant source of stress.
6. After transsphenoidal surgery:
   a. Encourage deep-breathing exercises.

    b. Caution the patient to avoid coughing and sneezing postoperatively to prevent leakage of CSF.

    c. Check incision within inner aspect of upper lip for drainage or bleeding.

    d. Note frequency of nasal dressing changes and character of drainage. Prepare the patient for packing removal 1 to several days postoperatively.

    e. Encourage the use of a humidifier to prevent drying from mouth breathing.

    f. Report appearance of persistent clear fluid from nose and increasing headache; could signal CSF leak.

Education and Health Maintenance

1. Advise patient about temporary limitations in activities outlined by surgeon.
2. Teach the patient the nature of hormonal deficiencies after treatment and the purpose of replacement therapy.
3. Instruct the patient in the early signs and symptoms of cortisol or thyroid hormone deficiency or excess and the need to report them.
4. Describe and demonstrate the correct method of administering prescribed medications.
5. Teach the patient the need for frequent initial follow-up and lifelong medical management when on hormonal therapy.
6. If applicable, advise patient on the need for postsurgery radiation therapy and periodic follow-up MRI and visual field testing.
7. Teach the patient to notify health care provider if signs of thyroid or cortisol imbalance become evident.
8. Advise patient to wear medical alert tag.

PNEUMONIA

Pneumonia is inflammation of the terminal airways and alveoli caused by acute infection by various agents. Pneumonia can be divided into three groups, which guide management: community acquired, hospital or nursing home acquired (nosocomial), and pneumonia in an immunocompromised person. Causes include bacteria (*Streptococcus, Staphylococcus, Hae-*

mophilus influenzae, Klebsiella, Legionella); virus; fungi; atypical organisms (*Mycoplasma* or *Chlamydia*); and *Pneumocystis carinii* associated with human immunodeficiency virus.

Bacterial pneumonia occurs when host resistance is altered by viral infection or underlying diseases (cancer, drug abuse, acquired immunodeficiency syndrome) or therapies (immunosuppressants, chemotherapy, radiation therapy). Such persons may develop an overwhelming infection. Recurring pneumonia often indicates underlying disease such as cancer of the lung and chronic obstructive lung disease.

Aspiration pneumonia is an acute inflammatory condition that results from aspiration of oropharyngeal secretions or stomach contents into the lungs. Patients at risk include those with loss or impairment of swallowing or coughing reflexes caused by altered state of consciousness, alcohol or drug overdose, or motor disease of the esophagus; those undergoing nasogastric (NG) or endotracheal intubations, or childbirth; or those with GI conditions, such as hiatal hernia or intestinal obstruction.

Complications of pneumonia include pleural effusion, septic shock, pericarditis, bacteremia, meningitis, delirium, atelectasis, and delayed resolution.

Assessment

In most cases of bacterial pneumonia:

1. Sudden onset; shaking chill; rapidly rising fever of 101° to 105° F (38.3° to 40.5° C). Aspiration pneumonia produces a fever, but no chills.
2. Cough, usually with purulent sputum. In aspiration pneumonia, sputum is pink, frothy, and foul-smelling, resembling that of acute pulmonary edema.
3. Pleuritic chest pain, aggravated by respiration and coughing.
4. Tachypnea, respiratory grunting, nasal flaring, use of accessory muscles of respiration. Cyanosis is evident in aspiration pneumonia.
5. Anxious, flushed appearance, splinting of affected side, hypoxia, confusion, disorientation; may indicate worsening condition.

6. Auscultation shows crackles overlying affected lung; bronchial breath sounds when *consolidation* (filling of airspaces with exudate) is present.
   a. In aspiration pneumonia, rhonchi and wheezing are also present.
   b. Absent breath sounds caused by atelectasis from mucous plugs.
7. Mental status changes, indicating hypoxemia.

GERONTOLOGIC ALERT Pneumonia may present as mental status change and cough in elderly patients without fever or leukocytosis. Presentation may be subtle or dramatic. People older than age 65 have a high mortality.

8. Predisposing factors that may interfere with normal lung drainage include tumor, general anesthesia and postoperative immobility, central nervous system depression, intubation or respiratory instrumentation, and neurologic disease, increasing risk of aspiration.

Diagnostic Evaluation

1. Chest X-rays detect infiltrates, atelectasis, and consolidation. In aspiration pneumonia, films may be clear initially, but later show consolidation and other abnormalities.
2. Sputum specimens for Gram stain and culture and sensitivity studies detect infectious agent.
3. Arterial blood gas (ABG) analysis evaluates oxygenation and acid-base status.
4. Blood cultures detect bacteremia.
5. Blood, sputum, and urine samples for immunologic tests detect microbial antigens.
6. Laryngoscopy or bronchoscopy determine if airways are blocked by solid material.

Collaborative Management
Therapeutic Interventions

1. Oxygen therapy if patient has inadequate gas exchange (see *Table P-3*):
   a. Avoid high oxygen concentrations in patients with chronic obstructive pulmonary disease (COPD); use of

TABLE P-3	Oxygen Administration

METHOD/FiO$_2$	NURSING CONSIDERATIONS
Nasal cannula: 40% or less	• Delivers low gas flow. • Requires nose breathing. • Drying to mucous membranes.
Face mask: 40–60%	• Delivers moderate gas flow to nose and mouth. • Aerosol can be added (all mask systems).
Venturi mask 24–60%	• Delivers high gas flow. • Eliminates CO_2 rebreathing.
Partial rebreather mask: 50–75%	• Must maintain high enough gas flow so the bag does not collapse during inspiration (would allow CO_2 rebreathing).
Non-rebreathing mask: 60–90%	• Must maintain high enough gas flow so the bag does not collapse during inspiration (would lower FiO$_2$).
Transtracheal catheter	• Surgical procedure required to create tract for removable catheter that delivers O_2 most efficiently. • Lower gas flow is required than other methods.
CPAP mask: 21–100%	• Provides end expiration and inspiration positive pressure. • Increases risk of aspiration.
T-piece (Briggs) adapter: 21–100%	• Attaches to tracheostomy or endotracheal tube for patient who is breathing spontaneously. • Gas flow must be suffucient to maintain mist from end piece, even during inspiration.

PQ

high oxygen may worsen alveolar ventilation by removing the patient's remaining ventilatory drive.

b. Mechanical ventilation may be necessary if adequate ABG values cannot be maintained.

2. Intercostal nerve block to obtain pain relief
3. In aspiration pneumonia, clear the obstructed airway to prevent further aspiration.
4. Fluid volume replacement

Pharmacologic Interventions

1. Appropriate antimicrobial therapy, based on culture and sensitivity when possible
2. Cough suppressants when coughing is nonproductive, debilitating, or when coughing paroxysms cause serious hypoxemia.
3. Analgesics to relieve pleuritic pain. However, use opioids cautiously in patients with a history of COPD.

GERONTOLOGIC ALERT Sedatives, opioids, and cough suppressants are used cautiously in elderly patients because of their tendency to suppress cough and gag reflexes and respiratory drive. Expectorants and bronchodilators may be more helpful.

EMERGENCY ALERT Restlessness, confusion, aggressiveness may be caused by cerebral hypoxia; if so, do not treat with sedatives.

Nursing Diagnoses
49, 57, 73, 119

Nursing Interventions
Monitoring

1. Monitor temperature, pulse, respiration, blood pressure, and oxygen saturation at regular intervals to assess the patient's response to therapy.
2. Follow results of ABG analysis to determine oxygen need and acid-base balance.
3. Employ special nursing surveillance for patients with the following conditions:
   a. Alcoholism, immunosuppression, heart failure
   b. COPD; it is difficult to detect subtle changes in condition because the patient may have seriously compromised pulmonary function
   c. The elderly may have little or no fever and subtle presentation

4. Monitor for unusual behavior, confusion, alterations in mental status, or stupor, which indicate hypoxemia.

5. Assess for signs of heart failure indicating decompensation because of increased work of the heart due to dyspnea, fever, or infection.

6. Assess for resistant or recurrent fever, indicating bacterial resistance to antibiotics.

7. In aspiration pneumonia, closely monitor for worsening condition indicating lung abscess, empyema, and necrotizing pneumonia.

Supportive Care

1. Place the patient in Fowler's position to obtain greater lung expansion and improve aeration. Encourage frequent position changes to prevent pooling of secretions.

2. Encourage the patient to cough; provide suction as needed. If patient is intubated, administer extra oxygenation before and after suctioning.

3. Demonstrate to the patient how to splint the chest while coughing, and advise against suppressing a productive cough.

4. Encourage increased fluid intake or provide aggressive I.V. fluids, unless contraindicated, to thin mucus, promote expectoration, and replace fluid losses from fever, diaphoresis, dehydration, and dyspnea. Also humidify room air or oxygen therapy.

5. Employ chest wall percussion and postural drainage when appropriate, to loosen and mobilize secretions. (See *Figure P-2*, page 740.)

6. Auscultate the chest for crackles to gauge effectiveness of percussion and drainage.

7. Apply heating pad to chest and administer analgesics as directed to relieve pleuritic pain; assist with intercostal nerve block as indicated.

8. Encourage modified bed rest during febrile period; light ambulation with extra rest when afebrile to mobilize secretions.

9. Watch for abdominal distention or ileus, which may be caused by swallowing of air during intervals of severe dys-

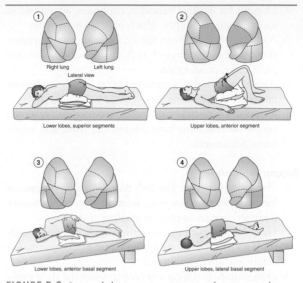

FIGURE P-2 Postural drainage positions and corresponding anatomic segment of the lung.

pnea. Insert NG or rectal tube as directed, to relieve distention.

10. Be aware of those at risk for aspiration pneumonia, feed patients with impaired swallowing slowly, and ensure that no food is retained in mouth after feeding. Give enteral feedings if indicated.

   a. Give tube feedings slowly, with patient sitting up in bed.

   b. Check position of tube in stomach before feeding.

   c. Check seal of cuff of tracheostomy or endotracheal tube before feeding.

11. Keep the patient with aspiration pneumonia in a fasting state before anesthesia (at least 8 hours).

EMERGENCY ALERT Morbidity and mortality of aspiration pneumonia remain high even with optimum treatment. Prevention is the key to the problem.

Education and Health Maintenance

1. Encourage chair rest after fever subsides; gradually increase activities to bring energy level back to pre-illness stage.

2. Encourage breathing exercises to clear lungs and promote full expansion and function after the fever subsides.

3. Advise patient to stop smoking. Cigarette smoking destroys mucociliary action and inhibits function of alveolar scavenger cells (macrophages).

4. Advise patient to keep up natural resistance with good nutrition and adequate rest. A single episode of pneumonia may predispose the patient to recurring respiratory infections.

5. Instruct the patient to avoid sudden extremes in temperature and excessive alcohol intake, which lower resistance to pneumonia.

6. Encourage yearly influenza immunization and immunization for *Streptococcus pneumoniae*, if indicated (major cause of bacterial pneumonia).

PQ

7. Tell the patient to avoid persons who have upper respiratory infections for several months after pneumonia and to practice frequent hand washing, especially after contact with other people and objects.

8. Advise patient to contact health care provider for return of fever, increased fatigue, dyspnea, or productive cough. Follow-up is often necessary 4 to 6 weeks after acute illness to evaluate lungs for clearing and to detect occult tumor that may have been the underlying cause of pneumonia.

PNEUMOTHORAX

Pneumothorax is accumulation of air in the pleural space that occurs spontaneously or as a result of trauma. In patients with chest trauma, it usually follows laceration of the lung parenchyma, tracheobronchial tree, or esophagus. If left untreated, acute respiratory failure may ensue. See *Table P-4*, page 742, for additional chest injuries.

TABLE P-4   Chest Injuries

INJURY/DESCRIPTION	MANAGEMENT
Rib fracture May interfere with ventilation due to pain; may lacerate liver or lung	• Provide anagesics; encourage deep breathing and coughing; intercostal nerve block or epidural anesthesia may be necessary (for multiple rib fractures)
Hemothorax Blood in pleural space due to blunt or penetrating trauma; may cause significant blood loss and shock	• Thoracentesis and/or chest tube insertion; I.V. fluid and blood replacement
Flail chest Loss of stability of chest wall due to multiple rib and possibly sternum fractures. Ventilation is compromised because detached portion of chest wall is pulled inward on inspiration and pushed outward on expiration (paradoxical chest movement)	• Chest wall is stabilized with hands, sand bag, or pressure dressing, patient is turned on affected side until intubated and mechanically ventilated • Epidural analgesia or surgical stabilization in some patients
Pulmonary contusion Leakage of blood and fluid into alveolar and interstitial space over 24 to 72 hours after injury; causes pleuritic chest pain and copious secretions.	• Mechanical ventilation for moderate to severe contusion; diuretic to relieve pulmonary edema; sodium bicarbonate to relieve acidosis; pumonary artery pressure monitoring
Cardiac tamponade Compression of heart by accumulation of fluid in pericardium due to penetrating injury; causes falling blood pressure, distended neck veins, elevated central venous pressure, muffled heart sounds, pulsus paradoxus, dyspnea, and cyanosis	• Emergency pericardiocentesis to improve hemodynamic function; thoracotomy to control bleeding and repair injury; I.V. fluid and blood replacement; support of vital functions

In *spontaneous pneumothorax*, air suddenly enters the pleural space, deflating the lung on the affected side (see *Figure P-3*). Usually caused by rupture of a subpleural bleb, it may occur secondary to chronic respiratory diseases or idiopathically. It may also strike healthy patients (risk is high in thin, white males and those with family history of pneumothorax).

In *open pneumothorax* (sucking chest wound), trauma to the chest wall creates an opening large enough for air to pass freely between the thoracic cavity and the outside of the body. With each attempted respiration, part of the tidal volume moves back and forth through the open wound instead of the trachea.

In *tension pneumothorax*, air builds up under pressure in the pleural space, which interferes with filling of both the heart and lungs. Cardiovascular collapse may occur.

Assessment

1. Mild to moderate dyspnea and chest discomfort with spontaneous pneumothorax
2. Air hunger, agitation, hypotension, and cyanosis with open or tension pneumothorax

PQ

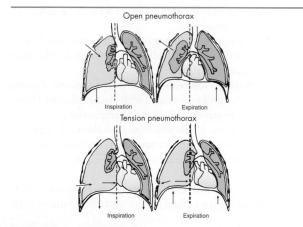

Open pneumothorax

Inspiration Expiration

Tension pneumothorax

Inspiration Expiration

FIGURE P-3 Pneumothorax.

3. Reduced mobility of affected half of thorax and possible tracheal deviation away from affected side (tension pneumothorax)
4. Diminished breath sounds and hyperresonance

Diagnostic Evaluation

1. Chest X-rays confirm presence of air in pleural space, evaluate possible lung collapse, and check for tracheal deviation away from affected side.

Collaborative Management
Therapeutic Interventions

1. In spontaneous pneumothorax:
   a. Observe and allow for spontaneous resolution for less than 50% pneumothorax in otherwise healthy patient.
   b. With greater than 50% pneumothorax, needle aspiration or chest tube drainage if needed to reexpand collapsed lung.
2. In tension pneumothorax:
   a. Immediate decompression with thoracentesis, thoracostomy, or chest tube insertion to vent trapped air and prevent cardiovascular collapse.
   b. Basic and advanced life support if cardiovascular collapse occurs.
   c. Maintenance of chest tube drainage with underwater-seal suction, to allow full lung expansion and healing.
3. In open pneumothorax:
   a. Immediate closure of wound with a pressure dressing (petrolatum gauze secured with elastic adhesive) to restore adequate ventilation and respiration.
   b. The patient should inhale and exhale gently against a closed glottis (Valsalva maneuver) as pressure dressing is applied. This maneuver helps to expand a collapsed lung.
   c. Chest tube insertion and underwater-seal suction, to permit escape of fluid and air and allow lung to reexpand.

Surgical Interventions
1. For recurrent spontaneous pneumothorax:
   a. Pleurodesis: intrapleural instillation of a chemical irritant causing the visceral and parietal pleura to adhere
   b. Thoracotomy with resection of apical blebs
2. For traumatic pneumothorax, repair chest trauma

Nursing Diagnoses
3, 57, 75

Nursing Interventions
Monitoring
1. Monitor vital signs and respiratory status continuously until lung has been reinflated.
2. Monitor oxygenation with oximetry and regular arterial blood gas readings.
3. Monitor chest tube patency and drainage.

Supportive Care
1. Maintain patent airway and provide oxygen via nasal cannula or mask as needed; suction as needed.
2. Maintain patency of chest tubes.
   a. Check tubing connections and prevent kinking of tube.
   b. Milk the tube periodically if directed.
   c. Ensure fluctuation in the water seal chamber until lung is reexpanded.
   d. Report excessive bubbling in water seal chamber, which may indicate leak in system.
3. Position the patient upright if possible, to allow greater chest expansion.
4. Help patient to splint chest while turning or coughing, and administer pain medications as needed.
5. Instruct and encourage patient to use an inspiratory spirometer to improve lung expansion.
6. Provide care for patient on mechanical ventilation, if necessary.

PQ

Education and Health Maintenance

1. Instruct patient to continue use of the inspiratory spirometer at home.
2. Patients with spontaneous pneumothorax are at risk for repeat occurrence; encourage these patients to report sudden onset of dyspnea immediately.

POISONING, ACUTE INGESTED

Poisoning by ingestion refers to the oral intake of a harmful substance that, even in small amounts, can damage tissues, disturb bodily functions, and possibly cause death. Immediate injury results when the poison excoriates soft tissues, as with a strong acid or alkali. A delayed response occurs when the poison is absorbed into the bloodstream and causes systemic symptoms.

Substances commonly ingested include over-the-counter medications (such as acetaminophen or iron supplements; see *Table P-5*), household cleaning products, or parts of houseplants. Ingested poisoning may be accidental or intentional. Permanent multiorgan damage may result from initial loss of airway, breathing, and circulation, and from specific organ toxicity.

PEDIATRIC ALERT Children younger than age 6 are unlikely to develop significant acetaminophen toxicity even with large doses because of their ability to metabolize; adolescents have higher incidence of toxicity.

PEDIATRIC ALERT Sixty-five percent of all poisonings occur in persons younger than age 20, and 90% of poisonings occur in the home.

Assessment

1. Altered level of consciousness, other neurologic signs common in poisonings that affect the nervous system

EMERGENCY ALERT Be prepared to initiate emergency respiratory and circulatory support at any time.

2. GI symptoms common in metallic acid, alkali, and bacterial poisoning include nausea and vomiting, diarrhea, abdominal pain or cramping, and anorexia.

| TABLE P-5 | Two Commonly Ingested Poisons |

POISON	CLINICAL MANIFESTATIONS
Acetaminophen • Common drug poisoning agent in chldren because of its availability and palatability. • Ingestion by adolescents is frequently intentional. • Results in necrosis of the liver.	*First 24 hours after ingestion* • May be asymptomatic or anorexia, nausea, vomiting, diaphoresis, malaise, pallor *Second 24 hours after ingestion* • Above symptoms diminish or disappear. Development of right upper quadrant pain, elevated liver function tests, oliguria *Days 3 to 5 after ingestion* • Peak liver function abnormalities; anorexia, nausea, vomiting, and malaise may reappear. • Jaundice, hypoglycemia, coagulopathy, and encephalopathy if severe liver failure *Day 5+ after ingestion* • Liver failure with overwhelming toxicity or recovery with blood chemistry return to normal
Iron • Occurs frequently in children because of prevalence of iron-containing preparations. • Severity is related to the amount of elemental iron absorbed. • The range of potential toxicity is approximately 50 to 60 mg/kg.	*30 minutes to 2 hours after ingestion* • Local necrosis and hemorrhage of GI tract; nausea and vomiting (including hematemesis). abdominal pain, diarrhea (often bloody), severe hypotension; symptoms subside after 6 to 12 hours. *6 to 24 hours after ingestion* • Period of apparent recovery *24 to 40 hours after ingestion* • Systemic toxicity with cardiovascular collapse, shock metabolic acidosis, hepatic amd renal failure, seizures, coma, and possible death *2 to 4 weeks after ingestion* • Pyloric and duodenal stenosis, hepatic cirrhosis

PQ

3. Seizures (especially with central nervous system [CNS] depressants such as alcohol, chloral hydrate, barbiturates) and behavioral changes. Dilated or pinpoint pupils may be noted.
4. Dyspnea (especially with aspiration of hydrocarbons) and cardiopulmonary depression or arrest. Cyanosis, especially in cyanide and strychnine ingestion.
5. Skin irritation; rash; burns to the mouth, esophagus, and stomach; eye inflammation; stains or odor around the mouth; lesions of the mucous membranes.

Diagnostic Evaluation
1. Blood and urine toxicology screening
2. Gastric contents may also be sent for toxicology screening in serious ingestions.
3. Liver function and renal function testing

Collaborative Management
Therapeutic Interventions
1. Emergency measures:
   a. Identify the poison when possible.
   b. Call the nearest poison control center to identify the toxic ingredient and obtain recommendations for emergency treatment.
   c. Save vomitus, stool, and urine for analysis.
   d. Maintain an open airway, because some ingested substances may cause soft tissue swelling and constrict the airway.
   e. If needed, obtain venous access, maintain safety during seizure activity, and treat shock.
2. Gastric lavage, forced diuresis, hemoperfusion, dialysis, or exchange transfusions may be necessary.

Pharmacologic Interventions
1. Administration of antidotes if known such as charcoal.
2. N-acetylcysteine is given as an antidote for acetaminophen poisoning.
3. Deferoxamine is an iron-chelating agent used in severe iron poisoning.

Nursing Diagnoses
6, 24, 92, 130, 136

Nursing Interventions
Monitoring
1. Continue to monitor airway, breathing, and circulation.
2. Monitor level of consciousness, pupil reactivity, and motor activity.
3. Monitor patient's vital signs.
4. Monitor for fluid and electrolyte imbalance after vomiting or diuresis.

Supportive Care
1. Call the poison control center with the following information or instruct family to do so if the patient is at home.
   a. Name, address, and telephone number of caller
   b. Immediate severity of the situation
   c. Age, weight, and signs and symptoms, including neurologic status
   d. Route of exposure
   e. Name of the ingested product, approximate amount ingested, and the time of ingestion
   f. Brief medical history
   g. Caller's relationship to victim
2. Clear the child's mouth of any unswallowed poison.
3. Identify what treatments have already been initiated.
4. Perform or advise appropriate emergency actions based on facility protocol and type of poison ingested.
   a. To remove poison from the body, dilute with 6 to 8 oz (177 to 237 mL) of water, based on poison.
   b. For skin or eye contact, remove contaminated clothing and flush with water for 15 to 20 minutes.
   c. For inhalation poisons, remove patient from the exposure site.
5. Instruct the parents to save vomitus, unswallowed liquid or pills, and the container and to bring them to the hospital as aids in identifying the poison.

PQ

6. While assisting with emergency care in the acute care facility, reassure child and family that therapeutic measures are being taken immediately.

7. Discourage anxious parents from holding, caressing, and overstimulating the child.

8. Avoid administering sedatives or opioids to avoid CNS depression and masking of symptoms.

9. Have artificial airway and tracheostomy set available in case respiratory depression develops.

10. Administer oxygen as directed.

11. Maintain I.V. therapy as directed to prevent shock.

12. Assist with gastric lavage and other treatments.

13. Avoid hypothermia or hyperthermia because control of body temperature is impaired in many types of poisoning.

14. Counsel parents, who usually feel guilty about the accident.

15. Involve the young child in therapeutic play to determine how he or she views the situation. Explain the child's treatment and correct misinterpretations in a manner appropriate for age.

16. Initiate a community health nursing referral. A home assessment should be made so underlying problems are recognized and appropriate help is provided.

Education and Health Maintenance

1. Teach measures to prevent accidental poisonings in the home.
   a. Keep medicines and chemicals out of reach and climbing ability of children; use childproof containers, locked cabinets, and high shelves.
   b. Keep potentially toxic substances in original containers away from food.
   c. Teach children not to taste unfamiliar substances.
   d. Read all labels carefully before each use.
   e. Never refer to drugs as candy or bribe children with such inducements.
   f. Teach adults not to take drugs in front of children, because children mimic behavior.

2. Reinforce the need for supervision of infants and young children.
3. Instruct parents and family to have regional poison control center number readily available in the home.

POLYCYTHEMIA VERA

Polycythemia vera is a chronic myeloproliferative disorder of unknown cause involving hyperplasia of all bone marrow elements. This causes overproduction of all three blood cell lines, most notably red blood cell mass, blood volume, and blood viscosity all increase. Hyperviscosity may also lead to complications such as deep vein thrombophlebitis; myocardial and cerebral infarction; pulmonary embolism; and thrombotic occlusion of the splenic, hepatic, portal and mesenteric veins. Other complications include heart failure, gout, spontaneous hemorrhage, and, possibly, myelofibrosis or acute leukemia in late stages of the disorder.

PQ

Assessment
1. Headache, fullness in head, dizziness, visual abnormalities, weakness, and fatigue
2. Reddish-purple hue of skin and mucosa; pruritus
3. Painful fingers and toes from arterial and venous insufficiency
4. Altered mentation from disturbed cerebral circulation
5. Splenomegaly and hepatomegaly
6. Bleeding tendency

Diagnostic Evaluation
1. Complete blood count (CBC) shows elevated red blood cells, hemoglobin, and hematocrit (greater than 60%); elevated platelets.
2. Bone marrow aspiration and biopsy check for hyperplasia.
3. Increased serum uric acid due to increased formation and destruction of erythrocytes and increased metabolism of nucleic acids.

Collaborative Management
Therapeutic Interventions
1. Phlebotomy (withdrawal of blood) is performed to treat hyperviscosity at intervals determined by CBC results, to reduce red cell mass. Generally, 8.5 to 17 oz (250 to 500 mL) is removed at a time.

Pharmacologic Interventions
1. Myelosuppressive therapy for marrow hyperplasia
   a. I.V. radioactive phosphorus (^{32}P)
   b. Alkylating agent such as hydroxyurea
2. Allopurinol to treat hyperuricemia
3. Antihistamines and other oral and topical drugs to treat pruritus

Nursing Diagnoses
88, 135

Nursing Interventions
Monitoring
1. Monitor for signs of bleeding or thromboembolism.
2. Monitor for hypertension and signs and symptoms of heart failure, including shortness of breath and distended neck veins.
3. Monitor CBC results.

Supportive Care and Education
1. Encourage or assist with ambulation.
2. Educate the patient about risk of thrombosis; encourage maintenance of normal activity patterns and avoiding long periods of bed rest.
3. Advise the patient to avoid taking hot showers or baths because rapid skin cooling worsens pruritus; use skin emollients; take antihistamines as directed.
4. Instruct the patient to take only prescribed medications.
5. Encourage the patient to report at prescribed intervals for follow-up blood studies (hematocrit).

PREMENSTRUAL SYNDROME

Premenstrual syndrome (PMS) is a group of symptoms related to onset of menstruation. The cause is unclear but may be linked to hormonal imbalances; prostaglandins; endorphins; psychological factors, such as attitudes and beliefs related to menstruation; and environmental factors, such as nutrition and pollution. PMS occurs most commonly in women in their 30s and is usually self-limiting without complications.

Assessment

1. Symptoms may begin 7 to 14 days before onset of menstrual flow; diminish 1 to 2 days after menses begins.
2. Physical: edema of extremities, abdominal fullness, breast swelling and tenderness, headache, vertigo, palpitations, acne, backache, constipation, thirst, weight gain.
3. Behavioral: irritability, fatigue, lethargy, depression, anxiety, crying spells.
4. Diagnosis based on clinical manifestations; usually no diagnostic evaluation necessary.

PQ

Collaborative Management
Therapeutic Interventions

1. Restrict sodium, caffeine, tobacco, alcohol, and refined sweets.
2. Aerobic exercise daily during symptomatic period helps reduce tension.
3. Counseling to help reduce emotional and behavioral symptoms.

Pharmacologic Interventions

1. Vitamin B_6 supplements may help reduce tension and irritability.
2. Progesterone replacement therapy may relieve symptoms.
3. Prostaglandin inhibitors such as ibuprofen are used.
4. Diuretics decrease fluid retention and weight gain.
5. Anxiolytic agents may be necessary.

6. Fluoxetine and other selective serotonin reuptake inhibitors help with control of the psychological symptoms of PMS.
7. Calcium supplementation of 1,200 mg elemental calcium per day has been shown to decrease mood swings, irritability, depression, and anxiety.

Nursing Diagnoses
6, 78, 139

Nursing Interventions
Supportive Care
1. Provide emotional support for patient and significant others.
2. Encourage patient to keep a diary for several consecutive months including dates, cycle days, stressors, and symptoms and their severity to determine if therapy is effective.

Education and Health Maintenance
1. Instruct patient in the use and adverse effects of prescribed medications.
2. Teach patient possible causes of PMS and nonpharmacologic methods to alleviate distress, such as dietary modifications, exercise, and rest.
3. Teach stress reduction techniques, such as imagery and deep breathing.
4. Refer for counseling and to support groups as needed.

PRESSURE SORES

Pressure sores (decubitus ulcers) are localized ulcerations of the skin and deeper structures. They most commonly result from prolonged periods of bed rest; however, they may develop within hours in a compromised individual. Pressure of 70 mm Hg applied for longer than 2 hours can produce tissue destruction. Friction (causing abrasion of the stratum corneum) and shearing (sliding of adjacent surfaces causing rupture of capillaries) forces contribute to the destructive mechanism of

pressure. Risk factors for pressure sores include bowel or bladder incontinence, malnutrition or significant weight loss, edema, anemia, hypoxia, hypotension, neurologic impairment,
immobility, and altered mental status. Complications include
tissue loss, infection, and sepsis.

Assessment

1. Presence of risk factors.
2. Frequent observation of the skin, especially over pressure
   points (see *Figure P-4*).
3. Staging of the pressure sore to initiate appropriate treatment:
   a. Stage I—nonblanching macule that may appear red
      or violet
   b. Stage II—skin breakdown as far as the dermis
   c. Stage III—skin breakdown into subcutaneous tissue
   d. Stage IV—penetrates bone, muscle, or joint

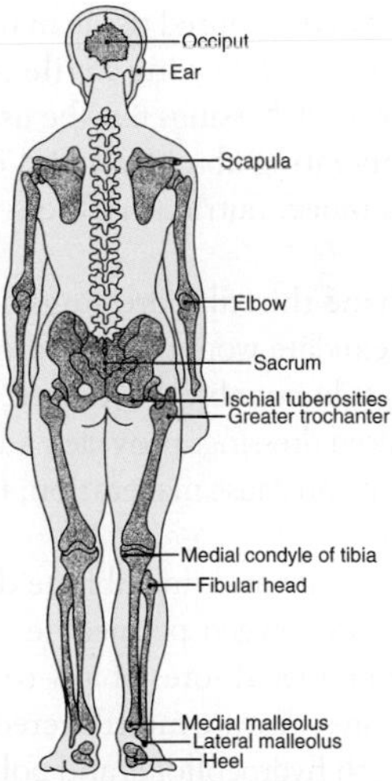

PQ

FIGURE P-4 Areas susceptible to pressure sores.

4. For stage IV pressure sores, assess for depth of ulcer and presence of tunneling; measure the entire diameter and depth of the ulcer.

Diagnostic Evaluation

1. No testing is usually indicated.
2. Wound cultures are usually inaccurate due to bacterial contamination and colonization, but may be done to guide antibiotic therapy when signs of infection are present.

Collaborative Management

Therapeutic Interventions

1. Pressure must be relieved and maceration, friction, and shearing forces avoided for wound healing to take place.
2. Normal saline is used for routine cleansing once to several times daily depending on amount of wound drainage, unless a protective dressing is used.
3. Wet-to-dry dressings may be used to assist with mechanical debridement.
4. Debridement of devitalized tissue may be necessary using scissors and scalpel following sterile technique.
5. Protective wound dressings may be used to minimize disruption of migrating fibroblasts and epithelial cells and to provide a moist, nutrient-rich environment for healing.
   a. Polyurethane thin film dressings are used for superficial, low-exudate wounds; they are air and water permeable but do not absorb exudate.
   b. Hydrocolloid dressings provide padding to stage I to II wounds but can cause maceration; they are not oxygen permeable.
   c. Polyurethane foam or membrane dressings absorb exudate and are oxygen permeable; used for skin tears, blisters, and stage II sores of low to moderate exudate.
   d. Hydrogel dressings are multilayered and include properties of both hydrocolloids and polyurethane; used for stage I to III sores.

Pharmacologic Interventions
1. Debriding enzymes may be used for stage III to IV ulcers; may damage healthy tissue and are not appropriate for hard eschar.
2. Topical antibiotics may be used to treat signs of local wound infection.
3. Analgesics are usually needed, particularly 30 to 60 minutes before wound care.

Nursing Diagnoses
3, 51, 63, 135, 136

Nursing Interventions
Monitoring
1. Monitor for signs of local infection (erythema around edges, foul odor, purulent exudate, poor healing) as well as sepsis (fever, cellulitis around wound, increased pain, decreased blood pressure, tachycardia, altered level of consciousness).
2. Assess size of pressure sore weekly in response to therapeutic measures; document the largest diameter, not just the surface diameter, and document at the greatest depth.
3. Monitor pain level and response to pain medication; in unresponsive patient, look for agitation, tachycardia, and increased blood pressure to indicate pain.
4. Monitor nutritional status through diet log and analysis, and serum albumin and prealbumin levels to ensure that healing can take place.

Supportive Care
1. Use pressure-reducing surface to help prevent pressure sores, but they are not effective in treating established pressure sores.
2. Avoid elevating head of bed more than 30 degrees to prevent shearing force as the patient slides downward against mattress.
3. Encourage activity and ambulation as much as possible.

PQ

4. Teach patient how to frequently shift weight and raise buttocks from chair every 30 minutes to relieve pressure and help prevent pressure sores.
5. Turn and reposition patients every 2 hours.
6. For established pressure sores, ensure that pressure is completely relieved from wound through positioning or use of special bed such as air-fluidized bed.
7. Bathe patient as needed with a bland soap, rinse, and blot dry with a soft towel.
8. Lubricate skin at least twice daily with a bland cream or gel, especially over pressure points.
9. Employ bowel and bladder programs to prevent incontinence.
10. Avoid plastic coverings and poorly ventilated chair or mattress surfaces.
11. Ensure that high-protein, nutritious diet is provided; utilize supplements as necessary and ensure adequate fluids to hydrate skin.
12. Provide pain medication as appropriate, particularly 30 to 60 minutes before wound care.
13. Clean pressure sore, as directed or per protocol; use normal saline or prescribed solution, irrigate as necessary to remove exudate, but do not disrupt healing tissue.
14. Facilitate debridement by applying wet-to-dry dressings as ordered, or apply enzymatic ointment, or assist with surgical debridement.
15. Apply gauze dressing or occlusive dressing as directed to protect pressure sore and aid in healing.

Education and Health Maintenance

1. Teach pressure-relieving methods for use at home for all patients who are not fully ambulatory.
2. Teach good skin care to prevent pressure sores.
3. Teach diet rich in protein, iron, and vitamin C to aid in full healing.
4. Educate family to identify stage I pressure sores and institute early treatment measures, and to report any stage II or greater pressure sore to the health care provider.

PROSTATE CANCER

See *Cancer, Prostate*.

PROSTATE SURGERY

Prostate surgery may be done to treat benign prostatic hyperplasia (BPH) or prostate cancer. The surgical approach depends on the size of the gland, severity of obstruction, the patient's age and underlying health, and the nature of the disease. There are two basic procedures.

Transurethral resection of the prostate (TUR or TURP) is the most common procedure. In TURP, the prostate is accessed and superficial lesions (early carcinomas, benign papillomas) are removed using a scope inserted through the urethra.

Open prostatectomy includes three approaches. Suprapubic prostatectomy (incision into the suprapubic area and through the bladder wall) is commonly used to treat BPH. Perineal prostatectomy (incision between the scrotum and rectal area) is used to treat prostate cancer. Because it has the highest incidence of urinary incontinence and impotence, it is usually used in patients who are no longer sexually active and who are at poor surgical risk for TURP. Retropubic prostatectomy (incision at level of symphysis pubis) is done for BPH and for prostate cancer; this approach preserves innervation related to sexual function in 50% of patients.

PQ

Potential Complications

1. Urinary incontinence
2. Retrograde ejaculation and sexual dysfunction
3. Wound infection and dehiscence
4. Urinary obstruction and infection
5. Hemorrhage
6. Thrombophlebitis and pulmonary embolism

Nursing Diagnoses

3, 6, 69, 135, 156, 163

Collaborative Management

Preoperative Care

1. Make sure that optimal cardiac, respiratory, and circulatory status have been achieved to decrease risk of complications.
2. Explain the nature of the procedure and the expected postoperative care, including catheter drainage, irrigation, and monitoring of hematuria.
3. Discuss complications of surgery and how patient will cope.
   a. Incontinence or dribbling of urine for up to 1 year after surgery; perineal (Kegel) exercises help regain urinary control.
   b. Retrograde ejaculation: seminal fluid released into bladder and eliminated in the urine rather than through prostatic fluid during intercourse.
   c. Impotence is usually not a complication of TURP but is commonly a complication of open prostatectomy.
4. Administer preoperative bowel preparation as prescribed, or instruct the patient in home administration and fasting after midnight.
5. Administer prophylactic antibiotics as ordered.

Postoperative Care

1. Maintain patency of urethral catheter placed after surgery.
   a. Monitor flow of three-way closed irrigation and drainage system if used.
   b. Using aseptic technique, perform manual irrigation with 1.7 oz (50 mL) irrigating fluid. Avoid overdistending the bladder, which could lead to hemorrhage.
2. Administer anticholinergic drugs, as ordered, to reduce bladder spasms.

 DRUG ALERT Anticholinergics are contraindicated in patients with narrow-angle glaucoma and paralytic ileus.

3. Assess degree of hematuria and any clot formation; drainage should become light pink within 24 hours.
   a. Report any arterial bleeding (bright red, with increased viscosity); surgical intervention may be required.

    b. Report any increase in venous bleeding (dark red); catheter traction may be needed to apply pressure to the prostatic fossa with inflated catheter balloon.

    c. Prepare for blood transfusion if bleeding persists.

4. Administer I.V. fluids as ordered and encourage oral fluids when tolerated to ensure hydration and urine output.

5. Maintain bed rest for the first 24 hours; frequently monitor vital signs, intake and output, and observe condition of incisional dressing, if present (no incision in TURP).

6. After 24 hours, encourage ambulation to prevent venous thrombosis, pulmonary embolism, and hypostatic pneumonia.

7. Observe urine for cloudiness or odor and obtain urine for evaluation of infection as ordered.

8. Report testicular pain, swelling, and tenderness, which could indicate epididymitis from spreading infection.

9. Assist with perineal care if perineal incision is present to prevent contamination by feces.

10. Administer pain medication or monitor patient-controlled analgesia as directed.

11. Position for comfort and tell the patient to avoid straining, which will increase pelvic venous congestion and may cause hemorrhage.

12. Administer stool softeners to prevent discomfort from constipation.

13. Make sure catheter is well secured to the patient's thigh to prevent traction on catheter, which will cause pain and potential hemorrhage.

EMERGENCY ALERT Avoid rectal temperatures, enemas, or rectal tubes postoperatively to prevent hemorrhage or disruption of healing.

Education and Health Maintenance

1. Tell patient to avoid sexual intercourse, straining at stool, heavy lifting, and long periods of sitting for 6 to 8 weeks after surgery, until prostatic fossa is healed.

2. Advise follow-up visits after treatment because urethral stricture may occur, and regrowth of prostate is possible

PQ

after TURP; prostate-specific antigen levels will be monitored every 3 to 6 months for prostate cancer patients.

3. Reassure patient that urinary incontinence, frequency, urgency, and dysuria are expected after the catheter is removed, and that these effects should gradually subside.

   a. If the patient is sent home catheterized, advise that catheter will be removed in about 3 weeks, when cystogram confirms healing.

   b. Discuss the use of absorbent products to contain urine leakage.

   c. Advise that incontinence is more pronounced when abdominal pressure is increased, such as coughing, laughing, or straining.

4. Teach pelvic floor exercises to regain urinary control.

   a. Have patient contract pelvic floor muscle as if to stop stream of urine or flatus; abdomen should be relaxed.

   b. Hold contraction for 5 seconds, then relax for 5 to 10 seconds.

   c. Practice this 15 to 20 times, three times per day.

5. Reinforce the surgeon's discussion of risk of impotence. Remind patient that erectile function may not return for as long as 6 months.

6. Encourage patient to express fears and anxieties related to potential loss of sexual function, and to discuss concerns with partner.

7. Advise that options, such as penile implant, are available to restore sexual function if impotence persists.

PROSTATIC HYPERPLASIA, BENIGN

Benign prostatic hyperplasia (BPH) is enlargement of the prostate that constricts the urethra, causing urinary symptoms. One of every four men who reach age 80 will require treatment for BPH. This disorder results from the effects of aging and the presence of circulating androgens. As prostatic tissue increases, nodules form and the outer capsule becomes thick and spongy. The effects of prolonged obstruction cause trabeculation (formation of cords) of the bladder, decreasing elasticity. Complications of BPH may include involuntary bladder contractions, bladder diverticula, cystolithiasis, vesicoureteral reflux, hydronephrosis, and urinary tract infection.

Assessment

1. In early or gradual prostatic enlargement, there may be no symptoms because the detrusor musculature can initially compensate for increased urethral resistance.
2. Obstructive symptoms include hesitancy, diminution in size and force of urinary stream, terminal dribbling, sensation of incomplete emptying of the bladder, and urinary retention.
3. Irritative voiding symptoms include urgency, frequency, and nocturia.
4. Enlarged prostate on rectal examination

Diagnostic Evaluation

1. Urinalysis rules out hematuria and infection.
2. Serum creatinine and blood urea nitrogen evaluate renal function.
3. Serum prostate-specific antigen (PSA) rules out cancer; however, PSA may also be elevated in BPH.
4. Additional diagnostic studies for further evaluation:
   a. Urodynamics measure peak urine flow rate, voiding time, and volume, and evaluate the bladder's ability to effectively contract.
   b. Measurement of postvoid residual urine by ultrasound or by catheterization
   c. Cystourethroscopy inspects the urethra and bladder and evaluates prostate size.

Collaborative Management
Therapeutic Interventions

1. Patients with mild symptoms (in the absence of significant bladder or renal impairment) are followed annually; BPH does not necessarily worsen in all men.
2. Balloon dilation of the prostatic urethra provides temporary relief of symptoms.

PQ

Pharmacologic Interventions

1. Alpha-adrenergic blockers, such as tamsulosin, doxazosin, or terazosin, to relax smooth muscle of bladder base and prostate to facilitate voiding.

 DRUG ALERT Alpha-adrenergic blockers (except tamsulosin) also have an antihypertensive effect. The medication should be started in a reduced dose and given at bedtime, then titrated up to prevent orthostatic hypotension.

2. Finasteride may be ordered for its antiandrogen effect on prostatic cells, which can reverse or prevent hyperplasia.

 DRUG ALERT Finasteride is present in semen and can have deleterious effects on the fetus of a pregnant woman.

Surgical Interventions

1. Transurethral resection of the prostate or transurethral incision of the prostate
2. Open prostatectomy (usually by suprapubic approach) may be required to remove a very large prostate.
3. Newer approaches include laser surgery; needle ablation, electrovaporization, insertion of prostatic stents or coils, and microwave hyperthermia treatments.

Nursing Diagnoses

69, 135

Nursing Interventions

Also see *Prostate Surgery*, page 759.

Supportive Care

1. To facilitate urinary elimination, provide privacy and time for the patient to void.
2. Assist with catheter insertion by way of guidewire or suprapubic cystotomy as indicated, and maintain catheter patency.
3. Monitor intake and output and postvoid residual as indicated.
4. Administer medications as ordered; teach the patient about adverse effects:

    a. Alpha-adrenergic blockers: hypotension, orthostatic hypotension, syncope (especially after first dose); impotence; blurred vision; rebound hypertension if discontinued abruptly

    b. Finasteride (Proscar): hepatic dysfunction; impotence; interference with PSA testing

5. Assess for and teach patient to report hematuria, signs of infection.

6. Be aware of and teach patient about drugs that may exacerbate urinary retention as BPH worsens — antidepressants, anticholinergics, decongestants, calcium channel blockers, tranquilizers, and alcohol.

Education and Health Maintenance

1. Tell patient to report urinary retention or signs of infection immediately.

ALTERNATIVE INTERVENTION

PQ

Saw palmetto is an herbal product that appears to be safe and somewhat effective in treating BPH. Advise patients that it may cause GI adverse effects and they should discuss its use with their health care providers.

---

2. After surgery, teach the patient to perform perineal (Kegel) exercises to help gain control over voiding:

    a. Contract the perineal muscle as if to stop stream of urine or control flatus, hold for 5 seconds, then relax.

    b. Repeat approximately 15 times (one set); do three sets per day.

3. Advise the patient that irritative voiding symptoms do not immediately resolve after obstruction is relieved, but that symptoms diminish over time.

4. Tell the patient to avoid sexual intercourse, straining at stool, heavy lifting, and long periods of sitting for 6 to 8 weeks after surgery until prostatic fossa is healed.

5. Advise follow-up visits after treatment because urethral stricture may occur and regrowth of prostate is possible after transurethral resection.

PULMONARY EDEMA

Pulmonary edema is the presence of excess fluid in the lung, either in the interstitial spaces or in the alveoli. Fluid accumulation in the alveoli impairs gas exchange, especially oxygen movement into pulmonary capillaries. This disorder is a common complication of cardiac disorders, including acute left ventricular failure, myocardial infarction, aortic stenosis, severe mitral valve disease, hypertension, and heart failure.

Pulmonary edema may also result from lung injuries, such as smoke inhalation, shock lung, pulmonary embolism, or infarct; from central nervous system injuries, such as stroke or head trauma; from allergies; and from infection (such as infectious pneumonia) and fever. It can also follow circulatory overload resulting from transfusions and infusions; adverse drug reactions, drug hypersensitivity, opioid overdose, or poisoning; it may also be a complication in patients who have undergone cardioversion, anesthesia, or cardiopulmonary bypass procedures. The disorder may progress to arrhythmias or respiratory failure.

 EMERGENCY ALERT Acute pulmonary edema is a true medical emergency, a life-threatening condition.

Assessment

1. Premonitory symptoms of cough and restlessness
2. Dyspnea, orthopnea, labored and rapid respirations, use of accessory muscles and retractions
3. White- or pink-tinged frothy sputum, inspiratory and expiratory wheezing, and bubbling sounds with respirations
4. Anxiety and panic because of suffocating feeling
5. Cyanosis with profuse perspiration, distended neck veins, and tachycardia
6. Inspiratory and expiratory wheezes, fine crackles beginning in the lung bases and progressing upward
7. Auscultation of the heart may reveal a third heart sound (S_3 gallop).

Diagnostic Evaluation

1. Chest X-ray shows interstitial edema.

2. Echocardiogram detects underlying valvular disease.
3. Pulmonary artery catheterization and measurement of pulmonary artery wedge pressure help differentiate cause.
4. Additional testing such as blood cultures, cardiac enzymes, and so forth determine cause; electrolytes, renal function tests, arterial blood gas (ABG) analysis, and so forth monitor effects of condition.

Collaborative Management
Therapeutic Interventions
1. Oxygen, in high concentration, relieves hypoxia, hypoxemia, and dyspnea.
2. Intubation and ventilatory support may be necessary to improve hypoxemia and prevent hypercarbia.

Pharmacologic Interventions
1. Morphine I.V. in small, titrated, intermittent doses, to reduce anxiety, promote venous pooling of blood in the periphery, and reduce vascular resistance and cardiac workload
   a. *Do not* give morphine if pulmonary edema is caused by stroke or occurs in the presence of chronic pulmonary disease or cardiogenic shock.
   b. Have morphine antagonist available to treat respiratory depression.
2. Diuretics I.V. to reduce blood volume and pulmonary congestion by producing prompt diuresis
3. Vasodilators, such as nitroglycerin or nitroprusside, to reduce amount of blood returning to the heart and the resistance against which the heart pumps
4. Positive inotropic agents, such as digoxin and dopamine, to enhance myocardial contractility and reduce fluid backup into the lungs
5. Aminophylline to prevent bronchospasm associated with pulmonary congestion, which may enhance myocardial contractility

PQ

Nursing Diagnoses
6, 57, 130

Nursing Interventions
Monitoring

1. Auscultate lung fields frequently and monitor progression or recession of wheezes, rhonchi, and moist, fine crackles.
2. Monitor for signs and symptoms of hypoxia, including restlessness, confusion, and headache.
3. Monitor hemodynamic status in response to therapy. Check blood pressure frequently and pulmonary artery pressure and cardiac output, as indicated; continuously monitor electrocardiogram for arrhythmias.

> **EMERGENCY ALERT** Watch for decreasing blood pressure, increasing heart rate, and decreasing urinary output — indications that the total body circulation is not tolerating diuresis and that hypovolemia may develop.

4. Monitor oxygen saturation and ABG levels as directed.
5. Monitor for respiratory depression and hypotension during morphine therapy.
6. Monitor potassium levels, daily weights, and intake and output while on diuretic therapy.

Supportive Care

1. Place the patient in upright position, with head and shoulders up, feet and legs hanging down, to favor pooling of blood in dependent extremities and decrease venous return.
2. Help reduce the patient's anxiety by remaining with and reassuring the patient. Explain in a calm manner all therapies administered and the reason for their use. (Arterial vasoconstriction diminishes when anxiety is relieved.)
3. Explain to the patient importance of wearing oxygen mask to improve breathing, but be aware of fear of suffocation.
4. Evaluate for headache due to vasodilator therapy and medicate as needed.
5. Continually evaluate the patient's response to therapy and report findings.
6. Allow the family to visit with patient for short periods and keep them informed of patient's condition; allow family time to express concerns and ask questions.

Education and Health Maintenance

1. Teach the patient about the pathogenesis of pulmonary edema to help prevent recurrence.
2. Help the patient to recognize and promptly report early symptoms of acute pulmonary edema.
3. If productive (wet) coughing develops, advise the patient to sit upright with legs dangling over the bedside to reduce symptoms.
4. See additional measures for heart failure, page 424.

PULMONARY EMBOLISM

Pulmonary embolism is obstruction of one or more pulmonary arteries by thrombi that are dislodged and carried to the lungs from their usual sites in the deep leg veins or in the right side of the heart. The obstruction restricts or cuts off blood flow, causing ventilation-perfusion ($\dot{V}/\dot{Q}$) mismatch and possible pulmonary infarction. Pulmonary emboli vary in size and seriousness of consequences; massive pulmonary embolism is a life-threatening emergency. Respiratory failure is the primary complication.

PQ

> **EMERGENCY ALERT** Be aware of risk factors for pulmonary embolism — immobilization, trauma to pelvis (especially surgical) and lower extremities (especially hip fracture), obesity, use of drugs (such as estrogen), history of thromboembolic disease, varicose veins, phlebitis, pregnancy, heart failure, myocardial infarction, malignant disease, postoperative period, estrogen therapy, and advancing age.

Assessment

1. Sudden onset of dyspnea.
2. Signs of hypoxia — headache, restlessness, apprehension, pallor, cyanosis, behavioral changes, tachypnea.
3. Pleuritic chest pain (worsens with coughing and deep breathing). Pain is accompanied by apprehension and a sense of impending doom when most of the pulmonary artery is obstructed.
4. Pleural friction rub, crackles, rhonchi, and wheezing.
5. Splitting of second heart sound, indicating increased right ventricular workload.

> ⚡ **EMERGENCY ALERT** Have a high index of suspicion for pulmonary embolus if there is a subtle deterioration in the patient's condition and unexplained cardiovascular and pulmonary findings.

6. Cyanosis, distended neck veins, tachyarrhythmias, syncope, and circulatory collapse in massive pulmonary embolism.

Diagnostic Evaluation

1. Arterial blood gas (ABG) analysis show decreased PaO_2 caused by abnormal lung perfusion.
2. Chest X-ray may show a possible wedge-shaped infiltrate.
3. $\dot{V}/\dot{Q}$ lung scan to evaluate regional blood flow and presence of perfusion defects. Ventilation may be abnormal with large perfusion defects.
4. Pulmonary angiography (most definitive test) in which emboli are shown as "filling defects."

Collaborative Management

Therapeutic Interventions

1. Emergency measures in massive pulmonary embolism, to stabilize cardiorespiratory status
   a. Oxygen to relieve hypoxemia, respiratory distress, and cyanosis
   b. I.V. to open a route for drugs and fluids
   c. Mechanical ventilation may be necessary

> ⚡ **EMERGENCY ALERT** Massive pulmonary embolism is a medical emergency; the patient's condition tends to deteriorate rapidly. There is a profound decrease in cardiac output, with an accompanying increase in right ventricular pressure.

Pharmacologic Interventions

1. Vasopressors, inotropic agents such as dopamine, or antiarrhythmic agents, to support circulation if the patient is unstable.
2. Small doses of morphine I.V. to relieve anxiety, alleviate chest discomfort (which improves ventilation), and ease adaptation to mechanical ventilator, if this is necessary.
3. After stabilization, heparin is given I.V. to stop further thrombus formation.

   a. I.V. loading dose is followed with continuous pump or drip infusion or give intermittently every 4 to 6 hours.
   b. Dosage is adjusted to maintain activated partial thromboplastin time at 1.5 to 2 times pretreatment value (if the value was normal).
   c. Protamine sulfate may be given to neutralize heparin in event of severe bleeding.
4. Thrombolytic agents such as streptokinase may be used if patient has massive pulmonary embolism.
   a. Give I.V. in a loading dose followed by constant infusion.
   b. Bleeding may result from fibrinolysis.
   c. Newer clot-specific thrombolytics (tissue plasminogen activator, streptokinase activator complex, single-chain urokinase) activate plasminogen only within thrombus itself rather than systematically, thus minimizing generalized fibrinolysis and subsequent bleeding.

EMERGENCY ALERT Discontinue thrombolytic therapy in the event of severe, uncontrolled bleeding.

5. Oral anticoagulant for follow-up anticoagulant therapy.
   a. Control dosage by monitoring serial prothrombin time and international normalized ratio of 2.0 to 3.0 as desired level.

GERONTOLOGIC ALERT Consider the patient's age and other medications in dosing of anticoagulation therapy — usually will need a decreased dosing regimen.

Surgical Interventions

1. Indications for surgery include contraindications to anticoagulation, recurrent embolization, or serious complications from drug therapy.
2. Embolectomy is the removal of embolus obstructing the pulmonary vasculature.
3. Prophylactic procedures include interruption of inferior vena cava (reducing size of vena cava by ligation or clipping) or placement of filter in vena cava (done transvenously usually through femoral vein).

Nursing Diagnoses
3, 6, 75, 88, 136

Nursing Interventions
Monitoring
1. Monitor vital signs, cardiac rhythm, oximetry, and ABG levels for adequacy of oxygenation.
2. Monitor for signs of shock; these include decreasing blood pressure; tachycardia; cool, clammy skin; and decreasing urine output.
3. Monitor for bleeding related to anticoagulant or thrombolytic therapy. Perform stool guaiac test and monitor platelet count to detect heparin-induced thrombocytopenia.
4. Monitor patient's response to I.V. fluids or vasopressors.

Supportive Care
1. Prepare the patient for assisted ventilation when hypoxemia occurs.
2. Position the patient with the head of bed slightly elevated (unless contraindicated by shock) and with chest splinted for deep breathing and coughing.
3. Correct dyspnea and relieve physical discomfort to help reduce anxiety. Give prescribed morphine and oxygen therapy and monitor for pain relief and signs of respiratory depression.

> **EMERGENCY ALERT** Assess for hypoxemia before administering sedative when increased anxiety or restlessness occurs. Look for cyanosis, circumoral pallor, and increased respiratory rate and obtain oxygen saturation.

4. Minimize risk of bleeding by performing essential ABG analysis on upper extremities or through arterial line. Apply digital compression at puncture site for 30 minutes, apply pressure dressing to previously involved sites, check site for oozing.
5. Maintain patient on strict bed rest during thrombolytic therapy and avoid unnecessary handling to reduce risk of rebleeding.

Education and Health Maintenance
1. Advise patient about the possible need to continue taking anticoagulant therapy for 6 weeks up to an indefinite period.
2. Teach about signs of bleeding, especially of gums, nose, bruising, or blood in urine and stools.
3. Warn patient against taking medications unless approved by health care provider because many drugs interact with anticoagulants.
4. Instruct patient to tell dentist about taking an anticoagulant.
5. Warn patient against inactivity for prolonged periods or sitting with legs crossed to prevent recurrence.
6. Warn patient against sports or activities that may cause injury to legs and predispose to a thrombus.
7. Encourage patient to wear a medical alert bracelet that identifies him or her as an anticoagulant user.
8. Instruct patient to lose weight if applicable; obesity is a risk factor for women.
9. Discuss contraceptive methods with patient, if applicable; advise female patients to avoid taking hormonal contraceptives.

PQ

PYELONEPHRITIS

Pyelonephritis is an acute inflammation and infection of the renal pelvis, tubules, and interstitial tissue. The disease typically results from infection by enteric bacteria (most commonly *Escherichia coli*) that have spread from the bladder to the ureters and kidneys secondary to vesicoureteral reflux. Other predisposing factors include urinary obstruction, recurrent infection, trauma, bloodborne infection, other renal disease, pregnancy, and metabolic disorders. Complications include renal insufficiency and possible chronic renal failure, hypertension, renal abscess, or perinephric abscess.

Assessment
1. Fever, chills, nausea, and vomiting
2. Costovertebral angle tenderness, flank pain (with or without radiation to groin)

PEDIATRIC ALERT Infants may display vomiting, irritability, and failure to thrive.

GERONTOLOGIC ALERT Elderly patients may exhibit GI or pulmonary symptoms or confusion only and not show the usual febrile response to pyelonephritis.

Diagnostic Evaluation

1. Urinalysis identifies leukocytes, bacteria, or pus in urine, gross or microscopic hematuria.
2. Urine culture identifies antibody-coated bacteria in urine. Bacteria invading the kidney induce an antibody response that coats the bacteria; this differentiates renal infection from bladder infection, in which bacteria are not coated.
3. I.V. urography and other urologic tests may be ordered to evaluate urinary tract obstruction and other causes.

Collaborative Management
Pharmacologic Interventions

1. Organism-specific antimicrobial therapy:
   a. Usually begun immediately to cover prevalent gram-negative pathogens, then adjusted according to urine culture results (taken before antibiotic is started).
   b. Treatment for 2 weeks or more is needed.
   c. Follow-up urine culture after completion of therapy.
2. Inpatient treatment with parenteral antimicrobial therapy if the patient cannot tolerate oral intake and is dehydrated or acutely ill.
3. Percutaneous drainage or prolonged antibiotic therapy is needed to treat renal or perinephric abscess.
4. Maintenance therapy for chronic or recurring infections to preserve renal function:
   a. Continuous treatment with urine-sterilizing agents after initial antibiotic treatment.
   b. Continue for months to years until there is no evidence of inflammation, causative factors have been treated or controlled, and renal function is stabilized.
   c. Serial urine cultures and evaluation studies must be done for an indefinite period.

d. Blood counts and serum creatinine determinations are required during long-term therapy.

Nursing Diagnoses
3, 49, 107

Nursing Interventions
Monitoring
1. Assess vital signs frequently for impending sepsis if patient is elderly or acutely ill.
2. Monitor intake and output.
3. Monitor renal function through urinalysis and serum blood urea nitrogen and creatinine.

Supportive Care
1. Administer or teach self-administration of antibiotics and analgesics as prescribed and monitor for effectiveness and adverse effects.
2. Administer antiemetic medications to control nausea and vomiting, and give antipyretics, as indicated.
3. Take measures to decrease body temperature if indicated (cooling blanket, application of ice to armpits and groin, and so forth).
4. Use comfort measures, such as positioning and heat, to locally relieve flank pain.
5. Correct dehydration by replacing fluids orally, if possible, or I.V.

Education and Health Maintenance
1. Explain to the patient possible causes of pyelonephritis and its signs and symptoms; also review signs and symptoms of lower urinary tract infection.
2. Review antibiotic therapy and stress importance of completing prescribed treatment regimen and having follow-up urine cultures.
3. Encourage follow-up (may be for 2 years after acute infection) to ensure eradication of infection and stabilization of kidney function.

PQ

4. Explain to the patient and family preventive measures including adequate fluid intake, healthy personal hygiene measures, and voiding habits.

PYLORIC STENOSIS, HYPERTROPHIC

Hypertrophic pyloric stenosis is congenital, progressive hypertrophy of the muscle of the pylorus, which causes narrowing or obstruction of the pyloric lumen. Constriction of the lumen dilates the stomach, delaying gastric emptying and leading to vomiting after feeding. The disorder has no known cause and is the second most common condition (after inguinal hernia) that requires surgery during the first 2 months of life. Rarely occurs before age 2 weeks or after age 5 months. It is more common among males and Caucasians. Severe cases may lead to dehydration, severe electrolyte imbalance, hematemesis, and starvation.

PEDIATRIC ALERT There may be a link between erythromycin use and the development of pyloric stenosis. Therefore, erythromycin is used very cautiously in infants younger than age 1 month.

Assessment
1. Onset is within the first 2 months after birth, usually at about age 3 to 6 weeks.
2. Vomiting — onset may be gradual and intermittent, vomiting after feeding, or sudden and forceful. May be occasional and nonprojectile, gradually increasing in frequency and intensity; or projectile vomiting, not bile stained.
3. Decreased quantity of stools.
4. Loss of weight or failure to gain weight if diagnosis is delayed.
5. Visible gastric peristaltic waves, left to right.
6. Excessive hunger — willingness to eat immediately after vomiting.
7. Dehydration — electrolyte disturbance with alkalosis if diagnosis delayed.
8. Palpable pyloric mass ("olive") in upper right quadrant of abdomen, to the right of the umbilicus, and best felt during feeding or immediately after vomiting.

Diagnostic Evaluation

1. Palpation shows pyloric mass in conjunction with persistent, projectile vomiting.
2. Radiographs of abdomen show dilated, air-filled stomach; nondilated pyloric canal.
3. Barium swallow shows narrowed pyloric canal, delayed gastric emptying, enlarged stomach, increased peristaltic waves, and gas distal to stomach.
4. Ultrasound evaluation shows thick hyperechoic ring in the region of the pylorus.

Collaborative Management
Therapeutic Interventions

1. Initial treatment if infant is dehydrated or in metabolic alkalosis aims to rehydrate to correct electrolytes, correct metabolic alkalosis.
2. Replacement of body fat and protein stores depends on severity of depletion and may require total parenteral nutrition for several days or weeks before surgery to improve surgical risk.

PQ

Surgical Interventions

1. Pyloromyotomy (Rammstedt procedure)
   a. Hypertrophy of the pyloric muscle regresses to normal size by approximately 12 weeks postoperatively.
   b. Gastroesophageal reflux may be a complication of surgery.

Nursing Diagnoses
3, 6, 23, 51, 104

Nursing Interventions
Monitoring

1. Carefully observe output, including amount and characteristics of urine (including specific gravity), also emesis and stools.
2. Accurately measure daily weight as a guide for calculating need for parenteral fluid.
3. Monitor laboratory data for serum electrolytes.

4. Monitor vital signs as indicated by condition. Watch for tachycardia, hypotension, and change in respirations.
5. Monitor blood glucose levels to prevent hypoglycemia.
6. Observe for drainage or signs of inflammation at surgical incision site.

> **EMERGENCY ALERT** Some postoperative vomiting is expected but should decrease over 48 hours. If persistent, a contrast study should be done to rule out gastric leak, fluid collection obstructing the gastric outlet, or other causes of obstruction.

Supportive Care
Preoperative Care

1. Administer I.V. therapy as ordered to treat dehydration, metabolic alkalosis, and electrolyte deficiency.
2. Position the infant to prevent interference with fluid therapy.
3. Maintain NPO status with indwelling nasogastric (NG) tube as ordered. Ensure proper functioning of tube and note drainage. Provide infant with a pacifier.
4. If oral feedings are to be continued, do the following:
   a. Provide small, frequent feedings; give slowly.
   b. Bubble frequently, before, during, and after feeding.
   c. Thicken formula if ordered.
   d. Allow breast-feeding as tolerated.
5. Prop the patient in upright position.
   a. Elevate head of bed, mattress, or infant seat at 75- to 80-degree angle.
   b. Place slightly on right side to aid gastric emptying.
6. Provide mouth care and wet lips frequently if NPO.
7. Provide for physical contact or nearness without excessive stimulation.
8. Provide for audio and visual stimulation that may be soothing.
9. Assess parents' understanding of diagnosis and plan of care. Provide specific information and clarify any misconceptions.
10. Prepare the parents for the surgery of their child; prepare them for the expected postoperative appearance of the infant.

11. Allow the parents to hold the infant to maintain bonding.
12. Reassure the parents that surgery is considered curative, and normal feeding should resume shortly afterward.

Postoperative Care

1. Elevate head slightly.
2. Maintain patent NG tube to prevent gastric distention. Record losses.
3. Administer I.V. fluids until adequate intake has been established.
4. When order is made to restart feedings (usually 6 hours after surgery), start with small, frequent feedings of glucose water and slowly advance to full-strength formula and regular diet, as tolerated.
5. Report vomiting — the amount and characteristics. Feeding schedule may be withheld 4 hours and then restarted.
6. Feed infant slowly and bubble frequently.
7. Increase the amount of feeding because the time between feedings is lengthened.
8. Allow breast-feeding to resume as tolerated (if cleared with surgeon); begin with limited nursing of 5 to 8 minutes and gradually increase.
9. Continue to elevate the infant's head and shoulders after feeding for 45 to 60 minutes, for several feedings after surgery. Place on right side to aid gastric emptying.
10. Expect that regurgitation may continue for a short period after surgery.
11. Administer analgesics as ordered and as indicated by behavior of infant.
12. Involve parents in care of infant postoperatively to prepare them for care after discharge.

Education and Health Maintenance

1. Teach parents proper care of the operative site, including watching for signs of infection. Provide specific care of site as ordered by health care provider.

PQ

2. Teach parents feeding technique to be continued at home; length of feeding technique varies, depending on wound healing, nutritional status, and growth. Advise parents that poor nutritional status may delay wound healing.

3. Provide written and verbal instructions regarding infant's care and follow-up schedule.

4. Review with family when medical attention is needed and appropriate resource:
   a. Signs of infection
   b. Frequent vomiting or poor feeding with signs of dehydration
   c. Abdominal distention

R

RAYNAUD'S DISEASE

Raynaud's disease (vasospastic disorder) refers to a condition of intermittent arteriolar vasoconstriction due to increased or unusual sensitivity to cold or emotional factors. Vasospasm results in coldness, numbness, and pallor, then cyanosis of the fingertips or toes. The cause of Raynaud's disease is unknown, but symptoms must last at least 2 years to confirm the diagnosis. If the disorder is primary, it is called Raynaud's disease; if it is secondary to connective tissue disorders, such as polymyositis, systemic lupus erythematosus, and scleroderma, it is called *Raynaud's phenomenon* or *Raynaud's syndrome*. Complications of Raynaud's disease include atrophy of skin and ulceration of involved digits.

Assessment

1. Characteristic color changes (white to blue to red):
   a. White: blanching, dead-white appearance if vasospasm is severe
   b. Blue: cyanotic, relatively stagnant blood flow due to prolonged vasoconstriction
   c. Red: a reactive hyperemia on rewarming; may be accompanied by pain
2. Changes in sensation: initial coldness is replaced by numbness, and finally paresthesias and pain as spasm resolves.
3. Ulcerations on fingertips or toes may be present.
4. Warmth brings about symptom relief, but it may be delayed.

Diagnostic Evaluation

1. Immunologic tests, such as antinuclear antibody, to rule out connective tissue diseases
2. Arterial Doppler study to rule out acute arterial occlusion if vasospasm is severe

Collaborative Management
Therapeutic Interventions
1. Smoking cessation; smoking increases vasoconstriction
2. Protection of extremities from cold
3. Optimal management of underlying disorder

Pharmacologic Interventions
1. Calcium channel blockers to prevent or reduce vasospasm
2. Nitroglycerin or sympatholytics, such as reserpine or prazosin, to cause vasodilation. Adverse effects include headache, dizziness, and orthostatic hypotension, which may necessitate discontinuation.
3. Antiplatelet agents, such as aspirin or ticlopidine, or the xanthine derivative pentoxifylline to prevent total occlusion.

ALTERNATIVE INTERVENTION

Biofeedback has been used successfully to alter the Raynaud's response in some patients.

Surgical Interventions
1. Sympathectomy (removal of the sympathetic ganglia or division of their branches) in selected cases to maintain vasodilation

Nursing Diagnoses
3, 24, 134

Nursing Interventions
Monitoring
1. Monitor condition of toes and fingertips for ulceration and infection.
2. Monitor for orthostatic hypotension if vasodilators or sympatholytics are used.

Supportive Care and Education
1. Administer and teach the patient about drug therapy.

a. Stress importance of taking prescribed drugs every day to prevent or minimize symptoms.

b. Advise patient to prevent orthostatic hypotension by changing positions slowly if taking sympatholytics.

2. Explain to the patient that pain may be experienced when spasm is relieved — hyperemic phase.

3. Administer or teach self-administration of analgesics.

4. Advise patient that a vasospastic episode may be stopped by placing the hands (or feet) in warm water.

5. Reassure the patient that pain is temporary. However, advise the patient to report persistent pain, ulceration, or signs of infection.

6. Help the patient learn to avoid triggers or aggravating factors of vasoconstriction.

a. Prevent exposure to cold — wear gloves while outside, turn on heater in car before traveling, use insulated cups for cold beverages, and wear gloves while shopping for frozen food.

b. Stop smoking, especially outdoors when cool.

c. Avoid stressful situations; use stress management techniques.

7. Advise patient to avoid injuring fingers and hands (eg, needle pricks, knife cuts), which may introduce infection and cause impaired healing.

RECTOCELE/ENTEROCELE

Rectocele is displacement (protrusion) of the rectum into the vagina. *Enterocele* is displacement of a segment of the intestine into the vagina. These conditions may result from weakening of the posterior vaginal wall caused by obstetric trauma and childbirth, pelvic surgery, or aging. They may result in total fecal incontinence if left untreated.

Assessment

1. Pelvic pressure or heaviness, backache, perineal burning; aggravated by standing for long periods

2. Constipation — may have difficulty in fecal evacuation; the patient may insert fingers into vagina to push feces up so defecation may take place.

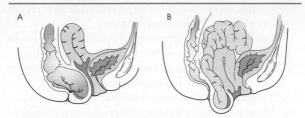

FIGURE R-1 **(A)** Rectocele. **(B)** Enterocele and prolapsed uterus.

3. Fecal incontinence and flatus may occur with tear between rectum and vagina.
4. Visible protrusion into vagina when patient bears down or stands. (See *Figure R-1*.)

Diagnostic Evaluation
1. Vaginal examination detects condition
2. May use Sims' speculum to uplift cervix and fully evaluate condition

Collaborative Management
Therapeutic and Pharmacologic Interventions
1. Vaginal pessary to insert into vagina to temporarily support pelvic organs
   a. Prolonged use may lead to necrosis and ulceration
   b. Should be removed and cleaned every 1 to 2 months
2. Estrogen therapy after menopause to decrease genital atrophy

Surgical Interventions
1. If rectocele is large and interferes with bowel functioning, may do posterior colpoplasty (perineorrhaphy) — repair of posterior vaginal wall

Nursing Diagnoses
3, 122, 135

Nursing Interventions
Also see *Gastrointestinal or Abdominal Surgery*, page 381.

Supportive Care
1. Encourage periods of rest with legs elevated to relieve pelvic strain, and teach Kegel exercises.
2. Encourage use of mild analgesics as needed.
3. Provide postoperative care.
   a. Suggest low-Fowler's position to reduce edema and discomfort.
   b. Administer perineal care to the patient after each voiding and bowel movement to prevent infection.
   c. Use a heat lamp to help dry the incision line and enhance the healing process.
   d. Apply ice packs locally to relieve congestion and discomfort.
   e. Administer analgesics and stool softeners as ordered.
4. Teach the patient to increase fluid and fiber in diet.
5. Encourage use of stool softeners or bulk laxatives to make passage of stool easier.
6. Enema may be necessary to prevent straining.

Education and Health Maintenance
1. Advise the patient to avoid straining and obesity, which may cause return of rectocele or enterocele.
2. Encourage patient to follow up and report bowel problems.

REGIONAL ENTERITIS
See *Crohn's Disease*.

RENAL CELL CARCINOMA
See *Cancer, Renal Cell*.

RENAL FAILURE, ACUTE
Acute renal failure (ARF) is a sudden decline in renal function, usually marked by increased concentrations of blood urea nitrogen (BUN; azotemia) and creatinine; oliguria (less than 17 oz [500 mL] urine in 24 hours); hyperkalemia; and sodium

R

retention. ARF has many causes, which are classified as prerenal, postrenal, and intrarenal. Prerenal failure results from conditions that interrupt the renal blood supply, thereby reducing renal perfusion (hypovolemia, shock, hemorrhage, burns, impaired cardiac output, diuretic therapy). Postrenal failure results from obstruction of urine flow. Intrarenal failure results from injury to the kidneys themselves (ischemia, toxins, immunologic processes, systemic and vascular disorders).

Whatever the cause, ARF progresses through three clinically distinct phases (oliguric–anuric, diuretic, and recovery), distinguished primarily by changes in urine volume and BUN and creatinine levels. The disorder can be reversed with medical treatment. Complications of ARF include dysrhythmias, increased susceptibility to infection, electrolyte abnormalities, GI bleeding due to stress ulcers, and multiple organ failure. Untreated ARF can also progress to chronic renal failure, end-stage renal disease, and death from uremia or related causes.

Assessment

1. Oliguric–anuric phase: urine volume less than 400 mL per 24 hours; increase in serum creatinine, urea, uric acid, organic acids, potassium, and magnesium; lasts 3 to 5 days in infants and children, 10 to 14 days in adolescents and adults.
2. Diuretic phase: begins when urine output exceeds 500 mL per 24 hours, ends when BUN and creatinine levels stop rising; length is variable.
3. Recovery phase: asymptomatic; lasts several months to 1 year; some scar tissue may remain
4. In prerenal disease — decreased tissue turgor, dryness of mucous membranes, weight loss, flat neck veins, hypotension, tachycardia
5. In postrenal disease — difficulty in voiding; changes in urine flow
6. In intrarenal disease, presentation varies; usually have edema, may have fever, skin rash.
7. Nausea, vomiting, diarrhea, and lethargy may also occur.

Diagnostic Evaluation

1. Urinalysis shows proteinuria, hematuria, casts. Urine chemistry distinguishes various forms of ARF (prerenal, postrenal, intrarenal).
2. Serum creatinine and BUN levels are elevated; arterial blood gas (ABG) levels, serum electrolytes may be abnormal.
3. Renal ultrasonography estimates renal size and rules out treatable obstructive uropathy.

Collaborative Management

Therapeutic and Pharmacologic Interventions

See Box R-1.

BOX R-1	Prevention of Renal Failure

- Identify patients with preexisting renal disease.
- Initiate adequate hydration before, during, and after operative procedures.
- Avoid exposure to various nephrotoxins. Be aware that most drugs or their metabolites are excreted by the kidneys. Ensure that dosages are adjusted to the degree of renal impairment of individual patients.
- Avoid chronic analgesic abuse — causes interstitial nephritis and papillary necrosis.
- Prevent and treat shock with blood and fluid replacement. Prevent prolonged periods of hypotension.
- Monitor urinary output and central venous pressure hourly in critically ill patients to detect onset of renal failure at the earliest moment.
- Schedule diagnostic studies requiring dehydration so there are "rest days," especially in elderly patients who may not have adequate renal reserve.
- Pay special attention to draining wounds, burns, and so forth, which can lead to dehydration, sepsis, and progressive renal damage.
- Avoid infection; give meticulous care to patients with indwelling catheters and I.V. lines.
- Take every precaution to ensure that the right person receives the right blood to avoid severe transfusion reactions that can precipitate renal complications.

1. Surgical relief of obstruction may be necessary
2. Correction of underlying fluid excesses or deficits
3. Correction and control of biochemical imbalances
   a. Hyperkalemia: Give glucose and insulin to shift potassium into cells; cation exchange resin orally or by enema to promote rectal excretion of potassium.
   b. Acidosis: Give sodium bicarbonate; be prepared for mechanical ventilation.
4. Restoration and maintenance of blood pressure through I.V. fluids and vasopressors
5. Maintenance of adequate nutrition: Low-protein diet with supplemental amino acids and vitamins
6. Initiation of hemodialysis, peritoneal dialysis, or continuous renal replacement therapy for patients with progressive azotemia and other life-threatening complications

Nursing Diagnoses
35, 42, 51, 135

Nursing Interventions
Monitoring
1. Monitor 24-hour urine volumes to follow clinical course of the disease.
2. Monitor BUN, creatinine, and electrolytes.
3. Monitor for signs and symptoms of hypovolemia or hypervolemia because regulating capacity of kidneys is inadequate.
4. Monitor urine specific gravity; measure and record intake and output, including urine, gastric suction, stools, wound drainage, perspiration (estimate). Specific gravity fixed at 1.010 indicates the kidneys' inability to concentrate urine.
5. Monitor electrocardiogram for dysrhythmias and changes associated with electrolyte imbalance, and report signs and symptoms of hyperkalemia (see page 351).
6. Monitor ABG levels as necessary to evaluate acid-base balance.

7. Weigh the patient daily to provide an index of fluid balance; expected weight loss is ½ to 1 lb (0.3 to 0.5 kg) daily.

8. Measure blood pressure at various times during the day with patients in supine, sitting, and standing positions.

9. Monitor for signs of infection. Be aware that patients with renal failure do not always have fever and leukocytosis.

10. Watch for and report mental status changes, including somnolence, lassitude, lethargy, and fatigue progressing to irritability, disorientation, twitching, and seizures.

Supportive Care

1. Adjust fluid intake to avoid volume overload and dehydration.
   a. Fluid restriction is not usually initiated until renal function is quite low.
   b. Give only enough fluids to replace losses during oliguric-anuric phase (usually 13.5 to 17 oz [400 to 500 mL] every 24 hours plus measured fluid losses).
   c. Fluid allowance should be distributed throughout the day.
   d. Restrict sodium and water intake if there is evidence of extracellular excess.

EMERGENCY ALERT Avoid restricting fluids for prolonged periods for laboratory and radiologic examinations because dehydrating procedures are hazardous to patients who cannot produce concentrated urine.

2. Watch for cardiac dysrhythmias and heart failure from hyperkalemia, electrolyte imbalance, or fluid overload. Have resuscitation equipment available in case of cardiac arrest.

PEDIATRIC ALERT Give I.V. fluids very slowly to prevent heart failure; monitor for bounding pulse, dyspnea, third heart sound, and pulmonary crackles.

3. Treat hyperkalemia as ordered: administer sodium bicarbonate or glucose and insulin to drive potassium into cells; and administer cation exchange resin enema to absorb potassium through rectal and colon wall.

4. If ordered, prepare for dialysis when rapid lowering of potassium is needed. If blood transfusions are ordered, administer during dialysis to prevent hyperkalemia from stored blood.

5. Watch for signs of urinary tract infection, and remove bladder catheter as soon as possible.

6. Employ intensive pulmonary hygiene because incidence of pulmonary edema and infection is high.

7. Provide meticulous wound care.

8. Work with the dietitian to regulate protein intake according to the type of renal impairment. Protein and potassium are usually restricted. Be aware that food and fluids containing large amounts of sodium and phosphorus may need to be restricted.

9. Offer high-carbohydrate feedings because carbohydrates have a greater protein-sparing power and provide additional calories.

10. Prepare for hyperalimentation when adequate nutrition cannot be maintained through the GI tract. Nutrients can also be added through dialysate.

11. To prevent or treat gastric bleeding caused by stress ulcers:
    a. Examine all stools and emesis for gross and occult blood.
    b. Administer histamine-2 (H_2) receptor antagonists or antacids as prophylaxis for gastric stress ulcers. If H_2-receptor antagonist is used, care must be taken to adjust the dose for the degree of renal impairment.
    c. Prepare for endoscopy if GI bleeding occurs.

12. Institute seizure precautions. Provide padded side rails and have airway and suction equipment at the bedside.

13. Encourage and assist the patient to turn and move because drowsiness and lethargy may reduce activity.

Education and Health Maintenance

1. Explain that the patient may experience residual defects in kidney function for a long time after acute illness.

2. Encourage the patient to report for routine urinalysis and follow-up examinations.

3. Advise patient to avoid any medication unless specifically prescribed.
4. Recommend resuming activity gradually because muscle weakness will be present from excessive catabolism.

RENAL FAILURE, CHRONIC

Chronic renal failure (CRF; end-stage renal disease [ESRD]) is a progressive deterioration of renal function, which ends fatally in uremia (an excess of urea and other nitrogenous wastes in the blood) and its complications unless dialysis or kidney transplantation is performed. Typically, the disease produces few signs and symptoms until approximately 75% of renal function (glomerular filtration) has already been lost.

Causes of CRF include prolonged, severe hypertension; diabetes mellitus; glomerulopathies and hereditary renal disease (common causes in children ages 5 to 15); interstitial nephritis; obstructive uropathy; and developmental or congenital disorders (common causes in children younger than age 5).

As renal function deteriorates, the disease may progress through four stages: (1) decreased renal reserve; (2) renal insufficiency; (3) renal failure; and (4) ESRD, leading to uremia. Decreased glomerular filtration rate stimulates renin-angiotensin system and aldosterone secretion, which causes retention of sodium and water and raises blood pressure. The kidneys are unable to concentrate hydrogen ions, causing metabolic acidosis and increased production of ammonia.

Assessment

1. Cardiovascular manifestations: Hyperkalemic electrocardiogram (ECG) changes (see "Monitoring," page 793), hypertension caused by increased aldosterone secretion, heart failure, pericarditis, pericardial effusion, pericardial tamponade
2. Respiratory manifestations: pulmonary edema, pleural effusions, pleural friction rub
3. GI manifestations: anorexia, nausea, vomiting, hiccoughs, ulceration of GI tract, hemorrhage

4. Neuromuscular manifestations: fatigue, sleep disorders, headache, lethargy, muscular irritability, peripheral neuropathy, seizures, coma
5. Metabolic and endocrine manifestations: glucose intolerance, hyperlipidemia, and sex hormone disturbances causing decreased libido, impotence, amenorrhea
6. Fluid, electrolyte, and acid-base balance: usually salt and water retention but may be sodium loss with dehydration, acidosis, hyperkalemia, hypomagnesemia, hypocalcemia (see page 351)
7. Dermatologic manifestations: pallor, hyperpigmentation, pruritus, ecchymoses, uremic frost
8. Skeletal manifestations: renal osteodystrophy resulting in osteomalacia
9. Hematologic manifestations: anemia caused by reduced erythropoietin from kidney; reduced platelet quality, increased bleeding tendencies
10. Alterations in psychosocial functions: personality and behavior changes, alteration in cognitive processes
11. Developmental manifestations: growth retardation, delayed sexual maturation

Diagnostic Evaluation
1. Complete blood count shows anemia
2. Elevated serum creatinine, blood urea nitrogen, and phosphorus levels
3. Decreased serum calcium, bicarbonate, and proteins, especially albumin
4. Arterial blood gas (ABG) analysis shows metabolic acidosis: low pH, high carbon dioxide

Collaborative Management
Therapeutic Interventions
1. Reversible causes of renal failure are treated, such as diabetes and hypertension.
2. Fluid restriction and diet therapy:
   a. Low-protein diet supplemented with essential amino acids or their keto-analogs to minimize uremic toxicity and prevent wasting and malnutrition.

> **PEDIATRIC ALERT** Children need adequate protein for growth and development; see that 1 to 1.5 g/kg of protein is included in the diet daily.

    b. Potassium intake is limited.

    c. Dietary phosphorus is reduced (chicken, milk, legumes, carbonated beverages).

3. Maintenance dialysis or kidney transplantation when symptoms can no longer be controlled with conservative measures.

Pharmacologic Interventions

1. Anemia is treated with recombinant human erythropoietin, a synthetic kidney hormone that enhances red blood cell formation.
2. Acidosis is treated with oral or I.V. sodium bicarbonate to replace bicarbonate stores.
3. Cation exchange resin to promote enteric excretion of potassium.
4. Phosphate-binding agents because they bind phosphorus in the intestinal tract.
5. Calcium supplements and vitamin D to increase calcium absorption.
6. Growth hormone administration to treat growth retardation in children.

Nursing Diagnoses
15, 16, 34, 42, 51, 63, 86, 136

Nursing Interventions
Monitoring

1. Evaluate for signs and symptoms of hyperkalemia and monitor serum potassium levels.
    a. Notify health care provider of value above 5.5. mEq/L.
    b. Watch for dysrhythmias and ECG changes indicating hyperkalemia: tall, tented T waves; depressed ST segment; wide QRS complex.
2. Monitor ABG levels as necessary to evaluate acid-base balance.
3. Weigh the patient daily and maintain intake and output.

4. Monitor for edema and respiratory compromise from fluid volume excess.
5. Monitor hemoglobin and hematocrit.
6. Monitor for all signs of infection. Be aware that renal failure patients do not always demonstrate fever and leukocytosis.

Supportive Care

1. Administer parenteral nutrition or oral supplements if unable to maintain adequate diet.
2. Keep skin clean while relieving itching and dryness caused by excretion of nitrogenous waste through sweat (uremic frost).
   a. Basis brand soap
   b. Sodium bicarbonate added to bath water
   c. Oatmeal baths
   d. Adding bath oil to bath water
3. Apply ointments or creams for comfort and to relieve itching.
4. Keep nails short and trimmed to prevent excoriation.
5. Keep hair clean and moisturized.
6. Administer oral antipruritics, if indicated.
7. To prevent constipation caused by phosphate binders, encourage high-fiber diet, bearing in mind the potassium content of some fruits and vegetables.
   a. Commercial fiber supplements (Fiberall; Fiber-Med) may be recommended.
   b. Use stool softeners as prescribed.
   c. Avoid laxatives and cathartics that cause electrolyte toxicities (compounds containing magnesium or phosphorus).
   d. Increase activity as tolerated.
8. To help ensure safe activity level, assess patient's gait, range of motion, and muscle strength. Provide assistance with care and ambulation as needed.
9. Administer analgesics, as ordered, and provide massage for severe muscle cramps.
10. Increase activity as tolerated; avoid immobilization because it increases bone demineralization.

11. Explore alternatives that may reduce or eliminate adverse effects of treatment.
    a. Adjust schedule so rest can be achieved after dialysis.
    b. Smaller, more frequent meals to reduce nausea and facilitate medication taking.
12. Contract with the patient for behavioral changes if patient is nonadherent to therapy or control of underlying condition. Support the family in adjustment to chronic illness of a member.

Education and Health Maintenance

1. To promote adherence to the therapeutic program, teach the following:
   a. Weigh every morning to avoid fluid overload.
   b. Drink limited amounts *only* when thirsty.
   c. Measure allotted fluids and save some for ice cubes; sucking on ice is thirst quenching.
   d. Eat food before drinking fluids to alleviate dry mouth.
   e. Use hard candy or chewing gum to moisten mouth.
   f. Teach how to read labels and avoid foods that are high in potassium and sodium.
2. Encourage strict follow-up for blood work, dialysis, and health care provider visits.
3. Advise patient of financial and other support through social service agencies.

RESPIRATORY DISTRESS SYNDROME

Respiratory distress syndrome (RDS; hyaline membrane disease) is a progressive and frequently fatal respiratory failure resulting from lack of alveolar surfactant, a lipoprotein that functions to maintain alveolar patency. The syndrome occurs most frequently in premature infants weighing between 1,000 and 1,500 g (2.2 and 3.3 lb) and between 28 and 37 weeks' gestation; incidence increases with the degree of prematurity.

Respiratory distress syndrome is self-limiting for some infants; those who are moderately ill or those who do not require assisted ventilation usually show slow improvement by approximately 48 hours and rapid recovery over the next 3 to 4 days with few complications. However, severely ill and very premature infants who require some ventilatory assistance usually demonstrate rapid deterioration. Ventilatory assistance may be required for several days, and complications, including pneumothorax, disseminated intravascular coagulation, patent ductus arteriosus with heart failure, and chronic lung disease, are common. For some infants, alveolar collapse leads to atelectasis, hypoxia, acidosis, and death.

Assessment

1. Symptoms of RDS are usually observed soon after birth.
2. Retractions (sternal, suprasternal, substernal, and intercostal), progressing to paradoxical seesaw respirations.
3. Tachypnea (more than 60 breaths/minute), nasal flaring.
4. Expiratory grunting or whining sounds when not crying (indicates an attempt to maintain positive end-expiratory pressure [PEEP] and prevent alveoli from collapsing).
5. Cyanosis with room air.
6. Diminished breath sounds and presence of dry "sandpaper" breath sounds.
7. As the disease progresses: marked abdominal protrusion on expiration, peripheral edema, decreased muscle tone, increasing cyanosis, hypothermia, apnea, bradycardia, pale and grayish skin color.
   a. Lethargic or listless
   b. Activity and response to stimuli

Diagnostic Evaluation

1. Arterial blood gas (ABG) analysis reveals: elevated PCO_2 and low PO_2 and low pH
2. Decreased serum calcium
3. Chest X-ray shows diffuse, fine granularity reflecting fluid-filled alveoli and atelectasis of some alveoli, surrounded by hyperdistended bronchioles (Pulmonary interstitial emphysema is due to overdistention of distal airways.)
4. Pulmonary function studies may be done to evaluate stiff lung with reduced effective pulmonary blood flow
5. Prenatal assessment of amniotic fluid to assess lung maturity

Collaborative Management
Therapeutic Interventions
Supportive

1. Maintenance of oxygenation: PaO_2 at 60 to 80 mm Hg to prevent hypoxia; frequent pH and ABG measurements
2. Maintenance of respiration with ventilatory support if necessary — mechanical ventilation plus PEEP, or continuous positive airway pressure (CPAP)
3. Maintenance of normal body temperature
4. Constant observation for complications

Aggressive

1. High-frequency ventilation: mechanical ventilation that uses rapid rates (can be greater than 900 breaths per minute) and tidal volumes near and often less than anatomic dead spaces
   a. Jet ventilator delivers short burst of gases at high flow with passive exhalation. Necrotizing tracheitis is a significant complication.
   b. Oscillator ventilator delivers gases by vibrating columns of air with active exhalation. The child appears to shake on the bed, which may be frightening for parents.
2. Extracorporeal membrane oxygenation (ECMO): modified heart-lung bypass machine used to allow gas exchange outside the body
   a. Blood is removed from the venous system by a catheter placed in the internal jugular vein or right atrium.
   b. Oxygen is added and carbon dioxide removed with a membrane oxygenator.
   c. Oxygenated blood is returned by way of the right common carotid (in venoarterial ECMO) or the femoral vein (in venovenous ECMO).
   d. The infant must be heparinized for the procedure, increasing the risk of intraventricular hemorrhage. Thus, very-low-birth weight (VLBW) infants or infants of decreased gestational age are usually not candidates for the procedure.

R

Pharmacologic Interventions
Supportive
1. Maintenance of fluid, electrolyte, and acid-base balance — sodium bicarbonate is given to buffer metabolic acidosis
2. Nutrition maintained with I.V. dextrose 10%
3. Antibiotics as needed to treat infection

Aggressive
1. Administration of exogenous surfactant into lungs early in the disease
   a. Especially beneficial in the VLBW infant
   b. May be given preventatively to VLBW infants at birth
   c. Available preparations: bovine (Survanta) and synthetic (Exosurf) surfactant
   d. Administered into the endotracheal tube; suction avoided for a few hours after instillation

Nursing Diagnoses
51, 57, 61, 87

Nursing Interventions
Monitoring
1. Institute cardiorespiratory monitoring to continuously monitor heart and respiratory rates.
2. Monitor for complications related to respiratory therapy:
   a. Air leak: pneumothorax, pneumomediastinum, pneumopericardium, and pneumoperitoneum
   b. Pneumonia, especially gram-negative organisms
   c. Pulmonary interstitial emphysema
3. Measure and record oxygen concentration with mechanical ventilation every hour.
4. Monitor ABG levels as appropriate. Obtain sample through indwelling catheter (usually placed in the umbilical artery), arterial puncture, or capillary puncture.
5. Institute pulse oximetry for continuous monitoring of oxygen saturation of arterial blood.
   a. Avoid using adhesive to secure the sensor when infant is active. Wrap the sensor snugly enough around the

foot to reduce sensitivity to movement but not tight enough to constrict blood flow.

  b. If transcutaneous PO_2 monitoring is used, reposition the probe every 3 to 4 hours to avoid burns caused when the probe is heated to achieve sufficient vasodilation.

6. Observe the infant's response to oxygen.

  a. Observe for improvement in color, respiratory rate and pattern, and nasal flaring.

  b. Note response by improvement in arterial pH, PaO_2, $PaCO_2$, or capillary blood gas.

  c. Observe closely for apnea.

EMERGENCY ALERT Stimulate infant if apnea occurs. If infant is unable to produce spontaneous respiration within 15 to 30 seconds of stimulation, initiate resuscitation.

7. If umbilical artery catheter is in place, monitor for bleeding.

8. When providing I.V. fluids or enteral nutrition, observe infusion rate closely to prevent fluid overload. Also monitor for hypoglycemia, which is especially common during stress. Maintain serum glucose greater than 45 mg/dL.

9. Monitor intake and output closely and weigh infant daily.

Supportive Care

1. Have emergency resuscitation equipment readily available for use in the event of cardiac or respiratory arrest.

2. Administer supplemental oxygen.

  a. Incubator with oxygen at prescribed concentration

  b. Plastic hood with oxygen at prescribed concentration when using radiant warmer

  c. CPAP, if indicated, by way of face mask, nasal prongs, or endotracheal tube

3. Assist with endotracheal intubation and maintain mechanical ventilation as indicated.

4. Position the infant to allow for maximal lung expansion and change position frequently.

  a. Prone position provides for a larger lung volume because of the position of the diaphragm; decreases energy expenditure; and increases time spent in quiet sleep.

b. May be contraindicated when umbilical artery catheter is in place.

c. Prone positioning increases the risk of sudden infant death syndrome, but the infant will be continually monitored.

PEDIATRIC ALERT Although the prone position is preferred for neonates and infants with RDS, it may present several problems. Turning head to side can compromise upper airway and increase air flow resistance; observation of chest is obstructed, retractions are more difficult to detect, and abdominal distention is more difficult to recognize.

5. Suction as needed because the gag reflex is weak and cough is ineffective.

6. Try to minimize time spent on procedures and interventions, and monitor effects on respiratory status. (Infants undergoing multiple procedures lasting 45 minutes to 1 hour have shown a moderate decrease in PaO_2.)

7. Provide adequate caloric intake (80 to 120 kcal/kg/ 24 hours) through nasojejunal tube (best tolerated by VLBW infants), nasogastric tube, or parenteral nutrition.

8. Provide a neutral thermal environment to maintain the infant's abdominal skin temperature between 97° and 98° F (36° and 36.7° C) to prevent hypothermia, which may result in vasoconstriction and acidosis.

9. Adjust Isolette or radiant warmer to obtain desired skin temperature.

a. For the infant weighing less than 1,250 g (44 oz), the radiant warmer should be used with caution because of increased water loss and potential for hypoglycemia.

b. Prevent frequent opening of Isolette.

10. Ensure that O_2 is warmed to 87.6° to 93.2° F (31° to 34° C) with 60% to 80% humidity.

11. Allow the parents to hold the infant as soon as possible and participate in care.

12. If the mother plans to breast-feed, assist her with pumping; use the breast milk to feed the infant when enteral feedings are initiated.

13. If the infant has been transported to a tertiary care center immediately after birth, prepare the parents for the neonatal intensive care unit, and update them on the infant's condition until they are able to visit.
14. If the infant has siblings, advise the parents on how to discuss the infant's illness with them.
15. Help the parents work through their grief at the birth of a premature infant.

Education and Health Maintenance

1. Prepare the family for long-term follow-up as appropriate. Infants with bronchopulmonary dysplasia may eventually go home on oxygen therapy.
2. Stress to the parents the importance of regular health care, periodic eye examinations, and developmental follow-up.
3. Make sure that the family receives information on routine well-baby care.
4. Before discharging, parents should feel comfortable in their abilities to care for infant, referrals for visiting nurses should be completed, and physician for follow-up care should be identified and appointment should be made.

RESPIRATORY FAILURE

Respiratory failure is an alteration in the function of the respiratory system that causes the PaO_2 to decrease to below 50 mm Hg (hypoxemia) or the $PaCO_2$ to increase to above 50 mm Hg (hypercapnia), as determined by arterial blood gas (ABG) analysis.

This complex condition is more a dysfunction than a disease, and occurs in several recognized forms. *Acute respiratory failure* occurs rapidly, usually within minutes to hours or days, and is marked by hypoxemia or hypercapnia and acidemia (pH less than 7.35); *chronic respiratory failure* occurs over a period of months to years, allowing compensatory mechanisms to operate; it is marked by hypoxemia or hypercapnia with a normal pH (7.35 to 7.40). *Combined acute and chronic respiratory failure* may occur after an acute upper respiratory infection or pneumonia (or without obvious cause) and is marked by an abrupt increase in hypoxemia or hypercapnia in patients with preexisting chronic respiratory failure.

Respiratory failure results from three physiologic conditions that increase the work of breathing and decrease respiratory drive: oxygenation failure, ventilatory failure in normal lungs, and ventilatory failure in intrinsic lung disease.

Oxygenation failure results from damage to the alveolar-capillary membrane that causes leakage of fluid into the interstitial space or alveoli. Causes of oxygenation failure include cardiogenic pulmonary edema and adult respiratory distress syndrome from shock of any cause, infections, trauma, near drowning, inhaled toxins, severe hematologic conditions, and metabolic disorders.

Ventilatory failure results from insufficient respiratory center stimulation or chest wall movement, causing alveolar hypoventilation. Causes of ventilatory failure in normal lungs include opioid overdose, general anesthesia, cerebral vascular insufficiency, brain tumor or trauma, increased intracranial pressure, neuromuscular disease, chest wall trauma (multiple fractures), or spinal cord trauma.

Ventilatory failure in intrinsic lung disease is characterized by hypercapnia because damage to lung parenchyma or airway obstruction limits the amount of carbon dioxide removed from the lungs. Causes include chronic obstructive pulmonary disease (COPD), cystic fibrosis, and severe asthma.

Complications of respiratory failure include oxygen toxicity from the prolonged high fractional inspired oxygen (FIO_2) required, barotrauma from mechanical ventilation, and death.

Assessment

1. Increased work of breathing signaled by diaphoresis, rapid shallow breathing, abdominal paradox (inward movement of abdominal wall during inspiration), and intercostal retractions.
2. Breath sounds may be diminished or absent indicating inability to ventilate the lungs sufficiently to prevent atelectasis; crackles caused by secretions and interstitial fluid; wheezing indicating bronchospasm; rhonchi indicating secretions in larger airways.

3. Confusion, restlessness, agitation, disorientation, delirium, and loss of consciousness signify hypoxemia; headache, somnolence, dizziness, and confusion signify hypercapnia.

Diagnostic Evaluation

1. ABG analysis shows deviations in Pao_2, $Paco_2$, and pH from patient's normal; or Pao_2 less than 50 mm Hg, $Paco_2$ greater than 50 mm Hg, and pH less than 7.35.
2. Pulse oximetry detects decreasing Sao_2.
3. End-tidal CO_2 monitoring (capnography) shows increase.
4. Complete blood count, serum electrolytes, urinalysis, and cultures (blood, sputum) determine underlying cause and patient's condition.
5. Chest X-ray may show underlying disease.

Collaborative Management
Therapeutic Interventions

1. Oxygen therapy to maintain Pao_2 of 60 mm Hg or Sao_2 greater than 90%. Use aerosol mask, partial rebreathing mask, or non-rebreathing mask to provide high oxygen concentration.

R

EMERGENCY ALERT Avoid high concentration of oxygen (Fio_2 of 100%) in patients with COPD because this may obliterate their usual hypoxic drive to breathe.

2. Mechanical ventilation may be necessary. Noninvasive positive-pressure ventilation using a face mask has been used in some patients.
3. Chest physical therapy and hydration to mobilize secretions.

Pharmacologic Interventions

1. Antibiotics, cardiac drugs, and diuretics to treat underlying disorder
2. Bronchodilators to reduce bronchospasm and corticosteroids to reduce airway inflammation; given orally, I.V., or by nebulization

3. Neuromuscular blockade with pancuronium to facilitate ventilation in some cases; heightened monitoring, sedation, and analgesia are required in these cases
4. I.V. fluids and mucolytics to reduce sputum viscosity

Nursing Diagnoses
6, 51, 57, 73

Nursing Interventions
Monitoring
1. Monitor fluid balance by measuring intake and output, urine specific gravity, daily weights, and pulmonary artery wedge pressure to detect hypovolemia or hypervolemia.
2. Monitor vital capacity (VC), respiratory rate, and negative inspiratory force (NIF). Values indicating need for mechanical ventilation:
   a. VC less than 10 to 15 mL/kg
   b. Respiratory rate greater than 35 breaths/minute
   c. NIF less than 20 to 25 cm H_2O
3. Monitor ABG levels and compare with previous values.
   a. If the patient cannot maintain a minute ventilation sufficient to prevent CO_2 retention, the pH will decrease.
   b. Mechanical ventilation may be needed if the pH decreases to less than 7.30.

EMERGENCY ALERT Obtain ABG levels whenever the history or signs and symptoms suggest the patient is at risk for developing respiratory failure. Initial and subsequent values should be recorded on a flow sheet so comparisons can be made over time. The need for ABG analysis can be reduced by using an oximeter to continuously monitor Sao_2.

4. If patient is paralyzed due to neuromuscular blockade, monitor autonomic signs of anxiety and pain, such as increased blood pressure, tachycardia, increased lacrimation, and diaphoresis.

Supportive Care

1. Provide measures to prevent atelectasis and promote chest expansion and secretion clearance, such as chest physiotherapy, pursed-lip breathing, and incentive spirometry.
2. Frequently assess oxygen-delivery devices for correct setting, functioning, and use by patient. Drain collected water from tubing, which may interfere with FIO_2 delivery.
3. Position the patient for maximal comfort and chest expansion, such as semi-Fowler's position. Turn and reposition frequently to prevent pooling of secretions and atelectasis.
4. If the patient becomes increasingly lethargic, cannot cough or expectorate secretions, cannot cooperate with therapy, or if pH decreases to below 7.30, despite use of the above therapy, report and prepare to assist with intubation and initiation of mechanical ventilation.
5. Suction frequently to prevent buildup of secretions that will interfere with oxygenation, but avoid prolonged episodes of suctioning while on mechanical ventilation to prevent hypoxia.
6. Provide meticulous care while intubated to prevent infection.
7. Provide frequent mouth and skin care.
8. Provide calm, confident care and reassurance during the weaning process to prevent dependence on mechanical ventilation.

ALTERNATIVE INTERVENTION

Music therapy has been shown to reduce anxiety (including blood pressure and respiratory rate) in mechanically ventilated patients.

9. Provide enteral or parenteral feedings as needed during acute stage.

Education and Health Maintenance

1. Instruct patient with preexisting pulmonary disease to seek early intervention for infections to prevent acute respiratory failure.

2. Encourage patients at risk, especially those who are elderly and those with preexisting lung disease, to get yearly influenza and one-time pneumococcal pneumonia immunizations.
3. Teach patient about medication regimen and use of oxygen devices at home.

COMMUNITY CARE CONSIDERATIONS

Pneumococcal vaccine is indicated for people older than age 2 with the following risk factors: chronic heart disease, COPD, diabetes, alcoholism, chronic liver disease, cerebrospinal leaks, asplenia, immunodeficiency, Inuits, some Native American populations, and residents of long-term care facilities.

RESPIRATORY INFECTIONS IN CHILDREN

Respiratory tract infections are a common cause of acute illness in infants and children. Many pediatric infections are seasonal. Response of the child to the infection will vary based on the child's age and general health, causative organism, and the existence of chronic medical conditions as well as the degree of contact with other children. Information about specific respiratory infections, including bacterial pneumonia, viral pneumonia, *Pneumocystis* pneumonia, *Mycoplasma* pneumonia, bronchiolitis, croup, and epiglottitis may be found in *Table R-1.*

Assessment

1. Infants: poor feeding, sleep pattern disrupted, vomiting, diarrhea, fever, tachypnea, grunting, nasal flaring, retractions, cough
2. Older children: runny nose, headache, anorexia, fever, dry cough
3. Possible sore throat and earache
4. Possible adventitious lung sounds

(*Text continues on page 810.*)

TABLE R-1	Respiratory Infections in Children

CONDITION AND DESCRIPTION	TREATMENT
Pneumococcal pneumonia • Caused by gram-positive *Streptococcus pneumoniae*. • Infants and young children present with history of upper respiratory infection (URI) for several days followed by sudden onset of high fever, lethargy, vomiting, poor appetite, fine crackles on lung examination. • Older children present like adults. • Winter and spring.	1. Penicillin G, amoxicillin, azithromycin, co-trimoxazole, or I.M. ceftriaxone if severe infection. 2. Avoid cough suppressants. 3. Monitor for response to antibiotics; signs of complications (bacteremia, meningitis, hemolytic uremic syndrome, pleural effusion, empyema)
Streptococcal pneumonia • Caused by gram-positive group A beta-hemolytic *Streptococcus*. • Ages 3 to 5, rare but serious. Sudden onset high fever, chills, increasing cough, respiratory distress, signs of shock. May also be milder illness or present as toxic shock syndrome (TSS).	1. Penicillin G. 2. Provide humidified oxygen as needed, rest, monitor intake and output. 3. Monitor for complications (empyema, TSS, respiratory compromise).
Staphylococcal pneumonia • Caused by gram-positive *Staphylococcus aureus*. • Most common in age-group 6 to 12 months. • October through May. • Predisposing factors: cystic fibrosis, immunodeficiency, maternal infection. • Presents like pneumococcal pneumonia.	1. Thoracentesis. 2. Nafcillin, oxacillin, methicillin, cefazolin, clindamycin, vancomycin. 3. Rapid treatment important. 4. Monitor for signs of tension pneumothorax. 5. Monitor response to therapy; methicillin-resistance may occur.

(continued)

R

Respiratory Infections in Children (continued)

CONDITION AND DESCRIPTION	TREATMENT

Haemophilus influenzae, type B

- Most common in ages 4 or younger; prevalent in winter and spring in the unimmunized.
- Preceded by a URI then insidious onset of cough, fever, tachypnea, respiratory distress.

1. Second- or third-generation cephalosporins, azithromycin, co-trimoxazole, amoxicillin potassium clavulanate.
2. Respiratory isolation until 24 hours after antibiotics begun.
3. Monitor for signs of complications (bacteremia, pericarditis, cellulitis, empyema, meningitis).
4. Encourage immunization of all children.

Viral pneumonia

- Most common causes are respiratory syncytial virus (RSV), para-influenza virus types 1, 2, and 3, adenoviruses types 1, 2, 3, 5, 6, 7, 11, 21 and influenza A and B.
- Occurs more often in winter months; peak ages 2 to 3.
- Presents with gradual onset of URI symptoms, low-grade fever, cough, wheeze, followed by increased respiratory distress.
- RSV subgroup A most common cause of pneumonia, bronchiolitis and hospitalizations in infants ages 2 to 7 months.
- Severity decreased with age and subsequent infections.

1. Amantadine for influenza A.
2. Racemic epinephrine for bronchiolitis.
3. Monitor hydration status.
4. Monitor for signs of complications, particularly in children with cardiopulmonary disease, cystic fibrosis, bronchopulmonary dysplasia, and neurovascular disease.
5. For infants with RSV, may consider ribavirin.
6. Contact isolation to prevent nosocomial spread.
7. RSV can be life-threatening, particularly in infants with comorbid conditions. Monitor closely for respiratory failure.

Respiratory Infections in Children *(continued)*

CONDITION AND DESCRIPTION	TREATMENT

Pneumocystis pneumonia
- Caused by *Pneumocystis carinii*. Predisposing factors: debilitated infant, cystic fibrosis, immunosuppression.
- Slow onset of tachypnea, retractions, cyanosis; peak incidence is 3 to 6 months.

1. Co-trimoxazole.
2. Pentamidine I.V. or aerosol.
3. Monitor for adverse reactions to therapy (nausea, vomiting, rash pancreatitis, renal failure).

Mycoplasma pneumonia
- Caused by *M pneumoniae*.
- Frequently occurs in 5- to 18-year-old children in fall and winter.
- Onset is slow with low-grade fevers, cough, mild chest pain, coryza.

1. Erythromycin or azithromycin doxycycline (children older than age 8).
2. Secretion precautions.
3. Monitor fever, signs of systemic infection.

Bronchiolitis
- Caused by *Mycoplasma* or a virus such as RSV, adenovirus, parainfluenza, influenza.
- Occurs in children ages 3 months to 2 years in late winter or early spring.
- Onset associated with URI, low-grade fever, wheezing.

1. Humidified oxygen, ventilatory assistance as needed.
2. Bronchodilators may be used.
3. Avoid high-density humidity.
4. Contact and respiratory isolation.
5. Prophylactic RSV immune globulin may be considered.

Croup
- Caused by same viruses as bronchiolitis with parainfluenza being the most common in all age groups.
- Occurs in children ages 3 months to 5 years in fall or winter.

1. If mild symptoms, home management with cool mist humidifier, rest, fluids.
2. Moderate symptoms, racemic epinephrine or nebulized L-epinephrine and/or steroids.

(continued)

Respiratory Infections in Children *(continued)*

CONDITION AND DESCRIPTION	TREATMENT
Croup *(continued)* • Onset preceded by URI, then barking cough, hoarseness, worse at night.	3. Monitor for severe airway edema, which may require intubation.
Epiglottitis • Caused by *Haemophilus influenzae* type B or GABHS. • Markedly decreased incidence due to the Hib vaccine. • Onset abrupt with severe sore throat, fever, toxicity, drooling, dysphagia, respiratory distress.	1. Hospital management required. 2. Prepare for intubation or tracheotomy. 3. Keep child and family as calm as possible. 4. I.V. third-generation cephalosporin or vancomycin. 5. Monitor and support respiratory status.
Bacterial tracheitis • Caused by *Staphylococcus aureus, Haemophilus influenzae, Streptococcus* group A or B, *Escherichia coli, Klebsiella, Moraxella catarrhalis, Pseudomonas, Chlamydia,* or diphtheria in an unvaccinated patient, usually children younger than age 6. • Onset is acute, preceded by a URI, high fever, toxic appearing.	1. Antibiotic therapy, usually a cephalosporin. 2. Oxygen and humidification. 3. Ventilatory assistance may be required. 4. Frequent suctioning.

Diagnostic Evaluation

1. Chest radiograph shows patchy or disseminated infiltrate with pneumonia.
2. Sputum cultures may isolate organism.

3. Complete blood count may show increased white blood cells of predominantly neutrophils or lymphocytes based on cause.
4. Lateral neck radiograph shows subglottic edema in croup, severely narrowed airway and pseudomembrane in bacterial tracheitis, and epiglottic edema in epiglottitis.

Nursing Diagnoses
6, 23, 43, 49, 73, 75, 94, 123

Nursing Interventions
Monitoring
1. Monitor for inspiratory stridor and retractions, tripod position, drooling in epiglottis, and report immediately.
2. Monitor for increasing respiratory difficulty signifying need for oxygen, intubation, and respiratory support.
3. Observe the child's response to antibiotic therapy, including drug sensitivity.
4. Check temperature regularly to determine effectiveness of antipyretic medications.
5. Record the child's intake and output and monitor urine specific gravity to identify dehydration.

R

Supportive Care
1. Provide a humidified environment enriched with oxygen to combat hypoxia and to liquefy secretions. Mist tents are no longer recommended.
2. Place the child in a comfortable position to promote easier ventilation.
   a. Semi-Fowler's: use pillows, infant seat, or elevate head of bed.
   b. Occasional side or abdominal position will aid drainage of liquefied secretions.
   c. Do not place the child in severe respiratory distress in a supine position; allow the child to assume a position of comfort.
3. Provide measures to improve ventilation of affected portion of the lung.
   a. Change position frequently.

b. Provide postural drainage if directed.

c. Relieve nasal obstruction that contributes to breathing difficulty. Instill saline solution or prescribed nose drops, and apply nasal suctioning.

d. Quiet prolonged crying, which can irritate the airway, by soothing the child; however, crying may be an effective way to ventilate the lungs.

e. Realize that coughing is a normal tracheobronchial cleansing procedure, but temporarily relieve coughing by allowing the child to sip water; use extreme caution to prevent aspiration.

f. Insert a nasogastric tube as ordered to relieve abdominal distention, which can limit diaphragmatic excursion.

EMERGENCY ALERT To minimize spasm and sudden blockage of airway, avoid having the child lie flat, forcing the child to drink, and looking down the child's throat.

4. For cases of severe respiratory distress, assist with intubation or tracheostomy and mechanical ventilation.

a. Tracheostomy tubes are generally not cuffed for infants and small children because the tube itself is big enough relative to the size of the trachea to act as its own sealer.

b. Position the infant with a tracheostomy with neck extended by placing a small, rolled towel under the shoulders to prevent occlusion of the tube by the chin. Support the head and neck carefully when moving the infant to avoid dislodging the tube.

c. When feeding, cover the tracheostomy with a moist piece of gauze, or use a bib for older infants or young children.

5. To promote hydration, administer I.V. fluids at the prescribed rate.

6. To prevent aspiration, withhold oral food and fluids if the child is in severe respiratory distress.

7. Offer the child small sips of clear fluid when respiratory status improves.

a. Note vomiting or abdominal distention after the oral fluid is given.

    b. As the child begins to take more fluid by mouth, notify the health care provider and modify the I.V. fluid rate to prevent fluid overload.

    c. Do not force the child to take fluids orally because this may cause increased distress and possibly vomiting. Anorexia will subside as condition improves.

8. To provide adequate rest, disturb the child as little as possible by organizing nursing care, and protect child from unnecessary interruptions.

9. Encourage the parents to stay with the child as much as possible to provide comfort and security for the child.

10. Provide opportunities for quiet play as the child's condition improves.

11. Provide a quiet, stress-free environment.

Education and Health Maintenance

1. Advise parents to use humidifier or vaporizer at home and encourage fluids as tolerated. Instruct about the need to keep equipment clean and free from bacteria, mold, or mildew.

2. Teach the importance of good hygiene. Include information on hand washing and appropriate ways to handle respiratory secretions at home.

3. Teach methods to isolate sick from well children in the home. Teach the family when it is appropriate to keep the child home from school (fever, coughing up secretions, significant runny nose in a toddler or younger-age child).

4. Teach methods to keep the ill child well hydrated.

    a. Provide small amounts of fluids frequently.

    b. Offer clear liquids such as Pedialyte.

    c. Avoid juices with a high sugar content.

5. Teach ways to assess the child's hydration status at home.

    a. Decreased number of wet diapers or number of voidings in a day

    b. Decreased activity level

    c. Dry lips and mucous membranes

    d. No tears when the child cries

R

6. Teach parents when to contact their health care provider: signs of respiratory distress, recurrent fever, and decreased appetite and activity.
7. Teach about medications and follow-up.
8. If tracheostomy was required, teach home care of the tracheostomy.

RETINAL DETACHMENT

Retinal detachment results from separation of the sensory layer of the retina containing the rod and cones from the pigmented epithelial layer beneath. It may occur spontaneously because of degenerative changes in the retina (as in diabetic retinopathy) or vitreous humor, trauma, inflammation, tumor, or loss of a lens to a cataract. Rare in children, the disorder most commonly occurs after age 40. Untreated retinal detachment results in loss of a portion of the visual field.

Assessment

1. Initially, the patient complains of flashes of light, floating spots or filaments in the vitreous, or blurred, "sooty" vision. Most of these phenomena result from traction between the retina and the vitreous.
2. If detachment progresses rapidly, the patient may report a veil-like curtain or shadow obscuring portions of the visual field. The veil appears to come from above, below, or from one side; the patient may initially mistake the obstruction for a drooping eyelid or elevated cheek.
3. Straight-ahead vision may be unaffected in early stages but, as detachment progresses, there will be loss of central as well as peripheral vision.

Diagnostic Evaluation

1. Ophthalmoscopy or slit-lamp examination with full pupil dilation shows retina as gray or opaque in detached areas. The retina is normally transparent.

Collaborative Management
Therapeutic Interventions
1. Preoperatively, sedation, bed rest, and eye patches may be used to restrict eye movements.

Surgical Interventions
1. Surgical intervention aims to reattach the retinal layer to the epithelial layer and has a 90% to 95% success rate. Techniques include:
   a. Photocoagulation, in which a laser or xenon arc "spot welds" the retina to the pigment epithelium
   b. Electrodiathermy, in which a tiny hole is made in the sclera to drain subretinal fluid, allowing the pigment epithelium to adhere to the retina
   c. Cryosurgery or retinal cryopexy, another "spot weld" technique that uses a supercooled probe to adhere the pigment epithelium to the retina
   d. Scleral buckling, in which the sclera is shortened to force the pigment epithelium closer to the retina; commonly accompanied by vitrectomy

Nursing Diagnoses
33, 44, 135, 136

R

Nursing Interventions
Also see *Ocular Surgery*, page 677.

Supportive Care
1. Prepare the patient for surgery.
   a. Instruct the patient to remain quiet in prescribed (dependent) position, to keep the detached area of the retina in dependent position.
   b. Patch both eyes.
   c. Wash the patient's face with antibacterial solution.
   d. Instruct the patient not to touch eyes to avoid contamination.
   e. Administer preoperative medications as ordered.
2. Take measures to prevent postoperative complications.
   a. Caution the patient to avoid bumping head.

b. Encourage the patient not to cough or sneeze or to perform other strain-inducing activities that will increase intraocular pressure.

c. Assist the patient with activities as needed.

3. Encourage ambulation and independence as tolerated.

4. Administer medications for pain, nausea, and vomiting as directed.

5. Provide quiet diversional activities, such as listening to a radio or audio books.

Education and Health Maintenance

1. Teach proper technique for giving eye medications.

2. Suggest applying a clean, warm, moist washcloth to eyes and eyelids several times per day for 10 minutes, to provide soothing and relaxing comfort.

3. Advise patient to avoid rapid eye movements for several weeks as well as straining and bending the head below the waist.

4. Advise patient that driving is restricted until cleared by ophthalmologist and that light activities are resumed gradually within 3 weeks; heavier activities and athletics may be restricted up to 6 weeks.

5. Teach the patient to recognize and immediately report symptoms that indicate recurring detachment, such as floating spots, flashing lights, and progressive shadows.

6. Advise patient to follow up. The first follow-up visit to the ophthalmologist should take place in 2 weeks, with other visits scheduled thereafter.

RETINOBLASTOMA

Retinoblastoma is a malignant, genetically inherited tumor arising in the retina of one or both eyes. Retinoblastoma occurs in approximately 1 in 18,000 live births and is usually diagnosed by age 2. Endophytic retinoblastomas arise in the internal nuclear layers of the retina and grow forward into the vitreous cavity. Exophytic tumors arise in the external nuclear layer and grow into the subretinal space, causing retinal detachment. Most retinoblastomas occur as a combination of these two types. The overall survival rate is high (90%); however, if untreated, the tumor may extend into the choroid, sclera, and optic nerve. Hematogenous spread of the tumor may occur to the bone marrow, skeleton, lymph nodes, and liver.

Assessment

1. "Cat's-eye" reflex (most common sign) is a whitish appearance of the pupil caused by the appearance of the tumor through the lens when light strikes the tumor mass.
2. Strabismus is the second most common sign.
3. Other occasional signs include orbital inflammation, hyphema, fixed pupil, and heterochromia iridis (different colors of each iris, or in the same iris).
4. Vision loss is not a symptom because young children do not complain of unilaterally decreased vision.

Diagnostic Evaluation

1. Bilateral indirect ophthalmoscopy under general anesthesia to evaluate tumor
2. Ultrasonography, CT scanning, or MRI may be done to visualize tumor.
3. Bone marrow aspiration and lumbar puncture under anesthesia determine metastasis.

Collaborative Management
Therapeutic Interventions

1. Unilateral tumors in stages I, II, or III are usually treated with external beam irradiation to eradicate the tumors and preserve useful vision. Radiation is usually administered over a 3- to 4-week period.
2. Radioactive applicators, light coagulation, and cryotherapy are sometimes used to treat small, localized tumors.

Pharmacologic Interventions

1. Chemotherapy is used to treat extraocular regional or distant metastases.

R

Surgical Interventions

1. Enucleation is the treatment of choice for advanced tumor growth, especially with optic nerve involvement.
2. Bilateral disease often requires enucleation of the severely diseased eye and irradiation of the least affected eye.
   a. Every attempt is made to salvage remaining vision.
   b. Bilateral enucleation is indicated with extensive bilateral retinoblastoma if vision cannot be salvaged.

Nursing Diagnoses

3, 6, 30, 33, 44, 67

Nursing Interventions

Also see *Ocular Surgery*, page 677.

Monitoring

1. Monitor for postoperative complications, including hemorrhage, infection, or implant extrusion.

Supportive Care

1. Sedate the child for irradiation, if necessary.
2. Observe for possible adverse effects of irradiation and prepare the parents for their occurrence, including skin changes at the temples, loss of lashes, fat atrophy with ptosis, delayed wound healing, dry eye, permanent radiation dermatitis, and impaired bone growth.
3. To prevent irritation of irradiated skin, use soap sparingly in these areas, avoid exposure to the sun, and apply a nonirritating lubricant.
4. Encourage the parents to "room in" and participate in the child's care to minimize separation anxiety.
5. Describe the surgery and anticipated postoperative appearance of the child. Draw pictures or use a doll if available.
   a. A ball implant is put in at the time of enucleation.
   b. An eyelid conformer is inserted to maintain integrity of the lids.
   c. The child's face may be edematous and ecchymotic after the procedure.

d. 4 to 6 weeks after surgery, the patient will receive an ocular prosthesis.

6. Offer the family the opportunity to talk with another parent who has gone through the experience or to see pictures of another child with an artificial eye.

7. Explain that the prosthesis will be made for the child and will resemble the removed eye.

8. Tell parents to expect the child to grieve the loss and to help the child by talking about it, but treating the child as the same person.

9. Provide postoperative care.
   a. Instill medications, usually antibiotic and steroid ointments, to prevent infection.
   b. Apply pressure or ice dressings, as ordered, to reduce swelling.
   c. Irrigate eyelid conformer area to reduce mucus.
   d. Clean eyelid to reduce chance of infection.

10. To minimize the effect of vision loss, maintain a safe, uncluttered environment for the child.

11. Assist patient in adjusting to monocular vision, especially with loss of peripheral vision and depth perception.
   a. Hold the child frequently and stand close, within his or her field of vision, while speaking or providing care.
   b. Encourage the use of touch and other senses for exploring.

12. Set environmental limits so the child feels safe and can obtain help easily.

13. Suggest genetic counseling if applicable.
   a. Risk for parents ranges from approximately 1% to 10% for having another affected child, and risk for patient's offspring is 1% to 50%, depending on family history and whether the affected child had unilateral or bilateral disease.
   b. Among affected offspring, there is a high probability (greater than 50%) of bilateral disease.

Education and Health Maintenance
1. Teach care of the orbit.

2. Teach care of the prosthesis. Initial instructions are provided by the ocularist and should be reinforced by the nurse.
   a. Inspecting eye and lid
   b. Instilling medication
   c. Irrigating site to remove mucus
   d. Removing and inserting the prosthesis
3. Advise protection of the remaining eye from accidental injury, such as wearing safety glasses for sports, keeping sharp objects away from eye, and treating eye infections promptly.
4. Encourage maintenance of routine checkups for eye and medical care.
5. Stress need to have subsequent children carefully evaluated for retinoblastoma and refer for genetic counseling as indicated.
   a. An ophthalmologic examination under anesthesia is usually recommended at about age 2 months.
   b. The child should receive frequent examinations thereafter until judged safe from developing retinoblastoma, usually about age 3.
6. Refer for information and support to Candlelighters, *www.candlelighters.org*.

RHEUMATIC FEVER, ACUTE

Acute rheumatic fever (ARF) is a systemic disease characterized by inflammatory lesions of connective tissue and endothelial tissue, primarily affecting the heart and joints. The pathogenesis is thought to be an autoimmune response to group A beta-hemolytic streptococcus. There is cross-reactivity between cardiac tissue antigens and streptococcal cell wall components. The unique pathologic lesion of rheumatic fever is the Aschoff body, a collection of reticuloendothelial cells surrounding a necrotic center on some structure of the heart.

ARF is commonly seen in children ages 5 to 15 but may occur in adults and during winter months. There is a high recurrence rate, and 75% of those with ARF progress to rheumatic heart disease in adulthood. Complications include significant heart failure, pericarditis, pericardial effusions, aortic or mitral valve insufficiency, and permanent cardiac damage.

Assessment

1. History of streptococcal pharyngitis or upper respiratory infection 2 to 6 weeks before onset of illness
2. Jones criteria established by the American Heart Association: presence of two major manifestations, or one major and two minor manifestations, plus evidence of a preceding streptococcal infection, are required to establish a diagnosis.
3. Major manifestations:
   a. Carditis: manifested by significant murmurs, signs of pericarditis, cardiac enlargement, heart failure.
   b. Polyarthritis: almost always migratory and manifested by swelling, heat, redness and tenderness, pain and limitation of motion of two or more joints.
   c. Chorea, a central nervous system disorder that lasts 1 to 3 months: purposeless, involuntary, rapid movements commonly associated with muscle weakness, involuntary facial grimaces, speech disturbances, emotional lability.
   d. Erythema marginatum: an evanescent, nonpruritic, pink rash. The erythematous areas have pale centers and round or wavy margins, vary greatly in size, and occur mainly on the trunk and extremities. Erythema is transient, migrates from place to place, and may be brought out by the application of heat.
   e. Subcutaneous nodules: firm, painless nodules seen or felt over the extensor surface of certain joints, particularly elbows, knees, and wrists, in the occipital region, or over the spinous processes of the thoracic and lumbar vertebrae; the skin overlying them moves freely and is not inflamed.
4. Minor manifestations:
   a. History of previous rheumatic fever or evidence of preexisting rheumatic heart disease

R

b. Arthralgia: pain in one or more joints without evidence of inflammation, tenderness to touch, or limitation of motion

c. Fever: temperature in excess of 100.4° F (38° C).

d. Erythrocyte sedimentation rate (ESR) — elevated

e. C-reactive protein — positive

f. Electrocardiogram (ECG) changes — mainly PR interval prolongation

g. White blood cell count — elevated (leukocytosis)

Diagnostic Evaluation

1. Throat culture for group A beta-hemolytic streptococci and blood sample for titer of streptococcal antibodies (antistreptolysin O, or ASO titer) to support evidence of recent streptococcal infection.

2. Complete blood count, ESR, and C-reactive protein for changes described above.

3. Baseline ECG and echocardiogram may be done to evaluate valve function.

4. Chest X-ray for cardiomegaly or heart failure.

Collaborative Management
Pharmacologic Interventions

1. Antibiotics to treat streptococcal infection — generally I.M. penicillin or erythromycin in penicillin allergy

2. Corticosteroids for patients with carditis complicated by heart failure to prevent permanent cardiac damage

3. Salicylates or nonsteroidals for patients with arthritis (but not while on high-dose corticosteroids because of risk of GI bleeding) and antipyretics to control fever, after diagnosis has been established

4. Phenobarbital, diazepam if chorea present

5. Prophylactic antibiotics for at least 5 years after ARF

Nursing Diagnoses
3, 13, 19, 43, 135, 136

Nursing Interventions
Monitoring

1. Monitor temperature frequently, and patient's response to antipyretics.
2. Monitor the patient's pulse frequently, especially after activity to determine degree of cardiac compensation.
3. Auscultate the heart periodically for development of new heart murmur or pericardial or pleural friction rub.
4. Observe for adverse effects of salicylate or nonsteroidal anti-inflammatory drug (NSAID) therapy, such as stomach upset, tinnitus, headache, GI bleeding, and altered mental status.
5. Monitor salicylate blood levels as directed.
6. Monitor for adverse effects of corticosteroid therapy, such as emotional disturbance, weight gain, hypertension caused by sodium retention, cushingoid appearance, and GI bleeding.
7. Monitor the patient's response to long-term activity restriction.

Supportive Care

1. Administer salicylates or NSAIDs with food to reduce stomach irritation.
2. Prepare the family for expected adverse effects of steroid therapy, such as rounding facial contour, acne, excessive hair, and weight gain.
3. Restrict sodium and fluids and obtain daily weights as indicated.
4. Know that steroids diminish the patient's resistance to infection and may mask symptoms of infection.

PEDIATRIC ALERT Do not place a child with an infectious disease in the room with the child with rheumatic fever. Restrict visitors and personnel with infectious diseases from contact with the child on steroid therapy.

5. Administer medications punctually and at regular intervals to achieve constant therapeutic blood levels.
6. Explain the need for rest (usually prescribed for 4 to 12 weeks, depending on the severity of the disease and health care provider's preference) and assure the patient that bed

rest will be imposed no longer than necessary (usually until the ESR returns to normal).

7. Organize nursing care to provide periods of uninterrupted rest and assure the child that needs will be met by responding to call light promptly.

8. Assist the patient to resume activity very gradually once asymptomatic at rest and indicators of acute inflammation have become normal.

9. Provide comfort measures, such as using a bed cradle over painful joints, supporting inflamed joints, providing meticulous skin care, maintaining good body alignment, changing positions frequently to decrease stiffness and prevent skin breakdown, and elevating the back of the bed and support the arms with pillows when patient is dyspneic.

10. Provide a safe, supportive environment for the child with chorea.

 a. Place the child in a bed with padded side rails, especially if uncontrolled body movements are severe.

 b. Feed the child slowly and carefully because of incoordinate movements of the head, mouth, and swallowing muscles. Avoid the use of sharp eating utensils, and do not use straws.

 c. Provide frequent feedings that are high in calories, protein, vitamins, and iron because constant movements cause the child to burn calories at a rapid rate.

 d. Spend time talking with the child even though speech may be defective. If severe, use other methods of communication.

 e. Assess the need for sedation.

 f. Keep the environment calm and provide increased periods of rest because movements increase with fatigue and increased excitement.

11. Observe for the development or disappearance of any major or minor manifestations of the disease and report signs of increased rheumatic activity as salicylates or steroids are being tapered.

Education and Health Maintenance

1. Explain rheumatic fever in age-appropriate terminology. Reassure patient that he or she has not had a heart attack.

   PEDIATRIC ALERT Have the child listen to the heart with a stethoscope to understand that the heart is still functioning.

2. Make sure that the child's school has been notified and that some tutoring will be available. Initiate referrals for home nursing or social services as indicated.

3. To prevent a recurrence or an additional case of rheumatic fever within the family, advise all family members to have throat cultures, be treated if necessary, and be alert to specific symptoms of streptococcal infections.

4. Encourage continuous prophylactic antimicrobial therapy (throughout the childhood years and well into adult life, usually indefinitely) to prevent recurrence.

RHEUMATOID ARTHRITIS

Rheumatoid arthritis (RA) refers to an autoimmune, inflammatory disease of the joints and various organ systems. In this disorder, synovial inflammation produces antigens and inflammatory by-products leading to destruction of joint cartilage, edema, and production of granulation tissue (pannus; see *Figure R-2*). The pannus forms adhesions on joint surfaces and

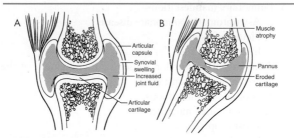

FIGURE R-2 Pathophysiology of rheumatoid arthritis. **(A)** Joint structure with synovial swelling and fluid accumulation in joint. **(B)** Pannus, eroded articular cartilage with joint space narrowing, muscle atrophy, and ankylosis.

supporting structures such as ligaments and tendons, causing contractures and ruptures that degrade joint structure and mobility. Bilateral symmetric arthritis affects any diarthrodial joint but most often involves the hands, wrists, knees, and feet.

The cause of RA is unknown, but it may result from a combination of environmental, demographic, infectious, and genetic factors. An infectious agent has not been identified, but many infectious processes can produce a polyarthritis similar to RA. Women are affected more commonly than men.

Assessment

1. Warm, tender, painful joints with stiffness lasting longer than 30 minutes after arising
2. Fever, fatigue, weight loss
3. Skin manifestations
   a. Rheumatoid nodules: elbows, occiput, sacrum
   b. Vasculitic changes: brown, splinterlike lesions in fingers or nail folds
4. Cardiac manifestations
   a. Acute pericarditis
   b. Conduction defects
   c. Valvular insufficiency
   d. Coronary arteritis
   e. Cardiac tamponade (rare)
5. Pulmonary manifestations
   a. Asymptomatic pulmonary disease
   b. Pleural effusion
   c. Interstitial fibrosis
   d. Laryngeal obstruction caused by involvement of the cricoarytenoid joint (rare)
6. Neurologic manifestations
   a. Mononeuritis multiplex
   b. Wrist drop
   c. Foot drop
   d. Carpal tunnel syndrome
   e. Compression of spinal nerve roots
7. Presence of deformities

a. Swan neck: proximal interphalangeal (PIP) joints hyperextend
b. Boutonniere: PIP joints flex
c. Ulnar deviation: fingers point toward ulna
8. Altered functional status

Diagnostic Evaluation

1. Complete blood count (CBC) — decreased hemoglobin and hematocrit with normal indices.
2. Rheumatoid factor — positive in a large percentage of patients.
3. Erythrocyte sedimentation rate — elevated.
4. Synovial fluid analysis — turbid, yellow color; white blood cell count 2,000 to 75,000/mm^3; low viscosity.
5. X-rays:
   a. Hands and wrists: marginal erosions of the PIP, metacarpophalangeal, and carpal bones, generalized osteopenia
   b. Cervical spine: erosions producing atlantoaxial subluxation
6. MRI scan — shows spinal cord compression resulting from C1-C2 subluxation and compression of surrounding vascular structures.
7. Bone scan — shows "increased uptake" in the joints involved.
8. Synovial biopsy — may be done to rule out other causes of polyarthritis by noting the absence of other pathologic findings.

Collaborative Management
Therapeutic Interventions

1. Application of heat and cold to relieve pain and inflammation
2. Use of splints to prevent contractures
3. Use of transcutaneous electrical nerve stimulation (TENS) unit to treat chronic pain
4. Iontophoresis (delivery of medication through the skin using direct electrical current) to relieve pain
5. Behavior modification, biofeedback, and relaxation techniques

R

Pharmacologic Interventions
1. Nonsteroidal anti-inflammatory drugs to relieve pain and inflammation
2. Disease-modifying antirheumatic drugs to reduce disease activity, such as oral or injectable gold, hydroxychloroquine, penicillamine, leflunomide, and etanercept
3. Corticosteroids to reduce inflammatory process

Surgical Interventions
1. Synovectomy
2. Arthrodesis (joint fusion)
3. Total joint replacement

Nursing Diagnoses
3, 13, 24, 43, 84, 108

Nursing Interventions
Monitoring
1. Monitor length of stiffness on arising.
2. Monitor pain control measures.
3. Monitor for signs and symptoms indicating adverse reaction to medications, such as rash, visual symptoms, GI distress, injection site reaction, renal toxicity, and liver dysfunction.
4. Monitor functional ability.

Supportive Care
1. Apply local heat or cold to affected joints for 15 to 20 minutes three to four times daily.
   a. Avoid temperatures likely to cause skin or tissue damage by checking temperature of warm soaks or covering cold packs with a towel.
2. Administer or teach self-administration of pharmacologic agents. Advise the patient about when to expect pain relief based on mechanism of action of the drug.
3. Encourage use of adjunctive pain control measures.
   a. Progressive muscle relaxation
   b. TENS
   c. Biofeedback

4. Encourage warm bath or shower in the morning on arising to decrease morning stiffness and improve mobility.
5. Encourage measures to protect affected joints.
   a. Perform gentle range-of-motion exercises.
   b. Use splints.
   c. Assist with activities of daily living, if necessary.
6. Encourage exercise consistent with degree of disease activity.
7. Refer to physical therapy and occupational therapy.
8. Provide pain relief before self-care activities.
9. Schedule adequate rest periods.
10. Help the patient obtain appropriate assistive devices, such as raised toilet seats, special eating utensils, and zipper pulls.
11. Be aware of potential problems in job, child care, maintenance of home, and social and family functioning that may result from RA.
12. Encourage the patient to express problems and feelings.
13. Assist with problem-solving approach to explore options and gain control of problem areas.
14. Refer to social worker or mental health counselor as needed.

Education and Health Maintenance

1. Instruct the patient and family in the nature of disease.
2. Advise that there is no cure for RA; avoid "miracle cures" and quackery.
3. Educate about pharmacologic agents.
   a. Medication must be taken consistently to achieve maximum benefit.
   b. Most medications used in the treatment of RA require periodic laboratory testing to monitor for potential adverse reactions.
   c. Advise the patient of possible adverse reactions of medications and need to report these to health care provider.
4. Advise frequent follow-up for monitoring of CBC and urinalysis while on gold and penicillamine therapy; ophthalmologic examinations while taking hydroxychloroquine; and liver function tests while taking etanercept.

5. Reinforce to the patient the need for lifelong treatment.

RHEUMATOID ARTHRITIS, JUVENILE

Juvenile rheumatoid arthritis (JRA) is a chronic, inflammatory, systemic disease of unknown cause that involves the joints, connective tissues, and various organs throughout the body. Genetic, infectious, or autoimmune factors are thought to play a role in this disorder, which begins in children younger than age 16.

The disease causes inflammation involving the synovial membranes, joint capsules, and ligaments. Eventually, the articular cartilage is destroyed; inflamed and overgrown synovial tissue eventually fills the joint space, leading to narrowing, fibrous ankylosis, and bony fusion. Adjacent tendons, tendon sheaths, and muscles may also become involved. Complications of JRA include crippling bony deformities from progressive polyarthritis; cervical spine and temporomandibular jaw problems; iridocyclitis leading to cataracts, glaucoma, or blindness; and pericarditis.

Three major forms of JRA are known: systemic (least common), polyarticular (five or more joints, mostly in girls), and pauciarticular (less than five joints).

Although JRA is a painful disease of long duration, the outlook for remission is good in 70% of cases.

Assessment

1. JRA is characterized by exacerbations and remissions. Infections, injuries, or surgical procedures often precipitate exacerbations.
2. Involved joints become inflamed with morning stiffness (gelling), swelling, warmth, pain, and impaired movement. This may occur gradually or suddenly.
3. In systemic JRA:
   a. High intermittent fever (102° F [39° C]), malaise
   b. Maculopapular rash
   c. Pleuritis
   d. Pericarditis
   e. Splenomegaly, hepatomegaly
   f. Lymphadenopathy

4. In polyarticular JRA:
   a. Minimal systemic signs, such as low-grade fever, malaise, and lymphadenopathy
   b. Severe arthritis
5. In pauciarticular JRA:
   a. Type I: chronic iridocyclitis (eye redness, pain, photophobia, decreased visual acuity, nonreactive pupils). May be unilateral or bilateral, and lead to blindness.
   b. May progress to polyarthritis in 20% of cases
   c. Type II: iridocyclitis, sacroiliitis
   d. May progress to ankylosing spondylitis
6. Rheumatoid nodules are uncommon in children.

Diagnostic Evaluation

1. C-reactive proteins are elevated in all types.
2. Erythrocyte sedimentation rate is elevated in all types.
3. Anemia and leukocytosis in systemic JRA.
4. Rheumatoid factor-negative in all types except in some forms of polyarticular JRA.
5. Serum antinuclear antibodies may or may not be positive.
6. Possible alteration in serum proteins (increased alpha and gamma; decreased albumin)
7. X-rays show changes in bone; initially nonspecific
8. Slit-lamp examinations of eye to rule out iridocyclitis

R

Collaborative Management

Therapeutic Interventions

1. There is no specific cure; treatment is supportive.
2. Physical therapy is used to promote joint movement.

Pharmacologic Interventions

1. The goal of drug therapy is to reduce inflammation and relieve pain.
2. Anti-inflammatory analgesics include aspirin and non-steroidal anti-inflammatory drugs (NSAIDs), such as ibuprofen and naproxen. Aspirin is the drug of choice, preferably enteric coated to avoid GI complications.

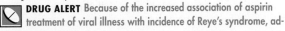 **DRUG ALERT** Because of the increased association of aspirin treatment of viral illness with incidence of Reye's syndrome, ad-

vise the family to contact the health care provider when the child has a viral illness. Aspirin may be discontinued and another treatment for JRA substituted until the viral illness is over.

3. Disease-modifying antirheumatic drugs (DMARDs), such as methotrexate or hydroxychloroquine, may be added to the regimen when NSAIDs have been ineffective.

   a. Methotrexate is given orally or by subcutaneous injection once per week along with daily folic acid supplement to prevent anemia.

   b. Hydroxychloroquine or chloroquine may cause gastric upset, retinal toxicity, and corneal and retinal changes leading to blindness.

4. Immunosuppressant drugs, such as cyclophosphamide, azathioprine, chlorambucil, and cyclosporine, are reserved for patients with severe debilitating disease and those who have responded poorly to NSAIDs and DMARDs.

5. Biologic therapies may be tried, including etanercept (a tumor necrosis factor) and adalimumab (a monoclonal antibody).

6. Corticosteroids, the most potent anti-inflammatory agents available, are used for life-threatening disease, incapacitating systemic disease not responsive to other anti-inflammatory therapy, and iridocyclitis.

   a. Administered in the lowest effective dose orally or I.V., on alternate days (rather than daily). Steroid use does not prevent complications of severe arthritis or influence ultimate prognosis.

   b. Tuberculin test should be done before starting steroid therapy, because corticosteroids can blunt skin test results.

   c. Ophthalmic drops or injections into the eye for severe uveitis.

7. Gamma globulin has been used with good effect on some children with systemic type JRA.

Surgical Interventions

1. Synovectomy may be used to maintain function when extensive synovitis develops, especially around wrists.

2. Joint replacement may be needed in severe destructive arthritis (ankylosing spondylitis).

Nursing Diagnoses
3, 13, 62, 80, 135, 136

Nursing Interventions
Monitoring
1. Monitor serum levels of aspirin (maintain 20 to 30 mg/dL) for anti-inflammatory effectiveness and to avoid toxicity. Therapeutic response may take weeks or even months. Signs of toxicity may include rapid or deep breathing or tinnitus.
2. Monitor corticosteroid use for glucosuria and other adverse effects, such as weight gain, edema, acne, and fatigue.
3. Monitor for adverse reactions to methotrexate (nausea, stomatitis, diarrhea, leukopenia, liver toxicity) and check laboratory tests every 4 to 8 weeks (complete blood count, liver function tests).

Supportive Care
1. Administer and teach parents to administer analgesic and anti-inflammatory drugs as prescribed and based on child's response.
2. Provide daytime heat to joints with tub baths, whirlpools, paraffin baths, and warm, moist pads; nighttime warmth with a sleeping bag, thermal underwear, or heated waterbed.
3. Immobilize acutely inflamed joints with pillows, splints, or slings.
4. Encourage compliance with physical therapy regimen to strengthen muscles and mobilize joints. Assist with range-of-motion exercises as indicated.
5. Splint joints to maintain proper position (joint extension) and to decrease pain and deformity.
6. Encourage prone position with thin or no pillow and firm mattress.

7. Encourage therapeutic play (eg, swimming, throwing, riding bike).
8. Encourage child to do own activities of daily living (ADLs) to maintain joint mobility.
9. Refer to occupational therapy for provision of adaptation devices to facilitate completion of ADLs (eg, Velcro closures, utensils, and self-care implements with enlarged handles).
10. Positively reward child for task completion.
11. Schedule rest periods to maximize energy; discourage bed rest and lengthy inactivity because it increases stiffness.
12. Offer pain medications and treatments before ADLs.
13. Encourage child and family to verbalize feelings.
14. Refer to community resources and support groups.
15. Encourage school attendance as much as possible, participation in activities, and socialization with peers.
16. Remind parents to devote time to other children, themselves, and each other because this disease affects the whole family.

Education and Health Maintenance

1. Educate and motivate parents and child in continuing program of treatment at home. Compliance with prescribed treatment will minimize crippling and allow the child to grow and develop to full potential.
2. Teach the family that daily exercises such as swimming help to maintain full range of motion. Avoid exercises that cause overtiring and joint pain.
3. Urge the parents to keep the school nurse informed of child's condition to ensure continuity of care even at school. Tell the parents to inform child's teacher of need for hourly movement, adverse effects of medications, and application of special equipment.
4. Teach the family about a nutritionally balanced diet to prevent obesity, which puts additional stress on joints.
5. Stress the need for routine follow-up care, ophthalmologic evaluation, and prompt attention to infections or other illness that may prompt exacerbations.

COMMUNITY CARE CONSIDERATIONS

Review child's immunization record to make sure health maintenance needs have not been overlooked. Advise to get flu vaccine
each year to decrease stress caused by the flu and risk of Reye's
syndrome from salicylate intake during viral illness. Do not give live
vaccines to patients on corticosteroids or biologic therapies because immunosuppression may lead to illness by vaccine.

6. Refer the family to agencies such as the American Juvenile Arthritis Foundation, www.jraworld.arthritisinsight.com,
   and the Arthritis Foundation, *www.arthritis.org*.

RHINITIS, ALLERGIC

Allergic rhinitis is an inflammation of the nasal mucosa caused
by an allergen. Airborne allergens, such as pollen (seasonal)
or dust, mold, or animal dander, (perennial) cause a type I hypersensitivity reaction with local vasodilation and increased
capillary permeability. Allergic rhinitis affects 8% to 10% of
the population. Other types of rhinitis include *nonallergic rhinitis,* also called *vasomotor rhinitis, drug-induced (rebound) rhinitis), rhinitis of pregnancy,* and *infectious rhinitis*. They have similar, but often milder, presentations and do not respond to
antihistamines. Sinusitis is a complication of rhinitis due to
obstruction.

Assessment
1. Mucous membrane congestion, edema, and itching; rhinorrhea, sneezing
2. Conjunctival edema, itching, and burning; increased
   lacrimation; dark circles under eyes (allergic shiners)
3. Itching and congestion of ears
4. Itching of palate and throat; nonproductive cough

Diagnostic Evaluation
1. Increased eosinophils on nasal smear
2. Skin testing confirms hypersensitivity to specific allergens.

R

3. Radioallergosorbent test: measurement of immunoglobulin (Ig) E antibodies in serum samples after a panel of allergens has been added

Collaborative Management
Therapeutic Interventions
1. Minimize contact with offending allergens.

Pharmacologic Interventions
1. Antihistamines block the effects of histamine and relieve symptoms.
2. Topical or oral decongestants shrink mucous membranes by causing vasoconstriction.
3. Intranasal cromolyn sodium, a mast cell stabilizer, hinders the release of chemical mediators and prevents acute symptoms.
4. Corticosteroids used intranasally or orally for short course reduces inflammation; also works for nonallergic rhinitis.
5. Immunotherapy: serial injections of increasing amounts of specific allergens to decrease sensitivity and reduce symptoms.

 EMERGENCY ALERT Immunotherapy should not be given to patients taking beta-adrenergic blockers because they may mask a systemic reaction.

Nursing Diagnoses
24, 75

Nursing Interventions
Supportive Care
1. Reassure patient that suffocation will not occur because of nasal obstruction; mouth breathing will occur.
2. Use a bedside humidifier and increase oral fluids to prevent drying of mucous membranes from mouth breathing.
3. Observe patient after immunotherapy injection for 30 minutes for severe local or systemic reaction.

EMERGENCY ALERT Always have epinephrine 1:1,000 available for injection should anaphylaxis occur after allergy shot.

Education and Health Maintenance

1. Teach patient the proper use of nasal inhalers: clear mucus from nose first, exhale, then inhale while releasing medication.
2. Advise patient to use caution when driving and in other situations that require alertness while taking potentially sedating antihistamines.
3. Advise patient to limit use of over-the-counter nasal decongestants to 2 to 3 days to prevent rebound effect causing mucosal edema.
4. Instruct patient on environmental control measures.
   a. Use nonallergenic bedding materials and cover mattress and pillows with plastic covers.
   b. Use washable curtains and throw rugs.
   c. Avoid stuffed animals and other dust-collecting items.
   d. Damp-dust daily and wear a mask while doing it.
   e. Keep windows closed and use an air conditioner while allergens are prevalent outside.
   f. Change furnace filter frequently and use air-filtering system if possible.
   g. If allergic to animal dander, keep pets outside, or at least out of bedroom.
   h. Keep damp areas well cleaned and dehumidified to avoid mold.

RUPTURED DISC
See *Herniated Intervertebral Disc (Ruptured Disc)*.

S

SCHIZOPHRENIA, SCHIZOPHRENIFORM, AND DELUSIONAL DISORDERS

Schizophrenia, schizophreniform, and *delusional disorders* are defined by psychotic symptoms. Psychotic symptoms are produced by a loss of ego boundaries and severe impairment of reality testing, and include prominent hallucinations and delusions, disorganized speech, and grossly disorganized or catatonic behavior.

Schizophrenia may result from a complex combination of genetic, neurobiological, and psychological factors. The American Psychological Association recognizes five types of schizophrenia: paranoid, disorganized, residual, catatonic, and undifferentiated. Symptoms in each of these forms must be evident for at least 6 months. *Schizophreniform disorder* is a syndrome that resembles schizophrenia in many respects, but lasts less than 6 months. Schizophrenia may affect up to 2% of the general population, and it occurs primarily during adolescence or early adulthood. *Schizoaffective disorder* is characterized by an uninterrupted period of illness in which there was a major depressive, manic, or mixed episode with concurrent symptoms of schizophrenia.

In a *delusional disorder*, there are no symptoms of schizophrenia, but tactile and olfactory hallucinations may be present and are related to the delusional theme. The patient manifests false beliefs (delusions) that may have a plausible basis in reality, and functioning is not greatly impaired. The delusions do not result from another mental disorder, medical condition, or drug. Little has been established about the cause of delusional disorders; there is no demonstrated genetic linkage. It is possible that psychosocial stressors play a role in some persons. Delusional disorders are more common in middle-aged or older patients.

Complications of these psychotic disorders are substance abuse, homelessness, neglect of medical conditions, and suicide.

Assessment

Positive symptoms of schizophrenia: These symptoms reflect aberrant mental activity and are usually present early in the first phase of the schizophrenic illness.

1. Delusion: false, fixed belief that is not amenable to change by reasoning. The most frequently elicited delusions include ideas of reference, delusions of grandeur, delusions of jealousy, delusions of persecution, and somatic delusions.
2. Loose associations: the thought process becomes illogical and confused.
3. Neologisms: made-up words that have a special meaning to the delusional person.
4. Concrete thinking: an overemphasis on small or specific details and an impaired ability to abstract.
5. Echolalia: pathologic repeating of another's words.
6. Clang associations: the meaningless rhyming of a word in a forceful way.
7. Word salad: a mixture of words that are meaningless to the listener.
8. Hallucinations: sensory perceptions that have no external stimulus; the most common are auditory, visual, gustatory, olfactory, and tactile.
9. Loss of ego boundaries: the patient lacks a sense of the body and how he or she relates to the environment.
   a. Depersonalization is a nonspecific feeling or sense that a person has lost his or her identity or is unreal.
   b. Derealization is the false perception by a person that the environment has changed.
10. Bizarre behavioral patterns
    a. Motor agitation or restlessness
    b. Automatic obedience or robotlike movement
    c. Negativism
    d. Stereotyped behaviors
    e. Stupor

    f. Waxy flexibility

11. Agitated or impulsive behavior

Negative symptoms of schizophrenia: these symptoms reflect a deficiency of mental functioning.

1. Alogia: inability to speak
2. Anergia: inability to react
3. Anhedonia: inability to experience pleasure
4. Avolition: inability to choose or decide
5. Poor social functioning
6. Poverty of speech
7. Social withdrawal
8. Thought blocking

Diagnostic Evaluation

1. Clinical diagnosis is developed on historical information and thorough mental status examination.
2. No laboratory findings have been identified that are diagnostic of schizophrenia.
3. Routine battery of laboratory tests may be useful in ruling out possible organic causes, such as a complete blood count, thyroid function tests, tests for syphilis, test for human immunodeficiency virus, and ceruloplasmin.
4. Rating scale assessment.
   a. Scale for the Assessment of Negative Symptoms (SANS)
   b. Scale for the Assessment of Positive Symptoms (SAPS)

Collaborative Management
Therapeutic Interventions

1. Psychosocial treatments in schizophrenia or schizophreniform disorder include:
   a. Supportive individual psychotherapy that is reality oriented and pragmatic
   b. Structured group psychotherapy
   c. Family therapy
   d. Psychoeducation group
   e. Support groups in community
   f. Community-based partial hospitalization programs
   g. Psychiatric home care nursing

2. Vocational and social skills education
3. In delusional disorders, individual psychotherapy most helpful
4. Hospitalization for comprehensive assessment for diagnostic purposes or if suicidal or homicidal

Pharmacologic Interventions

1. Antipsychotics (neuroleptic agents)
   a. Typical neuroleptics include haloperidol, chlorpromazine, and thioridazine.
   b. Atypical neuroleptics have fewer adverse effects and are more effective than typical neuroleptics in controlling negative symptoms; these include risperidone, olanzapine, and clozapine.
2. Anticholinergic agents, such as benztropine, to counteract extrapyramidal effects of neuroleptic medications
3. Adjunctive pharmacologic agents, such as anxiolytics, lithium, antidepressants, propranolol, and carbamazepine

Nursing Diagnoses

1, 35, 78, 136, 139, 146, 159

Nursing Interventions

Monitoring

1. Monitor and document the patient's response to antipsychotic medication regimen.
2. Monitor patient for increased anxiety.
3. Frequently monitor the restrained patient within the guidelines of the facility's policy on restrictive devices, and assess the patient's level of agitation.
4. Monitor patient for adverse effects of neuroleptics, such as orthostatic hypotension, dry mouth, blurred vision, constipation, urinary retention, and extrapyramidal reactions.
   a. Short-term extrapyramidal reactions include motor agitation, weakness, dystonias, and parkinsonian effects.
   b. Tardive dyskinesia is a long-term extrapyramidal reaction that involves abnormal, involuntary movements of the head, limbs, and trunks.

c. Report significant orthostatic hypotension, blurred vision, urinary retention, and extrapyramidal reactions; dose may be adjusted.

Supportive Care

1. Encourage the patient to talk about feelings.
2. Provide the patient with honest and consistent feedback in a nonthreatening manner.
3. Avoid challenging the content of the patient's behaviors.
4. Focus interactions on the patient's behaviors.
5. Use simple and clear language when speaking with the patient.
6. Explain all procedures, tests, and activities to the patient before starting them, and provide written or video material for learning purposes.
7. Provide opportunities for socialization and encourage participation in group activities.
8. Be aware of the patient's personal space and use touch in a judicious manner.
9. Assist the patient to identify behaviors that alienate significant others or family members.
10. Collaborate with the patient and occupational and physical therapy specialists to assess the patient's ability to perform activities of daily living (ADLs).
11. Collaborate with the patient to establish a daily, achievable routine within any physical limitations.
12. Teach strategies to manage adverse effects of antipsychotics:
    a. Change positions slowly.
    b. Gradually increase physical activities.
    c. Limit overexertion in hot, sunny weather.
    d. Use sun precautions.
    e. Rinse mouth frequently, brush teeth after meals, drink fluids between meals, and suck on sugarless hard candy or chew gum to minimize dry mouth.
    f. Increase fluids and fiber in diet and maintain activity to relieve constipation.
    g. Void at regular intervals in relaxed, private setting to overcome urinary retention.

    h. Use caution in activities if extrapyramidal symptoms develop.

13. Encourage the patient to explore adaptive behaviors that increase the patient's abilities and success in socializing and accomplishing ADLs.
14. Decrease environmental stimuli.
15. Collaborate with the patient to identify anxious behaviors as well as the causes.
16. Tell the patient that you will help him or her maintain control.
17. Establish consistent limits on the patient's behaviors and clearly communicate these limits to the patient, family members, and health care providers.
18. Secure all potential weapons and articles that could be used to inflict an injury from the patient's room and the unit environment.
19. To prepare for possible continued escalation, form a psychiatric emergency assist team and designate a leader to facilitate an effective and safe aggression management process.
20. Determine the need for external control, including seclusion or restraints. Communicate the decision to the patient and put plan into action.
21. When the patient's level of agitation begins to decrease and self-control is regained, establish a behavioral agreement that identifies specific self-control behaviors against re-escalating agitation.

Education and Health Maintenance

1. Teach the patient about the disease process and how to recognize and cope with relapse symptoms.
2. Instruct the patient about the uses, actions, and adverse effects of any prescribed medications.
3. Advise patient about community resources, support groups, and possible use of psychiatric home care nursing.

COMMUNITY CARE CONSIDERATIONS

Patients with these disorders may be in supportive housing, such as halfway houses, foster homes, and board and care homes. Psychiatric home care nursing is important for medication management and as part of the treatment team to teach independent living skills.

4. For additional information and support, refer to National Alliance for Research on Schizophrenia and Depression (NARSAD), *www.narsad.org*.

SCLERODERMA

Scleroderma (systemic sclerosis) is a generalized connective tissue disorder of unknown cause characterized by hardening or thickening of the skin, blood vessels, synovium, skeletal muscles, and internal organs. Fibrotic, degenerative, and inflammatory changes including vascular insufficiency are most likely caused by overproduction of collagen by fibroblasts. The disorder affects three to four times as many women as men.

Complications include skin ulcers, malabsorption, esophageal adenocarcinoma, pulmonary hypertension, renal failure, heart failure, and death.

Assessment

1. Skin-related manifestations:
   a. Bilateral symmetric swelling of the hands and sometimes the feet.
   b. Hardening and thickening of skin after edematous phase.
   c. Digits, dorsum of hand, neck, face, and trunk are involved.
   d. Normal landmarks in skin are absent (no skin folds).
   e. Increased or decreased skin pigmentation.
   f. Skin changes may regress after several years.
   g. Telangiectasias on tongue, face, fingers, and lips.
   h. Areas of calcinosis in late disease.
   i. Raynaud's phenomenon.
2. GI manifestations:

a. Esophageal dysmotility resulting in reflux and esophagitis.

b. Distal esophageal dilation and esophagitis.

c. Barrett's metaplasia may predispose to adenocarcinoma of the esophagus.

d. Duodenal atrophy and dilation may cause postprandial abdominal pain, malabsorption, diarrhea, and abdominal distention.

e. Colonic hypomotility resulting in constipation.

3. Musculoskeletal manifestations:

a. Joint pain

b. Polyarthritis (large and small joints affected)

c. Carpal tunnel syndrome

d. Flexion contractures

e. Inflammatory muscle atrophy

4. Cardiac manifestations:

a. Left ventricular dysfunction

b. Heart failure and atrial and ventricular arrhythmias

c. Right ventricular involvement secondary to pulmonary disease

5. Pulmonary manifestations:

a. Interstitial fibrosis

b. Restrictive lung disease

c. Pulmonary hypertension

6. Renal manifestations:

a. Scleroderma renal crisis — rapid malignant hypertension with encephalopathy

7. CREST syndrome: **C**alcinosis, **R**aynaud's phenomenon, **E**sophageal dysmotility, **S**clerodactyly, **T**elangiectasia.

8. Linear and morphea scleroderma: localized scleroderma with lesions appearing as streaks or bands in linear scleroderma, or purple-bordered lesions of several centimeters in diameter in morphea scleroderma. There is generally no visceral involvement.

Diagnostic Evaluation

1. Complete blood count and erythrocyte sedimentation rate are usually normal.

2. Rheumatoid factor is positive in approximately 30% of patients.
3. Antinuclear antibodies are generally present.
4. Scl 70 positive in diffuse cutaneous disease.
5. Anticentromere antibody highly specific for limited cutaneous disease.
6. X-rays of hands and wrists show muscle atrophy, osteopenia, and osteolysis.
7. Barium swallow shows esophageal dysmotility.
8. Multigated angiogram scans may be done to determine left ventricular function.
9. Pulmonary function tests show decreased diffusion capacity and vital capacity, restrictive lung disease.
10. Endoscopy may be done to obtain biopsy specimen for Barrett's metaplasia.
11. Esophageal manometry may be done to determine contractile capacity of esophageal muscles.

Collaborative Management
Therapeutic Interventions
1. Application of prescribed skin lubricants
2. Avoidance of factors associated with exacerbation of Raynaud's phenomenon
3. Use of biofeedback
4. Stem cell transplantation (under investigation)

Pharmacologic Interventions
1. Penicillamine to decrease disease activity
2. Calcium channel blockers for Raynaud's phenomenon
3. Nonsteroidal anti-inflammatory drugs to control pain of arthralgias and polyarthritis
4. Histamine-2 blockers and omeprazole for reflux
5. Antibiotics for malabsorption and bacterial overgrowth
6. Antihypertensive agents
7. Metoclopramide for intestinal dysmotility

Nursing Diagnoses
13, 60, 66, 134

Nursing Interventions
Monitoring
1. Monitor and report serious adverse reactions of penicillamine therapy, such as optic neuritis; thrombocytopenia; agranulocytosis; anemia; jaundice; abdominal pain due to pancreatitis; pruritus and rash, which may lead to exfoliative dermatitis; hematuria; and proteinuria.
2. Monitor nutritional intake and weigh the patient weekly.
3. Inspect the skin daily for cracking, ulceration, and signs of infection.

Supportive Care
1. Teach the patient to recognize Raynaud's phenomenon and to reduce factors associated with it, such as exposure to cold, smoking, and emotional stress.
2. Protect ulcerated digits and observe for signs of infection.
3. Apply moisturizers to skin daily.
4. Advise patient to avoid use of drying soaps and detergents.
5. Use protective padding (eg, elbow pads) to protect the skin from friction or trauma.
6. Provide small, frequent, well-balanced meals.
7. Encourage the patient to remain upright after meals for 45 to 60 minutes and raise head of bed during sleep to avoid reflux and aspiration.
8. Encourage good oral hygiene and frequent dental visits.
9. Advise patient to use lubricating agents, if necessary, to treat dry mouth and teach stretching exercises of mouth to maintain aperture.
10. Refer to social worker for supportive services and for counseling as needed.

Education and Health Maintenance
1. Explain to the patient diagnostic tests and their purpose in detecting GI, pulmonary, renal, or cardiac involvement.
2. Teach the patient about drug treatments, including adverse reactions.

3. Advise patient about fluid and sodium restriction if heart failure has been identified.

4. Advise patient to modify activity and use oxygen to prevent dyspnea caused by restrictive lung disease.

5. Encourage regular follow-up and prompt attention to worsening symptoms.

6. For more information, refer the patient to Scleroderma Foundation, *www.scleroderma.org*.

SCOLIOSIS

Scoliosis is a lateral curvature of the spine resulting from rotation and deformity of vertebrae. Three forms of structural scoliosis are recognized. *Idiopathic scoliosis* is the most common form and is classified into three groups: infantile, which presents from birth to age 3; juvenile, which presents from ages 3 to 10; and adolescent, which presents after age 10 (most common age). *Congenital scoliosis* results in the malformation of one or more vertebral bodies. In *neuromuscular scoliosis*, the child has a neuromuscular condition (such as cerebral palsy, spina bifida, or muscular dystrophy) that directly contributes to the deformity. Additional but less common causes of scoliosis include osteopathic conditions, such as fractures, bone disease, arthritic conditions, and infections.

In all types of scoliosis, the vertebrae rotate to the convex side of the curve that rotates the spinous processes to the concavity. Vertebrae become wedge shaped, and disc shape is also altered. In severe scoliosis, progressive changes in the thoracic cage may cause respiratory and cardiovascular compromise.

Assessment

1. Poor posture, uneven shoulder height.

2. One hip more prominent than the other.

3. Scapular prominence.

4. Uneven waistline (pelvis) or hemline.

5. Spinal curve observable or palpable both upright and bent forward.

6. Back pain may be present but is not a routine finding in idiopathic scoliosis.

7. Leg length discrepancy.

▣ **PEDIATRIC ALERT** The adolescent who presents with back pain and scoliosis warrants close consideration to rule out other conditions, such as a tumor, disk pathology, or intraspinal anomalies.

Diagnostic Evaluation

1. X-rays of the spine in the upright position, preferably on one long 36-inch (91-cm) cassette, show characteristic curvature.
2. MRI, myelograms, or CT scan with or without three-dimensional reconstruction may be indicated for children with severe curvatures who have a known or suspected spinal column anomaly, before management decisions are made.
3. Pulmonary function tests for compromised respiratory status.
4. Evaluate for renal abnormalities in children with congenital scoliosis (high correlation between the two).

Collaborative Management

Therapeutic Interventions

1. Curves that are less than 10 degrees are considered spinal asymmetry, not true scoliosis, and are managed by observation on routine well-child visits.
2. Curves measuring 10 to 25 degrees are followed by close observation every 3 to 4 months, particularly during growth spurts.
3. In curves that are observed to be progressing (more than 6 degrees on X-ray measurement or any change on examination) or curves measuring 25 to 40 degrees, brace management may be required either full time or nighttime.
   a. Requires child's faithful compliance to succeed.
   b. Some curves progress despite brace wear.
4. Types of braces include:
   a. Boston orthosis for low thoracic and thoracolumbar curves. This is an underarm molded orthosis.
   b. Milwaukee brace for thoracic or double major curves. Standard brace has neck ring with chin rest.

S

    c. Charleston bending brace has been tried for nighttime use in selected patients. Results have been positive in some centers, but brace is not yet widely accepted.

5. Exercise therapy has been promoted to help maintain spinal flexibility and prevent muscle atrophy during prolonged bracing.

Surgical Interventions

1. Stabilization of the spinal column is usually accomplished with a spinal fusion and one of several methods of instrumentation.
   a. Harrington instrumentation and posterior spinal fusion
   b. Multiple-level (segmental fixation) systems, such as the Texas Scottish Rite Hospital (TSRH) or Cotrel-Dubousset Systems
   c. Luque technique, which includes dual rods with sublaminar wire segmental fixation (usually reserved for children with preexisting neurologic compromise because of increased risk of neurologic damage from sublaminar wires)
   d. Anterior procedures, which include staple and cable or rod systems such as the Dwyer or Anterior TSRH

2. Indications for surgical correction vary, but generally include the following:
   a. Progression of the curve over a short period in a curve greater than 40 degrees despite bracing
   b. Skeletal immaturity
   c. Bracing not possible

3. Preoperative traction or casting may be used to help gain correction and increase flexibility.

4. Postoperative protection of the fusion mass by means of a cast or brace is usually required.

Nursing Diagnoses
30, 80, 134, 136

Nursing Interventions
Supportive Care
1. Prepare the child for casting or immobilization procedure by showing materials to be used and describing procedure in age-appropriate terms.
2. Promote comfort with proper fit of brace or cast.
3. Provide opportunity for the child to express fears and ask questions about deformity and brace wear.
4. Assess skin integrity under and around the brace or cast frequently.
5. Provide good skin care to prevent breakdown around any pressure areas.
6. Care of child undergoing surgery is similar to care of patient with herniated disc (see page 459).

Education and Health Maintenance
1. Instruct the patient to examine brace daily for signs of loosening or breakage. An orthotist should be contacted for necessary repairs.
2. Instruct patient to wear cotton shirt under brace to avoid rubbing.
3. Instruct patient about which previous activities can be continued in the brace. Usually all but contact sports and certain gymnastic activities can be continued.
4. Provide a peer support person when possible so the child can associate positive outcomes and experiences from others.

SEIZURE DISORDER

Seizures (also known as *convulsions*, *epileptic seizures*, and, if recurrent, *epilepsy*) are defined as sudden alterations in normal brain activity that cause distinct changes in behavior and body function. They are thought to result from abnormal, recurrent, uncontrolled electric discharges of neurons in the brain. The pathophysiology of seizures is poorly understood but seems to be related to metabolic and electrochemical factors at the cellular level. Predisposing factors include head or brain trauma; tumors; cranial surgery; metabolic disorders (hypocalcemia, hypoglycemia or hyperglycemia, hyponatremia, anoxia); central nervous system infection; circulatory disorders; drug toxicity; drug withdrawal states (alcohol, barbiturates); and congenital neurodegenerative disorders.

Seizures are classified as *partial* or *generalized* by the origin of the seizure activity and associated clinical manifestations. Simple partial seizures manifest motor, somatosensory, and psychomotor symptoms without impairment of consciousness. Complex partial seizures manifest impairment of consciousness with or without simple partial symptoms. Simple partial seizures can progress to complex partial seizures, and complex partial seizures can secondarily become generalized.

Generalized seizures manifest a loss of consciousness with convulsive or nonconvulsive behaviors and include tonic-clonic, myoclonic, atonic, and absence seizures.

Seizures affect all ages. Most cases of epilepsy are identified in childhood, and several seizure types are particular to children. Complications include status epilepticus (see *Box S-1*), cerebral impairment caused by anoxia with generalized seizures, and injuries caused by falls.

Assessment

1. Generalized tonic-clonic (grand mal) seizure
   a. May be preceded by an aura such as a peculiar sensation or dizziness; then sudden onset of seizure with loss of consciousness
   b. Rigid muscle contraction in tonic phase with clenched jaw and hands; eyes open with pupils dilated; lasts 30 to 60 seconds
   c. Rhythmic, jerky contraction and relaxation of all muscles in clonic phase with incontinence and frothing at the lips; may bite tongue or cheek; lasts several minutes
   d. Sleeping or dazed postictal state for up to several hours
2. Absence (petit mal) seizure
   a. Loss of contact with environment for 5 to 30 seconds
   b. Appears to be daydreaming or may roll eyes, nod head, move hands, or smack lips
   c. Resumes activity and is not aware of seizure
3. Myoclonic seizure (infantile spasm)

| BOX S-1 | **Emergency Management of Status Epilepticus** |

Status epilepticus (acute, prolonged, repetitive seizure activity) is a series of generalized seizures without return to consciousness between attacks. The term has been broadened to include continuous clinical or electrical seizures lasting at least 5 minutes, even without impairment of consciousness.

Status epilepticus is considered a serious neurologic emergency. It has a high mortality and morbidity rate (permanent brain damage; severe neurologic deficits).

Factors that precipitate status epilepticus include medication withdrawal, fever, metabolic or environmental stresses, alcohol withdrawal, and sleep deprivation, in patients with preexisting seizure disorder.

INTERVENTIONS

- Establish an airway and maintain blood pressure.
- Obtain blood studies for glucose, blood urea nitrogen, electrolytes, and anticonvulsant drug levels to determine metabolic abnormalities and serve as a guide for maintenance of biochemical homeostasis.
- Administer oxygen. There is some respiratory arrest at height of each seizure, which may produce venous congestion and hypoxia of brain.
- Establish I.V. lines and keep open for blood sampling, drug administration, and infusion of fluids.
- Administer I.V. anticonvulsants slowly (diazepam, phenytoin) to ensure effective brain tissue and serum concentrations.
  - Additional anticonvulsants given as directed.
  - Anticonvulsant drug levels monitored regularly.
- Monitor the patient continuously; depression of respiration and blood pressure induced by drug therapy may be delayed.
- Use of mechanical ventilation as needed.
- If initial treatment is unsuccessful, general anesthesia may be required.
- Assist with search for precipitating factors.
  - Monitor vital and neurologic signs on a continuing basis.
  - Use electroencephalographic monitoring to determine nature and abolition (after diazepam administration) of epileptic activity.
  - Determine (from family member) if there is a history of epilepsy, alcohol or drug use, trauma, or recent infection.

S

a. Seen in children or infants, caused by cerebral pathology, often with mental retardation.

b. Infantile spasms usually disappear by age 4, but child may develop other types of seizures.

c. Brief, sudden, forceful contractions of the muscles of the trunk, neck, and extremities.

d. Extensor type — infant extends head, spreads arms out, bends body backward in "spread eagle" position.

e. Mixed flexor and extensor types may occur in clusters or alternate.

f. May cause children to drop or throw something.

g. Infant may cry out, grunt, grimace, laugh, or appear fearful during an attack.

4. Partial (focal) motor seizure

a. Rhythmic twitching of muscle group, usually hand or face

b. May spread to involve entire limb, other extremity, and face on that side; known as *jacksonian seizure*

5. Partial (focal) somatosensory seizure

a. Numbness and tingling in a part of the body

b. May also be visual, taste, auditory, or olfactory sensation

6. Partial psychomotor (temporal lobe) seizure

a. May be aura of abdominal discomfort or bad odor or taste.

b. Auditory or visual hallucinations, déjà vu feeling, or sense of fear or anxiety.

c. Repetitive purposeless movements (automatisms) may occur, such as picking at clothes, smacking lips, chewing, and grimacing.

d. Lasts seconds to minutes.

7. Complex partial seizures: begin as partial seizures and progress to impairment of consciousness or impaired consciousness at onset

8. Febrile seizure

a. Generalized tonic-clonic seizure with fever over 101.8° F (38.8° C).

b. Occurs in children younger than age 5.

c. Treatment is to decrease temperature, treat source of fever, and control seizure.

d. Long-term treatment to prevent recurrent seizures with fever is controversial.

Diagnostic Evaluation

1. EEG, with or without video monitoring, locates epileptic focus, spread, intensity, and duration; helps classify seizure type.
2. CT scanning or MRI identifies lesion that may be cause of seizure.
3. Single photon emission CT scanning (SPECT) or positron emission tomography (PET) identifies seizure foci.
4. Neuropsychological studies evaluate for behavioral disturbances.
5. Serum electrolytes, glucose, and toxicology screen determine cause of first seizure.
6. Lumbar puncture and blood cultures may be necessary if fever is present.

Collaborative Management
Therapeutic Interventions

1. Maintain good nutrition and sleep hygiene and avoid stress to help decrease frequency of seizures.
2. A ketogenic diet has been used for seizure control in some patients, when medications fail or adequate dosage of medication causes toxicity.
   a. Diet consists of precisely calculated portions of protein and fat without carbohydrates. As fats are metabolized for energy, ketones are formed, which are thought to inhibit seizures.
   b. I.V. fluids should be dextrose free, and all medications should be in sugar-free suspensions.
3. Biofeedback may help prevent seizures in the patient with reliable auras.

Pharmacologic Interventions

1. Antiepileptic drugs (AEDs) may be used singly or in combination to increase effectiveness, treat mixed seizure types, and reduce adverse effects. (See *Table S-1*.)
   a. It may take several months to titrate drugs to obtain the desired clinical effect. Dosage changes are made slowly.
   b. Most AEDs are not considered safe in pregnancy unless the benefit outweighs the risk, therefore women of childbearing age should use a reliable form of contraception. Pregnant women should not discontinue AEDs abruptly.
2. A wide variety of adverse reactions may occur, including hepatic and renal dysfunction, vision disturbances, drowsiness, ataxia, anemia, leukopenia, thrombocytopenia, psychotic symptoms, skin rash, stomach upset, and idiosyncratic reactions.

PEDIATRIC ALERT There is some evidence that long-term treatment of children with some anticonvulsants may cause intellectual impairment. Therefore, medication may be withdrawn if child is seizure free for 2 years.

Surgical Interventions

1. Surgical treatment of brain tumor or hematoma may relieve seizures caused by these.
2. Temporal lobectomy, extratemporal resection, corpus callosotomy, or hemispherectomy may be necessary in medically intractable seizure disorders.

Nursing Diagnoses
78, 88, 93, 119, 136

Nursing Interventions
Monitoring

1. Monitor the entire seizure event, including prodromal signs, seizure behavior, and postictal state.
2. Monitor serum levels for therapeutic range of medications.

TABLE S-1	Select Antiepileptic Drugs

DRUG/USE	NURSING CONSIDERATIONS
Phenytoin (Dilantin) Partial and generalized seizures (except absence seizures)	Encourage good oral hygiene; therapeutic range is 10 to 20 mcg/mL; administer I.V. with normal saline, do not exceed 0.5 mg/kg/minute; interacts with many drugs; administer with food
Phenobarbital (Luminal) Partial and generalized seizures	Contraindicated in hepatic or renal dysfunction; therapeutic range is 20 to 40 mcg/mL; avoid use with other central nervous system (CNS) depressants; may cause dependence; I.V. rate should not exceed 1 mg/kg/minute. Interactions with valproic acid, theophylline, oral contraceptives, anticoagulants, beta-adrenergic blockers, doxycycline, metronidazole, and other drugs.
Valproic acid (Depakene)/Divalproex sodium (Depakote) Sole therapy for absence seizures and adjunct therapy for partial and generalized seizures	Liver function tests and platelet count should be monitored monthly for at least first 6 months; take with food to minimize GI adverse effects; therapeutic range is 50 to 100 mcg/mL; administer I.V. over 60 minutes, not more than 20 mg/minute; avoid use with other CNS depressants
Carbamazepine (Tegretol) Refractory partial and generalized seizures	Use cautiously in patients with existing cardiac, renal, or liver problems; therapeutic range is 4 to 12 mcg/mL; many drug interactions exist; give with food; periodic eye examinations and laboratory testing for liver function, complete blood count (CBC), and renal function may be ordered

(continued)

S

Select Antiepileptic Drugs *(continued)*

DRUG/USE	NURSING CONSIDERATIONS
Gabapentin (Neurontin) Adjunct treatment of partial and secondarily generalized seizures	Take first dose at night and avoid activities that require alertness until effects are known; serum levels not necessary
Primidone (Mysoline) Partial seizures, refractory generalized seizures	CBC and liver function tests every 6 months; therapeutic range is 5 to 12 mcg/mL; avoid other CNS depressants; avoid activities that require alertness until effects are known; may interfere with concentration of other antiepileptic medications

EMERGENCY ALERT Noncompliance as well as toxicity of antiepileptic medications can increase seizure frequency. Review serum drug levels before implementing medication changes.

3. Monitor patient for adverse reactions of medications.
4. Monitor complete blood count, urinalysis, and liver function studies for toxicity caused by medications.
5. Monitor emotional and intellectual development in children with seizures.

Supportive Care

1. Provide a safe environment by padding side rails and removing clutter.
2. Place the bed in a low position.
3. Do not restrain the patient during a seizure.

COMMUNITY CARE CONSIDERATIONS

Make sure that the home environment is safe, especially for children. Remove toys with sharp edges or parts and small pieces that could be choked on, and cover hard surfaces that the child could fall against.

4. Do not put anything in the patient's mouth during a seizure.
5. Maintain a patent airway until the patient is fully awake after a seizure. An oral airway may be placed at the start of a seizure or the airway suctioned if necessary.
6. Provide oxygen during the seizure if the patient becomes cyanotic.
7. Place the patient on side during a seizure to prevent aspiration.
8. Protect the patient's head during a seizure. Provide a helmet to the patient who may fall during a seizure.
9. Stay with the patient who is ambulating or in a confused state during a seizure.
10. Consult with a social worker for community resources for vocational rehabilitation, counselors, and support groups.
11. Teach stress-reduction techniques that will fit into the patient's lifestyle.
12. Initiate appropriate consultation for management of behavior problems that may arise with chronic epilepsy.

Education and Health Maintenance

1. Encourage the patient to determine existence of trigger factors for seizures, such as skipped meals, lack of sleep, and emotional stress.
2. Remind the family of the importance of following medication regimen and maintaining regular laboratory testing, immunizations, medical checkups, and dental and visual examinations.
3. Tell the patient to avoid alcohol because it interferes with metabolism of AEDs and adds to sedation.
4. Encourage the patient and family to discuss feelings and attitudes about epilepsy.
5. Encourage the patient to wear a medical alert card or bracelet.
6. Advise patient that because many other medications share drug interactions with AEDs, check with the health care provider and pharmacist before taking any other prescription or over-the-counter medications.

S

> **DRUG ALERT** Many AEDs interfere with the effectiveness of oral contraceptives. Another reliable form of contraception should be used.

7. Encourage patient to follow a moderate lifestyle routine, including exercise, mental activity, and nutritious diet.
8. Correct myths about epilepsy and reassure family that epilepsy is not contagious, not proven to be hereditary, and not associated with insanity.
9. For the surgical candidate, reinforce instructions related to surgical outcome of the specific surgical approach.
10. Refer the patient and family to Epilepsy Foundation, *www.efa.org*.

SENILE DEMENTIA OF THE ALZHEIMER TYPE

See *Alzheimer's Disease*.

SEVERE ACUTE RESPIRATORY SYNDROME AND OTHER EMERGING INFECTIONS

Severe acute respiratory syndrome (SARS) was first recognized in China in the fall of 2002 and progressed to a global health threat by spring of 2003. It is caused by a previously unrecognized coronavirus, SARS-CoV. The virus can affect humans and animals and is believed to be transmitted through droplet and aerosol routes. Isolation procedures have brought this infection under control; however, the mosquito-borne illness, West Nile virus, has taken over as a threat to elderly persons that are infected.

SARS and West Nile virus join several other viral illnesses that have emerged in the past decade. None has proven as devastating to the world, however, as the human immunodeficiency virus and acquired immunodeficiency syndrome (see page 477). For most of these emerging infections, prompt identification, isolation precautions, and support care can reduce the morbidity and mortality. (See *Table S-2*.)

For the latest recommendations, see *www.cdc.gov/ncidod/dvrd/spb/index.htm*.

TABLE S-2   Emerging Infections

DISEASE, CAUSE, TRANSMISSION	NURSING IMPLICATIONS

Hantavirus pulmonary syndrome or hemorrhagic fever

- Hantavirus spread through direct contact with infected rodents, their droppings, or aerosolized rodent excreta
- Not transmitted person to person

- Phases may be overlapping and include: febrile, hypotensive, oliguric, diuretic, and convalescent.
- Intensive care for 24 to 48 hours is critical; morbidity is 50% with pulmonary syndrome.
- Prevention through rodent control, wet-mop cleaning to avoid aerosolization, and disinfection with 10% bleach solution.

Ebola-Marburg viral diseases causing clinical hemorrhagic fever

- Marburg virus or Ebola virus, both filoviruses, are spread through direct contact with humans or primates who are infected, through blood, secretions, organs, or semen

- Patient presents with sudden onset of fever, myalgias, headache; followed by pharyngitis, vomiting, diarrhea, and maculopapular rash.
- May lead to hepatic and renal failure, involvement of central nervous system, shock, and multiorgan failure.
- Mortality is 25% with Marburg, 50% to 90% with Ebola, virtually 100% if due to needle contamination; strict adherence to standard and respiratory precautions are critical.

West Nile meningoencephalitis

- West Nile virus is transmitted through the bite of an infected mosquito to animals and humans, not transmitted person to person
- First appeared in the United States in 1999 and has been reported in more than 40 states.

- Presents as febrile illness with rash, arthritis, myalgias, weakness, lymphadenopathy, meningeal irritability, and encephalitis.
- Condition deteriorates quickly; mortality 50% in the elderly.
- Prevention through mosquito control, protective clothing, use of repellent.

(continued)

S

Emerging Infections *(continued)*

DISEASE, CAUSE, TRANSMISSION	NURSING IMPLICATIONS
SARS; SARS-CoV (corona virus variant)	
• Transmitted via large droplets, possibly aerosol from an infected person	• Patient presents with fever greater than 100.4° F (38° C), cough, dyspnea • Chest X-ray shows pneumonia • Outbreaks can be contained by strict adherence to use of gloves, gown, mask, and eye protection and quarantine of known contacts.
Avian (bird) flu, avian influenza (H5N1)	
• Occurs in outbreaks primarily in Asia in domesticated birds, such as chickens and turkeys, on poultry farms and can be spread to humans through direct contact with infected poultry and contaminated surfaces from their excretions • Person-to-person spread is rare	• Fever, cough, sore throat, muscle aches usually occur, with possible conjunctivitis, pneumonia, and acute respiratory distress. Supportive care is given similar to other types of influenza. • Travelers to Asia should be cautioned to avoid live poultry in farms and markets, and avoid areas that may be contaminated by excretions.

SEXUALLY TRANSMITTED DISEASES

Sexually transmitted diseases (STDs) include a wide variety of viral, bacterial, and other infections transmitted through sexual contact, usually through genital secretions and direct contact with lesions. STDs include gonorrhea, chlamydia, genital herpes, genital warts, syphilis, trichomonas (see page 953), human immunodeficiency virus and acquired immunodeficiency syndrome (see page 477), viral hepatitis (see page 448), scabies, and pubic lice. Rarer STDs include chancroid, lymphogranuloma venereum, and granuloma inguinale. *Table*

S-3, pages 864 and 865, describes common STDs and their clinical manifestation.

Diagnostic Evaluation and Collaborative Management

1. Herpes genitalis
   a. Diagnostic tests include Tzanck smear, viral culture, and antibody tests.
   b. No cure, but symptomatic period is diminished by acyclovir or valacyclovir started with each recurrence; or recurrences reduced or prevented by continuous therapy.
   c. Analgesics and sitz baths promote comfort.
2. Condyloma acuminatum
   a. Diagnosed by appearance, Papanicolaou smear, or biopsy.
   b. Topical therapy with podofilox 0.5%, podophyllin 10% to 25%, or trichloroacetic acid 80% to 90% — may require multiple applications.
   c. Cryotherapy, electrodissection, electrocautery, carbon dioxide laser, or surgical excision may be necessary.
3. Syphilis
   a. Venereal Disease Research Laboratory (VDRL) or rapid plasma regain blood test with confirmation by specific treponemal antibody test.
   b. Preferred treatment is benzathine penicillin G 2.4 million units in single dose.
   c. Oral doxycycline, tetracycline, or erythromycin may be used.
4. Gonorrhea
   a. Diagnosed by Gram stain, culture, or antigen detection test.
   b. I.M. or oral antibiotic therapy with penicillinase-resistant penicillins, some cephalosporins, and quinolones; one large dose treatment is effective for cervicitis and urethritis.
5. Chlamydia
   a. Antigen detection tests.
   b. One dose of azithromycin, or 7-day antibiotic therapy, usually with doxycycline.

S

TABLE S-3 Sexually Transmitted Diseases

DISORDER, CAUSE, INCUBATION	CLINICAL MANIFESTATIONS
Herpes genitalis • Caused by herpes simplex virus, type II in most cases • Incubation is 5-20 days.	• Clustered vesicles on erythematous, edematous base that rupture, leaving shallow, painful ulcer that eventually crusts, mild lymphadenopathy; recurrent and may be brought on by sunburn, fever, stress, infection, menses, pregnancy
Condyloma acuminatum (Genital warts) • Caused by human papilloma virus • Incubation is 3 weeks to 3 months, possibly years before grossly visible	• Single or multiple, soft, fleshy, flat or vegetating, nonpainful growths that may occur on external genitalia, anal area, or internally in the vagina, cervix, or urethra
Syphilis • Caused by the spirochete *Treponema pallidum* • Incubation is 10-90 days for primary, up to 6 months after chancre for secondary	• *Primary:* Nontender, shallow, indurated, clean, dry ulcer; mild regional lymphadenopathy • *Secondary:* Maculopapular rash including palms and soles; mucous patches and condalomatous lesions, fever, generalized lymphadenopathy
Gonorrhea • Caused by *Neisseria gonorrhoeae* • Incubation is 2-5 days	• *Urethritis in men:* Dysuria, yellow discharge; may develop into epididymitis or prostatis. • *Cervicitis in females:* Asymptomatic or mucopurulent discharge, dysuria, pelvic pain; may progress to pelvic inflammatory disease (PID). • *In both sexes:* Pharyngitis, conjunctivitis, proctitis, or disseminated arthritis and skin lesion.

DISORDER, CAUSE, INCUBATION	CLINICAL MANIFESTATIONS
Chlamydia • Caused by *Chlamydia trachomatis* • Incubation period is 7-10 days or longer	• *Urethritis in men:* Asymptomatic or clear to whitish discharge, dysuria, may progress to epididymitis. • *Cervicitis:* Asymptomatic or clear to creamy discharge, bleeding, dysuria, pelvic discomfort; may progress to PID or infertility.

Nursing Diagnoses
3, 24, 135, 136

Nursing Interventions and Patient Education

1. Explain transmission of STDs and preventive measures, such as male or female condoms, abstinence, and mutual monogamy.

2. Stress the need for sexual abstinence or the use of condoms until treatment of both patient and partner is complete and follow-up has determined cure. In recurrent herpes genitalis, intercourse should be avoided from the first sign of outbreak to complete resolution of symptoms; however, asymptomatic shedding still occurs in many patients.

3. Encourage women to have routine Papanicolaou smears because herpes simplex virus and human papillomavirus may cause cervical changes leading to cancer.

4. Make sure that pregnant women are tested and treated for STDs because risk to fetus occurs during pregnancy and delivery.

5. For further information and support, refer the patient and family to STD National Hotline 800-227-8922 or the American Social Health Association, *www.ashastd.org*.

SHOCK

Shock is inadequate tissue perfusion that occurs as a result of failure of one or more of the following: the heart as a pump, blood volume, arterial resistance vessels, and the capacity of venous beds. Shock is classified as:

Hypovolemic shock occurs when a significant amount of fluid (blood, plasma, electrolytes) is lost from the intravascular space; may result from hemorrhage, burns, or shifts in fluids.

Cardiogenic shock occurs when the heart fails as a pump, primarily because of myocardial infarction, serious cardiac arrhythmias, and depressed myocardial contractility. Secondary causes include mechanical restriction or venous obstruction, as in cardiac tamponade, vena cava obstruction, or tension pneumothorax.

Septic shock occurs as a result of bacteria and their toxins, primarily vasoactive mediators released by gram-negative bacteria. Any infection has the potential to produce septic shock and compromise every physiologic system.

Neurogenic shock occurs as a result of failure of arterial resistance caused by loss of thoracic spinal nerve control, as in spinal cord injury or spinal anesthesia. Other types of shock include anaphylactic shock and hypoglycemic shock.

No matter the cause of shock, inadequate tissue perfusion can lead to multiorgan systems failure, cardiac arrest, and death.

Assessment

1. Decreased level of consciousness
   a. Early signs: confusion, irritability, anxiety, and inability to concentrate
   b. Progresses to lethargy, obtundation, and coma
2. Cool, pale extremities and capillary refill greater than 2 seconds
3. Change in blood pressure
   a. May initially increase because of compensation
   b. Narrow pulse pressure seen early because of increase in diastolic pressure
   c. Decrease in systolic pressure eventually occurs: deviation from normal or systolic below 80 mm Hg or mean arterial pressure below 60 mm Hg
4. Tachycardia, weak thready pulse, tachypnea

5. Decreased urine output: less than 25 mL/hour in adults; less than 1 mL/kg/hour in children

Diagnostic Evaluation

1. Condition is diagnosed by clinical signs, and treatment is begun immediately.
2. Diagnostic testing is done to determine cause of sepsis (cultures of blood, urine, wounds, sputum) as well as body's response to shock (electrolytes, complete blood count, kidney function tests).

Collaborative Management
Therapeutic Interventions

1. Oxygen therapy by nonrebreather face mask to augment oxygen-carrying capacity of arterial blood
2. Intubation and assisted ventilation if necessary
3. Fluid resuscitation for hypovolemic shock, preferably through two large-bore or central lines, initially with lactated Ringer's solution
4. Blood product replacement as indicated
5. Hemodynamic monitoring with Swan-Ganz catheter, especially for cardiogenic shock
6. Hypothermia blanket in septic shock to cool patient

Pharmacologic Interventions

1. Vasopressors, such as dopamine, norepinephrine, and metaraminol, to cause vasoconstriction and raise blood pressure.
2. Positive inotropic agents in cardiogenic shock, such as isoproterenol, digoxin, dobutamine, and amrinone, to increase cardiac contractility and raise cardiac output.
3. Diuretics may be given in cardiogenic shock to decrease pulmonary congestion.
4. Broad-spectrum antibiotics and antipyretics in septic shock.

Nursing Diagnoses
19, 23, 26, 88

S

Nursing Interventions

Monitoring

1. Maintain ongoing monitoring of blood pressure, oxygen saturation, heart rate, central venous pressure, and cardiac rhythm.
2. Monitor respiratory rate, effort, and breath sounds.
3. Monitor patient's temperature in septic shock.
4. Monitor pulmonary artery pressure, pulmonary artery wedge pressure, and cardiac output in cardiogenic shock.
5. Monitor at least hourly urinary output by way of urinary catheter.
6. Monitor arterial blood gas values for acidosis associated with poor perfusion.
7. Monitor hemoglobin level and hematocrit to assess hemorrhage.

Supportive Care

1. Maintain patient in supine position with legs elevated.

 EMERGENCY ALERT Trendelenburg's position for shock is no longer recommended because of potential for respiratory compromise from pressure of abdominal organs.

2. Infuse I.V. fluids at a rapid rate based on the degree of hypovolemia. Large volumes of normal saline are given cautiously because hyperchloremic acidosis may result.
3. Infuse blood replacement in hemorrhagic shock and administer antibiotics in septic shock.

 EMERGENCY ALERT Warm the blood before infusion of multiple units to prevent cardiac arrhythmias. Additional platelets and clotting factors are also necessary.

4. Report changes in blood pressure and clinical condition immediately.
5. Maintain NPO status until condition is stable and patient is fully alert with good bowel sounds.
6. Titrate vasopressors to desired blood pressure and within prescribed parameters.
7. Stay with patient and provide reassurance. Keep family informed of patient's condition.
8. After stabilization, provide for periods of uninterrupted rest.

Education and Health Maintenance

1. Explain effects of shock on all body systems so patient understands seriousness of illness.
2. Ensure the proper follow-up for underlying cause as well as residual effects of shock (such as renal impairment).
3. Teach patient about medications he or she may be maintained on, such as antibiotics or digoxin.
4. Encourage follow-up blood work for hemoglobin level and hematocrit, electrolytes, kidney function tests, digoxin level, and other tests as indicated.

SICKLE CELL DISEASE

Sickle cell disease (sickle cell anemia) is a severe, chronic, hemolytic anemia occurring in people who are homozygous for the hemoglobin-S (sickle) gene. (See *Table S-4.*) The clinical course is marked by episodes of pain caused by the occlusion of small blood vessels by "sickled" red blood cells (RBC). People heterozygous for the sickling gene (about 8% of blacks) are said to possess *sickle cell trait*, which does not progress to sickle cell anemia.

Sickled RBCs are fragile and rapidly destroyed in the circulation; they live 6 to 20 days versus 120 days for normal RBCs. Anemia results when the rate of destruction of RBCs is greater than the rate of production. Increased sequestration

TABLE S-4	Transmission of Sickle Cell Disease		
GENOTYPE OF PARENTS	**PROBABILITY OF ABNORMAL HEMOGLOBIN IN OFFSPRING**		
	Normal	*Trait*	*Disease*
One parent with trait	50%	50%	0
Both parents with trait	25%	50%	25%
One parent with trait; one parent with disease	0	50%	50%
Both parents with disease	0	0	100%

of RBCs also occurs in the spleen. Premature death may occur from overwhelming sepsis or RBCs sequestration.

Assessment

1. Children do not become symptomatic until late in the first year of life, then symptoms are sporadic.
2. Anemia may last 1 to 2 weeks and subside spontaneously. The child may have a hemoglobin level of 6 to 9 g/dL with loss of appetite, pallor, weakness, fever, irritability, and jaundice.
3. Crisis may be precipitated by dehydration, infection, trauma, strenuous physical exertion, extreme fatigue, cold exposure, hypoxia, or acidosis.
4. Vaso-occlusive (painful) crisis—most common form of crisis:
   a. Osteoporosis or ischemic necrosis of bones due to hyperplasia of bone marrow
   b. Bone pain; painful and swollen large joints
   c. Dactylitis ("hand-foot" syndrome): aseptic infarction of metacarpals and metatarsals causing symmetric swelling and pain; often first vaso-occlusive crisis seen in infants and toddlers
   d. Abdominal pain and splenomegaly
   e. Cerebral occlusion causing stroke, hemiplegia, retinal damage leading to blindness, seizures
   f. Pulmonary infarction
   g. Altered renal function: enuresis, hematuria
   h. Impaired liver function
   i. Priapism: abnormal, recurrent, prolonged, painful erection of the penis
5. Splenic sequestration crisis: spleen becomes massively enlarged because of pooling of blood.
   a. Sudden decrease in RBC count.
   b. Signs of circulatory collapse develop rapidly.
   c. Frequent cause of death in infant with sickle cell disease.
6. Aplastic crisis: bone marrow ceases to produce RBCs.
   a. Low reticulocyte count
   b. Pallor, lethargy, dyspnea

c. Possible coma
7. Chronic symptoms related to organ damage:
   a. Jaundice
   b. Gallstones
   c. Progressive impairment of kidney function
   d. Fibrotic spleen resulting in high susceptibility to *Haemophilus influenzae*, *Streptococcus pneumoniae*, osteomyelitis, and pneumococcal septicemia
   e. Growth retardation of the long bones and spine deformities
   f. Aseptic necrosis of bones, especially the femoral and humoral heads
   g. Delayed puberty
   h. Cardiac decompensation related to chronic anemia
   i. Chronic, painful leg ulcers related to decreased peripheral circulation and unrelated to injury; may take months to heal or may not heal without intense therapy, including blood transfusions and grafting
   j. Shortened life span

Diagnostic Evaluation
1. Sickle cell preparation (sickling test)
   a. Blood from heel or fingerstick is deoxygenated and observed under the microscope for evidence of sickled RBCs.
   b. Test does not distinguish between people with sickle cell trait and disease or other sickle hemoglobinopathies.
2. Sickledex test
   a. Combines blood sample in test tube with solution containing a chemical reducing agent. Clouded solution indicates hemoglobin-S.
   b. Also does not distinguish between people with sickle cell trait and disease or other sickle hemoglobinopathies.
3. Hemoglobin electrophoresis
   a. Requires venipuncture.
   b. Hemoglobin is subjected to an electric current that separates the various types and determines the amounts present.

S

    c. Used to diagnose both sickle cell trait and sickle cell disease if two types of hemoglobin are demonstrated in approximately equal amounts.

    d. A person is diagnosed as having sickle cell disease if most of his or her hemoglobin is S-type. The test may also diagnose other sickle hemoglobinopathies, including sickle-C, sickle-G thalassemia, or other hemoglobin variants.

4. Antenatal diagnosis is available to the high-risk group through amniocentesis with DNA analysis.

5. Complete blood count indicates decreased RBCs, elevated white blood cells, elevated platelets, decreased erythrocyte sedimentation rate, increased serum iron, decreased RBC survival time, and low or normal hemoglobin.

Collaborative Management
Therapeutic Interventions

1. Prevention of sickling by promoting adequate oxygenation and hemodilution.

    a. Encourage increased fluid intake: 150 mL/kg/day or 2,250 mL/m^2/day.

    b. Avoid high altitudes and other low-oxygen environments or extreme temperature environments.

    c. Avoid strenuous physical exertion.

    d. Administer oxygen for pulse oximetry of 90% or less.

2. *Aplastic episode:* usually requires a blood transfusion starting at 10 mL/kg.

3. *Splenic sequestration:* usually requires a blood transfusion to release trapped RBCs in severe cases. Plasma volume expanders may also be used to correct hypovolemia.

4. *Hemolytic episode:* usually requires only hydration. May occur with splenic sequestration, aplastic, and painful episodes, which are then treated accordingly. Transfusions are required if there is a significant decrease in hemoglobin.

5. *Vaso-occlusive (painful) episode:* must be distinguished from underlying illness (infection) or other inflammatory condition.

a. Hydration is provided by increased oral and parenteral fluid intake of up to one and one-half or twice fluid maintenance needs.

b. Electrolytes and acid-base balance must be maintained.

6. In vaso-occlusive episode, adjunct pain management techniques may include behavior modification programs, relaxation therapy, hypnosis, and transcutaneous electrical nerve stimulation.

Pharmacologic Interventions

1. Analgesics: administered on fixed schedule, not to extend beyond the duration of the pharmacologic effect.

a. I.V. opioids, such as morphine, are preferred for severe pain, either as a continuous infusion or on a patient-controlled analgesia pump to reach desired effects.

b. Other agents, such as nonsteroidal anti-inflammatory drugs and acetaminophen, are used for milder pain or to increase the analgesic effects of opioids.

2. Investigational drugs include alpha butyrate and hydroxyurea, which increase fetal hemoglobin, thereby preventing sickling.

3. Prevention of infection — major cause of morbidity and mortality — is accomplished through regular immunizations as well as pneumococcal, influenza, and hepatitis immunizations.

4. Antibiotics may be given prophylactically.

Surgical Interventions

1. One or more episodes of splenic sequestration may require splenectomy.

Nursing Diagnoses

1, 3, 23, 88, 108, 135, 136

Nursing Interventions
Monitoring

1. Obtain pulse oximetry reading frequently. Arterial blood gas analysis should be done for correlation and to evaluate acid-base status.

2. Monitor pain relief and adjust dose or time interval for adequate control.
3. Monitor for respiratory depression, hypotension, and drowsiness with opioid analgesics.
4. Monitor fluid intake and output, daily weight, and urine specific gravity to determine fluid balance and hydration status.

Supportive Care

1. Use effective pain relief measures, such as:
   a. Carefully position and support painful areas.
   b. Hold or rock the infant; handle gently.
   c. Distract the child by singing, reading stories, or providing play activities.
   d. Provide familiar objects; encourage visits by familiar persons.
   e. Bathe the child in warm water, applying local heat or massage.
   f. Maintain bed rest during crisis.

PEDIATRIC ALERT Be aware that some children may deny pain to avoid I.M. injection; use alternate route of analgesia. Also, do not give analgesics mixed with aspirin because it enhances acidosis.

2. Share effective methods of reducing pain with other staff members and family.
3. Administer oxygen by way of tent, face mask, or nasal cannula, depending on age of patient.
4. Give meticulous care to leg ulcers and other open wounds.
5. Use good hand-washing and fastidious technique in all procedures.
6. Maintain adequate hydration before and after surgery, and observe the child closely for signs of infection postoperatively, especially of the respiratory tract, to prevent crisis.
7. Maintain bed rest during crisis, then increase activity gradually to increase endurance.
8. Encourage good eating habits, sleep, and relaxation.
9. Provide emotional support to the child and family.
10. Help the child and family to express their feelings of fear and anxiety about what is happening.

11. Assure adolescents that, although sexual development is delayed, they will eventually catch up with their peers.
12. Stress the normalcy of the child despite sickle cell.
    a. Disease does not affect intelligence; the child should go to school and keep up with class work while stable.
    b. Between periods of crisis, the child can usually participate in peer group activities, with the exception of some strenuous sports.
    c. The child needs discipline and limit setting, as do other children in family.

Education and Health Maintenance

1. Discuss the genetic implications of sickle cell disease and offer genetic counseling to the family.
2. Instruct parents in ways that they can help their child to avoid precipitating factors of sickling episodes.
3. Encourage parents to seek prompt treatment of cuts, sores, and mosquito bites, and to notify the health care provider if the child is exposed to a communicable disease.
4. Encourage good dental hygiene and frequent dental checkups to avoid dental infections.

COMMUNITY CARE CONSIDERATIONS

Make sure that patient receives preventive care, including all of the normal childhood immunizations, pneumococcal vaccine, a tuberculin test every 2 to 3 years, trivalent influenza (yearly) vaccine; and dental care every 6 months.

5. Teach the child to avoid undue emotional stress.
6. Warn against trips to the mountains or in not well-pressurized airplanes that will decrease oxygen concentration.
7. Provide sexually active adolescents with information on contraception and sexually transmitted diseases.
8. Teach parents to recognize and manage a mild crisis. Hospitalization may be required for the child if pain becomes severe or if I.V. hydration is required.
9. Teach the signs of severe crisis and whom to notify. Immediately report fever of 102° F (38.9° C).

10. Instruct parents to have emergency information available to those involved in the child's care (school nurse, teacher, baby-sitter, family members, and so forth).
11. Stress the benefit of wearing a medical alert tag.
12. For additional information and support, refer the patient and family to Sickle Cell Foundation of California, *www.scdfc.org*.

SINUSITIS

Sinusitis is an inflammation of the mucous membranes of one or more paranasal sinuses (see *Figure S-1*). Occurring in acute and chronic forms, sinusitis is usually precipitated by congestion from a viral upper respiratory infection or nasal allergy, leading to obstruction of the sinus ostia and retention of secretions. *Chronic sinusitis* is a suppurative inflammation of the sinuses that produces irreversible changes in the mucous membranes. Complications of sinusitis include orbital cellulitis, cranial osteomyelitis, cavernous sinus thrombosis, meningitis, and brain abscess.

Assessment

1. Acute sinusitis:
   a. Stabbing or aching pain over the infected sinus. Pain in forehead intensified by bending forward indicates frontal sinusitis. Aching pain in facial region, and from inner canthus of the eye to the teeth, indicates maxil-

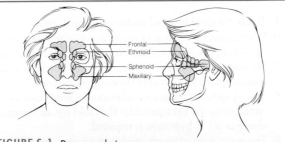

FIGURE S-1 Paranasal sinuses.

lary sinusitis. Frontal or orbital headache indicates ethmoid sinusitis. Headache referred to top of head and deep to the eyes indicates sphenoid sinusitis.
b. Nasal congestion, discharge, postnasal drip, and anosmia (lack of smell) may or may not be present.
c. Fever may be present.
d. Nasal mucosa appears red and edematous.
e. Percussion over involved sinus may produce tenderness, and transillumination will produce dullness.
2. Chronic sinusitis:
a. Persistent nasal obstruction; chronic nasal discharge, clear but becomes purulent when acutely infected
b. Feeling of facial fullness or pressure
c. Cough produced by chronic postnasal drip
d. Headache (more noticeable in the morning), fatigue

Diagnostic Evaluation

1. Sinus X-rays or CT scan may show air-fluid level, thickened mucous membranes, or complete opacification.
2. Antral puncture and lavage provide culture material to identify infectious organism; also a therapeutic modality to clear sinus of bacteria, fluid, and inflammatory cells (acute sinusitis).
3. Endoscopy of nose with CT scanning show mucosal changes in chronic sinusitis.

Collaborative Management
Therapeutic and Pharmacologic Interventions

1. Topical decongestant spray or systemic decongestants for mucosal shrinkage to enhance sinus drainage. Topical therapy should not be used for more than 3 successive days to prevent rebound effect.
2. In chronic sinusitis, nasal corticosteroids may be used to promote drainage, and antihistamines are used for underlying allergies.
3. Antibiotics, such as penicillinase-resistant penicillin, fluoroquinolones, macrolide preparations, or cephalosporins, are used for purulent sinusitis. Therapy may be extended for 6 weeks or more in chronic sinusitis.

S

4. Nasal irrigation with warmed saline solution by bulb syringe to clear nasal passages of crusted drainage and open sinus ostia to promote drainage of secretions from sinuses.

Surgical Interventions

1. Endoscopic sinus surgery — endoscopic removal of diseased tissue from affected sinus; used to treat chronic sinusitis of maxillary, ethmoid, and frontal sinuses
2. Nasal antrostomy (nasal-antral window) — surgical placement of an opening under inferior turbinate to provide aeration of the antrum and to allow drainage of purulent materials in chronic sinusitis

Nursing Diagnoses
3, 13, 24

Nursing Interventions
Monitoring

1. Be alert for possible extension of infection to the orbital contents and eyelids.

   EMERGENCY ALERT Watch for lid edema, edema of ocular conjunctiva, drooping lid, limitation of extraocular motion, and visual loss; these may indicate orbital cellulitis, which requires immediate treatment.

2. Monitor response to therapy and for adverse reactions to antibiotics.
3. After surgery, monitor for bleeding, fever caused by local infection, and aspiration.

Supportive Care

1. After surgery, keep head elevated at night to reduce swelling, and encourage fluids and use of humidifier while nasal packing in place and patient is mouth breathing.
2. Encourage use of cold compresses over incisional area or involved sinus to reduce bleeding and swelling.
3. Encourage frequent mouth care and change of any external dressings when saturated.

4. Advise follow-up for removal of packing approximately 48 hours after surgery.
5. Encourage blotting of nose with tissue rather than blowing or picking at crusts.

Education and Health Maintenance

1. Advise patient to use over-the-counter analgesics and warm compresses over sinuses to relieve acute pain.
2. Advise patient with chronic or recurrent sinusitis to adhere to treatment regimen of antihistamines, nasal corticosteroids, or other drugs and to promptly seek medical attention for acute sinus infection to prevent chronic sinus disease.
3. Discourage patient to swim or dive, which may cause contaminated water to be forced into a sinus (usually frontal).
4. Stress the importance of complying with antibiotic therapy; 2 to 3 weeks may be necessary for acute infection, longer for chronic infection.
5. Advise the patient with asthma that sinusitis has been associated with exacerbation of asthma symptoms; warn patient to seek treatment for increased wheezing, chest tightness, or cough.

SJÖGREN'S SYNDROME

Sjögren's syndrome is a chronic inflammatory autoimmune process of unknown cause that affects the lacrimal and salivary glands. It is thought that antibodies directed at exocrine glands are produced, causing lymphocytic infiltration and impairing function of the involved tissue. The disease occurs primarily in middle-aged women and can be primary or secondary. Secondary Sjögren's syndrome is seen most commonly in rheumatoid arthritis but can be seen in systemic lupus erythematosus (SLE) and some other connective tissue diseases.

The syndrome may cause a variety of complications, such as corneal disease, tooth loss, pulmonary fibrosis or hypertension, obstructive airway disease, chronic atrophic gastritis, chronic pancreatitis, abnormal liver or kidney function, and dementia.

Assessment

1. Decreased tear production leading to keratoconjunctivitis, photophobia
2. Dry mouth (xerostomia), mucosal ulcers, stomatitis, salivary gland enlargement (unilateral or bilateral), dysphagia
3. Nasal dryness, epistaxis, nasal ulcers
4. Dryness of bronchial tree, hoarseness, recurrent otitis media, pneumonia, and bronchitis
5. Skin dryness (xerodermia), urticaria, purpura
6. Pancreatitis, hypochlorhydria or achlorhydria, autoimmune liver disease
7. Renal tubular acidosis, nephrogenic diabetes insipidus
8. Trigeminal neuropathy (Bell's palsy), polymyopathy, sensory and motor neuropathy, seizures, multiple sclerosis-like syndrome
9. Autoimmune thyroiditis
10. Raynaud's phenomenon, vasculitis; infants born to mothers with Sjögren's syndrome may have congenital heart block
11. Vaginal dryness, dyspareunia
12. Nonerosive polyarthritis

Diagnostic Evaluation

1. Complete blood count shows mild anemia; leukopenia present in 30% of patients.
2. Erythrocyte sedimentation rate is elevated in 90% of patients.
3. Rheumatoid factor is positive in 75% to 90% of patients.
4. Antinuclear antibody is positive in 70% of patients; speckled and nucleolar patterns are most common.
5. Antibodies to SSA or SSB detect antibodies to specific nuclear proteins.
   a. SSA: positive in patients with Sjögren's syndrome and SLE.
   b. SSB: positive in 60% of patients with Sjögren's syndrome; can also be positive in patients with SLE.
   c. Organ-specific antibodies: antibodies directed against specific organ tissues, including gastric, thyroid, smooth

muscle, salivary glands, and lacrimal glands, have been found.
6. Salivary scintigraphy evaluates salivary gland function.
7. X-rays of affected joints rule out erosive arthritis.
8. Salivary gland biopsy may be done to determine lymphocytic infiltration of tissue.

Collaborative Management
Therapeutic Interventions
1. Provide symptomatic relief of dryness:
   a. Artificial tears and lubricants
   b. Saliva substitutes
   c. Frequent use of nonsugar liquids, gums, and candies
   d. Vaginal lubricants
   e. Use of occlusive goggles at bedtime to prevent drying
2. Encourage dental care — frequent brushing and flossing, topical fluoride treatments, and avoidance of high-sucrose foods

Pharmacologic Interventions
1. Corticosteroids and immunosuppressants such as cyclophosphamide are used in severe cases.
2. Antifungal agents therapeutically or prophylactically for superimposed fungal infections of mouth or vagina.
3. Cevimeline 30 mg t.i.d., a cholinergic agonist for treatment of dry mouth.

Nursing Diagnoses
51, 60, 107, 134, 156

Nursing Interventions
Supportive Care
1. Inspect oral mucosa for oral *Candida* infection, ulcers, saliva pools, and dental hygiene.
2. Instruct or assist patient in proper oral hygiene.
3. Encourage frequent intake of noncaffeinated, nonsugar liquids. Keep pitcher filled with cool water.
4. Instruct or assist patient in daily inspection of skin for areas of trauma or potential breakdown.

5. Apply lubricants to skin daily.
6. Avoid shearing forces and encourage or perform frequent position changes.
7. Increase liquid intake with meals.
8. Assist or instruct patient to avoid choosing spicy or dry foods from menu choices.
9. Suggest smaller, more frequent meals.
10. Weigh patient weekly and review diet history for basic nutrient deficiencies.
11. Advise patient on proper use of water-soluble vaginal lubrication.
12. Suggest alternate positioning and practices to prevent dyspareunia.
13. Teach the patient to recognize and report symptoms of vaginitis because infection may result from altered mucosal barrier.

Education and Health Maintenance

1. Advise patient of commercially available artificial saliva preparations, artificial tears, moisturizing nasal sprays, and artificial vaginal moisturizers.
2. Encourage frequent dental visits. Dental cavities are more frequent in patients with Sjögren's syndrome.
3. Advise patient to check with health care provider before using any medications because many cause mouth dryness (eg, diuretics, tricyclic antidepressants, antihistamines).
4. Advise patient to wear protective eyewear while outdoors.
5. Refer the patient and family to Sjögren's Syndrome Foundation, *www.sjogrens.org*.

SKIN CANCER

See *Cancer, Skin*.

SOMATOFORM DISORDERS

See *Anxiety, Somatoform, and Dissociative Disorders*.

SPINA BIFIDA

Spina bifida refers to malformations of the spine in which the posterior portion of the vertebral laminae fails to close. These malformations are thought to result from incomplete or defective closure of the neural tube during the fourth to sixth weeks of embryonic life. The etiology is unknown, but it is thought to have some genetic predisposition triggered by something in the environment.

Three major types of spina bifida are recognized (see *Figure S-2*). In *spina bifida occulta*, the most common type, the defect involves only the vertebrae; the spinal cord and meninges are normal. However, the spinal cord and its meninges may be connected with a fistulous tract extending to and opening onto the surface of the skin. Neurologic problems are rare.

In *meningocele*, the meninges protrude through the opening in the spinal canal, forming a cyst filled with cerebrospinal fluid (CSF) and covered with skin. The defect may occur anywhere on the spinal cord. Higher defects (from thorax and upward) are usually meningoceles. As in spina bifida occulta, neurologic problems are rare.

In *myelomeningocele*, both the spinal cord and meninges protrude through the defect in the vertebral column and are protected by a thin, membranous sac. Various forms of per-

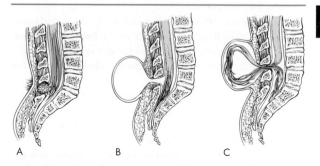

FIGURE S-2 Spina bifida. **(A)** Spina bifida occulta. **(B)** Spina bifida with meningocele. **(C)** Spina bifida with myelomeningocele.

manent neurologic deficit are present. The sac may leak in utero or may rupture after birth, allowing free drainage of CSF. This renders the child highly susceptible to meningitis. Myelomeningocele occurs four to five times more frequently than meningocele. In the absence of treatment, most infants with myelomeningocele die soon after birth.

Spina bifida is the most common developmental defect of the central nervous system and occurs in approximately 1 per every 1,000 live births in the United States. The condition may have other congenital anomalies associated with it, especially hydrocephalus.

Assessment

1. Spina bifida occulta
   a. Most patients have no symptoms. A dimple in the skin or hair growth may appear over the malformed vertebra.
   b. With growth, the child may develop foot weakness or bowel and bladder sphincter disturbances.
2. Meningocele
   a. Physical examination shows a saclike outpouching in the spinal cord, usually in the midline.
   b. Seldom evidence of weakness of the legs or lack of sphincter control.
3. Myelomeningocele
   a. Physical examination shows a round, raised, and poorly epithelialized area, usually in the lumbosacral area. Lesion may occur at any level of the spinal column.
   b. Loss of motor control and sensation below the level of the lesion.
   c. A low thoracic lesion may cause total flaccid paralysis below the waist.
   d. A small sacral lesion may cause only patchy spots of decreased sensation in the feet.
   e. Contractures may occur in the ankles, knees, or hips.
   f. Clubfoot commonly occurs; thought to be related to position of paraplegic feet in the uterus.

g. Urinary incontinence and retention and fecal incontinence and constipation occur because of impairment of sacral nerves.

Diagnostic Evaluation

1. Prenatal detection is possible through amniocentesis and measurement of alpha-fetoprotein. This testing should be offered to all women at risk (women who are affected themselves or have had other affected children).
2. Diagnosis is primarily based on clinical manifestations.
3. CT scan and MRI may be performed to further evaluate the brain and spinal cord.

Collaborative Management
Therapeutic Interventions

1. A coordinated team approach will help maximize the physical and intellectual potential of each affected child.
   a. The team may include a neurologist, neurosurgeon, orthopedic surgeon, urologist, primary care provider, social worker, physical therapist, a variety of community-based and hospital staff nurses, the child, and family.
   b. Numerous neurosurgical, orthopedic, and urologic procedures may be necessary to help the child achieve maximum potential.

Surgical Interventions

1. In meningocele and myelomeningocele, laminectomy and closure of an open lesion or removal of the sac usually can be done soon after birth.
2. Surgery is done to prevent further deterioration of neural function, to minimize danger of rupture of sac and meningitis, to improve cosmetic effect, and to facilitate handling of infant.

Nursing Diagnoses
16, 30, 44, 62, 69, 104, 134, 135, 136

S

Nursing Interventions
Monitoring

1. Monitor and report immediately signs of infection.
   a. Oozing of fluid or pus from the sac
   b. Fever
   c. Irritability or listlessness
   d. Seizure
2. Monitor urine elimination and report concentrated or foul-smelling urine, indicating a urinary tract infection (UTI).
3. Monitor for signs of hydrocephalus and report immediately.
   a. Irritability
   b. Feeding difficulty, vomiting, decreased appetite
   c. Temperature fluctuation
   d. Decreased alertness
   e. Tense fontanelle
   f. Increased head circumference
4. Frequently monitor temperature, pulse, respirations, color, and level of responsiveness postoperatively, based on the infant's stability.

Supportive Care
Preoperative Care in Neonatal Period

1. Use prone positioning with hips only slightly flexed to decrease tension on the sac; check position at least once every hour.
2. Do not place diaper or any covering directly over the sac.
3. Observe the sac frequently for evidence of irritation or leakage of CSF.
4. Place padding between the infant's legs to maintain the hips in abduction and to prevent or counteract subluxation.
5. Use a foam or fleece pad to reduce pressure of the mattress against the infant's skin.
6. Allow the infant's feet to hang freely over pads or mattress edge to avoid aggravating foot deformities.
7. Provide meticulous skin care to all areas of the body, especially ankles, knees, tip of nose, cheeks, and chin.

8. Provide passive range-of-motion exercises for those muscles and joints that the infant does not use spontaneously. Avoid hip exercises because of common hip dislocation, unless otherwise recommended.

9. Avoid pressure on infant's back during feeding by holding the infant with your elbow rotated to avoid touching the sac, or feeding while infant is lying on side or prone on your lap. Encourage parents to use these positions to provide infant stimulation and bonding.

10. Keep the buttocks and genitalia scrupulously clean; infection of the sac is most commonly caused by contamination by urine and feces.
    a. Do not use diapers for the infant if the defect is in the lower portion of the spine.
    b. Use a small plastic drape taped between the defect and the anus to help prevent contamination.

11. Apply a sterile dressing over the sac only as directed and change frequently to prevent adhesion to sac and to maintain sterility.

12. To promote urinary elimination, use Credé's method to empty the bladder (unless contraindicated by vesicoureteral reflux), and teach parents the technique. Continue the procedure as long as urine can be manually expressed.

13. Straight catheterize the patient as needed.

14. Ensure fluid intake to dilute the urine.

Postoperative Care in Infancy and Childhood

1. Use an Isolette or infant warmer to prevent temperature fluctuation.

2. Prevent respiratory complications.
   a. Periodically reposition the infant to promote lung expansion.
   b. Watch for abdominal distention, which could interfere with breathing.
   c. Have oxygen available.

3. Maintain hydration and nutritional intake.
   a. Administer I.V. fluids as ordered; keep accurate intake and output log.
   b. Administer gavage feedings as ordered.

c. Begin bottle feeding when infant responsive and tolerating feedings.
4. Be aware that children with spina bifida are susceptible to latex allergy. Symptoms include hives, itching, wheezing, and anaphylaxis. Incidence increases with time and may be related to repeated exposure.
   a. Limit or prevent direct contact of child with such products as blood pressure cuffs, tourniquets, tape, Foley catheters, gloves, and I.V. tubing injection ports.

COMMUNITY CARE CONSIDERATIONS

Toys and equipment for children, such as nipples, pacifiers, and elastic on the legs of some clothing, also contain latex. The home environment should be surveyed for latex and substitute products obtained, if possible. Teach the parents how to recognize latex allergy and notify the child's health care provider.

5. Teach parents that continence can usually be achieved with clean, intermittent self-catheterization.
   a. Children can generally be taught to catheterize themselves by age 6 or 7.
   b. Parents can catheterize younger children.
   c. Red rubber catheters are used rather than latex catheters.

COMMUNITY CARE CONSIDERATIONS

The family can be taught to clean and reuse urinary catheters. The catheter should be washed in warm, soapy water and rinsed well in warm water. The catheter should be air-dried and, when completely dried, placed in a clean jar or plastic bag. A catheter should be replaced when it becomes dry, cracked, stiff, or if the child develops a UTI.

6. Teach the signs of UTI (concentrated, foul-smelling urine, burning, and fever) and the proper administration of antibiotics either prophylactically or when prescribed for infection.

7. Assist with bowel training program, including high-fiber, high-fluid diet, bowel medication, and regular elimination time.
8. To foster positive body image in an older child, emphasize rehabilitation that uses the child's strengths and minimizes disabilities.
9. Continually reassess functional abilities and offer suggestions to increase independence. Periodically consult with physical or occupational therapists to help maximize function.
10. Encourage the use of braces and specialized equipment to enhance ambulation, while minimizing the appearance of the equipment.
11. Encourage patient to participate with peer group and in activities that build on strengths, such as cognitive abilities, interest in music, or art.
12. Periodically reassess bowel and bladder programs. The ability to stay dry for reasonable intervals is one of the greatest factors in enhancing self-esteem and positive body image.

Education and Health Maintenance

1. Teach special techniques that may be required for holding and positioning, feeding, caring for the incision, emptying the bladder, and exercising muscles.
2. Alert the parents to safety needs of the child with decreased sensation, such as protection from prolonged pressure, risk of burns from bath water that is too warm, and avoidance of trauma from contact with sharp objects.
3. Reinforce that parents need to notify the health care provider for signs of associated problems such as hydrocephalus, meningitis, UTI, and latex sensitivity.
4. Urge continued follow-up and health maintenance, including immunizations and evaluation of growth and development.
5. Advise parents that children with paralysis are at risk for becoming overweight because of inactivity, so they should provide a low-fat, balanced diet; control snacking; and encourage as much activity as possible.

S

6. For additional resources, refer family to agencies such as the Spina Bifida Association of America, *www.sbaa.org.*

SPINAL CORD INJURY

Spinal cord injury may result from trauma, vascular disruption, infection, tumors, and other insults. The injury may be partial or complete and vary from a mild cord concussion with transient numbness to complete cord transection causing immediate and permanent tetraplegia. The most common sites

TABLE S-5	Incomplete Spinal Cord Clinical Syndromes
SYNDROME, AFFECTED SITE	**DEFICIT**
Central cord Central cervical spinal cord	More motor deficit in upper extremities than lower extremities caused by medial damage of corticospinal tract
Brown-Sequard Hemisection of spinal cord	Ipsilateral motor function and fine touch, vibration, and proprioception (posterior tract); contralateral sensory function pain and temperature (spinothalamic tract)
Anterior cord Main anterior spinal artery of anterior spinal cord affecting anterior two-thirds of spinal cord	Variable motor deficit; variable sensory deficit of pain and temperature (spinothalamic tract)
Conus medullaris Conus and lumbar nerve roots in spinal cord	Variable motor deficit; bowel, bladder, and lower extremity reflexes (flaccid)
Cauda equina Lumbosacral nerve roots in spinal cord	Variable motor deficit; bowel, bladder, and lower extremity reflexes (flaccid)

of injury are the cervical areas C5, C6, and C7, and the junction of the thoracic and lumbar vertebrae, T12 and L1.

Clinical manifestations vary with the location and severity of cord damage. In general, complete transection causes loss of all function below the level of the lesion, and incomplete cord damage results in a variety of regional deficits (see *Table S-5*). Complications include shock, respiratory or cardiac arrest, thromboembolism, infections, and autonomic dysreflexia.

Assessment

1. Motor and sensory deficits indicate the level of the spinal cord lesion (see *Figure S-3*). Widening deficits may be attributable to edema and hemorrhage.

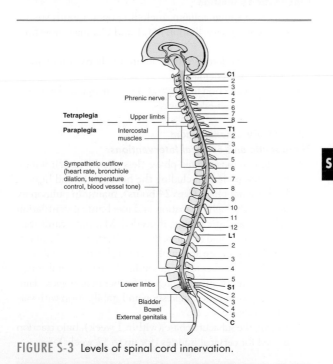

FIGURE S-3 Levels of spinal cord innervation.

   2. Signs of autonomic dysfunction:
      a. Respirations: unusual patterns, distress, signs of hypoxia. Diaphragmatic or abdominal breathing may indicate cervical spine injury.
      b. Cardiovascular function: hypotension caused by vasodilation and blood pooling in lower extremities; bradycardia from unopposed vagal influence.
   3. Decreased rectal sphincter tone and bowel and bladder dysfunction.
   4. Pain due to vertebral fractures, which may be simple, compressed, dislocated, subluxed (partially dislocated over another vertebrae), comminuted (shattered), or teardrop (chipped).

Diagnostic Evaluation
   1. X-rays of spinal column, including open mouth studies for adequate visualization of C1 and C2, may show fracture.
   2. Spinal MRI detects soft tissue injury, bony injury, hemorrhage, and edema.
   3. Nerve conduction testing and electromyogram determine function of neural pathways.

Collaborative Management
Therapeutic and Surgical Interventions
   1. Immediate posttrauma phase (less than 1 hour): immobilize the patient, including the head, body, and hips.
   2. In the acute phase (1 to 24 hours), maintain pulmonary stability through intubation and mechanical ventilation or diaphragmatic pacing, if needed. Maintain cardiovascular stability and ensure perfusion of spinal cord by restoring blood pressure and implementing localized cord cooling. The spinal cord is immobilized with skeletal tongs. Surgical intervention to prevent further neurological damage may include decompression and stabilization with various hardware.
   3. During the subacute phase (within 1 week), halo traction is used for cervical injuries (for up to 12 weeks).

4. During chronic phase (beyond 1 week), emphasis is on rehabilitation, including physical therapy, urologic evaluation, and occupational therapy.

Pharmacologic Interventions

1. Methylprednisolone is given I.V. as soon as possible to reduce spinal cord edema.
2. GM-1 ganglioside sodium salt I.V., begun 72 hours after injury, and continued for 18 to 32 days to enhance neuronal regeneration.
3. Histamine-2 receptor blockers are given to prevent gastric irritation and hemorrhage.
4. Anticoagulants are given in small doses to reduce risk of thrombophlebitis and pulmonary emboli.
5. Management of spasticity with muscle relaxants such as baclofen and diazepam.

Nursing Diagnoses
3, 8, 13, 16, 62, 75, 97, 134, 136, 156, 162, 166

Nursing Interventions
Monitoring

1. For patients with high-level lesions, continuously monitor respirations and maintain a patent airway. Be prepared to intubate if respiratory fatigue or arrest occurs.
2. Monitor results of arterial blood gas analysis, chest X-rays, and sputum cultures for possible respiratory infections.
3. Monitor fluid intake and output.
4. Monitor neurologic changes; report change in skin sensation, loss or gain of muscle strength, which may indicate worsening or resolving lesion.
5. Monitor for spinal shock — may cause loss of all reflex, motor, sensory, and autonomic activity below the level of the lesion; eventually resolves.
6. Monitor for autonomic dysreflexia (exaggerated autonomic response to stimuli below the level of the lesion in patients with lesions at or above T6).

 EMERGENCY ALERT Autonomic dysreflexia is a medical emergency that may result in seizures and death without prompt treatment. Be alert to such signs as pounding headache, profuse sweating, nasal congestion, piloerection (goose bumps), bradycardia, and severe hypertension. Immediately place the patient in a sitting position to help lower blood pressure and diminish intracranial pressure. Remove possible causative stimuli; administer antihypertensive medication as ordered; and monitor blood pressure every 3 to 5 minutes until the condition resolves.

7. Monitor blood pressure with position changes in a patient with lesions above midthoracic area to prevent orthostatic hypotension.

Supportive Care

1. Frequently assess cough and vital capacity. Teach effective coughing if the patient is able.
2. Provide fluids and humidified air or oxygen to loosen secretions. Implement chest physiotherapy to assist pulmonary drainage and prevent infection.
3. Suction as needed; observe for vagal response, which causes bradycardia (should be temporary).
4. Turn the patient frequently, maintaining alignment, or transfer the patient to a turning table or rotating bed when stable. Never attempt to reposition a patient by grasping a halo or other stabilization device.
5. Keep skin clean, dry, and well-lubricated. Inspect for pressure sore development every 2 hours when turning patient, including the back of head, ears, heels, and elbows.
6. Provide meticulous skin care at pin sites of skull tongs or halo device to prevent infection.
7. Perform range-of-motion exercises to prevent contractures and maintain rehabilitation potential. Encourage physical therapy and practicing of exercises as tolerated.
8. Encourage weight-bearing activity to prevent osteoporosis and risk of kidney stones.
9. Apply elastic support hose, sequential compression device, and administer anticoagulants as ordered, to reduce the risk of thrombophlebitis.
10. Replace an indwelling catheter with intermittent catheterization as soon as possible to minimize risk of infection. Avoid overdistention of the bladder.

    a. If reflex voiding is present, monitor for urinary retention by percussing the suprapubic area for dullness, or catheterizing for residual urine after voiding.

    b. Train the patient in reflex voiding by encouraging fluids at 2-hour intervals, then applying pressure to the suprapubic area 30 minutes later in attempt to void. Avoid giving fluids in the evening to prevent nocturnal dribbling and overdistention.

11. Assess bowel sounds and note abdominal distention. Paralytic ileus is common immediately after injury.

    a. Initiate nasogastric suction as necessary.

    b. Encourage high-calorie, high-protein, and high-fiber diet when bowel sounds return and the patient tolerates food.

12. Institute a bowel care program as early as possible to manage defecation. (See *Box S-2.*) Observe for loose stool ooz-

---

BOX S-2   Reflexic Bowel Care

- Schedule bowel care at the same time every day or every other day based on usual time of defecation to develop a predictable outcome.
- Help stimulate the gastrocolic reflex 30 minutes before toileting by giving food or liquid or plan bowel care after a meal.
- Insert a glycerin suppository or provide manual rectal stimulation with a gloved and lubricated finger within 30 minutes before toileting.
- Position the patient on a commode, toilet, or bowel chair with adequate support and safety measures in place. If necessary, position the patient on his or her left side in bed with the head raised 30 to 45 degrees.
- Encourage the patient to perform deep breathing, sip warm fluids, lean forward, contract abdominal muscles, or provide abdominal massage to enhance success.
- Record characteristics of stool, time from stimulation to defecation, and patient's tolerance of the procedure. Adjust subsequent care based on the results.
- For patients with lower motor neuron lesions (involving the spinal nerve roots) or any part of the sacral spinal cord, perform reflexic bowel care by removing stool manually.

S

ing from rectum and check for fecal impaction; remove if necessary.

13. Protect the patient from possible stimuli for autonomic dysreflexia, including:
    a. Bowel or bladder distention caused by fecal impaction, urinary retention, or a kinked indwelling catheter.
    b. Abnormal skin stimulation, such as lying on wrinkled sheets, hot or cold stimulation, or pain from constricting clothing.
    c. Distention or contraction of visceral organs, such as gastric distention or emptying an overdistended bladder too fast.
    d. Infection, especially of the urinary tract.

COMMUNITY CARE CONSIDERATIONS

Alert caregivers that autonomic dysreflexia is a complication that may occur for 5 to 6 years after a spinal cord injury. Teach patient and caregivers how to prevent autonomic dysreflexia, identify it, and implement emergency measures.

14. Praise patient for accomplishments; minimize deficits.
15. Ensure adequate rest and discuss stress management techniques, such as relaxation therapy, counseling, and problem solving.

Education and Health Maintenance
1. Teach the patient and family about the physiology of nerve transmission and how spinal injury has affected normal function.
2. Reinforce that rehabilitation is lengthy and involves adherence to therapy to increase bodily function.
3. Explain that spasticity may develop 2 weeks to 3 months after injury and may interfere with routine care and activities of daily living.
    a. Teach measures to manage spasticity, such as maintaining a calm, stress-free environment; allowing plenty of time for activities; performing range of motion

slowly and smoothly; and avoiding temperature extremes.
   b. Advise that spasms should be reported to the health care provider for possible treatment with muscle relaxants.
4. Teach protection from pressure ulcer development by frequent inspection of skin, repositioning while in bed, weight shifting and lift-offs every 15 minutes while in a wheelchair, and avoidance of shear forces and friction.
5. Encourage sexual counseling, if indicated, to promote satisfaction in personal relationships.

SPINAL CORD TUMOR

Tumors of the spinal cord and canal cause compression of the spinal cord and nerves, progressing to paralysis if untreated. Spinal tumors vary widely in type and location. They may be extradural (existing outside the dural membranes), including chondroma and osteoblastoma, and may spread to the vertebral bodies; intradural-extramedullary (within the subarachnoid space), including meningiomas and schwannomas; or intramedullary (within the spinal cord), including astrocytomas, ependymomas, and oligodendrogliomas. Spinal cord tumor may occur at any age and may be primary or secondary to malignancy of the lung, breast, prostate, or other tumors. Abnormal cell growth results in spinal nerve or cord compression. Complications include spinal cord infarction, hydrocephalus, and infection.

Assessment
1. Back pain may be localized or radiating, depending on location and type of tumor.
2. Weakness of extremities, abnormal reflexes, and sensory changes.
3. Abnormal autonomic function relative to level of lesion — abnormal pupillary responses, orthostatic hypotension, or bladder or bowel dysfunction indicates tumor in the cauda equina.

Diagnostic Evaluation

1. Plain X-ray or CT scan shows vertebral fracture, collapse, or destruction from a mass.
2. MRI shows tumor location.
3. CT myelography with lumbar puncture before surgery more fully evaluates tumor.

Collaborative Management

Therapeutic and Pharmacologic Interventions

1. Radiation therapy with or without surgery.
2. Corticosteroids may be used before radiation to improve ambulation rate.

Surgical Interventions

1. Surgical excision of the tumor via an anterior approach (most common) or posterolateral approach (for thoracic tumors). Intraoperative motor and somatosensory evoked potentials can be used to help reduce neurologic deficits postoperatively by mapping the motor and sensory tracts within the spinal cord.
2. Special techniques, such as microsurgical laser, ultrasound, X-ray, and coagulation, are used intraoperatively.

Nursing Diagnoses

3, 6, 13, 33, 69, 135, 136

Nursing Interventions

Monitoring

1. Monitor neurologic deficits and make sure safety needs are being met.
2. Monitor intake and output to evaluate urine retention.
3. After surgery, monitor site for bleeding, drainage of cerebrospinal fluid, and signs of infection.

Supportive Care

1. Administer analgesics or instruct the patient how to use patient-controlled analgesia, as directed.

2. Provide periods of rest with reduced environmental stimulation and allow patient and family time to ask questions and discuss their fears.

3. Instruct the patient with painful paresthesias in appropriate use of ice, massage, exercise, or rest.

4. Instruct the patient in relaxation techniques, such as deep breathing, distraction, or imagery.

5. Instruct the patient with sensory loss to visually scan the extremity during use to avoid injury related to lack of tactile input. Pad the bed rails or chair to prevent injury.

6. Encourage fluid intake to maintain urinary elimination pattern. Teach Credé's maneuver or self-catheterization as indicated.

7. Assess for urine retention by percussing the bladder for dullness or catheterizing for residual after voiding.

8. Support the weak or paralyzed extremity in a functional position, to prevent contractures.

9. Refer patient to physical therapy for assistance with activities of daily living and ambulation.

10. Promote periods of rest to enhance coping skills.

11. Reassure the postoperative patient that the degree of sensory or motor impairment may decrease during the recovery period as surgical edema decreases.

12. Keep surgical dressings clean and dry, and clean surgical site as ordered.

13. Position the patient to keep pressure off postoperative surgical site.

Education and Health Maintenance

1. Encourage the patient with motor impairment to use adaptive devices.

2. Demonstrate proper positioning and transfer techniques.

3. Instruct the patient with sensory losses about dangers of extreme temperatures, and the need for adequate foot protection at all times.

4. Refer the patient and family to cancer and spinal cord lesion support groups as needed.

SPRAINS, STRAINS, AND CONTUSIONS

A *sprain* is an injury to ligamentous structures surrounding a joint; it is usually caused by a wrench or twist resulting in a decrease in joint stability. A *strain* is a microscopic tearing of muscle or tendon caused by excessive force, stretching, or overuse. A *contusion* is an injury to the soft tissue produced by a blunt force (blow, kick, or fall).

Assessment
1. *Sprain:* rapid swelling caused by extravasation of blood within tissues; pain on passive movement of joint; increasing pain during first few hours caused by continued swelling
2. *Strain:* swelling, tenderness; pain with isometric contraction; may be associated spasm
3. *Contusion:* hemorrhage into injured part (ecchymosis); pain, swelling; hyperkalemia may be present with extensive contusions, resulting from destruction of body tissue and loss of blood

Diagnostic Evaluation
1. X-ray of affected part may be done to rule out fracture.

Collaborative Management
Therapeutic Interventions
1. Immobilize the affected part in splint, elastic wrap, or compression dressing to support weakened structures and control swelling.
2. Apply ice first 24 hours.

Pharmacologic Interventions
1. Analgesics usually include nonsteroidal anti-inflammatory drugs.

Surgical Interventions
1. Severe sprains may require surgical repair or cast immobilization.

Nursing Diagnoses
3, 62, 141

Nursing Interventions
Supportive Care
1. Elevate the affected part. Maintain splint or immobilization as prescribed.
2. Apply cold compresses for the first 24 hours (20 to 30 minutes at a time) to produce vasoconstriction, decrease edema, and reduce discomfort.
3. Apply heat to affected area after 24 hours (20 to 30 minutes at a time) four times per day to promote circulation and absorption.
4. Assess neurovascular status of distal extremity if significant swelling occurs.
5. Ensure correct use of crutches or other mobility aid with or without weight bearing as prescribed.

Education and Health Maintenance
1. Instruct the patient about the use of pain medication as prescribed.
2. Educate patient on need to rest injured part for about 1 month to allow for healing.
3. Teach patient to resume activities gradually.
4. Advise patient to avoid excessive exercise of injured part.
5. Teach patient to avoid reinjury by "warming up" before exercise.

STATUS ASTHMATICUS
See *Asthma*.

STOMACH CANCER
See *Cancer, Gastric*.

STROKE
Stroke or *cerebrovascular accident* (also called *brain attack*) results from sudden interruption of blood supply to the brain, which precipitates neurologic dysfunction lasting longer than 24 hours. Strokes are either ischemic, caused by partial or complete occlusion of a cerebral blood vessel by cerebral thrombosis or embolism or hemorrhage (leakage of blood from a vessel causes compression of brain tissue and spasm of adjacent vessels). Hemorrhage may occur outside the dura (extradur-

al), beneath the dura mater (subdural), in the subarachnoid space (subarachnoid), or within the brain substance itself (intracerebral).

Risk factors for stroke include transient ischemic attacks (TIAs) — warning sign of impending stroke — hypertension, arteriosclerosis, heart disease, elevated cholesterol, diabetes mellitus, obesity, carotid stenosis, polycythemia, hormonal use, I.V. drug use, arrhythmias, and cigarette smoking. Complications of stroke include aspiration pneumonia, dysphagia, contractures, deep vein thrombosis, pulmonary embolism, depression, and brain stem herniation.

Assessment

1. Headache may be sign of impending cerebral hemorrhage or infarction, but is not always present.
2. Clinical manifestations of stroke depend on the vascular territory affected (see *Table S-6*).
   a. Numbness, (paresthesia), weakness (paresis), or loss of motor ability (plegia), on one side of the body
   b. Difficulty in swallowing (dysphagia)
   c. Speech or communication impairment (aphasia)
   d. Visual difficulties: loss of half of visual field, double vision
   e. Altered cognitive abilities and psychological effects
3. Tone of muscles and presence of deep tendon reflexes change from initial flaccid period to later spastic period.
4. Incontinence and self-care deficits.

Diagnostic Evaluation

1. CT scan, MRI, and CT angiography determine cause and location of stroke.
2. Cerebral angiography determines extent of cerebrovascular insufficiency.
3. Positron emission tomography (PET) and MRI with diffusion weighted images scans may be done to localize ischemic damage.
4. Transcranial Doppler evaluates and monitors cerebral perfusions.

TABLE S-6	Clinical Manifestations Related to Vascular Territory

AREA INVOLVED	SIGNS AND SYMPTOMS*
Anterior cerebral artery	
Frontal lobe	Paralysis of contralateral foot or leg; impaired gait; paresis of contralateral arm; contralateral sensory loss over toes, foot, and leg; problems making decisions or performing acts voluntarily; lack of spontaneity, easily distracted; slowness of thought; aphasia depends on the hemisphere involved; urinary incontinence; cognitive and affective disorders
Middle cerebral artery	
Lateral hemisphere and deeper structures	Contralateral hemiplegia (face and arm); contralateral sensory impairment; aphasia; homonymous hemiplegia; altered consciousness (confusion to coma); inability to turn eyes toward paralyzed side; denial of paralyzed side or limb (hemiattention); possible acalculia, alexia, finger agnosia and left-right confusion; vasomotor paresis and instability
Posterior cerebral artery (PCA)	
Occipital lobe; anterior and medial portion of temporal lobe	Homonymous hemianopia and other visual defects such as color blindness, loss of central vision, and visual hallucinations; memory deficits; perseveration (repeated performance of same verbal or motor response)
PCA	
Thalamus involvement	Loss of all sensory modalities; spontaneous pain; intentional tremor; mild hemiparesis; aphasia
PCA	
Cerebral peduncle involvement	Oculomotor nerve palsy with contralateral hemiplegia

(continued)

S

Clinical Manifestations Related to Vascular Territory *(continued)*

AREA INVOLVED	SIGNS AND SYMPTOMS*
Basilar and vertebral arteries	
Cerebellum and brain stem	Visual disturbance such as diplopia, dystaxia, vertigo, dysphagia, dysphonia

*Dependent on hemisphere involved and adequacy of collaterals.

Collaborative Management

Therapeutic Interventions

1. In the acute phase (first 48 to 72 hours), maintain the patient's airway, breathing, oxygenation, and circulation.
2. Physical therapy and rehabilitation program are initiated as soon as patient is medically stable.

Pharmacologic Interventions

1. During acute phase:
   a. I.V. therapy with colloid and albumin to facilitate reperfusion and hemodilution
   b. Thrombolytics (tissue plasminogen activator) to reverse occlusion in embolic stroke — must be started I.V. within 3 hours of onset of symptoms, 6 hours if given transarterially
   c. Diuretics to reduce cerebral edema, which peaks 3 to 5 days after infarction
   d. Nimodipine for vasodilation and other calcium channel blockers to reduce blood pressure and prevent cerebral vasospasm
2. Provide additional treatment after the acute phase:
   a. Anticoagulants for nonhemorrhagic stroke
   b. Antiplatelet agents such as ticlopidine or aspirin
   c. Antispasmodic agents for spastic paralysis
   d. Antidepressants to treat poststroke depression

Nursing Diagnoses
8, 28, 35, 36, 45, 46, 51, 62, 69, 134, 136

Nursing Interventions
Monitoring
1. Maintain a neurologic flow sheet during the acute phase (48 to 72 hours after onset of stroke).
   a. Frequently assess the patient's respiratory status, vital signs, heart rate and rhythm to maintain and support vital functions.
   b. Assess for voluntary and involuntary movements, muscle tone, response to stimulation, deep tendon reflexes.
2. Monitor bowel and bladder function.
3. Frequently assess the patient's level of function and psychosocial response to condition. Look for signs of post-stroke depression.
4. Monitor for bleeding with thrombolytic, anticoagulant, and antiplatelet therapy.
5. Assess for skin breakdown, contractures, and other complications of immobility (see *Pressure Sores*, page 754).

> **EMERGENCY ALERT** Prothrombin time levels are reported in International Normalized Ratio (INR). Oral anticoagulants are adjusted to maintain an INR at 2.0 or 3.0 to prevent stroke. Report INR that is elevated to reduce the risk of bleeding, or decreased levels so that therapy may be adjusted to be more effective.

Supportive Care
1. During the acute phase:
   a. Maintain bed rest with head of bed slightly elevated and side rails in place.
   b. Administer oxygen as ordered to maximize cerebral oxygenation.
   c. Perform intermittent or indwelling bladder catheterization.
2. Position the patient and align the extremities carefully, to prevent complications of immobility:
   a. Apply a trochanter roll from the crest of the ileum to the mid-thigh to prevent external rotation of the hip.

b. Place a pillow in the axilla of the affected side to prevent adduction of the shoulder.

c. Place the affected extremity slightly flexed on pillow supports with each joint positioned higher than the preceding one to prevent edema and fibrosis; alternate elbow flexion and extension.

d. Avoid excessive pressure on ball of foot after spasticity develops (do not use footboard) but try to avoid plantar flexion.

e. Avoid having the patient sit up in a chair for long periods to prevent knee and hip flexion contractures; place the patient in prone position for short periods, if tolerated.

f. Try to maintain a relaxed, neutral position of affected extremities and exercise them passively through range of motion four to five times per day to maintain joint mobility and enhance circulation; encourage active range-of-motion exercise as able and have the patient do as much as safely possible.

3. Apply splints and braces as indicated to support flaccid extremities or reduce spasticity.

COMMUNITY CARE CONSIDERATIONS

Hemiplegic deformities resulting from stroke commonly include "frozen" shoulder; adduction and internal rotation of arm with flexion of elbow, wrist, and fingers; and external rotation of the hip with flexion of the knee and plantar flexion of the ankle. Instruct the patient and family in range-of-motion exercises. Reinforce that these muscle and ligament deformities resulting from stroke can be prevented with daily stretching and strengthening exercises.

4. Prepare for ambulation cautiously. Check for orthostatic hypotension as you elevate head of bed and progress to dangling of legs; assist physical therapist who will assess the patient's standing balance. Help the patient begin walking as soon as standing balance is achieved; ensure safety with a patient waist belt.

5. Participate in cognitive retraining program (reality orientation, visual imagery, cueing procedures) as outlined by occupational or rehabilitation therapist.

6. To facilitate communication, speak slowly, using visual cues and gestures, be consistent and repeat as necessary. Allow the patient plenty of time to respond; reinforce correct responses. Minimize distractions. Alternatively, use nonverbal methods of communication (see *Box S-3*, pages 908 and 909).

7. Help restore the patient's feelings of independence and set realistic goals.

   a. Teach the patient to use unaffected side for activities of daily living, but not to neglect affected side. To help the patient with visual deficits avoid injury, teach how to scan the environment.

   b. Encourage the family to provide clothing that is a size larger than the patient wears, with front closures, Velcro, and stretch fabric; teach the patient to dress while sitting to maintain balance.

   c. Make sure that personal care items, urinal, commode, and so forth, are nearby and that the patient obtains assistance with transfers and other activities as needed.

8. Obtain a consultation with a speech therapist for swallowing evaluation before feeding.

   a. When cleared, help the patient relearn swallowing sequence. Place ice on tongue and encourage sucking; progress to Popsicle and small amounts of soft food.

   b. Progress diet from mechanical soft or puree diet as tolerated, based on the patient's ability to chew.

   c. Position the patient so he or she is sitting with 90 degrees of flexion at the hips and slight flexion at the neck. Use pillows behind the back and along the weak side to achieve correct position.

   d. Maintain position for 30 to 45 minutes after the meal to prevent regurgitation and aspiration.

   e. Teach the family how to assist the patient with meals to facilitate chewing and swallowing.

9. Help the patient regain bladder control:

BOX S-3 Aphasia

Aphasia is an acquired disorder of communication resulting from brain damage due to stroke, head injury, brain tumors, or brain cysts. It may involve impairment of the ability to speak, understand the speech of others, read, write, calculate, and understand gestures. Most aphasic people have difficulty with expression and comprehension to varying degrees. Fatigue will have adverse effect on speech.

To enhance your communication with the aphasic patient, keep the environment simple and relaxed, minimize distractions, and use multiple sensory channels. Refer the family to the American Speech-Language-Hearing Association, *www.asha.org*.

APHASIA SYNDROMES
- *Fluent aphasia:* Patient retains verbal fluency but may have difficulty in understanding speech.
- *Wernicke's aphasia:* Patient speaks readily, but speech lacks clear content, information, and direction; jargon frequently used.
- *Anomic or amnesic aphasia:* Speech is almost normal, but marred by word-finding difficulty.
- *Broca's aphasia:* Expressive aphasia; broken or dysarthric speech patterns.
- *Conduction aphasia:* Comprehension of language is good, but person has difficulty repeating spoken material.
- *Nonfluent aphasia:* Speech is sparse and produced slowly and with effort and poor articulation; usually has a relative preservation of auditory comprehension.
- *Global aphasia:* Severe disruption of all aspects of communication (verbal speech, written, reading, understanding).

NURSING INTERVENTIONS
- Speak at your normal rate and volume; the patient is not hard of hearing.
- Allow plenty of time for patient to answer.
- Do not ask questions that require complex answers.
- Rote phrases can be spontaneous.
- Provide pad and pen if the patient prefers and is able to write.
- Avoid forcing speech.
- Watch the patient for clues and gestures if his or her speech is jargon; make neutral statements.
- Ask for minimal word response.

Aphasia *(continued)*

- Encourage patient to speak slowly.
- Expect frustration and anger at inability to communicate.
- Keep environment simple.
- Use gestures as well as language.
- Allow patient to manipulate objects for additional sensory input.

---

    a. The patient will have been catheterized during the acute stage. Once bladder tone returns, establish regular schedule of voiding (every 2 or 3 hours).

    b. Assist with standing or sitting to void (especially males).

10. To help the family cope with patient care, teach stress management techniques such as relaxation exercises, use of community and church support networks, respite program, or other available resources in area.

Education and Health Maintenance

1. Teach the patient and family to adapt the home environment for safety and ease of use.
2. Emphasize importance of rest periods throughout day.
3. Reassure the family that it is common for poststroke patients to experience emotional lability and depression; treatment can be given.

COMMUNITY CARE CONSIDERATIONS

Educate all individuals about risk factors for stroke and ways to overcome those risks.

---

4. Assist family to obtain self-help aids for the patient.
5. Instruct the family in management of aphasia.
6. Refer the patient and family for more information and support to agencies such as National Stroke Association, *www.stroke.org.*

SUBDURAL HEMATOMA IN CHILDREN

Subdural hematoma refers to an accumulation of fluid, blood, and its degradation products between the dura mater and subarachnoid membrane. Hematoma results from direct or indirect trauma to the head, such as birth trauma; accidents; purposeful injury, as in cases of child abuse; or a disease process such as meningitis. Subdural hematomas may be acute (evident within 24 to 48 hours of injury) or chronic (most common, evident after days or weeks). It is often difficult to delineate the exact time and type of injury, because the precipitating episode may appear relatively insignificant. The lesion may arrest spontaneously at any point, or it may enlarge and, if unrelieved, ultimately cause cerebral atrophy or death of compression and herniation.

Treatment is usually successful and subsequent development is normal when the diagnosis is made early, before cerebral atrophy and a fixed neurologic deficit have occurred. With delayed treatment, complications include mental retardation, ocular abnormalities, seizures, spasticity, and paralysis. Mortality in massive, acute subdural bleeding is very high, even if promptly diagnosed.

Assessment
Acute Subdural Hematoma
1. Continuous unconsciousness from time of injury or lucid interval followed by unconsciousness
2. Progressive hemiplegia
3. Focal seizures
4. Signs of brain stem herniation: pupillary dilation, changes in vital signs, decerebrate posturing, and respiratory failure

> **EMERGENCY ALERT** Impending brain stem herniation is an absolute medical-surgical emergency requiring burr hole placement for relief of pressure, along with medical support of vital functions.

Chronic Subdural Hematoma
1. In infants, early signs include anorexia, difficulty feeding, vomiting, irritability, low-grade fever, retinal hemorrhages, and failure to gain weight.

2. In infants, later signs include enlargement of head, bulging and pulsation of anterior fontanelle, glossy scalp with dilated scalp veins, strabismus, pupillary inequality, hyperactive reflexes, seizures, and retarded motor development.
3. In older children, early signs include lethargy, anorexia, and signs of increased intracranial pressure (ICP), such as vomiting, irritability, headache, increased pulse pressure, and change in respirations.
4. In older children, later signs include seizures and coma.

Diagnostic Evaluation
1. CT scan, without contrast, is the procedure of choice for diagnosing subdural hematomas.
2. Bilateral subdural taps may provide the diagnosis as well as give immediate relief of increased ICP.
3. Skull and long bone X-rays may be obtained if abuse is suspected.

Collaborative Management
Surgical Interventions
1. In acute subdural hematoma, the clot is evacuated through a burr hole or craniotomy.
2. In chronic subdural hematoma, repeated subdural taps are done to remove the accumulating fluid.
   a. In infants, the needle can be inserted through the fontanelle or suture line.
   b. In older children, the needle is inserted through burr holes into the skull.
   c. The subdural taps may be the only treatment required if the fluid disappears entirely and symptoms do not recur.
   d. Concurrent treatment is instituted to correct anemia, electrolyte imbalance, and malnutrition.
3. A shunting procedure may be done if repeated taps fail to significantly reduce the volume or protein content of the subdural collections. Shunting is usually to the peritoneal cavity.

S

Nursing Diagnoses
3, 51, 62, 88, 104, 135, 136

Nursing Interventions
Monitoring
1. Monitor vital signs for changes indicating increased ICP. (See *Box B-1*, page 89.)
2. Monitor level of consciousness and behavior for changes.
3. Monitor urine output and specific gravity daily to ensure adequate hydration.
4. Monitor electrolyte and protein levels to prevent imbalances.
5. After subdural tap:
   a. Observe the child frequently for signs of shock.
   b. Observe for drainage from the site of the tap; report purulent drainage or frank bleeding.
   c. Monitor temperature frequently and monitor for signs of developing infection.
6. Monitor for signs of respiratory or urinary infection related to immobility.

Supportive Care
1. Maintain a quiet environment without sudden changes in position to avoid increased ICP.
2. Organize nursing activities to allow for long periods of uninterrupted rest.
3. Carefully regulate fluid administration to avoid danger of fluid overload.
4. Administer laxatives or suppositories to prevent straining during a bowel movement, which may increase ICP.
5. Assist with subdural taps.
   a. Hold the child securely to avoid injury caused by sudden movement.
   b. Apply firm pressure over the puncture sites for a few minutes after the tap has been completed, to prevent fluid leakage along the needle tract.
   c. Reinforce the dressing as needed to prevent contamination of the wound.
6. Have emergency equipment available for resuscitation.

7. Change the child's position frequently and provide meticulous skin care.

8. Perform passive range-of-motion exercises on all extremities and support the child's body in good alignment using splints as necessary to prevent contractures.

9. Apply suction as necessary to remove secretions in the mouth and nasopharynx.

10. Keep the child's eyes well lubricated to prevent corneal damage while unconscious.

11. Provide nutrition and fluids through nasogastric feedings as ordered. Observe for gastric distention.

12. Maintain good mouth care even if child is not eating.

13. Encourage the parents to care for and hold the child as much as possible.

14. Encourage the parents to bring diversional materials from home for the recovery period.

15. Provide emotional support to the parents; reassure them that the prognosis is favorable with adequate treatment.

16. Act nonjudgmentally in cases caused by intentional or accidental trauma.

> **PEDIATRIC ALERT** Make sure that cases of suspected child abuse have been reported to the appropriate agency and that parents have been referred for counseling.

Education and Health Maintenance

1. Reinforce explanations regarding the child's condition, causes of the child's specific symptoms, rationale for treatment, and postoperative recovery expectations.

2. Encourage parents to keep all follow-up appointments for medical evaluation and physical and occupational therapy.

3. Teach parents safety measures to prevent injuries in the future.

4. Have periodic developmental assessments done and report any delays.

5. Discuss return-to-play criteria in older children participating in sports; refer to *www.nata.org*.

SYSTEMIC SCLEROSIS

See *Scleroderma*.

T

TESTICULAR CANCER

See *Cancer, Testicular*.

THORACIC SURGERIES

Thoracic surgeries are operative procedures that are performed to aid in the diagnosis and treatment of certain pulmonary conditions. Procedures include thoracotomy, lobectomy (see *Figure T-1*), pneumonectomy, segmental resection, and wedge resection. Except with pneumonectomy, these procedures require chest drainage immediately after surgery. Chest drainage is usually not used after pneumonectomy because it is desirable that the empty hemithorax fill with an effusion, which eventually obliterates the space.

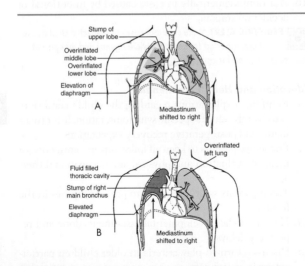

Stump of upper lobe

Overinflated middle lobe
Overinflated lower lobe

Elevation of diaphragm

A

Mediastinum shifted to right

Overinflated left lung

Fluid filled thoracic cavity

Stump of right main bronchus

Elevated diaphragm

B

Mediastinum shifted to right

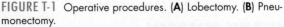

FIGURE T-1 Operative procedures. **(A)** Lobectomy. **(B)** Pneumonectomy.

Indications for thoracic surgeries include biopsy of suspicious masses, chest trauma, benign and malignant tumors, giant emphysematous blebs, bronchiectasis, fungal infections, abscesses, and extensive tuberculosis.

Potential Complications
1. Hypoxia
2. Postoperative bleeding
3. Atelectasis and pneumonia
4. Bronchopleural fistula from disruption of a bronchial suture or staple; bronchial stump leak
5. Cardiac arrhythmias (usually occurring on the third to the fourth postoperative day)
6. Myocardial infarction or heart failure

Nursing Diagnoses
3, 62, 75, 123

Collaborative Management and Interventions
Preoperative Care
Goal is to maximize respiratory function to improve the outcome postoperatively and reduce risk of complications.
1. Encourage the patient to stop smoking to restore bronchial ciliary action and to reduce the amount of sputum and likelihood of postoperative atelectasis or pneumonia.
2. Teach an effective coughing technique:
   a. Sit upright with knees flexed and body bending slightly forward (or lie on side with hips and knees flexed if unable to sit up).
   b. Splint the incision with hands or folded towel.
   c. Take three short breaths, followed by a deep inspiration, inhaling slowly and evenly through the nose.
   d. Contract abdominal muscles and cough twice forcefully with mouth open.
3. Humidify the air to loosen secretions.
4. Administer bronchodilators if bronchospasm occurs.
5. Administer antimicrobials to reduce risk of infection.
6. Encourage deep breathing with the use of incentive spirometer to prevent atelectasis postoperatively.

T

7. Teach diaphragmatic breathing.
8. Evaluate cardiovascular status for risk and prevention of complication.
9. Encourage activity to improve exercise tolerance.
10. Correct anemia or dehydration with blood transfusions and I.V. infusions, as indicated.
11. Orient the patient to events that will occur in the post-operative period — coughing and deep breathing, suctioning, chest tube and drainage bottles, oxygen therapy, ventilator therapy, pain control, leg exercises, and range-of-motion exercises for affected shoulder.
12. Make sure that the patient fully understands surgery and is emotionally prepared for it; verify that informed consent has been obtained.

Postoperative Care

1. Auscultate chest for adequacy of air movement — to detect bronchospasm, consolidation, atelectasis.
2. Obtain arterial blood gas values and pulmonary function measurements as directed.
3. Monitor level of consciousness and inspiratory effort closely. If patient is mechanically ventilated, begin weaning from ventilator as soon as possible.
4. Suction frequently using meticulous aseptic technique because tracheobronchial secretions are increased because of trauma to the tracheobronchial tree during operation, diminished lung ventilation, and diminished cough reflex.

EMERGENCY ALERT Look for changes in color and consistency of sputum. Colorless or white, fluid sputum is not unusual; change in color or thickening of sputum may mean dehydration or infection.

5. Elevate the head of the bed 30 to 40 degrees when patient is oriented and blood pressure is stabilized to improve movement of diaphragm.
6. Encourage coughing and deep-breathing exercises and use of an incentive spirometer to prevent bronchospasm, retained secretions, atelectasis, and pneumonia.
7. Watch for and report restlessness, tachycardia, tachypnea, and elevated blood pressure, indicating hypoxia.

EMERGENCY ALERT Sudden onset of respiratory distress or cough productive of serosanguineous fluid may indicate bronchopulmonary fistula or leak after pneumonectomy. Position with operative side down and report immediately. Prepare for immediate chest tube insertion or surgical intervention.

8. Monitor heart rate and rhythm with auscultation and electrocardiogram because arrhythmias are frequently seen after thoracic surgery.

9. Monitor central venous pressure, if indicated, for prompt recognition of hypovolemia and for effectiveness of fluid replacement. Also note restlessness, anxiety, pallor, tachycardia, and hypotension, which may indicate postoperative bleeding.

10. Monitor cardiac output and pulmonary artery systolic, diastolic, and wedge pressures if Swan-Ganz catheter is in place. Watch for subtle changes, especially in the patient with underlying cardiovascular disease.

11. Assess chest tube drainage for amount and character of fluid. (See *Box T-1*.)

BOX T-1 | Managing Chest Tube Drainage

- Make sure that tubing from pleural space is connected to tubing that leads to drainage bottle.
- Make sure that tubing does not loop, allowing dependent fluid to collect, which interferes with negative pressure.
- Milk the tubing in the direction of the drainage bottle, as directed, to prevent fibrin dots.
- Check for fluctuation (tidaling) of fluid level in the tube indicating communication between the pleural space and drainage bottle. Tidaling will stop when the lung has expanded, a dependent loop develops in the tubing, suction is not operating, or there is an obstruction.
- Observe for constant bubbling in the water seal bottle (chamber), which indicates an air leak.
- Assist with removal of a chest tube by administering pain medication 30 minutes before removal, clamping the tube close to the patient's chest, asking the patient to breathe quietly or performing the Valsalva maneuver, and securing a petroleum gauze dressing over the wound once the tube is removed.

T

    a. Chest drainage should progressively decrease after first 12 hours.

    b. Prepare for blood replacement and possible reoperation to achieve hemostasis if bleeding persists.

12. Maintain intake and output record, including chest tube drainage.

13. Monitor infusions of blood and parenteral fluids closely because patient is at risk for fluid overload if portion of pulmonary vascular system has been reduced (with pneumonectomy).

14. Give opioids (usually by continuous I.V. infusion or by epidural catheter) for pain relief, as directed, to permit patient to breathe more deeply and cough more effectively.

    a. Severity of pain varies with type of incision and patient's individual pain tolerance. Usually a posterolateral incision is the most painful.

    b. Be alert for respiratory and central nervous system depression caused by opioids; patient should be alert enough to cough.

15. Assist with intercostal nerve block or cryoanalgesia (intercostal nerve freezing) for pain control as ordered.

16. Position for comfort and optimal ventilation (head of bed elevated 15 to 30 degrees); this also helps residual air to rise in upper portion of pleural space, where it can be removed by the chest tube.

    a. Vary the position from horizontal to semierect to prevent retention of secretions in the dependent portion of the lungs.

17. Encourage splinting of incision with pillow, folded towel, or hands while turning.

18. Teach relaxation techniques, such as progressive muscle relaxation and imagery, to help reduce pain.

19. Begin range of motion of arm and shoulder on affected side immediately to prevent ankylosis of the shoulder ("frozen" shoulder).

    a. Perform exercises at time of maximal pain relief.

   b. Encourage patient to actively perform exercises three to four times daily, taking care not to disrupt chest tube or I.V. lines.

Education and Health Maintenance

1. Advise patient that there will be some intercostal pain for several weeks, which can be relieved by local heat and oral analgesia.
2. Advise patient that weakness and fatigability are common during the first 3 weeks after a thoracotomy, but exercise tolerance will improve with conditioning.
3. Suggest patient alternate walking and other activities with frequent short rest periods. Walk at a moderate pace and gradually extend walking time and distance.
4. Encourage patient to continue deep-breathing exercises for several weeks after surgery to attain full expansion of residual lung tissue.
5. Advise patient to avoid lifting more than 20 lb (9 kg) for several months until complete healing has taken place.
6. Warn patient to discontinue activity that causes undue fatigue, increased shortness of breath, or chest pain.
7. Encourage patient to receive annual influenza immunization and pneumococcal pneumonia vaccine. Also, tell patient to avoid respiratory irritants and persons with respiratory infections.
8. Encourage follow-up visits.

THROMBOCYTOPENIA

Thrombocytopenia is a decrease in circulating platelet count (less than $100,000/mm^3$) and is the most common cause of bleeding disorders. It may be congenital or acquired, and results from decreased platelet production, as in aplastic anemia, myelofibrosis, radiation therapy, or leukemia; increased platelet destruction, as in certain infections, drug toxicity, or disseminated intravascular coagulation; abnormal distribution or sequestration in spleen; or dilutional thrombocytopenia after hemorrhage or red blood cell transfusions. Severe thrombocytopenia may cause death as a result of blood loss or bleeding into vital organs.

An autoimmune form of thrombocytopenia, *idiopathic thrombocytopenic purpura (ITP)*, results from destruction of platelets by antiplatelet antibodies. Acute ITP typically follows a viral illness and is more common in children. Eighty to ninety percent of patients recover uneventfully. Chronic ITP (more than 6-month course) is most common at ages 20 to 40, and is more common in women than men.

Assessment
1. Asymptomatic until platelet count decreases to below 20,000/mm^3
2. Signs of bleeding
   a. Petechiae: occur spontaneously
   b. Ecchymoses: occur at sites of minor trauma
   c. Bleeding: from mucosal surfaces, gums, nose, respiratory tract
   d. Menorrhagia
   e. Hematuria
   f. GI bleeding
3. Excessive bleeding after surgical and dental procedures

Diagnostic Evaluation
1. Complete blood count and platelet count show decreased hemoglobin, hematocrit, platelets.
2. Bleeding time, prothrombin time, and partial thromboplastin time are prolonged.
3. Platelet aggregation test is positive for heparin-dependent platelets.

Collaborative Management
Therapeutic and Pharmacologic Interventions
1. Treat underlying cause, if possible.
2. Administer platelet transfusions and institute bleeding control.
3. Corticosteroids or I.V. immunoglobulins may be helpful in selected patients.

Surgical Interventions

1. Splenectomy may be done to decrease destruction of platelets in ITP.

Nursing Diagnoses

24, 136

Nursing Interventions

Monitoring

1. When administering blood products, monitor for signs and symptoms of allergic reactions, anaphylaxis, and volume overload.
2. Evaluate all urine and stool for gross and occult blood.
3. Monitor platelet count.
4. Monitor vital signs during acute bleeding episode.

Supportive Care

1. Institute bleeding precautions.
   a. Avoid use of plain razor, hard toothbrush or floss, I.M. injections, tourniquets, and rectal temperatures or suppositories.
   b. Administer stool softeners as necessary to prevent constipation.
   c. Discourage blowing of nose.
   d. Restrict activity and exercise when platelet count is less than 20,000/mm^3 or when there is active bleeding.
2. Monitor pad count and amount of saturation during menses; administer or teach self-administration of hormones to suppress menstruation as ordered.
3. Administer blood products as ordered.

Education and Health Maintenance

1. Teach patient bleeding precautions.
2. Tell patient to take only prescribed medications and to avoid aspirin, herbals, and nonsteroidal anti-inflammatory drugs, which may interfere with platelet function.
3. Demonstrate the use of direct, steady pressure at bleeding site if bleeding does develop.

4. Stress the importance of routine follow-up for platelet counts.

THROMBOPHLEBITIS AND RELATED CONDITIONS

Thrombophlebitis is a condition in which a clot forms in a vein secondary to phlebitis (inflammation of the vein wall) or because of partial obstruction of the vein. In general, the clotting is related to stasis of blood, injury to the vessel wall, and altered blood coagulation (Virchow's triad).

Deep vein thrombosis (DVT) refers to thrombosis of deep rather than superficial veins. Deep veins of the lower extremities are most commonly involved.

Phlebitis is an inflammation in the wall of a vein. The term is used clinically to indicate a superficial and localized condition that can be treated with application of heat.

Venous thrombosis can result from many conditions, such as venous stasis (after operations, childbirth, or prolonged bed rest or sitting); direct trauma to veins from I.V. injections or indwelling catheters; extension of nearby infection to the vein; a complication of varicose veins; continuous pressure on the vessel, as from a tumor, aneurysm, or heavy pregnancy; unusual activity in a person who has been sedentary; hypercoagulability associated with malignant disease; or blood dyscrasias. Venous thrombosis of the popliteal veins or above is most dangerous. Thrombi confined to the calf area below the popliteal vein are least dangerous. Complications include pulmonary embolism and postphlebitic syndrome.

Assessment

1. High-risk factors for thrombophlebitis include malignancy, previous venous insufficiency, conditions causing prolonged bed rest, leg trauma, general surgery (especially if the patient is older than age 40), obesity, estrogen therapy, smoking.
2. Patient may be asymptomatic or have severe calf and leg pain.
3. Fever and chills may occur with DVT.

4. Asymmetry of the legs, venous distention or edema, taut skin, hardness to the touch, warmth of extremity, and redness and induration along a vein (venous cord).

5. Calf pain may occur; however, Homans' sign has a low sensitivity for detecting thrombophlebitis and is no longer used in assessment.

6. Contrast with signs of arterial occlusion. (See *Arterial occlusive disease*, page 51.)

Diagnostic Evaluation

1. Venous duplex or color duplex ultrasound is a noninvasive test that can detect thrombus in the lower extremities.

2. Phlebography (venography), involving X-rays and injection of contrast medium, shows venous obstruction.

3. Plethysmography measures changes in calf volume corresponding to changes in blood volume caused by temporary venous occlusion with a high-pressure pneumatic cuff (will show slow decrease in impedance associated with thrombus).

4. ^{125}I fibrinogen uptake test detects clot formation with serial scanning and comparison of one leg with the other (most sensitive screen for acute calf vein thrombosis).

5. Coagulation profile, including prothrombin time (PT) or International Normalized Ratio (INR), partial thromboplastin time (PTT), platelet count, circulating fibrin, and other tests, is obtained before anticoagulant treatment is initiated to detect hidden bleeding tendencies.

Collaborative Management
Therapeutic Interventions

1. Conservative measures for superficial thrombophlebitis, and as an adjunct to anticoagulation with DVT:
   a. Dry heat to the affected area with warm water bottles, thermostatically controlled heat cradle, or ultrasound
   b. Moist heat using hydrotherapy, whirlpool baths, or warm compresses
   c. Pressure gradient therapy using compression devices and garments to promote venous return

T

    d. Bed rest during acute stage to prevent muscle contraction with walking that may dislodge the clot

    e. Elevation of the extremity above the level of the heart to promote venous return

Pharmacologic Interventions

1. To prevent embolization in DVT, heparin may be given subcutaneously (S.C.) or I.V.

2. S.C. enoxaparin therapy (a low-molecular-weight heparin) may be used instead of heparin and can be used on an outpatient basis; also used postoperatively and in immobilized patients to prevent DVT.

3. Oral anticoagulation with Coumadin is given for 3 to 6 months after heparin therapy to prevent recurrence and embolization. Heparin may be continued for 4 to 5 days after oral anticoagulant is started because of delayed onset of therapeutic effectiveness with oral anticoagulants.

⚡ **EMERGENCY ALERT** Drug interactions can alter the effect of anticoagulants. Review the effect of other medications the patient may be taking during anticoagulant therapy.

4. In severe cases of DVT with compromised blood flow, the patient will be hospitalized and streptokinase may be used to dissolve the clot.

Surgical Interventions

1. If the patient cannot tolerate prolonged anticoagulant therapy, a filter may be placed in the inferior vena cava to prevent pulmonary embolism.

2. Thrombectomy may be necessary for severely compromised venous drainage of the extremity.

Nursing Diagnoses
3, 62, 136

Nursing Interventions
Monitoring

1. Measure and record the patient's leg circumferences daily to monitor for venous obstruction.

2. With anticoagulant therapy, monitor PT or INR and PTT daily or as ordered and check results before giving next anticoagulant dose. Dosage may be adjusted to achieve desired elevation of these levels.
   a. PTT monitors heparin therapy — should be 1½ to 2 times the control.
   b. PT monitors oral anticoagulant therapy — INR should be 2.0 to 2.5, or higher based on condition being treated.
3. Monitor for signs of pulmonary embolism — chest pain, dyspnea, and apprehension — and report immediately.

Supportive Care

1. Identify preoperative patients at risk for DVT (major surgery; surgery in patients older than age 40; comorbid risk factors; surgery involving more than 30 minutes of general, orthopedic surgery; multiple traumas) and administer prophylaxis as directed. Elevate the patient's legs as directed to promote venous drainage, reduce swelling, and relieve pain.
2. Apply warm compresses or a heating pad as directed to promote circulation and reduce pain.

EMERGENCY ALERT Avoid massaging or rubbing the calf — this risks breaking up the clot, which can then circulate as an embolus.

3. Administer analgesic as prescribed and as needed. Avoid using aspirin and nonsteroidal anti-inflammatory drug-containing products during anticoagulant therapy to prevent further risk of bleeding.
4. Prevent venous stasis by proper patient positioning in bed. Support the full length of the legs when they are to be elevated.
5. Initiate active exercises, unless contraindicated, in which case, use passive exercises.
6. Encourage adequate fluid intake, frequent changes of position, effective coughing, and deep-breathing exercises to prevent complications of bed rest.

7. After the acute phase (5 to 7 days), apply elastic stockings, as directed. Remove twice per day and check for skin changes and calf tenderness.
8. Encourage ambulation when allowed (usually after 5 to 7 days when clot has fully adhered to vessel wall).

Education and Health Maintenance

1. Teach patient to recognize and immediately report signs of recurrent thrombophlebitis and pulmonary embolism.
2. Provide thorough instructions about oral anticoagulation therapy.

ALTERNATIVE INTERVENTION

Advise patient not to use ginkgo biloba, horse chestnut, or over-the-counter products to improve circulation while on anticoagulant therapy.

3. Teach patient to promote circulation and prevent stasis by applying elastic hosiery at home. Elastic hosiery has no role in managing the acute phase of DVT but is of value once ambulation has begun. Properly filling elastic hosiery will minimize or delay development of postphlebitic syndrome (venous insufficiency).
4. Advise patient against straining or any maneuver that increases venous pressure in the leg. Eliminate the necessity to strain at stool by increasing fiber and fluids in the diet.
5. Warn patient of the hazards of smoking and obesity: Nicotine constricts veins, decreasing venous blood flow, and extra pounds increase pressure on leg veins. Arrange a consultation with a dietitian, if necessary.

COMMUNITY CARE CONSIDERATIONS

Practice preventive measures for bedridden patients who are prone to develop thrombosis.

Have the patient lie in bed in the slightly reversed Trendelenburg's position because it is better for the veins to be full of blood than empty.

Place a footboard across the foot of the bed. Instruct the patient to press the balls of the feet against the footboard, as if rising up on toes.

Then have the patient relax the foot. Request that the patient do this 5 to 10 times per hour.

THYROID CANCER

See *Cancer, Thyroid.*

THYROIDECTOMY

Thyroidectomy involves the partial (one lobe or isthmus removed), subtotal (95% removed to leave parathyroid tissue intact), or complete removal of the thyroid gland to treat thyroid tumors, hyperthyroidism, or hyperparathyroidism.

Potential Complications

1. Hemorrhage, glottal edema, laryngeal nerve damage.
2. Hypothyroidism occurs in 5% of patients in first postoperative year; increases at rate of 2% to 3% per year.
3. Hypoparathyroidism occurs in approximately 4% of patients and is usually mild and transient. More severe cases require oral and I.V. calcium supplements.

Nursing Diagnoses
3, 6, 66, 123, 136

Collaborative Management and Interventions
Preoperative Care

1. Administer thionamides to control hyperthyroidism and make sure that the patient is euthyroid at time of surgery.
2. Administer iodide to increase firmness of gland tissue and reduce its vascularity to control bleeding during surgery.
3. Maintain a restful and therapeutic environment and provide nutritious diet to counteract effects of hypermetabolism. Make sure that the patient has a good night's rest preceding surgery.

T

4. Advise patient that speaking is minimized immediately after surgery and that oxygen and humidification may be administered to facilitate breathing.

5. Explain that, postoperatively, fluids may be given I.V. to maintain fluid, electrolyte, and nutritional needs; glucose may also be given I.V. before administration of anesthesia.

Postoperative Care

1. Administer humidified oxygen as directed to reduce irritation of airway and prevent edema.

2. Observe for signs of hemorrhage.
   a. Watch for repeated clearing of the throat or complaint of smothering or difficulty swallowing, which may be early signs of hemorrhage.
   b. Watch for irregular breathing, swelling of the neck, and choking — other signs pointing to the possibility of hemorrhage and tracheal compression.
   c. Observe for bleeding at sides and back of the neck, as well as anteriorly, when the patient is in dorsal position.
   d. Monitor vital signs frequently, watching for tachycardia and hypotension indicating hemorrhage (most likely between 12 and 24 hours postoperatively).

3. Be alert for voice changes, which may indicate damage to laryngeal nerve.

4. Have equipment available to treat respiratory difficulties: airway, suction equipment, and tracheostomy tray.

5. Move the patient carefully; provide adequate support to the head so no tension is placed on the sutures.

6. Place the patient in semi-Fowler's position with the head elevated and supported by pillows; avoid flexion of neck.

7. Reinforce dressing if indicated.

8. Watch for the development of hypocalcemic tetany caused by removal or disturbance of parathyroid glands. Progression of signs and symptoms includes:
   a. Patient is apprehensive; reports tingling of toes and fingers and around the mouth.

b. Positive *Chvostek's sign:* tapping the cheek over the facial nerve causes a twitch of the lip or facial muscles (see *Figure T-2A*).

c. Positive *Trousseau's sign:* carpopedal spasm induced by occluding circulation in the arm with a blood pressure cuff (see *Figure T-2B*).

9. Be prepared to treat tetany.

a. Monitor calcium levels: if level decreases to below 7 mg/100 mL (3 mEq) in 48 hours, administer calcium replacement (gluconate, lactate) I.V. Administer slowly through large vein to avoid extravasation and necrosis.

⚡ EMERGENCY ALERT Give I.V. calcium cautiously to a patient who has renal disease or who is receiving digoxin preparations; hypercalcemia may result.

b. Position the patient for optimal ventilation, with pillow removed to prevent the head from bending forward and compressing the trachea.

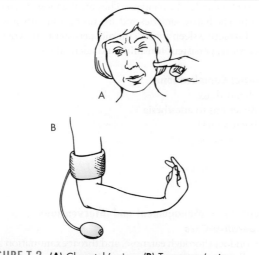

FIGURE T-2 **(A)** Chvostek's sign. **(B)** Trousseau's sign.

   c. Keep side rails padded and elevated, and position the patient to prevent injury if a seizure occurs. Avoid restraints because they only aggravate the patient and may cause muscle strain or fractures.

   d. Have cardiac arrest equipment available.

Education and Health Maintenance
1. Make sure that patient understands the importance of follow-up blood work in evaluating thyroid hormone and calcium balance.
2. Teach patient about thyroid hormone replacement. It may not be necessary immediately postoperatively, but may become necessary later.
3. Advise proper rest, relaxation, and nutrition to facilitate healing. He or she may resume usual activities as soon as swelling has resolved and incision has adequately healed.

TONSILLECTOMY AND ADENOIDECTOMY

Tonsillectomy and *adenoidectomy* are the surgical removal of the tonsillar and adenoidal structures, part of the lymphoid tissue that encircles the pharynx. They are the most frequently performed pediatric surgeries and are most commonly used to treat obstructive sleep apnea; chronic, persistent otitis media; and chronic, persistent tonsillitis and adenoiditis.

Potential Complications
1. Hemorrhage
2. Reactions to anesthesia
3. Bacteremia
4. Otitis media

Nursing Diagnoses
3, 44, 73, 119, 123, 135

Collaborative Management and Interventions
Preoperative Care
1. Conduct thorough ear, nose, and throat examination and collect appropriate cultures to determine presence and source of infection.

2. Obtain blood samples for preoperative studies to determine risk of bleeding: clotting time, platelet count, prothrombin time, and partial thromboplastin time.

3. Conduct preoperative assessment.

   a. Assess the child's psychological preparation for hospitalization and surgery.

PEDIATRIC ALERT The preschool child is especially vulnerable to psychological trauma as a result of surgical procedures or hospitalization.

   b. Obtain thorough nursing history from the parents to obtain pertinent information that would impact on the child's care, such as recent infections (the child should be free of respiratory infection for at least 2 to 3 weeks); recent exposure to any communicable diseases; presence of loose teeth that may pose the threat of aspiration; or bleeding tendencies in the child or family.

4. Assess hydration status.

5. Prepare the child specifically for what to expect postoperatively, using techniques appropriate to the child's developmental level (books, dolls, drawings).

6. Talk to the child about the new things to be seen in the operating room, and clear up misconceptions.

7. Help the parents prepare their child by talking at first in general terms about surgery and progressing to more specific information.

8. Assure parents that complication rates are low and that recovery is usually swift.

9. Encourage parents to stay with child and help provide care.

Postoperative Care

1. Assess pain on a frequent basis and administer analgesics as indicated.

2. Assess patient frequently for signs of postoperative bleeding; frequent swallowing or clearing of throat, pallor, restlessness, and increased pulse. Inspect back of throat with flashlight for oozing.

 EMERGENCY ALERT Notify surgeon immediately if bleeding occurs.

T

3. Have suction equipment, oxygen, and nasal-packing material readily available in case of emergency.

4. While the child is still under the effects of anesthesia, position the child prone or semiprone with head turned to the side to prevent aspiration.

5. Allow the child to assume a position of comfort when alert. (Parent may hold the child.)

6. The child may vomit old blood initially. If suctioning is necessary, avoid trauma to oropharynx.

7. Remind the child not to cough or clear throat unless necessary.

8. Provide adequate fluid intake; give ice chips 1 to 2 hours after awakening from anesthesia. When vomiting has ceased, advance to clear liquids cautiously.

9. Offer cool fruit juices without pulp at first because they are best tolerated; then offer Popsicles and cool water for first 12 to 24 hours.

10. There is some controversy regarding intake of milk and ice cream the evening of surgery. It can be soothing and reduce swelling, but it does coat the throat, which causes the child to clear throat more often, thus increasing risk of bleeding.

11. Provide ice collar to neck, if desired. (Remove ice collar if child becomes restless.)

12. Rinse mouth with cool water or alkaline solution.

13. Keep child and environment free from blood-tinged drainage to help decrease anxiety.

14. Encourage the parents to be with the child when the child awakens.

Education and Health Maintenance

1. Explain and provide written instructions for care of the child at home after discharge.

   a. Diet should still consist of large amounts of fluids as well as soft, cool, nonirritating foods.

   b. Eating helps promote healing because it increases the blood supply to tissues and prevents tightness of throat muscles.

    c. Maintain bed rest for 1 to 2 days, then daily rest periods for 1 week. Resume normal eating and activities within 2 weeks after surgery.

    d. Avoid contact with persons with infections.

    e. Discourage the child from blowing nose, frequent coughing, or clearing of throat.

    f. Avoid gargling. Mouth odor may be present for a few days after surgery; only mouth rinsing is acceptable.

2. Advise when to call health care provider. (Make sure that parents have the telephone number of health care provider and emergency department.)

    a. Earache accompanied by fever

    b. Any bleeding, often indicated only by frequent swallowing; most common about fifth to tenth day when membrane sloughs from surgical site

3. Teach about medications prescribed or suggested for pain relief.

4. Guide parents in helping the child think of the experience as a positive one once surgery is over, to make subsequent health care experiences easier.

TOTAL JOINT REPLACEMENT

See *Arthroplasty and Total Joint Replacement.*

TOXIC SHOCK SYNDROME

Toxic shock syndrome (TSS) is a rare, potentially life-threatening condition caused by a bacterial toxin secreted by *Staphylococcus aureus* in the bloodstream. The cause is uncertain, but 70% of cases are associated with menstruation and tampon use. Research suggests that magnesium-absorbing fibers in tampons may lower magnesium levels in the body, thereby providing ideal conditions for toxin formation.

    TSS has also occurred in nonmenstruating people with conditions such as cellulitis, surgical wound infection, vaginal infections, and subcutaneous abscesses, and with the use of contraceptive sponges, diaphragms, and tubal ligation. Death may result from cardiovascular collapse and renal failure caused by shock.

Assessment

1. Sudden onset of high fever greater than 102° F (39° C)
2. Vomiting and profuse, watery diarrhea
3. Rapid progression to hypotension and shock within 72 hours of onset
4. Mucous membrane hyperemia
5. Sometimes, sore throat, headache, and myalgia
6. Rash (similar to sunburn) that develops 1 to 2 weeks after onset of illness and is followed by desquamation, particularly of the palms and soles

Diagnostic Evaluation

1. Blood, urine, throat and vaginal or cervical cultures, and possibly cerebrospinal fluid culture, detect or rule out infectious organism.
2. Additional tests may be required to rule out other febrile illnesses: Rocky Mountain spotted fever, Lyme disease, meningitis, Epstein-Barr, or Coxsackie viruses.
3. Complete blood count, electrolytes, and renal function tests monitor condition.

Collaborative Management
Therapeutic Interventions

1. Fluid and electrolyte replacements to increase blood pressure and prevent renal failure
2. Supportive care to maintain cardiorespiratory functions

Pharmacologic Interventions

1. Vasopressors, such as dopamine, to treat shock
2. Antibiotics, such as penicillinase-resistant penicillins, or cephalosporins to decrease the rate of relapse
3. Antipyretics to treat fever
4. Use of corticosteroids and immunoglobulins is controversial

Nursing Diagnoses
23, 24, 44, 49, 63

Nursing Interventions

Monitoring

1. Monitor core body temperature frequently.
2. Perform hemodynamic monitoring as indicated (ie, arterial line, central venous pressure, or pulmonary artery pressure).
3. Maintain strict intake and output measurement.
4. Insert indwelling catheter to monitor hourly urine output.
5. Monitor respiratory status for pulmonary edema and respiratory distress syndrome caused by fluid overload from increased fluid replacement; diuretics may be necessary.

Supportive Care

1. Use cooling measures, such as sponge baths and hypothermia blanket, if indicated.
2. Administer I.V. fluids, antibiotics, and vasopressors as indicated.
3. Tell patient to expect desquamation of skin, as in peeling sunburn.
4. Protect skin and avoid using harsh soaps and alcohol, which cause drying.
5. Tell patient to apply mild moisturizer and avoid direct sunlight until healed.
6. Advise patient that reversible hair loss may occur 1 or 2 months after TSS.

Education and Health Maintenance

1. Tell patient to expect fatigue for several weeks to months after TSS.
2. Tell patient to avoid using tampons to reduce risk of recurrence.
3. Encourage follow-up visits for examination and cultures.
4. Teach prevention of TSS.
   a. Alternate use of pads with tampons; avoid superabsorbent tampons.
   b. Change tampons frequently and do not wear one longer than 8 hours; 4 hours maximum during heavy menses.

c. Be careful of vaginal abrasions that can be caused by some applicators.

d. Recognize and report symptoms of TSS.

TUBERCULOSIS

Tuberculosis is an infectious disease caused by the slow-growing bacteria that resembles a fungus, *Mycobacterium tuberculosis*, which are usually spread from person to person by droplet nuclei through the air. The lung is the usual infection site, but the disease can occur elsewhere in the body. Typically, the bacteria form a lesion (tubercle) in the alveoli. The lesion may heal, leaving scar tissue; may continue as an active granuloma, heal, then reactivate; or may progress to necrosis, liquefaction, sloughing, and cavitation of lung tissue. The initial lesion may disseminate bacteria directly to adjacent tissue, through the bloodstream, the lymphatic system, or the bronchi. Most people who become infected do not develop clinical illness because the body's immune system brings the infection under control. However, the incidence of tuberculosis (especially drug-resistant varieties) is rising. Alcoholics, the homeless and patients infected with the human immunodeficiency virus (HIV) are especially at risk. Complications of tuberculosis include pneumonia, pleural effusion, and extrapulmonary disease.

Assessment

1. Constitutional symptoms:
   a. Fatigue, anorexia, weight loss, low-grade fever, afternoon temperature elevation, night sweats, indigestion
   b. Some patients have acute febrile illness; chills; generalized, influenza-like symptoms
   c. Some patients may be asymptomatic or may have insidious symptoms that are ignored
2. Pulmonary signs and symptoms:
   a. Cough (insidious onset) progressing in frequency and producing mucoid or mucopurulent sputum
   b. Hemoptysis; pleuritic chest pain; dyspnea (indicates extensive involvement)
   c. Crackles on auscultation of lungs

3. Extrapulmonary forms of tuberculosis: lesions in any organ in the body including pleurae, lymph nodes, genitourinary tract, bones and joints, peritoneum, central nervous system

Diagnostic Evaluation

1. Tuberculin skin test (purified protein derivative or Mantoux) detects infection with *Mycobacterium tuberculosis* (past or present, active or inactive)
2. Sputum for smears and cultures confirm the infection with acid-fast bacilli; performed on first morning sputum on 3 consecutive days
3. Chest X-rays, bone X-ray, and other tests determine presence and extent of disease

Collaborative Management
Therapeutic Interventions

1. Standard precautions, if hospitalized, for all direct contact with the patient, lines, or articles in the room; use of negative pressure room to keep droplets from leaving the room; use of high-efficiency particulate air (HEPA) filter masks for respiratory procedures
2. Adequate nutrition and alcohol detoxification for the malnourished, alcoholic patient

Pharmacologic Interventions

1. Combination of drugs to which the organism is susceptible to destroy viable bacilli as rapidly as possible and to protect against the emergence of drug-resistant organisms.
   a. Current recommended regimen for treating uncomplicated pulmonary tuberculosis is 2 months of bactericidal drugs: isoniazid (INH), rifampin, ethambutol, and pyrazinamide followed by 4 months of INH and rifampin.
   b. Second-line drugs, such as capreomycin, kanamycin, ethionamide, para-aminosalicylic acid, and cycloserine, are used in patients with resistant strains, for retreatment, and in those intolerant to other agents. Pa-

T

tients taking these drugs should be monitored by health care providers experienced in their use.

DRUG ALERT Adverse reactions to tuberculosis drugs may be significant, and include rash, GI intolerance, liver dysfunction, neurotoxicity, hypersensitivity, and optic neuritis. Signs of hepatitis including nausea, vomiting, anorexia, jaundice, and abdominal pain should be reported immediately by patients taking INH, rifampin, and pyrazinamide.

2. Once treatment is instituted, sputum smears are obtained every 2 weeks until they are negative; sputum cultures do not become negative for 3 to 5 months.
3. Pyridoxine (vitamin B_6) is given to prevent peripheral neuropathy in patients taking INH.

Nursing Diagnoses
24, 49, 51, 75, 93

Nursing Interventions
Monitoring
1. Monitor breath sounds, respiratory rate, sputum production, respiratory effort, and fever.
2. Monitor compliance with long-term course of antibiotic therapy.
3. Monitor weekly weight to assess nutritional status.
4. Assess for liver dysfunction due to drug therapy.
   a. Ask the patient about loss of appetite, fatigue, joint pain, fever, abdominal pain, nausea and vomiting, rash, and dark urine.
   b. Monitor results of periodic liver function studies.

Supportive Care
1. Encourage rest and avoidance of exertion.
2. Provide supplemental oxygen as ordered.
3. Take measures to prevent spread of infection.
   a. Provide care for hospitalized patient in a negative-pressure room to prevent respiratory droplets from leaving room when door is opened.
   b. Enforce that all staff and visitors use standard dust, mist, or fume masks (class C) for any contact with patient.

    c. Use HEPA filter masks for high-risk procedures, such as suctioning, bronchoscopy, or pentamidine treatments.

    d. Use standard precautions for additional protection: gowns and gloves for any direct contact with patient, linens, or articles in room; and meticulous hand washing.

4. Teach the patient measures to control spread of infection through secretions.

5. Stress the importance of eating a nutritious diet to promote healing and improve defense against infection.

6. Provide small, frequent meals and liquid supplements during symptomatic period.

7. Participate in observation of medication taking, weekly pill counts, or other programs designed to increase compliance with treatment for tuberculosis.

COMMUNITY CARE CONSIDERATIONS

Patient compliance remains a major problem in eradicating tuberculosis. Therefore, it may be helpful or necessary to have the patient take medication in an observed setting throughout therapy.

8. Investigate living conditions, availability of transportation, financial status, alcohol and drug abuse, and motivation, which may affect compliance with follow-up and treatment. Initiate referrals to a social worker for interventions in these areas.

Education and Health Maintenance

1. Educate the patient about the disease and stress the importance of continuing to take medications for the prescribed time.

2. Review the adverse effects of drug therapy and tell patient to immediately report experiencing any of the following: GI intolerance causing noncompliance; rash; numbness and tingling of extremities (INH); visual changes (ethambutol); painful and swollen joint (pyrazinamide); signs of liver toxicity (INH and others).

T

3. Review symptoms of recurrence (persistent cough, fever, or hemoptysis). Urge the patient to report symptoms.

4. Advise patient to avoid job-related exposure to excessive amounts of silicone (working in foundry, rock quarry, sand blasting), which increases chance of reactivation.

5. Encourage the patient to report at specified intervals for bacteriologic (smear) examination of sputum to monitor therapeutic response and compliance.

6. Teach the patient about basic hygiene practices and investigate living conditions, because crowded conditions contribute to development and spread of tuberculosis.

7. Encourage follow-up chest X-rays for rest of life to evaluate for recurrence.

COMMUNITY CARE CONSIDERATIONS

Provide tuberculosis screening for people at risk, including people who have had direct contact with tuberculosis infection; people infected with HIV; people who are immunosuppressed; substance abusers; those with chronic illnesses, such as diabetes; immigrants from Asia, Africa, and Latin America; residents of long-term care facilities; health care workers; those with alcoholism or malnutrition; and those who are homeless or living in crowded conditions. A 5-mm reaction is considered positive in those with HIV or immunosuppression; 10 mm in most people at risk; and 15 mm in those who do not fall into a risk group.

8. Instruct on prophylaxis with INH for persons infected with the tubercle bacillus without active disease to prevent disease from occurring, or to people at high risk of becoming infected. Prophylaxis is recommended for the following groups:

   a. Household members and other close associates of potentially infectious tuberculosis cases

   b. Newly infected people (positive skin test within 2 years)

   c. People with past tuberculosis who have not received adequate therapy

   d. People with significant reactions to tuberculin skin test and who are in special clinical situations (silicosis, di-

abetes, B-cell malignancies, end-stage renal disease, severe malnutrition, immunosuppression, HIV positive)
e. Tuberculin skin reactors younger than age 35 with none of the aforementioned risk factors

U

ULCERATIVE COLITIS

Ulcerative colitis is a chronic inflammatory disease of the mucosa and, less frequently, the submucosa of the colon and rectum. Its exact cause is unknown, but theories include viral or bacterial infections, immune mechanisms, and genetic predisposition. The disease usually begins in the rectum and sigmoid and spreads upward, eventually involving the entire colon. There may be a defect in the intestinal barrier and defect in mucosal injury repair, which develop into a chronic condition. Multiple crypt abscesses develop in the mucosa, which may become necrotic and lead to ulceration. There is a tendency for the patient to experience remissions and exacerbations. It may also manifest as a systemic disease with inflammatory changes of connective tissues.

Complications of ulcerative colitis include perforation, hemorrhage, toxic megacolon, abscess formation, stricture and obstruction, anal fistula, malnutrition, anemia, and secondary colon cancer.

Assessment

1. Diarrhea is the prominent symptom; it may be bloody or contain pus or mucus. Tenesmus (painful straining), urgency, and cramping may be associated with bowel movements.
2. Crampy abdominal pain may be prominent and brought on by certain foods or dairy products.
3. May be increased bowel sounds, and left lower abdomen may be tender on palpation.
4. As the disease progresses, there may be anorexia, nausea and vomiting, weight loss, fever, dehydration, hypokalemia, and cachexia.
5. There may be associated systemic manifestations, such as arthritis, iritis, and skin lesions.

Diagnostic Evaluation

1. Stool evaluation for culture and ova and parasites rules out other causes of diarrhea. Tests for blood are positive during active disease.
2. Blood tests may show low hemoglobin and hematocrit caused by bleeding; increased white blood cells; increased erythrocyte sedimentation rate; and decreased potassium, magnesium, and albumin levels.
3. Proctosigmoidoscopy or colonoscopy with biopsy is necessary to confirm diagnosis.
4. Barium enema determines extent of disease and detects pseudopolyps, carcinoma, and strictures.

Collaborative Management
Therapeutic Interventions

1. During acute exacerbations, bed rest, I.V. fluids containing potassium and vitamins, and clear liquid diet are indicated.
2. For severe dehydration and excessive diarrhea, total parenteral nutrition may be necessary to rest the intestinal tract and restore nitrogen balance.

Pharmacologic Interventions

1. Iron supplements are necessary to treat anemia from chronic bleeding; blood replacement for massive bleeding.
2. Sulfasalazine is the mainstay drug for acute and maintenance therapy.
3. If patient does not tolerate sulfasalazine, oral salicylates such as mesalamine appear to be as effective as sulfasalazine.
4. Mesalamine enema is available for proctosigmoiditis; suppository for proctitis.
5. Corticosteroids may be used I.V., orally, or by enema to manage inflammatory disease and induce remission. Immunosuppressant agents may be indicated if patient is refractory or dependent on corticosteroids.
6. Antidiarrheal medications may be prescribed to control diarrhea, rectal urgency and cramping, and abdominal pain; however, their use is not routine.

U

Surgical Interventions

1. Surgery is recommended when patient fails to respond to medical therapy, if clinical status is worsening, for severe hemorrhage, or for signs of toxic megacolon. Noncurative procedures (possible curative procedure and reconstruction later) include:
   a. Temporary loop colostomy for decompression of toxic megacolon.
   b. Subtotal colectomy, ileostomy, and Hartman's pouch.
   c. Colectomy with ileorectal anastomosis.
2. Curative surgery aims to remove entire colon and rectum to cure patient of ulcerative colitis. Procedures include:
   a. Total proctocolectomy with end-ileostomy.
   b. Total proctocolectomy with continent ileostomy.
   c. Total colectomy with ileal reservoir–anal anastomosis (see *Figure U-1*).

Nursing Diagnoses

3, 13, 23, 51, 78, 135

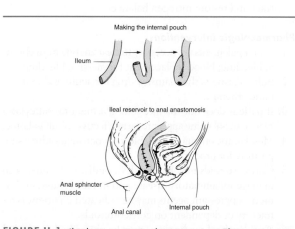

FIGURE U-1 Ileal reservoir–anal anastomosis. This reservoir is constructed of two loops of small intestine forming a J configuration (J pouch).

Nursing Interventions

Also see *Gastrointestinal or Abdominal Surgery*, page 381.

Monitoring

1. Monitor intake and output, including liquid stools.
2. Monitor serum or fingerstick glucose of patient on corticosteroids or hyperalimentation, and report elevations.
3. Weigh patient daily; rapid increase or decrease may relate to fluid imbalance, slower change related to nutritional status.
4. Monitor patient's response to therapy. Observe for adverse reactions. Dose-related adverse effects of sulfasalazine include vomiting, anorexia, headache, skin discoloration, and dyspepsia; oral mesalamine may cause nephrotoxicity.
5. Observe for complications such as sudden abdominal distention, pain, and fever, which may indicate perforation or toxic megacolon.
6. Observe for signs of dehydration — decreased skin turgor, dry skin, oliguria, weakness, and increased hematocrit, blood urea nitrogen, and urine specific gravity.

Supportive Care

1. Provide comfort measures and assess the need for sedatives and tranquilizers, to facilitate rest and slow peristalsis.
2. Observe for pressure sores caused by malnourishment and enforced inactivity, especially if patient is thin.
   a. Clean the skin gently after each bowel movement.
   b. Apply a protective emollient such as petroleum jelly, skin sealant, or moisture-barrier ointment.
3. Reduce physical activity to a minimum or provide frequent rest periods.
4. Provide commode or bathroom next to bed, because urgency of movements may be a problem.
5. Provide a well-balanced, low-residue, high-protein diet to correct malnutrition. Determine foods that agree with patient and those that do not. Avoid dairy products if the patient is lactose intolerant. Modify diet plan accordingly.

U

6. Avoid cold fluids and discourage smoking because they increase intestinal motility.
7. Administer I.V. fluids, vitamin supplements, and parenteral nutrition as indicated.
8. Encourage the patient to talk; listen and offer psychological support. Answer questions about the permanent or temporary ileostomy, if appropriate. Refer for psychological counseling, as needed.

Education and Health Maintenance

1. Teach the patient about chronic aspects of ulcerative colitis and each component of care prescribed.
2. Encourage self-care in monitoring symptoms, seeking annual checkup, and maintaining health.
3. Alert the patient to possible postoperative problems with skin care, aesthetic difficulties, and surgical revisions.
   a. Pouchitis is a late complication of continent restorative procedures causing increased stool output, cramps, and malaise; it can be treated with metronidazole.
   b. Food blockage may occur with permanent or temporary ileostomy in the first 6 weeks or later due to obstruction by undigested food at the level of the fascia; abdominal cramping, bloating, and stomal swelling may occur and the health care provider should be notified.
4. Warn patients to report immediately any early indications of relapse, such as bleeding or increased diarrhea, so that steroid treatment may be initiated.

ALTERNATIVE INTERVENTION

Advise patient with ulcerative colitis to avoid use of supplemental vitamins, herbal products, and homeopathic remedies for any condition without the recommendation of the health care provider. Many of these products affect bowel function and may exacerbate symptoms of ulcerative colitis.

5. Facilitate referral to local chapter of the United Ostomy Association or Crohn's and Colitis Foundation of America, *www.ccfa.org*.

URINARY TRACT INFECTION

A *urinary tract infection (UTI)* may occur in the bladder, where it is called *cystitis,* or in the urethra, where it is called *urethritis.* Upper tract infection results in pyelonephritis. Most UTIs result from ascending infections by bacteria that have entered through the urinary meatus but some may be caused by hematogenous spread. UTIs are much more common in females because the shorter female urethra makes them more vulnerable to entry of organisms from surrounding structures (vagina, periurethral glands, and rectum). During the first year of life, male and female rate of UTIs is the same, then the rate of male infections sharply drops until later in life. Predisposing factors include urinary stasis, obstruction (stones, prostatic hyperplasia, congenital anomaly), vesicoureteral reflux, catheterization, constipation, local inflammation (sexual activity, gynecologic conditions), infection elsewhere in the body, dysfunctional voiding, and other urologic or renal conditions. Acute infection is most often caused by organisms of the patient's own intestinal flora (*Escherichia coli*).

Recurrent UTIs may indicate relapse (recurrent infection with an organism that has been isolated during a prior infection) or reinfection (recurrent infection with an organism distinct from previous infecting organism). Untreated UTIs may lead to pyelonephritis, sepsis, and kidney damage, especially in the infant and young child.

PEDIATRIC ALERT A UTI in a child can cause renal scarring and permanent renal damage. Therefore, greater attention to symptoms and more aggressive diagnoses and treatment are required than in an adult; sexusl abuse should also be ruled out.

Assessment

1. Dysuria, frequency, urgency, nocturia, dribbling, enuresis
2. Suprapubic pain, mild low back pain, possible costovertebral angle tenderness
3. Fever, anorexia, malaise, irritability, vomiting in the child

GERONTOLOGIC ALERT The only sign of UTI in elderly patients may be mental status change.

U

Diagnostic Evaluation

1. Urine specimens for urine dipstick test may react positively for blood, white blood cells, and nitrates, indicating infection.
2. Urine microscopy shows red blood cells and many white blood cells per field without epithelial cells.
   a. Urinalysis showing many epithelial cells is likely contaminated by vaginal secretions in women and is, therefore, inaccurate in indicating infection.
   b. Urine culture may be reported as contaminated with mixed flora as well. Obtaining a clean-catch midstream specimen is essential for accurate results.
3. Obtain urine specimens for urine culture to detect presence of bacteria and for antimicrobial sensitivity testing. Bacteriuria (10^5 bacteria colonies per mL of urine or greater) generally indicates infection; if catheterized for urine specimen, 10^4 bacteria colonies per mL is positive.
4. In asymptomatic bacteriuria, organisms are found in urine, but the patient has no symptoms. Usually not treated unless the patient is pregnant or at risk for ascending infection.
5. Urologic workup with renal ultrasound, intravenous pyelogram, and voiding cystourethrogram, and other studies may be done to evaluate cause of recurrent infections.

Collaborative Management
Pharmacologic Interventions

1. Uncomplicated UTIs are usually treated with a 3-day course of antibiotics, such as amoxicillin, trimethoprim-sulfamethoxazole, or ciprofloxacin, or a 7-day course of nitrofurantoin.
2. A 7- to 10-day course of therapy is recommended for UTI with associated complications, such as obstruction, resistant pathogens, upper UTI, or urologic dysfunction; as well as in pregnant women, and in most cases of UTI in men and children.
3. Analgesic or antispasmodic if pain is severe.

4. Follow-up culture is recommended to prove effectiveness in pregnant women, children with severe or recurrent infection, and men.
5. Indwelling catheters should be changed at the start of antibiotic therapy.
6. Long-term antibiotic therapy is considered for patients with recurrent infections.

Surgical Interventions
1. Correction of underlying obstruction or congenital anomalies

Nursing Diagnoses
3, 6, 24, 69

Nursing Interventions
Supportive Care
1. Obtain first voided urine, if possible, for testing.
   a. Obtain a midstream, clean-catch specimen.
   b. Apply a urine collection bag for an infant or toddler, after cleaning the penis or perineum.
   c. Catheterize if necessary.
2. Administer or teach self-administration of prescribed antibiotic and antispasmodic.
3. Apply heat to the abdomen to relieve bladder spasms.
4. Encourage rest during the acute phase if symptoms are severe.
5. Encourage plenty of fluids to promote urinary output and to flush out bacteria from urinary tract.
6. Encourage frequent voiding (every 2 to 3 hours) and emptying the bladder completely. This enhances bacterial clearance, reduces urine stasis, and prevents reinfection.

COMMUNITY CARE CONSIDERATIONS

U

Patients with indwelling catheters or who intermittently self-catheterize are at increased risk for UTIs; review methods of handling catheters and drainage bags at home.

Education and Health Maintenance

1. For those with recurrent UTIs, give the following instructions on preventive measures:
   a. Minimize the spread of bacteria from the anal and vaginal areas to the urethra by cleaning the perineal area from the urethra backward toward the anus.
   b. Drink liberal amounts of water to lower bacterial concentrations in the urine.
   c. Avoid urinary irritants, such as coffee, tea, alcohol, and cola drinks.
   d. Decrease the entry of microorganisms into the bladder during intercourse by voiding immediately after sexual intercourse.
   e. Avoid external irritants, such as bubble baths and perfumed vaginal cleaners or deodorants.
   f. Encourage patient to follow a high-fiber diet to avoid constipation.
2. Advise patient with persistent bacteria who is on long-term antimicrobial therapy to:
   a. Take antibiotic at bedtime after emptying bladder to ensure adequate concentration of drug during overnight period because low rates of urine flow and infrequent bladder emptying predispose to multiplication of bacteria.
   b. Use self-monitoring tests (dipsticks) at home to monitor for UTI.
3. Encourage follow-up for recurrent or severe infections.

ALTERNATIVE INTERVENTION

Cranberry (juice or capsules) may help prevent cystitis by altering the chemical composition of urine, and it appears to be safe.

UTERINE CANCER

See *Cancer, Uterine*.

UTERINE PROLAPSE

Uterine prolapse refers to an abnormal position of the uterus, in which the organ herniates through the pelvic floor and protrudes into the vagina (prolapse) and possibly beyond the introitus (procidentia). This condition usually results from obstetric trauma and overstretching of musculofascial supports. Three degrees of uterine prolapse are recognized. In first-degree prolapse, the cervix appears at the introitus without straining or traction. In second-degree prolapse, the cervix extends over the perineum. In third-degree prolapse, the entire uterus (or most of it) protrudes. Complications of uterine prolapse include cervical or uterine necrosis.

Assessment
1. Backache or abdominal pain; pressure and heaviness in vaginal region
2. Symptoms aggravated by obesity, standing, straining, coughing, or lifting a heavy object because of increased intra-abdominal pressure
3. Bloody discharge caused by cervix rubbing against clothing or inner thighs
4. Protrusion and ulceration of cervix on examination

Diagnostic Evaluation
1. Pelvic examination identifies condition; spread labia gently, do not attempt to insert speculum.

Collaborative Management
Therapeutic Interventions
1. Vaginal pessary to insert into vagina to support pelvic organs if surgery cannot be done
   a. Prolonged use may lead to necrosis and ulceration.
   b. Should be removed and cleaned every 1 to 2 months.

Pharmacologic Interventions
1. Estrogen cream to decrease genital atrophy

U

Surgical Interventions

1. Surgical correction is recommended treatment with an anterior and posterior repair; effective and permanent.
2. Abdominal sacropexy may be done to anchor the vagina.
3. Hysterectomy may be necessary for necrosis.

Nursing Diagnoses

3, 67, 156

Nursing Interventions

Supportive Care

1. Encourage sitz baths to relieve discomfort.
2. Provide heating pad for low back or lower abdomen.
3. Administer pain medications as directed.
4. Increase fluid intake and encourage the patient to void frequently to prevent bladder infection.
5. For second- and third-degree prolapse, apply saline compresses frequently.
6. Provide postoperative care.
   a. Administer perineal care to the patient after each voiding and defecation.
   b. Employ a heat lamp to help dry the incision line and enhance healing process.
   c. If urine retention occurs, catheterize or use indwelling catheter until bladder tone is regained.
   d. Apply an ice pack locally to relieve congestion.
   e. Promote ambulation but prevent straining to reduce pelvic pressure.
7. Explain to the patient that sexual intercourse is possible with pessary; however, vaginal canal may be shortened.

Education and Health Maintenance

1. Reinforce surgeon's instructions postoperatively about waiting to have vaginal penetration.
2. Encourage the patient to explore with partner ways to engage in sexual activity without strain and with greatest comfort.
3. Instruct the patient on care of vaginal pessary — removal for cleaning every 1 to 2 months.

V

VAGINITIS

Vaginitis is inflammation of the vagina caused by infection from a variety of organisms, and is commonly marked by vaginal discharge and discomfort. Five major types of vaginitis are recognized.

In *simple (contact) vaginitis*, inflammation results from poor hygiene, irritation (eg, from contact allergens, tampons or diaphragm that has been retained in the vaginal canal for too long), and invading organisms.

In *bacterial vaginosis*, inflammation results from infection by *Gardnerella vaginitis*, a gram-negative bacillus that is not considered sexually transmitted. The infection is benign. (When discharge is wiped away, underlying tissue is healthy and pink.)

In *Trichomonas vaginitis*, inflammation results from infection by a protozoan, *Trichomonas vaginalis*, which thrives in alkaline environments and is sexually transmitted. This organism may spread to the urinary tract, where it is hard to eradicate. Men are usually asymptomatic carriers.

In *Candida vaginitis*, inflammation results from infection by a fungus, *Candida albicans*, a normal inhabitant of the GI tract. Because this fungus thrives in an environment rich in carbohydrates, it commonly occurs in patients with poorly controlled diabetes and in patients who have been on prolonged antibiotic or steroid therapy.

The last type, *atrophic vaginitis*, commonly occurs in postmenopausal women because of atrophy of the vaginal mucosa secondary to decreased estrogen levels.

Urethritis and vulvitis often accompany vaginitis because of the proximity to the vagina.

Assessment

1. Vaginal itching, irritation, burning
2. Odor, increased or unusual vaginal discharge

V

3. Dyspareunia, pelvic pain, dysuria
4. Possible history of unprotected intercourse with a new or infected partner

 GERONTOLOGIC ALERT In the postmenopausal woman, if vaginal bleeding occurs, it must be investigated promptly to determine if cancer is the cause.

Diagnostic Evaluation

1. Physical examination, including vaginal speculum examination, obtains vaginal discharge specimens
2. Wet smear for microscopic examination
   a. Saline slide: discharge mixed with saline; useful in detecting *Gardnerella* and *Trichomonas*.
   b. Potassium hydroxide (KOH): useful in detecting *C. albicans*. If fishy odor is noted when KOH mixed with discharge, suspect *Gardnerella*.
3. Vaginal pH — use Nitrazine paper:
   a. Normal pH: 4.0 to 4.5
   b. *Gardnerella*: 5.0 to 5.5
   c. *Trichomonas*: 5.5+
4. Papanicolaou smear may detect any type of vaginitis
5. Chlamydia and gonorrhea cultures or DNA probe rule out chlamydia or gonorrhea cervicitis

Collaborative Management
See *Table V-1.*

Nursing Diagnoses
3, 13, 24, 67, 156

Nursing Interventions
Supportive Care and Education

1. Instruct the patient to discontinue use of irritating agents, such as bubble baths and vaginal douches.
2. Suggest cool baths or sitz baths and pat dry or dry with hair dryer on low setting.
3. Encourage the patient to wear loose cotton undergarments.

TABLE V-1 Specific Types of Vaginitis

TYPE	MANAGEMENT
Simple (contact) vaginitis	1. Enhance natural vaginal flora by administering a weak acid douche — 15 mL vinegar to 1,000 mL water (1 tablespoon white vinegar to 1 quart water), as ordered. 2. Stimulate growth of lactobacilli (Döderlein's bacilli) by administering beta-lactamase vaginal suppository; this dissolves with body heat, and the sugar then acts. 3. Foster cleanliness by meticulous care after voiding and defecation. 4. Discontinue use of causative agent.
Gardnerella vaginitis	1. Metronidazole (Flagyl) taken orally for 7 days or topical clindamycin or metronidazole. 2. Alcohol intake should be avoided during Flagyl treatment to avoid severe reaction. 3. Treating partners is controversial unless the condition is recurrent.
Trichomonas vaginitis	1. Destroy infective protozoa by taking metronidazole (Flagyl) orally, usually single dose of 2 g. 2. Prevent reinfection by treating partner concurrently with Flagyl. 3. Avoid alcohol during treatment.
Candida vaginitis	1. Eradicate fungus by applying antifungal vaginal cream, or vaginal suppository for 3 or 7 nights as directed. 2. Treat the symptomatic or uncircumcised partner by applying antifungal cream under the foreskin nightly for 7 nights. 3. Oral fluconazole 150 mg in a single dose may be used. 4. For severe or recurrent cases, investigate underlying cause, such as diabetes or infection with human immunodeficiency virus.
Atrophic vaginitis	1. Vaginal estrogen replacement. 2. If infection also present, this is treated.

V

4. Teach the patient to clean perineum before topically applying medication. Demonstrate application of prescribed medication.

5. Emphasize importance of taking prescribed medication for full length of therapy and as directed; teach the patient adverse effects of medication.

 DRUG ALERT Flagyl is contraindicated in the first trimester of pregnancy.

6. Instruct the patient on the proper technique for douching (2 tsp white vinegar to 1 quart water), if desired; however, douching is generally discouraged.

7. Emphasize importance of abstinence until therapy is complete and sexual partner has been treated, if indicated.

8. Tell the patient that use of condoms may be protective but may produce irritation during treatment.

9. Instruct the patient in the use of water-soluble lubricant if vagina is dry and atrophic.

10. Teach causes of vaginitis and their symptoms so the patient can seek treatment promptly.

11. Teach the patient about all sexually transmitted diseases and means of prevention.

12. For recurrent *Candida* infections, encourage good control if patient has diabetes, or encourage the patient to be tested for diabetes. Teach all patients to eliminate concentrated carbohydrates from diet to prevent recurrence.

VALVULAR HEART DISEASE, ACQUIRED

Normal heart valves function to maintain the forward flow of blood from the atria to the ventricles and from the ventricles to the great vessels. *Valvular dysfunction* stems from three types of valvular damage: stenosis, or narrowing of the valve opening; incomplete valve closure, causing regurgitation; or prolapse, in which valve leaflets drop down into the heart chamber. Valvular disorders may progress to left-sided heart failure, possible right-sided heart failure, and various arrhythmias. Acquired valvular disease occurs in several forms.

In *mitral stenosis,* valve cusps become progressively thickened and contracted, which narrows the orifice and impairs forward blood flow. Acute rheumatic valvulitis is a common cause. Because of increased workload, the left atrium becomes dilated and hypertrophied. As pulmonary circulation becomes congested, pulmonary arterial pressure increases, leading to right-sided heart failure.

In mitral insufficiency or regurgitation, the mitral valve fails to close tightly during systole, which allows blood to flow back into the left atrium. Poor closure may be caused by valve distortion or damage to chordae tendineae or papillary muscles caused by mitral valve prolapse, chronic rheumatic heart disease, myocardial infarction, infective endocarditis, or trauma. Left atrial pressures increase because of backflow into the atrium, and left ventricular hypertrophy may develop because of inefficient emptying.

In *aortic stenosis*, the orifice between the left ventricle and the aorta is narrowed because of congenital anomalies, calcification, or rheumatic fever. Impaired aortic outflow increases left ventricular workload that results in hypertrophy and failure. Left atrial pressure also increases; the increased pulmonary vascular pressure may eventually cause right-sided heart failure.

In aortic insufficiency (regurgitation), poor valve closure during diastole allows blood to flow back from the aorta into the left ventricle. This condition may be caused by rheumatic or infective endocarditis, congenital malformation, Marfan's syndrome, Ehlers-Danlos syndrome, systemic lupus erythematosus, or by diseases that cause dilation or tearing of the ascending aorta (syphilis, rheumatoid spondylitis, dissecting aneurysm). The left ventricle contracts more forcefully to maintain adequate cardiac output and becomes hypertrophied as a result. Low aortic diastolic pressures result in decreased coronary artery perfusion.

In *tricuspid stenosis*, commissural fusion and fibrosis restrict the tricuspid valve orifice. This condition usually follows rheumatic fever, commonly accompanies mitral valve diseases, and can lead to right-sided heart failure.

In *tricuspid insufficiency* or regurgitation, valve leaflets allow blood to flow back from the right ventricle into the right atrium during ventricular systole. Commonly caused by a dilated right ventricle or rheumatic fever, this condition reduces

V

cardiac output and eventually leads to right-sided heart failure.

Assessment

1. Possible symptoms include fatigue, weakness, dyspnea, cough, orthopnea, and nocturnal dyspnea
2. Hemoptysis (from pulmonary hypertension) and hoarseness (from compression of left recurrent laryngeal nerve) in mitral stenosis
3. Hypotension, dizziness, syncope, angina, and heart failure in aortic stenosis
4. Arterial pulsations visible and palpable over precordium and visible in neck; widened pulse pressure, and water-hammer (Corrigan's) pulse (pulse strikes palpating finger with a quick, sharp stroke and then suddenly collapses) in aortic insufficiency
5. Right-sided heart failure (edema, ascites, hepatomegaly) in tricuspid stenosis and insufficiency
6. Characteristic heart sounds:
   a. *Mitral stenosis:* accentuated first heart sound, usually accompanied by an "opening snap" (caused by sudden tensing of valve leaflets), and a low-pitched diastolic murmur (rumbling murmur). Murmur best heard at apex, with bell of stethoscope, with patient in left lateral recumbent position.
   b. *Mitral insufficiency:* diminished first heart sound and blowing systolic murmur (pansystolic if mild insufficiency), commencing immediately after first heart sound at apex, and radiating to axilla and left infrascapular area.
   c. *Aortic stenosis:* prominent fourth heart sound, possible paradoxical splitting of second heart sound (suggestive of associated left ventricular dysfunction), and a midsystolic murmur heard best over the aortic area. Note harsh and rasping quality at base of heart and a higher pitch at apex of heart. Often associated with a palpable thrill.
   d. *Aortic insufficiency:* soft first heart sound and high-pitched blowing decrescendo diastolic murmur along left sternal border. Accentuated with patient in sitting

position leaning forward, and with patient holding breath at end of deep expiration.

e. *Tricuspid stenosis:* blowing diastolic murmur at the lower left sternal border (increases with inspiration); similar to that of rheumatic mitral disease.

f. *Tricuspid insufficiency:* third heart sound (may be accentuated by inspiration) and a pansystolic, usually high-pitched murmur at the lower left sternal border.

Diagnostic Evaluation

1. 12-lead electrocardiogram (ECG) detects arrhythmias
2. Echocardiogram shows structural or functional abnormalities of valves
3. Chest X-ray detects cardiomegaly and pulmonary vascular congestion
4. Cardiac catheterization and angiocardiography confirm diagnosis and determine severity of valvular disease

Collaborative Management
Pharmacologic Interventions

1. Antibiotic prophylaxis for endocarditis before invasive procedures (eg, cardiac catheterization) for mitral insufficiency, rheumatic heart disease, and prosthetic cardiac valves
2. Treatment of heart failure with diuretics, angiotensin-converting enzyme inhibitors, vasodilators, and cardiac glycosides (see page 424)

Surgical Interventions

1. Depending on condition, surgical procedures may include valvotomy, balloon valvuloplasty, annuloplasty (retailoring of the valve ring), or valve replacement with biologic or prosthetic valve (see page 178).

Nursing Diagnoses

1, 19, 108, 135

V

Nursing Interventions
Monitoring
1. Assess patient frequently for change in existing murmur or new murmur.
2. Monitor vital signs, shortness of breath, edema, jugular vein distention, weight, and hemodynamic parameters to assess for heart failure.
3. Maintain continuous ECG monitoring and watch for arrhythmias, as indicated.
4. After cardiac catheterization, monitor blood pressure and apical pulse closely; check peripheral pulses in affected extremity; watch for hematoma formation at puncture site; assess for chest, back, thigh, or groin pain; and keep the patient in bed until the following morning.
5. Monitor response to therapy.

Supportive Care
1. Maintain bed rest while symptoms of heart failure are severe.
2. Allow the patient to rest between interventions.
3. Assist with or perform hygiene needs for patient to reserve patient's strength for ambulation.
4. Begin activities gradually, such as sitting in a chair for brief periods.
5. Monitor intake and output and dietary sodium intake, and enforce restrictions, as indicated.
6. Instruct the patient regarding the specific valvular dysfunction, possible causes, and therapies implemented to relieve symptoms. Explain to the patient the surgical intervention selected, if applicable.

Education and Health Maintenance
1. Review activity restrictions and schedule with the patient and family.
2. Instruct the patient to report signs of impending or worsening heart failure, such as dyspnea, cough, increased fatigue, and swelling of ankles.
3. Review sodium or fluid restrictions.

4. Review medications: purpose, action, schedule, and adverse effects.
5. Advise patient of the need for antibiotic prophylaxis before some dental and other invasive procedures to prevent endocarditis.

COMMUNITY CARE CONSIDERATIONS

Refer the patient to appropriate counseling services, if indicated (vocational, social work, cardiac rehabilitation).

VARICOSE VEINS

Varicose veins result from poor venous valve function and dilation of weakened vein walls. This combination of vein dilation and valve incompetence produces the varicosity. The process is irreversible.

Primary varicose veins result from bilateral dilation and elongation of saphenous veins, whereas deeper veins are normal. Secondary varicose veins are obstructed deep veins. Most common in leg veins, varicose veins may occur elsewhere (eg, esophageal and hemorrhoidal veins) when blood flow or pressure is abnormally high. Complications of varicose veins include hemorrhage, ulceration, infection, and chronic venous insufficiency.

Telangiectasia (spider veins) are dilated superficial capillaries, arterioles, and venules that may be cosmetically unattractive, but do not impair circulation.

Assessment

1. Predisposing factors include hereditary weakness of vein walls or valves; pregnancy, obesity, or prolonged standing (may cause chronic venous distention); and elderly patient (loss of vessel elasticity with age).
2. Presenting symptoms include easy leg fatigue, feeling of heaviness in the legs, leg cramps, nocturnal muscle cramps, and increased pain during menstruation.
3. Discoloration of calves or ankles; dilated, tortuous vessels of extremities.

V

4. Manual compression test to assess severity. Place the fingertips of one hand on the dilated vein. With your other hand, compress firmly at least 8 inches (20 cm) higher on the leg. Feel for an impulse transmitted toward your lower hand. Competent saphenous valves should block the impulse. A palpable impulse indicates incompetent valves.

Diagnostic Evaluation

1. Walking tourniquet test demonstrates presence or absence of valvular incompetence of communicating veins
   a. A tourniquet is snugly fastened around the lower extremity just above the highest noted varicosities.
   b. The patient is directed to walk briskly for 2 minutes.
   c. Failure of varicosities to empty suggests valvular incompetence of communicating veins distal to tourniquet.
2. Doppler ultrasound rapidly detects presence or absence of venous reflux in deep or superficial vessels; noninvasive
3. Photoplethysmography shows venous flow hemodynamics by noting changes in the blood content of the skin; noninvasive
4. Venous outflow and reflux plethysmography detects deep venous occlusion; noninvasive
5. Ascending and descending contrast venography (an invasive test) demonstrates secondary venous occlusion and patterns of collateral flow in deep veins

Collaborative Management
Therapeutic Interventions

1. Conservative measures, such as encouraging weight loss if appropriate and avoiding activities that cause venous stasis by obstructing venous flow

Surgical Interventions

1. Surgery is considered to treat ulceration, bleeding, or for cosmetic purposes in selected patients, if patency of deep veins is ensured.

a. Ligation and stripping of the greater or lesser saphenous systems (most effective procedure).

b. Multiple vein ligation.

c. Laser therapy may be tried in some cases.

d. Venous reconstruction or venous valvular transplant.

2. Injection of a sclerosing agent to thicken and harden vessel walls. The sclerosed vessel is then compressed with a bandage for 6 weeks to bring inflamed endothelial surfaces together. Combined with ligation surgery or done for isolated varicosity.

Nursing Diagnoses
3, 67, 134, 135

Nursing Interventions
Monitoring
1. Postoperatively, monitor neurovascular status of feet (color, warmth, capillary refill, sensation, pulses) to prevent circulatory compromise caused by swelling.

2. Monitor for signs of bleeding (especially the first 24 hours), such as blood soaking through bandages, increased pain, hematoma formation, hypotension, and tachycardia.

Supportive Care
1. Maintain elastic compression bandages from toes to groin postoperatively.

2. Elevate legs approximately 30 degrees, providing support for the entire leg. Ensure that knee gatch is positioned for straight incline.

3. Encourage mostly bed rest the first day with legs elevated. The second day, encourage ambulation for 5 to 10 minutes every 2 hours.

4. Advise ambulatory patient to avoid prolonged standing or sitting, or crossing or dangling legs to prevent obstruction. (Crossing legs reduces circulation by 15%.)

5. If incisional bleeding occurs, elevate the leg above the level of the heart, apply pressure over the site, and notify the surgeon.

V

6. Be alert for complaints of pain over bony prominences of the foot and ankle; if the elastic bandage is too tight, loosen it. Later, have it reapplied.
7. Maintain I.V. infusion for fluids and antibiotics as ordered.
8. Administer analgesics as directed.
9. After removal of compression bandages (approximately 7 days postoperatively), observe and teach patient to observe for signs of cellulitis or incisional infection.

Education and Health Maintenance

Postoperatively, instruct the patient to:

1. Wear pressure bandages or elastic stockings as directed — usually for 3 to 4 weeks after surgery.
2. Elevate legs approximately 30 degrees and provide adequate support for entire leg during periods of rest.
3. Take analgesics for pain as ordered.
4. Report signs such as sensory loss, calf pain, or fever to the health care provider.
5. Avoid dangling the legs.
6. Walk as able.
7. Note that complaints of patchy numbness can be expected, but should disappear in less than 1 year.
8. Follow conservative management instructions to prevent recurrence.
   a. Avoid activities that cause venous stasis (sitting or standing for prolonged periods, crossing legs, wearing a girdle).
   b. Control excessive weight gain.
   c. Wear firm elastic support as prescribed, from toe to thigh when in upright position.
   d. Elevate the foot of the bed 6 to 8 inches (15 to 20 cm) for night sleeping, to encourage venous return.
   e. Avoid injuring legs.

VASOSPASTIC DISORDER

See *Raynaud's Disease*.

VON WILLEBRAND'S DISEASE

Von Willebrand's disease is an inherited (autosomal dominant) or acquired bleeding disorder characterized by decreased level of von Willebrand factor and prolonged bleeding time. Von Willebrand factor enhances platelet adhesion as the first step in clot formation, and also acts as a carrier of factor VIII in the blood. Von Willebrand's is the most common inherited bleeding disorder; it has various subtypes with varying degrees of severity. It occurs both in females and males and presents in children unless mild, in which case it may not present until adulthood. The acquired form is rare and generally appears late in life, often in association with lymphoma, leukemia, multiple myeloma, or autoimmune disorders. Severe blood loss or bleeding into vital organs may be life-threatening in untreated disease.

Assessment
1. Mucosal and cutaneous bleeding, such as bruising, gingival bleeding, and epistaxis
2. Menorrhagia (heavy menstrual bleeding)
3. Prolonged bleeding from cuts or after dental and surgical procedures
4. GI bleeding — bloody stools, hematemesis, or positive occult blood

Diagnostic Evaluation
1. Bleeding time — prolonged
2. Ristocetin cofactor — abnormal
3. von Willebrand factor — decreased
4. Factor VIII — generally decreased

Collaborative Management
Pharmacologic Interventions
1. Replacement of factor VIII through infusions of clotting factor precipitates, as needed.
2. Antifibrinolytic medication, specifically aminocaproic acid, to stabilize clot formation before dental procedures and minor surgery.

V

3. Desmopressin, a synthetic analog of vasopressin, may be given to manage mild to moderate bleeding.
4. Estrogen and progesterone stimulate production of von Willebrand factor and help control menorrhagia.

Nursing Diagnoses
24, 136

Nursing Interventions
Monitoring
1. Monitor replacement therapy for signs and symptoms of allergic reactions, anaphylaxis, and volume overload.
2. Monitor pad count and amount of saturation during menses.
3. Monitor hemoglobin and hematocrit for anemia caused by blood loss.

Supportive Care
1. Institute bleeding precautions: avoid use of plain razor, hard toothbrush or floss, I.M. injections, tourniquets, rectal temperatures, or suppositories; administer stool softeners as necessary to prevent constipation; and restrict activity and exercise when platelet count is less than $20,000/mm^3$ or when there is active bleeding.
2. Administer first aid for bleeding as indicated.
3. Administer or teach self-administration of hormones to suppress menstruation as prescribed.

Education and Health Maintenance
1. Teach bleeding precautions; also advise to avoid blowing nose, take only prescribed medications, avoid use of aspirin and nonsteroidal anti-inflammatory drugs, which may interfere with platelet function.
2. Demonstrate the use of direct, steady pressure at bleeding site if bleeding develops.
3. Encourage routine follow-up for laboratory screening.

VULVAR CANCER
See *Cancer, Vulvar*.

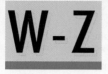

WILMS' TUMOR

Wilms' tumor is a malignant renal tumor. It accounts for 6% of all childhood cancers. It generally grows to a large size before it is diagnosed, usually before the child reaches age 5. In most cases, the tumor expands the renal parenchyma, and the capsule of the kidney becomes stretched over the surface of the tumor. Staging is from I (limited to kidney) to IV (metastasis) and stage V, which indicates bilateral involvement (rare). The tumor may metastasize to the lymph nodes, lungs, liver, and brain.

Assessment

1. A firm, nontender mass in the upper quadrant of the abdomen is usually the presenting sign; it may be on either side. (It is usually detected by the parents.)

EMERGENCY ALERT Avoid indiscriminate manipulation of the abdomen both preoperatively and postoperatively to decrease the danger of metastasis. Because the tumor is soft and highly vascular, seeding may occur because of excessive palpation or handling of the child's abdomen.

2. Abdominal pain, which is related to rapid growth of the tumor.
3. As the tumor enlarges, pressure may cause constipation, vomiting, abdominal distress, anorexia, weight loss, and dyspnea.
4. Less common manifestations are hypertension, fever, hematuria, and anemia.
5. Associated anomalies include aniridia (absence of the iris), hemihypertrophy of the vertebrae, and genitourinary anomalies.

Diagnostic Evaluation

1. Abdominal ultrasound detects the tumor and assesses the status of the opposite kidney.

2. Chest X-ray and CT scan may be done to identify metastases.
3. MRI or CT scan of the abdomen may be done to evaluate local spread to lymph nodes.
4. Urine specimens show hematuria; no increase in vanillylmandelic acid and homovanillic acid levels as occurs with neuroblastoma.
5. Complete blood count, blood chemistries, especially serum electrolytes, uric acid, renal function tests, and liver function tests, are done for baseline measurements and to detect metastasis.

Collaborative Management
Therapeutic Interventions
1. Radiation may be given preoperatively to patients with massive tumors or risky intravascular extension to reduce tumor burden.
2. The tumor bed is irradiated postoperatively to render nonviable all cells that have escaped locally from the excised tumor. Radiation is usually indicated for children who have stage III and IV tumors or an unfavorable histology.
3. Whole-lung radiation is used to treat stage IV tumors with lung metastasis.
4. Late effects of radiation therapy to the abdomen include scoliosis, underdevelopment of soft tissues, and possible organ dysfunction of local organs.

Pharmacologic Interventions
1. Chemotherapy is initiated postoperatively to achieve maximal killing of tumor cells. Drug combinations include vincristine and doxorubicin or vincristine and actinomycin D, depending on stage.

Surgical Interventions
1. Surgery is the gold standard of therapy. Also, accurate staging by the type of the tumor and the extent of invasiveness is performed.

Nursing Diagnoses
3, 6, 30, 51, 123, 135

Nursing Interventions
Monitoring

1. Observe the surgical incision for erythema, drainage, or separation. Report any of these changes.
2. Monitor for elevated temperature or sign of infection postoperatively.
3. Monitor I.V. fluid therapy and intake and output carefully, including nasogastric (NG) drainage.

Supportive Care

1. Encourage the parents to ask questions and to understand fully the risks and benefits of surgery.
2. Prepare the child for surgery; explain procedures at the appropriate developmental level.
3. Continue supporting the parents during the postoperative period. They may be frightened and upset by the appearance of their child.
4. Insert NG tube as ordered. Many children require gastric suction postoperatively to prevent distention or vomiting.
5. When bowel sounds have returned, begin administering small amounts of clear fluids.
6. Administer pain control medications as ordered in the immediate postoperative period.
7. Allow the child to participate in the selection of foods.
8. As the child recovers, encourage child to eat progressively larger meals.
9. If unable to eat because of radiation and chemotherapy, provide I.V. fluids, hyperalimentation, or tube feedings as indicated.
10. Prepare child and family for fatigue during recovery from surgery and with radiation treatments. Plan frequent rest periods between daily activities.
11. Prepare the child and parents for loss of hair associated with chemotherapy and encourage use of hat as desired; reassure that hair will grow back.

Education and Health Maintenance

1. Provide parents with written information about the child's needs — medications, activity, care of the incision, and follow-up appointments.
2. Teach the parents about radiation or chemotherapy treatments and their adverse effects.
3. Teach parents that children who have only one kidney should not play rough contact sports to avoid injuring the remaining kidney.
4. Inform parents to report if child has temperature over 101° F (38.3° C), any bleeding, any signs of infections, or any exposure to chickenpox if the child has not had them.
5. Teach measures to prevent infection while immunosuppressed because of chemotherapy and radiation therapy, such as hand washing and isolation from children with communicable diseases.
6. Refer families to resources such as Candlelighters, *www.candlelighters.org*.

PART TWO

Maternity Nursing

THE USUAL CHILDBEARING EXPERIENCE

PRENATAL CARE
Maternal Assessment
Duration of Pregnancy

1. Averages 10 lunar months (9 calendar months) or 40 weeks from the first day of the last normal menstrual period.
2. Duration may also be divided into three equal parts, or trimesters, of slightly more than 13 weeks or 3 calendar months each.
3. *Estimated date of confinement* (EDC) is calculated by adding 7 days to the date of the first day of the last menstrual period and counting back 3 months (*Nägele's rule*).
   a. For example, if a woman's last menstrual period began on 9/10/06, her EDC would be 9/10/06 plus 7 days = 9/17/06, minus 3 months = 6/17/07.

Obstetric History

1. The number of pregnancies (gravida-G) and deliveries (para-P) a woman has had is important to know. One method to summarize this is by using four digits after the P that correspond with the abbreviation TPAL:
   a. T represents full-term deliveries, 37 completed weeks or more.
   b. P represents preterm deliveries, 20 to less than 37 completed weeks.
   c. A represents abortions, either elective or spontaneous miscarriages.
   d. L represents the number of children living.
2. A woman's history that is summarized G 7, P 5-0-2-5 means that she has been pregnant 7 times, had 5 term deliveries, 0 preterm deliveries, 2 abortions, and 5 living children.

Health History

1. Age is important because adolescents have an increased incidence of anemia, pregnancy-induced hypertension, preterm labor, small-for-gestational-age (SGA) infants, cephalopelvic disproportion, and dystocia; older women have an increased incidence of hypertension, pregnancies complicated by underlying medical problems, and infants with genetic abnormalities.

2. Family history of congenital disorders, hereditary diseases, multiple pregnancies, diabetes, heart disease, hypertension, or mental retardation.

3. Woman's medical history:
   a. Childhood diseases, especially rubella
   b. Major illnesses, surgery; blood transfusions
   c. Drug, food, and environmental sensitivities
   d. Urinary infections, heart disease, diabetes, hypertension, endocrine disorders, anemias
   e. Use of oral or other contraceptives
   f. History of sexually transmitted diseases
   g. Menstrual history (menarche, length, and regularity of menstrual cycle)
   h. Use of medications, over-the-counter products, other drugs, alcohol, tobacco, and caffeine
   i. History of tuberculosis, hepatitis, group B beta-hemolytic streptococcus, or human immunodeficiency virus (HIV) infection

4. Woman's obstetric history:
   a. Problems of infertility, date of previous pregnancies and deliveries — infant weights; length of labors; types of deliveries; multiple births; abortions; maternal, fetal, and neonatal complications
   b. Woman's perception of past pregnancy, labor, and delivery for herself and impact on her family
   c. Gravidity, parity
   d. Date of last menstrual period
   e. Estimated date of birth: expected date of confinement
   f. Signs and symptoms of pregnancy include amenorrhea, breast changes, nausea and vomiting, fetal movement,

fatigue, urinary frequency, and changes in skin pigmentation

5. Psychosocial status: emotional changes she is experiencing; woman's and family's reactions to current pregnancy; support system: family's and friends' willingness to provide support; woman's current coping with lifestyle changes caused by the pregnancy.

Laboratory Data

1. Urinalysis for glucose and protein.
   a. Glucose may be present in small amounts, but should be investigated to rule out diabetes.
   b. Proteinuria (> 250 mg/dL) should be reported because it may be a sign of a hypertensive disorder of pregnancy or renal problems.
   c. If the urine is cloudy and bacteria or leukocytes (> 4/high-powered field) are present, a urine culture is done.
   d. Ketones in the urine should be reported because they may be a sign of excessive weight loss, dehydration, or electrolyte imbalance, often secondary to nausea and vomiting of pregnancy.
2. Hematocrit and hemoglobin levels and morphology of the red blood cells to find evidence of anemia.
3. Blood type, Rh factor, and antibody screen: if the woman is found to be Rh negative or have a positive antibody screen, her partner is screened and a maternal antibody titer is drawn as indicated.
   a. Coombs' test: retested at 28 weeks in the Rh-negative woman for detection of antibodies
   b. $Rh_o(D)$ immune globulin, RhoGAM, given at 28 weeks as indicated, as well as following chorionic villus sampling (CVS), amniocentesis, trauma, or placental separation.
4. Glucose: diabetic screening at 24 to 28 weeks using 1-hour 50-g glucose load test.
5. Maternal serum alpha-fetoprotein (AFP): done at 15 to 18 weeks. High maternal levels after 18 weeks may indi-

cate a neural tube defect in the fetus; however, this test has high false-positive results. Low levels are associated with Down syndrome. Inaccurate pregnancy dating may result in abnormal AFP.

6. Venereal Disease Research Lab (VDRL) or other tests for syphilis are done on the initial visit; repeated at 32 weeks as indicated.

7. Gonorrhea and chlamydia: cervical cultures or DNA test is usually done at the initial visit and when symptoms are present.

8. Herpes: all possible lesions are cultured, and the cervix is cultured weekly beginning 4 to 8 weeks before delivery if genital herpes is active.

9. Rubella titer: if nonimmune (less then 1:8), immunize postpartum.

10. Hepatitis B surface antigen: for chronic hepatitis and carrier state.

11. HIV: screening on high-risk women.

12. Other tests:
    a. Toxoplasmosis as indicated for women at risk
    b. Tuberculin skin tests as indicated
    c. Papanicolaou smear, unless recent results available
    d. Sickle cell screen to detect presence of sickle hemoglobin in at-risk women
    e. Group B beta-hemolytic streptococcus (cervical and pharyngeal swabs) to detect carriers or active infection

Physical Assessment

1. Ask the woman to empty her bladder before the examination so that during vaginal examination her uterus and pelvic organs may be readily palpated.

2. Evaluate the woman's weight and blood pressure.

3. Examination of eyes, ears, and nose: nasal congestion during pregnancy may occur as a result of peripheral vasodilation.

4. Examination of the mouth, teeth, throat, and thyroid: gums may be hyperemic and softened because of increased progesterone; thyroid may be slightly enlarged.

5. Inspection of breasts and nipples: breasts may be enlarged and tender; nipple and areolar pigment may be darkened.
6. Auscultation of heart for changes in heart sounds and murmurs.
7. Auscultation and percussion of the lungs.
8. Examination of the abdomen for scars or striations, diastasis, or umbilical hernia.
9. Palpation of the abdomen for height of the fundus.
10. Palpation of the abdomen for fetal outline and position — third trimester.
11. Check of fetal heart tone (FHT): FHTs are audible with Doppler after 10 weeks and at 18 to 20 weeks with a fetoscope.
12. Record fetal position, presentation, and FHTs.

Pelvic Examination

1. Assist woman to lithotomy position.
2. Inspect external genitalia.
3. Vaginal examination rules out abnormalities of the birth canal and to obtain cytologic smear.
4. Cervix is examined for position, size, mobility, and consistency.
5. Ovaries are identified for size, shape, and position.
6. Rectovaginal exploration identifies hemorrhoids, fissures, herniation, or masses.
7. Pelvic inlet is evaluated: anteroposterior diameter of the pelvis by measuring the diagonal conjugate (distance between the lower margin of the symphysis pubis and sacral promontory).
8. Midpelvis is evaluated for prominence of the ischial spines.
9. Pelvic outlet is evaluated: distance between ischial tuberosities.

Subsequent Prenatal Assessments

1. Uterine growth and estimated fetal growth (see *Maternity Figure 1*).
   a. A greater fundal height suggests multiple pregnancy, miscalculated due date, polyhydramnios (excessive amniotic fluid), hydatidiform mole (degeneration of villi

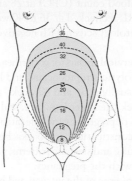

MATERNITY FIGURE 1 Height of fundus. (From Scott, J., DiSaia, P.J., Hammond, C., & Spellacy, W.N. *Danforth's Obstetrics and Gynecology,* 8th ed. Philadelphia: Lippincott Williams & Wilkins, 1999)

into grapelike clusters; fetus does not usually develop), or uterine fibroids.

   b. A lesser fundal height suggests intrauterine fetal growth retardation, error in estimating gestation, fetal or amniotic fluid abnormalities, intrauterine fetal death, or SGA.

2. FHTs: normal is 110 to 160 beats/minute.

3. Weight: major increase in weight occurs during second half of pregnancy; usually between ½ lb (0.2 kg)/week and 1 lb (0.5 kg)/week. Greater weight gain may indicate fluid retention and hypertensive disorder.

4. Blood pressure: should remain near the woman's normal baseline.

EMERGENCY ALERT Hypertensive disease affects 22% of women during pregnancy (termed "hypertensive disorders of pregnancy") and may result in maternal and fetal death. Severe headaches after 20 weeks' gestation that are accompanied by visual changes, elevated blood pressure, proteinuria, and facial edema should be evaluated immediately.

5. Urinalysis: for protein, glucose, blood, and nitrates (indicates infection).

6. Complete blood count (CBC) at 28 and 32 weeks' gestation; VDRL rechecked at 36 to 40 weeks' gestation.

7. Antibody serology screen if Rh negative at 36 weeks' gestation.

8. Vaginal or cervical smears for gonorrhea, chlamydia, group B beta-hemolytic streptococcus, and herpes simplex, if indicated, usually at 36 and 40 weeks' gestation.

9. Edema: check the lower legs, face, and hands.

10. Discomforts of pregnancy include fatigue, heartburn, hemorrhoids, constipation, and backache.

11. Evaluate eating and sleeping patterns, general adjustment and coping with the pregnancy.

12. Evaluate concerns of the woman and her family.

13. Evaluate preparation for labor, delivery, and parenting.

Nursing Diagnoses
1, 3, 6, 13, 16, 24, 31, 43, 51, 67, 69

Nursing Interventions and Education
Minimizing Pain (Backache and Leg Cramps)

1. Teach good body mechanics; wear comfortable, low-heeled shoes with good arch support; try the use of a maternity girdle if desired.

2. Encourage rest periods with legs elevated.

3. Encourage adequate calcium intake to decrease leg cramps.

4. Instruct on immediate relief of leg cramps: dorsiflex the foot while applying pressure to the knee to straighten the leg.

5. Suggest yoga or therapeutic touch for possible pain relief.

Maintaining Tissue Integrity (Breast Care)

1. Advise the woman to wear a fitted, supportive bra.

2. Instruct the woman to wash her breasts and nipples with water only.

3. Instruct the woman to apply vitamin E or lanolin cream to nipples. Lanolin is contraindicated for women with allergies to lamb's wool.

Minimizing Nausea, Maintaining Adequate Nutrition

1. Encourage low-fat, protein-containing foods and dry carbohydrates, such as toast and crackers, if nauseated.
2. Encourage small, frequent meals, eating slowly.
3. Advise the woman not to brush teeth soon after eating and to avoid strong odors.
4. Suggest getting out of bed slowly.
5. Encourage drinking liquids between meals to avoid stomach distention and dehydration.
6. Instruct the woman in the use of antacids; caution against the use of sodium bicarbonate because it results in the absorption of excess sodium and fluid retention.
7. Review the basic food groups with appropriate daily servings for balanced nutrition.
    a. 7 servings of protein foods, including 1 serving of a vegetable protein
    b. 3 servings of milk or milk products
    c. 7 servings of grain products
    d. 2 servings of vitamin C-rich vegetable or fruit
    e. 3 servings of other fruits and vegetables
    f. 3 servings of unsaturated fats
8. Teach about appropriate weight gain (25 to 35 lb [11 to 16 kg]): less for overweight women; and more for young adolescents, multiple pregnancy, and underweight women.
9. Advise the woman to limit her caffeine intake.
10. Inform the woman to limit or eliminate alcohol consumption during pregnancy; no safe level of intake has been established.
11. Stress that smoking should be eliminated or severely reduced during pregnancy; risk of spontaneous abortion, fetal death, low birth weight, and neonatal death increases with increased levels of maternal smoking.
12. Advise the woman that ingesting any drug during pregnancy may affect fetal growth and should be discussed with health care provider.

ALTERNATIVE INTERVENTION

There are many herbal remedies marketed for nausea and stomach upset. Encourage the woman to discuss these products with her health care provider. In general, red raspberry, peppermint, spearmint, and chamomile teas; ginger root; catnip; and fennel are safe if used in recommended doses.

Minimizing Urinary Frequency
1. Advise the woman to limit fluid intake in the evening.
2. Encourage the woman to void before going to bed and after meals.
3. Inform the woman that cranberry juice may be helpful in preventing urinary tract infections.

Avoiding Constipation
1. Instruct the woman to increase her fluid intake to at least 8 glasses of water a day; 1 to 2 quarts (1 to 2 L) of fluid per day is desirable.
2. Teach about foods high in fiber.
3. Encourage regular patterns of elimination.
4. Encourage daily exercise such as walking.
5. Discourage the use of over-the-counter laxatives; bulk-forming agents may be prescribed if indicated.

Maintaining Tissue Integrity (Varicose Veins)
1. Encourage frequent rest periods with legs elevated.
2. Advise the woman to use support stockings and to wear loose-fitting clothing for leg varicosities.
3. Instruct the woman to rest periodically with a small pillow under the buttocks to elevate the pelvis for vulvar varicosities.
4. Instruct the woman to avoid constipation, apply cold compresses, take sitz baths, and use topical anesthetics, such as witch hazel, for the relief of anal varicosities (hemorrhoids).
5. Provide reassurance that varicosities will totally or greatly resolve after delivery.

Reducing Anxiety and Providing Knowledge in Preparation for Labor, Delivery, and Parenthood

1. Encourage the woman and couple to discuss their knowledge, perceptions, and expectations of the labor and delivery process.
2. Provide information on childbirth education classes and encourage participation.
3. Facilitate a tour of the birth facility.
4. Discuss coping and pain control techniques for labor and birth.
5. Encourage the woman and couple to discuss their perceptions and expectations of parenthood and their "idealized child."
6. Discuss the infant's sleeping, eating, activity, and response patterns for the first month of life.
7. Discuss physical preparations for the infant, such as a sleeping space, clothing, feeding, changing, and bathing equipment.
8. Encourage discussion of feelings and concerns regarding the new role of mother and father.
9. Discuss physiologic causes for changes in sexual relationships, such as fatigue, loss of interest, and discomfort from advancing pregnancy.
10. Teach the woman and couple that there are no contraindications to sexual activity provided the woman's membranes are intact, there is no vaginal bleeding, and she has no current problems or history of premature labor.

Minimizing Fatigue

1. Advise 8 hours of rest at night. Inability to sleep may be caused by excessive fatigue during day.
2. Advise the woman that, in the latter months of pregnancy, sleeping on the side with a small pillow under the abdomen may enhance comfort.
3. Encourage frequent 15- to 30-minute rest periods during the day to avoid overfatigue.
4. Suggest the woman work while sitting with legs elevated whenever possible.

5. Discourage standing for prolonged periods, especially during the third trimester.
6. To promote placental perfusion, discourage the woman from lying flat on back — the left lateral position provides the best placental perfusion.

Promoting Exercise and Mobility

1. Explain that exercise during pregnancy should be in keeping with the woman's prepregnancy pattern and type of exercise.
2. Identify activities or sports that have a risk of bodily harm (eg, skiing, skating, horseback riding).
3. Explain that endurance during exercise may be decreased.
4. Recommend exercise classes for pregnant women that concentrate on toning and stretching to enhance physical condition, increase self-esteem, and provide socialization.

Fetal Assessment
Fetal Heart Tones

1. Audible by Doppler at approximately 10 weeks' fetal gestation; by fetoscope (fetal stethoscope) at approximately 18 to 20 weeks' fetal gestation. Electronic fetal monitoring may be done after 24 weeks.
2. Rate should be between 110 and 160 beats/minute.
3. Location of heart sounds varies with presentation of fetus.
4. Failure to hear FHTs at the expected time may be caused by maternal obesity, polyhydramnios, error in date calculation, or fetal death.
5. Nursing and patient care considerations:
   a. Explain the procedure and assist the woman to a side-lying or semi-Fowler's position; expose and drape the abdomen.
   b. Document findings on chart with date, time, activity level, medications, and so forth, and include monitor strip if applicable. Monitor tracings become part of the patient's chart and are legal documents.

Fetal Movement

1. Fetal movements or "kick counts" may be evaluated daily by the pregnant woman to provide reassurance of fetal well-being.
2. Cardiff Count-to-Ten:
   a. Assess fetal movement once per day at the same time each day.
   b. Less than 10 fetal movements in 10 hours for 2 consecutive days or no fetal movement in a 10-hour period must be reported.
3. Sadovsky:
   a. Assess fetal movement tid at the same time.
   b. Less than 4 fetal movements in 2 hours must be reported.
4. Nursing and patient care considerations:
   a. Instruct the woman to lie on her side, place her hands on the largest part of her abdomen, and concentrate on fetal movement.
   b. Instruct the woman to watch the time and record the movements felt.
   c. Instruct the woman that fetal movements are best assessed after meals, after or with light abdominal massage, and after short walks.
   d. Instruct the woman that the fetus can sleep for up to 40 minutes.

Ultrasound

1. Uses in the first trimester of pregnancy include:
   a. Early confirmation of pregnancy and determination of the EDC.
   b. Diagnosis of an ectopic pregnancy.
   c. Detection of an intrauterine device.
   d. Evaluation of placental location.
   e. Diagnosis of a multiple gestation.
2. Uses in the second trimester include:
   a. Evaluation of fetal growth, weight, and gestational age.
   b. Evaluation of the placenta for placenta previa or separation associated with vaginal bleeding.

    c. Evaluation of fetal presentation and position.

    d. Evaluation of fetal abnormalities and viability.

    e. Determination of the Biophysical Profile Score.

    f. Evaluation of amniotic fluid volume.

    g. Guidance for amniocentesis.

3. Nursing and patient care considerations:

    a. Explain the purpose and procedure to the woman, emphasizing the need to remain still.

    b. During early pregnancy, instruct the woman to drink 3 to 4 glasses of water to ensure full bladder before procedure.

    c. Remove the lubricant from the woman's abdomen and allow her to void after the procedure.

Amniocentesis

1. Usually performed between 16 and 18 weeks' gestation; involves placement of a needle through the abdominal and uterine walls and into the amniotic sac to remove fluid. It may also be done in late pregnancy to assess lung maturity.

2. In determination of genetic or metabolic diseases, the procedure is useful for women age 35 or older, family history of metabolic disease, previous child with a chromosomal abnormality, family history of chromosomal abnormality, patient or partner with a chromosomal abnormality, or a possible female carrier of an X-linked disease.

3. In determination of lung maturity, the lecithin/sphingomyelin (L/S) ratio is analyzed (should be 2:1 or greater).

4. The presence of phosphatidylglycerol (PG), one of the last lung surfactants to develop, is the most reliable indicator of fetal lung maturity. PG is not present until 36 weeks' gestation and is measured as being present or absent. PG is not affected by hypoglycemia, hypoxia, or hypothermia like L/S is.

5. In treatment of polyhydramnios (68 oz [2,000 mL] amniotic fluid or > 10 inches [25 cm] amniotic fluid index), amniocentesis may be performed to drain excess fluid and relieve pressure. Polyhydramnios is associated with spe-

cific fetal abnormalities, such as trisomy 18, anencephaly, spina bifida, and esophageal atresia or tracheoesophageal fistula.

6. Nursing considerations before the procedure:
   a. Reduce the parents' anxiety by determining their understanding of the procedure and the concerns they have about the procedure and the fetus.
   b. Correct misinformation they may have; make sure they know when the results will be available and how they may obtain the results as soon as possible.
   c. Assure woman that local anesthetic will be given.

7. Nursing considerations during the procedure:
   a. Have the woman empty her bladder if the fetus is more than 20 weeks' gestation to avoid injury to the woman's bladder. If the fetus is less than 20 weeks' gestation, the woman's full bladder will hold the uterus steady and out of the pelvis. The placenta is localized by ultrasound.
   b. Obtain maternal vital signs and a fetal heart rate (FHR) tracing to serve as a baseline to evaluate possible complications.
   c. Have the woman lie comfortably on her back with her hands and a pillow under her head. Relaxation breathing may help.
   d. Start I.V. fluids and administer tocolytics in accordance with facility policy.
   e. Monitor the woman during and after the procedure for signs of premature labor or bleeding.
   f. Tell the woman to report signs of bleeding, unusual fetal activity, abdominal pain, cramping, or fever while at home after the procedure.

Chorionic Villus Sampling

1. Assisted by ultrasonography, a catheter is passed vaginally into the woman's uterus, where a sample of chorionic villus tissue is snipped off or obtained by suction.
2. Can be performed earlier than amniocentesis — between 9 and 12 weeks of pregnancy.

3. Results from chorionic villus sampling are available in 1 or 2 weeks.
4. Complications include rupture of membranes, intrauterine infection, spontaneous abortion, hematoma, fetal trauma, or maternal tissue contamination.
5. Incidence of fetal loss is approximately 2% to 5%.
6. Nursing and patient care considerations:
   a. Obtain maternal vital signs.
   b. Instruct the woman to void.
   c. Inform the woman that a small amount of spotting is normal, but heavy bleeding or passing clots or tissue should be reported.
   d. Instruct the woman to rest at home for a few hours after the procedure.

Percutaneous Umbilical Blood Sampling

1. Percutaneous umbilical blood sampling or cordocentesis involves a puncture of the umbilical cord for aspiration of fetal blood under ultrasound guidance.
2. It is used in the diagnosis of blood incompatibilities, anemias, and genetic studies or for blood transfusion.
3. Nursing and patient care considerations:
   a. Explain the procedure and provide support during the procedure.
   b. Monitor the woman after the procedure for uterine contractions and the FHR for distress.

Nonstress Test

1. Used to evaluate FHR accelerations that normally occur in response to fetal activity. Accelerations are indicative of an intact central and autonomic nervous system.
2. Maternal indications include > 40 weeks, Rh sensitization, maternal age 35 or older, chronic renal disease, hypertension, collagen disease, sickle cell disease, diabetes, premature rupture of membranes (PROM), history of stillbirth, or vaginal bleeding in the second and third trimester.
3. Fetal indications include decreased fetal movement, intrauterine growth retardation, fetal evaluation after an amniocentesis, oligohydramnios, or polyhydramnios.

4. Criteria for a reactive nonstress test (NST) include two accelerations in a 20-minute period, each lasting at least 15 seconds with an FHR increased by 15 beats/minute above baseline in response to fetal activity (15 × 15 criteria).

5. In a nonreactive NST, the fetus may be compromised and needs further assessment with a biophysical profile or oxytocin challenge test.

6. Nursing and patient care considerations:
   a. Explain the procedure and monitoring equipment.
   b. Assist the woman to a semi-Fowler's position in bed and apply the external fetal and uterine monitors.
   c. Event markers are used when fetal movement is not observed on the fetal monitor. Instruct the woman to make a mark on the monitor strip each time fetal movement is felt (or the nurse does this).
   d. Evaluate the response of the FHR immediately after fetal activity.
   e. Monitor the woman's blood pressure and uterine activity for deviations during the procedure.

Acoustic Stimulation Test

1. Fetal acoustic and vibroacoustic stimulation, using an artificial larynx, is used to stimulate the fetus and assess its reaction to the sound.

2. Interpretation depends on facility guidelines, usually:
   a. Reactive—two accelerations meeting 15 × 15 criteria.
   b. Nonreactive—no accelerations.
   c. Equivocal—one acceleration or accelerations not meeting the 15 × 15 criteria or uninterpretable or unreadable fetal tracing.

3. Nursing and patient care considerations:
   a. Explain procedure and equipment to the woman.
   b. Assist the woman to a semi-Fowler's position in bed.
   c. Apply external fetal monitors to the woman.
   d. Observe for reactivity.

Oxytocin Challenge Test

1. Oxytocin challenge test (OCT) or contraction stress test (CST) are used to evaluate the ability of the fetus to withstand the stress of uterine contractions as would occur during labor.
   a. With OCT, endogenous oxytocin is given I.V.
   b. With CST, nipple stimulation produces endogenous oxytocin.
2. Contraindicated in woman with third-trimester bleeding, multiple gestation, incompetent cervix, PROM, placental previa, previous clonic uterine incision, hydramnios, and history of preterm labor.
3. Nursing and patient care considerations:
   a. Obtain maternal vital signs and instruct the woman to void.
   b. Assist the woman to a semi-Fowler's or side-lying position in bed.
   c. Obtain a 20-minute strip of FHR and uterine activity for baseline data.
   d. For an OCT, administer diluted oxytocin by an I.V. line infusion pump as indicated until three contractions occur within 10 minutes. This may take 1 or 2 hours.
   e. For a CST, apply warm packs to breasts for 10 minutes to increase blood flow. Instruct the woman on nipple stimulation for four cycles of 2 minutes of stimulation alternating with 2 minutes of nonstimulation.

Biophysical Profile

1. Uses ultrasonography and NST to assess five variables in determining fetal well-being.
   a. NST: looking for acceleration in relation to fetal movements
   b. Amniotic fluid volume: assessing for one or more pockets of amniotic fluid measuring 0.8 inch (2 cm) in two perpendicular planes
   c. Fetal breathing: one or more episodes lasting at least 30 seconds
   d. Gross body movements: three or more body or limb movements in 30 minutes

    e. Fetal tone: one or more episodes of active extension with return to flexion of spine, hand, or limbs

2. For each variable, if the criteria are met, a score of 2 is given. For an abnormal observation, a score of 0 or 1 is given. A score of 8 to 10 is considered normal, 6 is equivocal, and 4 or less is abnormal.

3. Nursing and patient care considerations:
    a. Explain the purpose and procedure to the woman.
    b. Instruct the woman to drink 3 or 4 glasses of water if the bladder is not full.
    c. Remove the lubricant from the woman's abdomen and allow her to void after the procedure.

LABOR AND DELIVERY

Assessment During Labor

Events Preliminary to Labor

1. *Lightening* (the settling of the fetus in the lower uterine segment) occurs 2 to 3 weeks before term in the primigravida and later, during labor, in the multigravida.
    a. Breathing becomes easier as the fetus falls away from the diaphragm.
    b. Lordosis of the spine is increased as the fetus enters the pelvis and falls forward. Walking may become more difficult; leg cramping may increase.
    c. Urinary frequency occurs because of pressure on the bladder.

2. Vaginal secretions may increase.

3. Mucus plug is discharged from the cervix along with a small amount of blood from surrounding capillaries; referred to as "show" or "bloody show."

4. Cervix becomes soft and effaced (thinned).

5. Membranes may rupture.

6. False labor contractions may occur (see *Maternity Table 1*, page 990).

7. Backache may increase.

8. Diarrhea may occur.

9. Weight loss of 1 to 3 lb (0.5 to 1.4 kg).

10. Sudden burst of energy is experienced by some women.

| MATERNITY TABLE 1 | True and False Labor Contractions |

TRUE LABOR CONTRACTIONS	FALSE LABOR CONTRACTIONS
Result in progressive cervical dilation and effacement	Do not result in progressive cervical dilation and effacement
Occur at regular intervals	Occur at irregular intervals
Interval between contractions decreases	Interval between contractions remains the same or increases
Frequency, duration, and intensity increases	Intensity decreases or remains the same
Located mainly in back and abdomen	Located mainly in lower abdomen and groin
Generally intensified by walking	Generally unaffected by walking
Not affected by mild sedation	Generally relieved by mild sedation

Stages of Labor

1. First stage of labor (stage of cervical dilation): begins with the first true labor contractions and ends with complete effacement and dilation of the cervix (10 cm dilation)
   a. Averages 13.3 hours for a nullipara and 7.5 hours for a multipara.
   b. Latent phase (early): dilation from 0 to 4 cm; contractions are usually every 5 to 20 minutes, lasting 20 to 40 seconds, and of mild intensity.
   c. Active phase: dilation from 4 to 7 cm; contractions are usually every 2 to 5 minutes; lasting 30 to 50 seconds, and of mild to moderate intensity.

d. Transitional phase: dilation from 8 to 10 cm; contractions are every 2 to 3 minutes, lasting 50 to 60 seconds, and of moderate to strong intensity. Some contractions may last up to 90 seconds.

2. Second stage of labor, or stage of expulsion: begins with complete dilation and ends with birth of the baby
   a. May last from 1 to 1½ hours in the nullipara and from 20 to 45 minutes in the multipara

3. Third stage of labor, or placental stage: begins with delivery of the baby and ends with delivery of the placenta
   a. May last from a few minutes up to 30 minutes

4. Fourth stage: begins after delivery of the placenta and ends when postpartum condition of the woman has become stabilized (usually 1 hour after delivery)

Fetal Monitoring

1. The purpose of fetal heart monitoring (FHM) during labor is both identification of the fetus experiencing well-being and identification of the fetus experiencing compromise.

2. *External monitoring* (indirect monitoring) uses separate transducers secured to the woman's abdomen: a tocodynamometer (tocotransducer) measures abdominal tension, and an ultrasonic transducer transmits fetal heart sounds into electrical signals that record on a graph chart.
   a. Apply ultrasonic transducer over the area of the abdomen where the sharpest FHT is heard and lubricate with a thin layer of ultrasonic gel to aid in the transmission of sounds.
   b. Readjust transducer when the fetus changes positions.
   c. Apply the tocodynamometer over the fundus and adjust as the uterus descends during labor.

EMERGENCY ALERT The external monitoring of uterine contractions is not accurate for intensity or resting tone. External monitoring of FHR is not accurate for short-term variability (STV).

3. *Internal monitoring* (direct monitoring) records intrauterine pressure and the FHR through internal measurements; it is more accurate than external monitoring.

a. Fetal spiral electrode: continuous FHR is detected by screwing a small spiral electrode into the presenting part. The membranes must be ruptured, the cervix dilated at least 2 to 3 cm, and the presenting part must be accessible and identifiable.

b. Uterine contractions are recorded by means of a sensor-tipped catheter placed in the uterine cavity behind the presenting part. A transducer converts the pressure values to millimeters of mercury (mm Hg).

c. Monitor strips record the fetal heart and uterine contraction simultaneously.

Interpretation

1. FHR is initially evaluated for the baseline rate when the fetus is not moving, between contractions, and when the fetus is not being stimulated. Fluctuations in the heart rate are either accelerations or decelerations.

2. Tachycardia is a FHR of 160 beats/minute or more, or more than 30 beats/minute above the normal baseline rate for at least 10 minutes. It may be caused by early fetal hypoxia, fetal immaturity, maternal fever, maternal hyperthyroidism, maternal ingestion of parasympatholytic and beta-sympathomimetic drugs, amnionitis, fetal anemia, fetal cardiac arrhythmias, and fetal heart failure.

3. Bradycardia is a baseline FHR less than 120 beats/minute for at least 10 minutes. Bradycardia may be caused by late or profound fetal hypoxia, maternal hypotension, prolonged umbilical cord compression, hypothermia, maternal ingestion of beta-adrenergic blockers, and anesthetics.

4. Variability refers to the beat-to-beat changes in FHR that result from the interplay between the sympathetic and parasympathetic nervous systems. It indicates normal neurologic function in relation to heart rate and also fetal reserve.

a. STV: the beat-to-beat change in the FHR.

b. Long-term variability (LTV): the rhythmic changes in the heart rate, usually 3 to 5 cycles/minute.

c. STV and LTV tend to increase and decrease together.

d. Variability is described as 0 to 2 beats/minute, absent variability; 3 to 5 beats/minute, minimal variability; 6 to 25 beats/minute, moderate variability (normal); more than 25 beats/minute, marked variability.

Periodic Fetal Heart Rate Changes or Patterns

1. Accelerations are increases in the FHR caused most often by fetal movements or fetal stimulation; also seen with breech presentations, occiput posterior presentations, and uterine contractions. No treatment indicated.
2. Early decelerations are decreases in FHR caused by head compression from uterine contractions, vaginal examination, or scalp stimulation; also frequently seen in women who are completely dilated. No treatment indicated.
3. Late decelerations occur late in the contraction and are caused by uteroplacental insufficiency.
   a. Treatment is aimed at increasing uteroplacental perfusion: change maternal position to left or right lateral position; correct any hypotension through increasing the maintenance I.V. fluids; stop oxytocin; give oxygen by face mask at 8 to 12 L/minute.
4. Variable decelerations are caused by cord compression that can result from maternal position, prolapsed cord, cord around a fetal part, a short cord, and a true knot in the cord.
   a. Configuration is variable and does not follow the uterine contraction; frequently are shaped like a "V," "U," or "W."
   b. Onset is variable, frequently preceded by an acceleration.
   c. Recovery occurs rapidly, often followed by an acceleration.
   d. Decrease in FHR below baseline is at least 15 beats/minute, lasting at least 15 seconds and 2 minutes from onset to return to baseline.
   e. Treatment involves changing of maternal position, performing vaginal examination for prolapsed cord, providing oxygen, and observing that the return occurs quickly and that there is no loss of variability.

5. Undulating patterns have a characteristic repetitive shape in the form of a sine wave. The baseline rate is usually within the normal range; referred to as "sinusoidal" or "pseudosinusoidal."

Sinusoidal:

a. Uniform wavelike pattern
b. Undulations smooth, uniform, and persistent
c. Characteristics: no STV, no accelerations, no response to uterine contractions
d. Serious pattern; associated with Rh isoimmunization, severe fetal anemia, abruptio placentae, severe fetal acidosis, or fetal-maternal hemorrhage

Pseudosinusoidal:

a. Less uniform wavelike pattern
b. Saw-toothed appearance and intermittent
c. Characteristics: periods of normal variability (STV or LTV), accelerations, shows periodic changes in response to uterine contractions
d. Associated with opioid ingestion, analgesic ingestion, or thumb sucking of the fetus in utero; cause unknown

Nursing Diagnoses
3, 6, 24, 67, 73, 78, 87, 123, 133, 135, 136

Nursing Interventions When Labor Begins
Obtaining History and Baseline Data

1. Introduce yourself; ask for name of woman's health care provider and if he or she has been notified that the woman was coming to the hospital or birth center.
2. Establish baseline information.
   a. Gravidity, parity, expected date of delivery or confinement
   b. When contractions began, how far apart they are, how long they last
   c. If the membranes have ruptured; if so, what is the color, consistency, and amount of fluid leakage
   d. Presence of bloody show
   e. Level of discomfort the woman is experiencing
   f. Any problems in this or past pregnancies

g. Blood type and Rh; RhoGAM treatment

h. Time of last meal or drink

i. Drugs — nonprescription, prescription, illicit

3. Establish baseline maternal and fetal vital signs.

a. Temperature: elevation suggests a possible infection or dehydration.

b. Pulse: evaluate between contractions; may be slightly elevated over the resting rate.

c. Respirations: evaluated between contractions.

d. Blood pressure: evaluated between contractions.

e. Assess the FHR: if a fetal monitor is to be used, run a 30-minute strip for baseline data.

f. Assess reflexes and clonus.

Assessing Fetal Heart Tones

1. Determine the position, presentation, and lie of the fetus by palpation. As internal rotation and descent occur, the location of the FHT changes, swinging gradually from the lateral to the medial area and dropping until immediately before birth, when it is above the pubic bone.

2. Place the fetoscope or Doptone on the abdomen over the back or chest of fetus. Avoid friction noises caused by fingers on the abdominal surface area.

3. Differentiate between FHT and other abdominal sounds.

a. *FHT:* rapid crisp or ticking sound.

b. *Uterine bruit:* soft murmur, caused by the passage of blood through dilated uterine vessels; is synchronous with maternal pulse.

c. *Uterine souffle:* hissing sound produced by passage of blood through the umbilical arteries; it is synchronous with the FHR.

4. Listen and count the rate for 1 minute; note the location and character when counting.

5. Check the rate before, during, and after a contraction to detect any slowing or irregularities.

6. Check the FHT immediately after the rupture of membranes; a sudden release of fluid may cause a prolapse of the umbilical cord.

EMERGENCY ALERT If decreases are heard in the FHR during auscultation, the patient should be turned to her side and placed on external electronic fetal monitoring (EFM) to verify the fetal tracing. Once placed on EFM, if the decreases are interpreted as variable or late deceleration patterns, notify the health care provider and continue with applicable interventions.

Assessing Uterine Contractions

1. Place fingertips gently on the fundus. As contraction begins, tension will be felt under the fingertips. Uterus will become harder, then slowly soften.
2. Describe the intensity as follows:
   a. Mild: uterine muscle is somewhat tense.
   b. Moderate: uterine muscle is moderately firm.
   c. Strong (hard): uterine muscle is so firm that it seems almost boardlike.
3. Determine frequency in minutes: represents the time from the beginning of one contraction until the beginning of the next.
4. Determine duration of a contraction: time from the moment the uterus first begins to tighten until it relaxes again.
5. Note the progression of labor: the character of the contractions changes and they last longer. When the cervix becomes completely dilated (the transition phase), the contractions become very strong, last for 60 seconds, and occur at 2- to 3-minute intervals.

EMERGENCY ALERT If any contraction lasts longer than 90 seconds and is not followed by a period of uterine muscle relaxation, notify the health care provider immediately. Uterine rupture and fetal hypoxia may occur if the pattern persists without intervention.

Performing Vaginal Examination

1. Place the woman in lithotomy position and conduct examination gently, under aseptic conditions.
2. Evaluate the condition of cervix:
   a. Hard or soft (in labor, cervix is soft)
   b. Effaced and thin or thick and long (in labor, cervix is thin and effaced)
   c. Easily dilatable or resistant

    d. Closed or open (dilated); degree of dilation

3. Determine presentation:
    a. Breech, cephalic (head), or shoulder
    b. Caput succedaneum (edema occurring in and under fe-
       tal scalp) present (small or large)
    c. Station: engaged or floating

4. Evaluate position: for cephalic presentation, identify sagittal suture and its direction; locate posterior fontanelle
   (see *Maternity Figure 2*).

5. Determine if membranes are intact or ruptured.
    a. If ruptured, determine time of drainage of fluid or pas-
       sage of meconium.

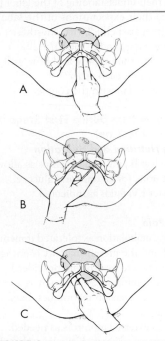

MATERNITY FIGURE 2 Vaginal examination. (**A**) Determining the station and palpating the sagittal suture. (**B**) Identifying the posterior fontanelle. (**C**) Identifying the anterior fontanelle.

b. Rupture usually increases frequency and intensity of uterine contractions.

c. Manual rupture of membranes is contraindicated in presence of vaginal bleeding, premature labor, or abnormal fetal presentation or position.

Assessing Mother's and Couple's Expectations and Concerns

1. What are their concerns?
2. How anxious are they?
3. What has been their preparation for labor (type, by whom, and when)?
4. What is their understanding of the labor process?
5. What are their expectations of the labor and delivery process (prepared childbirth, anesthesia, analgesics, use of birthing room, and so forth)?
6. How well are they coping and how well are they communicating with each other?
7. Review birth plan with the couple.

Nursing Interventions During First Stage of Labor: Latent Phase (0 to 3 cm)
Maintaining Nutrition and Hydration

1. Provide clear liquids and ice chips as allowed.
2. Evaluate urine for ketones and glucose.
3. Administer I.V. fluids as indicated.

Controlling Pain

1. Encourage ambulation as tolerated if membranes are not ruptured and the presenting part is engaged. (This may vary according to health care provider.)
2. Encourage comfort measures, such as a warm shower, relaxation and diversion techniques, back rubs, and position changes.
3. Reposition external monitors as needed.
4. Teach slow, paced breathing: relax, take one deep breath, and exhale slowly and completely. Breathe deeply, slowly, rhythmically throughout contraction. Follow with an-

other deep, complete breath. Take about 6 to 9 breaths per minute.

5. Teach modified, paced breathing: take one deep breath and exhale slowly and completely. Breathe regularly at more shallow level. When stronger contraction occurs, breathe more quickly with very light breaths. Then take deep breath and exhale slowly.

6. Teach patterned, paced breathing (most often used during transition): Concentrate on breathing in controlled manner. Take a deep breath, and exhale slowly and completely. At beginning of contraction, take a fairly deep breath. Then engage in modified paced breathing. After a certain number of breaths, the woman exhales with a more forceful puff or blow. The number of breaths before the more forceful exhalation can range between two and six, or the ratio of breaths to blows may be constant.

Relieving Anxiety and Monitoring Progress

1. Monitor temperature every 4 hours, unless elevated or membranes ruptured, then every 2 hours.

2. Obtain pulse rate and respirations every hour unless receiving pain medication, then every 15 to 30 minutes or as indicated.

3. Check blood pressure every hour unless hypertension or hypotension exists or woman has received pain medication or anesthesia. Then evaluate more frequently based on findings or as indicated.

4. Monitor the FHR. Frequency of monitoring is established by facility policy; may vary from every 1 or 2 hours depending on patient's condition, provider's orders, and facility policy.

5. Inform the woman and couple of maternal status, fetal status, and labor progress.

Nursing Interventions During First Stage of Labor: Active or Transition Phase
Monitoring Mother and Fetus to Ensure Safety

1. Monitor maternal temperature every 4 hours unless elevated or membranes ruptured, then every 2 hours.

2. Monitor blood pressure, pulse, and respirations every 30 minutes unless receiving pain medication or epidural anesthesia; then at least every 15 minutes or more frequently as indicated until stable.
3. Evaluate the FHR every 30 minutes if low-risk patient or every 15 minutes if high-risk patient regardless if monitoring is continuous or intermittent.

Relieving Anxiety and Providing Supportive Care

1. Provide intensive encouragement and support and involve the support person in the woman's care.
2. Assist the woman with breathing and relaxation techniques as needed.
3. Provide back, leg, and shoulder massage as needed.
4. Maintain I.V. fluids as indicated.
5. Encourage the woman to void at least 100 mL every 2 hours. Catheterize (in and out) if bladder becomes distended and unable to void.
6. Monitor intake and output.

Minimizing Pain

1. Assist with regional anesthesia (epidural) if needed.
2. Administer I.V. fluid bolus of Ringer's lactate before epidural catheterization as indicated.
3. Assist with positioning the woman.
4. Monitor the FHR during the procedure and assess for a nonreassuring pattern.
5. Monitor the woman's blood pressure, pulse, and respirations every 2 to 3 minutes after the procedure, then every 15 minutes thereafter or as indicated.
6. Observe for hypotension, nausea and vomiting, and lightheadedness after epidural is initiated. If these occur:
   a. Increase the rate of the I.V. fluid.
   b. Flatten the head of the bed and elevate legs if necessary.
   c. Turn the woman to left side.
   d. Administer oxygen face mask at 8 to 10 L/minute.
   e. Have ephedrine available.

Strengthening Coping

1. Provide comfort measures, which may include back and leg rubs; a cool cloth to face, neck, abdomen, or back; ice chips to moisten mouth; clean pads and linens as needed; and a quiet environment; and repositioning — either side is preferable — with pillow and blanket.
2. Administer prescribed analgesia after confirming that the woman has no known allergies to the drug.
   a. Evaluate maternal vital signs after drug administration.
   b. Evaluate FHR pattern. Decreased variability and a sinusoidal pattern are sometimes seen after opioid administration to the mother.
3. Encourage the woman to deal with one contraction at a time and to alter her breathing techniques to maintain control. Provide reassurance and encouragement during each contraction.
4. Provide information on the contractions' ascent, peak, and descent.
5. Encourage resting between contractions.
6. Encourage the woman not to push with feelings of rectal pressure until complete cervical dilation has occurred, to prevent cervical edema and lacerations. Assisting her with panting may be helpful.

Preventing Intrauterine Infection

1. Change the pads and linens when wet or soiled.
2. Provide perineal care after voiding and as needed.
3. Discourage the use of sanitary pads because they create a warm, moist environment for bacteria.
4. Minimize vaginal examinations.
5. Report elevated maternal temperature. Record every 2 hours if membranes not ruptured; record hourly if membranes have ruptured.
6. Observe for fetal tachycardia.
7. Obtain CBC as indicated.

Nursing Interventions During Second Stage of Labor
Monitoring Mother and Fetus
1. Monitor blood pressure every 5 to 30 minutes, depending on the woman's status.
2. Monitor pulse and respirations every 15 to 30 minutes.
3. Monitor temperature every 2 hours once membranes have ruptured.
4. Monitor FHR and uterine contractions every 15 minutes in low-risk women and every 5 minutes in high-risk women.
   a. Early decelerations and some fetal bradycardia may occur because of head compression.
   b. There is normally no loss of variability during pushing.
   c. Contractions may become less frequent, but intensity does not decrease.

Providing Supportive Care
1. Explain procedures and equipment during pushing and delivery.
2. Keep the woman and couple informed of status.
3. Provide frequent, positive encouragement. Use of a mirror typically allows the woman to see her progress.
4. Assist and instruct the woman in the pushing technique:
   a. Take a full cleansing breath, in through the nose and out through the mouth, at the beginning and end of each contraction.
   b. Push only during contractions.
   c. Push down toward the perineum with the abdominal muscles and try to keep the rest of the body relaxed.
   d. For each push, take a breath and push for 6 or 7 seconds while exhaling slightly.
5. Assist the woman to a comfortable position, such as left or right lateral, squatting, or semi-sitting position.
   a. Assist the woman with pulling her legs back so her knees are flexed.
   b. Teach the woman to put her chin to her chest so that her body forms a "C" shape while pushing.
6. Evaluate bladder fullness and encourage voiding or catheterize as needed.

Promoting a Safe Delivery

1. Prepare the birthing room or delivery room using aseptic technique, allowing ample time for setup before delivery.
2. Prepare the infant resuscitation area for delivery.
3. Prepare necessary items for neonate care.
4. Notify necessary personnel to prepare for delivery.
5. Transfer the primigravida to the delivery room when the fetal head is crowning. The multigravida is taken earlier, depending on fetal size and speed of fetal descent.
6. Place all side rails up before moving. Instruct the woman to keep her hands off the rails, and move from the bed to the delivery table between contractions.
7. Position the woman for delivery, using a large cushion for her head, back, and shoulders. Elevate the head of the bed. Stirrups or footrests may be used for leg or foot support. Pad the stirrups. Place both legs in the stirrups at the same time to avoid ligament strain, backache, or injury.
8. Clean the vulva and perineal areas once the woman is positioned for delivery.
   a. Clean from the mons to the lower abdomen.
   b. Then clean the groin to the inner thigh of each side.
   c. Then clean each labium.
   d. Finally, clean the introitus.
9. Guide the woman step by step during the delivery process.
   a. When the fetal head is encircled by the vulvovaginal ring, an episiotomy may be performed to prevent tearing.
   b. When the head is delivered, mucus is wiped from the face, and the mouth and nose are aspirated with a bulb syringe.
   c. If loops of umbilical cord are found around the infant's neck, they are loosened and slipped from around the neck. If the cord cannot be slipped over the head, it is clamped with two clamps and cut between the two clamps.
   d. After this step, the woman is asked to give a gentle push so the infant's body may be quickly delivered.

MATERNITY BOX 1 Emergency Delivery

- Provide reassurance and instruct the woman in a calm, controlled manner while assisting her to a lithotomy position.
- Wash hands and cleanse woman's perineum.
- Exert gentle pressure against the head of the fetus to control its progress and prevent too rapid a delivery.
  - Use a clean or sterile towel.
  - This prevents undue stretching of the perineum and sudden expulsion through the vulva with subsequent infant and maternal complications.
- Encourage the woman to pant at this time to prevent bearing down.
- If membranes have not ruptured by the time the head has been delivered, tear them at the nape of the infant's neck.
- Wipe the infant's face and mouth with a clean towel. Suction the mouth and nose with a bulb syringe if available.
- Check to see if the cord is wrapped around the infant's neck or other body part. If the cord is too tight to permit slipping it over the infant's head, it must be clamped in two places and cut between the clamps before the rest of the body is delivered.
- Hold the infant's head in both hands and gently exert downward pressure toward the floor, thus slipping the anterior shoulder under the symphysis pubis.
- Support the infant's body and head as it is born.
- Hold the infant with the head down to help drain mucus; wipe away excess mucus from the mouth and nose; gentle rubbing of the back may stimulate breathing.
- Place the infant on the mother's abdomen, where she can see him or her after the infant cries.
- Avoid touching the perineal area to prevent infection.
- Avoid pulling on the cord, which might break and cause hemorrhage.
- Watch for signs of placental separation.
- Do the following when the placenta is delivered:
  - Clamp the cord with a cord clamp when the cord stops pulsating. If a clamp is not available, tie off the cord with any suitable material several centimeters from the infant's abdomen.
  - Wrap the infant and placenta in a blanket; keep the infant warm and close to the mother.
- Check fundal contractions; massage if indicated. Putting the baby to the breast may help the uterus to contract.

Emergency Delivery (continued)

- Place identification of some kind on the mother and infant.
- Give the woman fluids.
- Assist the woman to a suitable environment if she is not in a bed or a place where she can lie down.
- Do not leave the woman alone.
- Teach the woman to massage her fundus; explain why the cord has not been cut.
- Record the time and date of birth.

    e. After delivery of the infant's body and cutting of the cord, the infant is shown to the parents and then placed on the maternal abdomen, or taken to the radiant warmer for inspection and identification procedures.
10. Practice standard precautions during entire labor and delivery process.
11. Remain calm during emergency delivery, if indicated (see *Maternity Box 1*).

Nursing Interventions During Third Stage of Labor
Assisting with Placental Delivery

1. Ask the woman to bear down gently, or fundal pressure may be applied to facilitate delivery of the placenta on signs of separation. These include:
   a. The uterus rises upward in the abdomen.
   b. The umbilical cord lengthens.
   c. Trickle or spurt of blood appears.
   d. The uterus becomes globular in shape.
2. Evaluate the placenta for size, shape, and cord site implantation.
3. Check to see that the placenta and membranes are complete.
4. Evaluate and massage the uterine fundus until firm.
5. Administer Pitocin as indicated to assist with maintaining uterine tone immediately after delivery of the placenta.
6. Evaluate vaginal bleeding. If bleeding continuously and uterus is boggy, prepare methylergonivine I.M. or carbo-

prost I.M. for injection. Administer as directed. Increase I.V. fluids. Monitor vital signs, especially blood pressure and pulse.

⚡ EMERGENCY ALERT Methylergonivine is contraindicated in women with hypertension. Carboprost is contraindicated in women with asthma.

7. If bleeding continues and uterus is firm, notify the health care provider for evaluation of lacerations or retained placental fragments.
8. If still no relief, prepare patient for possible surgery (dilatation and curettage or, rarely, hysterectomy).

Immediate Care of the Neonate
Promoting Airway Clearance and Transition
1. Wipe mucus from the face, mouth, and nose. Aspirate with a bulb syringe. If meconium is present before the delivery, mechanical suctioning of the nasopharynx with an 8 or 10 French catheter will be done by the birth attendant when the head is delivered. See *Maternity Box 2*, for neonate resuscitation.

MATERNITY BOX 2 | Neonate Resuscitation

- Call for assistance if needed.
- Place the infant in a warm radiant warmer in Trendelenburg's position.
- Suction the nose and mouth with a bulb syringe or wall suction.
- Dry off the trunk with warmed towels and attempt to keep the infant warm.
- Assess respiratory and cardiac status.
- Begin bag and mask ventilation.
  - Use an inspiratory pressure of 20 to 30 cm H_2O cm at a rate of 40 to 60 breaths/minute.
  - Observe chest movement and auscultate for air movement in all lung fields.
- Begin external cardiac massage at a rate of 100 to 120 compressions/minute if needed.
- Assist with endotracheal intubation if needed.
- Assist with insertion of an umbilical venous line for administration of medications and fluids if needed.

2. Assist with clamping the umbilical cord approximately 1 inch (2.5 cm) from the abdominal wall with a cord clamp (usually done by birth attendant). Count the number of vessels in the cord; fewer than three vessels have been associated with renal and cardiac anomalies.

3. Evaluate the neonate's condition by the Apgar scoring system (see *Maternity Table 2*) at 1 and 5 minutes after birth.
   a. Neonates scoring 7 to 10 are free of immediate stress.
   b. Neonates scoring 4 to 6 are moderately depressed.
   c. Neonates scoring 0 to 3 are severely depressed.
   d. Apgar scores below 7 at 5 minutes are to be repeated every 5 minutes until 20 minutes have passed, the infant is intubated, or two successive scores of over 7 occur.

Promoting Thermoregulation

1. Dry the neonate immediately after delivery. A wet, small neonate loses up to 200 cal/kg/minute in the delivery room through evaporation, convection, and radiation. Drying the infant cuts this heat loss in half.

MATERNITY TABLE 2	Apgar Scoring Chart		
SIGN	**0**	**1**	**2**
Heart rate	Absent	Slow (less than 100)	Over 100
Respiratory effort	Absent	Slow, irregular	Good, crying
Muscle tone	Flaccid	Some flexion of extremities	Active motion
Reflex irritability	No response	Cry	Vigorous cry
Color	Blue, pale	Body pink, extremities blue	Completely pink

2. Cover the neonate's head with a cotton stocking cap to prevent heat loss.
3. Wrap the neonate in warm blankets.
4. Place the neonate under a radiant heat warmer, or place the neonate on the mother's abdomen with skin-to-skin contact.
5. Provide a warm, draft-free environment for the neonate.
6. Take the neonate's axillary temperature. A normal temperature is between 97.5° and 99° F (36.4° and 37.2° C).

Preventing Infection and Ensuring Safety

1. Administer prophylactic treatment against ophthalmia neonatorum (gonorrheal or chlamydial) by applying erythromycin or tetracycline antibiotic ophthalmic ointment or drops.
   a. If the mother has a positive gonococcal or chlamydial culture, the neonate will require further treatment.
   b. Treatment is mandatory in all states.
2. Administer injection of vitamin K to prevent neonatal hemorrhage during the first few days of life before the neonate begins to produce its own vitamin K.
3. Place matching identification bracelets on the mother's and the neonate's wrists or ankles.
   a. The father or significant other may also wear a bracelet matching the mother's.
   b. Information includes the mother's name, hospital number, neonate's sex, race, and date and time of birth.
4. Obtain fingerprints of the mother and footprints of the neonate per facility policy. If footprints are to be done, remove all vernix from the foot before inking to improve the quality of the footprint.
5. Complete all identification procedures before the infant leaves the delivery room.
6. Weigh and measure the infant:
   a. Normal neonate weight is 6 to 9 lb (2,700 to 4,000 g).
   b. Normal neonate length is 19 to 21 inches (48 to 53 cm).
7. Administer hepatitis B vaccine for all infants born in the United States, recommended within 12 hours after birth

for the prevention of acute and chronic hepatitis B infection.
  a. If mother is hepatitis B positive, infant will also receive hepatitis B immunoglobulin (HBIG).
  b. Additional doses of HBIG will be given at age 1 month and 6 months.

Nursing Interventions During Fourth Stage of Labor
Preventing Hemorrhage

1. Monitor blood pressure, pulse, and respirations every 15 minutes for 1 hour, then every ½ hour to 1 hour until stable or transferred to the postpartum unit.
2. Take temperature every 4 hours unless elevated, then every 2 hours.
3. Evaluate uterine fundal tone, height, and position. The uterus should be firm around the level of the umbilicus, at the midline.
4. Evaluate amount of vaginal bleeding:
  a. Scant: only blood on tissue when wiped, or less than 1-inch (2.5-cm) stain on peripad within 1 hour
  b. Small or light: approximately 4-inch (10-cm) stain on peripad within 1 hour
  c. Moderate: approximately 6-inch (15-cm) stain on peripad within 1 hour
  d. Heavy: saturated peripad within 1 hour
5. Observe perineum for edema, discoloration, bleeding, or hematoma formation.
6. Check episiotomy for intactness and bleeding.

Maintaining Fluid Volume and Providing Supportive Care

1. Maintain I.V. fluids as indicated.
2. Provide oral fluids and a snack or meal as tolerated.
3. Apply a covered ice pack to the perineum for an episiotomy, perineal laceration, or edema.
4. Administer analgesics as indicated.
5. Assist the woman with a partial bath and perineal care, and change linens and pads as necessary.

6. Allow for privacy and rest periods between postpartum checks.

7. Provide warm blankets, and reassure the woman that tremors are common during this period.

8. Encourage voiding, and evaluate the bladder for distention. Provide privacy, the sound of running water, and the flow of water against the perineum, if necessary, to facilitate voiding.

9. Catheterize the woman (in and out) if the bladder is full and she is unable to void.
   a. Birth trauma, anesthesia, and pain from lacerations and episiotomy may reduce or alter the voiding reflex.
   b. Bladder distention may displace the uterus upward and to the side, resulting in improper contraction and risk of hemorrhage.

10. Evaluate mobility and sensation of the lower extremities if regional anesthesia was given.
    a. Remain with the woman and assist her out of bed for the first time. Evaluate her ability to support her weight and ambulate at this time.
    b. Be careful with hot water if sensation is decreased.

Promoting Parenting

1. Show the neonate to the mother and father or support person immediately after birth when possible.

2. Encourage the mother or father to hold the baby as soon as possible.

3. Teach the mother/parents to hold the neonate close to their faces, approximately 8 to 12 inches (20 to 30 cm) when talking to the baby.

4. Have the mother and parents look at and inspect the baby's body to familiarize themselves with their child.

5. Assist the mother with breast-feeding during the first 2 hours after birth. This is often a period of quiet alert time for the neonate, and he or she will often readily take to the breast.

6. Provide quiet alone time in a low-lit room for the family to become acquainted.

7. Observe and record the reaction of the mother or parents to the neonate.

POSTPARTUM AND NEONATAL CARE
Postpartum Assessment
The *puerperium* is the period beginning after delivery and ending when the woman's body has returned as closely as possible to its prepregnant state; lasts approximately 6 weeks.

Uterine Changes
1. Check firmness and height of fundus at regular intervals. The fundus is usually midline and approximately at the level of the woman's umbilicus after delivery. Within 12 hours of delivery, the fundus may be 0.4 inch (1 cm) above the umbilicus. After this, the level of the fundus descends approximately 1 fingerbreadth (or 0.4 inch [1 cm]) each day until, by the 10th day, it has descended into the pelvic cavity and can no longer be palpated.

> **EMERGENCY ALERT** The first hour after delivery of the placenta is a critical period; postpartum hemorrhage is most likely to occur at this time.

2. Inspect the perineum regularly for bleeding and discharge. A vaginal discharge known as lochia, consisting of fatty epithelial cells, shreds of membrane, decidua, and blood, is red (*lochia rubra*) for approximately 2 to 3 days after delivery. It then progresses to a paler or more brownish color (*lochia serosa*), followed by a whitish or yellowish color (*lochia alba*) in the 7th to 10th day. Lochia usually ceases by 3 weeks, and the placental site is completely healed by the 6th week.
3. Perform a pad count to determine how many maternity pads the woman is saturating in a 1-hour, 4-hour, or 8-hour period.

Breast Changes
1. Assess for breast engorgement and condition of the nipples if breast-feeding.
   a. *Colostrum*, a yellowish fluid containing more minerals and protein but less sugar and fat than mature breast

milk and having a laxative effect on the infant, is secreted for the first 2 days postpartum.

b. Mature milk secretion is usually present by the third postpartum day but may be present earlier if a woman breast-feeds immediately after delivery.

c. Breast engorgement with milk; venous and lymphatic stasis; and swollen, tense, and tender breast tissue may occur between the third and fifth postpartum days.

Emotional and Behavioral Changes

1. Assess for expected mood changes and realistic goal setting. After delivery, the woman may progress through Rubin's stages of "taking in" and "taking hold."

   a. "Taking in" may begin with a refreshing sleep after delivery. The woman exhibits passive, dependent behavior and is concerned with sleep and the intake of food, both for herself and for the infant.

   b. With "taking hold," the woman begins to initiate action and to function more independently.

2. Report any signs of postpartum depression. Some mothers may experience "postpartum blues" about the third postpartum day and exhibit irritability, poor appetite, insomnia, tearfulness, or crying. This is a temporary situation. Severe or prolonged depression is usually a sign of a more serious condition.

3. If a patient is Rh negative, evaluate the need for $Rh_o(D)$ immune globulin (RhoGAM). If indicated, administer the RhoGAM within 72 hours of delivery.

4. If the woman is not rubella immune, a rubella vaccination may be given, and pregnancy must be avoided for at least 3 months.

Changes in Blood Volume

1. Assess vital signs at least every 4 hours for first 24 hours, then every 8 to 12 hours, as indicated. Watch for changes in vital signs that may indicate unstable hemodynamics.

   a. Expect postpartum diuresis between the second and fifth days, as extracellular fluid accumulated during pregnancy is excreted.

b. Decreased respiratory rate less than 14 breaths/minute may occur after receiving epidural opioids or opioid analgesics.

c. Increased respiratory rate more than 24 breaths/minute may be attributable to increased blood loss, pulmonary edema, or a pulmonary embolus.

d. Increased pulse rate more than 100 beats/minute may be present with increased blood loss, fever, or pain.

e. Decrease in blood pressure 15 to 20 mm Hg below baseline pressures may indicate decreased fluid volume or increased blood loss.

2. Evaluate for orthostatic blood pressure changes, and have the woman lie in bed if symptoms exist.

3. Evaluate lower extremity sensory and motor function before ambulation if the woman had regional anesthesia.

4. Monitor hemoglobin and hematocrit as indicated.

Changes in Bowel and Bladder Function

EMERGENCY ALERT Hematuria immediately after normal spontaneous vaginal birth is usually indicative of bladder trauma; no treatment is necessary if it does not recur. However, hematuria occurring after the first 24 hours may indicate a urinary tract infection, requiring prompt treatment.

1. Palpate the abdomen for bladder distention if the woman is unable to void within 6 to 8 hours after delivery or complains of fullness after voiding.

a. Uterine displacement from the midline suggests bladder distention.

b. Frequent voidings of small amounts of urine suggest urinary retention with overflow.

2. Catheterize the woman (in and out) if indicated.

3. Instruct the woman to void every several hours and after meals to keep her bladder empty. An undistended bladder may help decrease uterine cramping.

4. Expect that bowel activity may be sluggish because of decreased abdominal muscle tone, anesthetic effects, effects of progesterone, decreased solid food intake during labor, and prelabor diarrhea. In addition, pain from hemorrhoids,

lacerations, and episiotomies may cause her to delay her first bowel movement.

5. Assess for constipation and encourage daily adequate amounts of fresh fruit, vegetables, fiber, and at least eight glasses of water.

Other Assessments

1. Inspect the legs for signs of thromboembolism — erythema, swelling, and unequal calf circumference; note pain and palpate for calf tenderness.
2. Assess incisions for signs of infection and healing.

Nursing Diagnoses

1, 3, 24, 43, 67, 74, 135, 136

Nursing Interventions During the Postpartum Period
Reducing Fatigue

1. Provide a quiet and minimally disturbing environment.
2. Organize nursing care to keep interruptions to a minimum.
3. Encourage the woman to minimize visitors and phone calls.
4. Encourage the woman to sleep while the baby is sleeping.

Minimizing Pain

1. Instruct the woman to apply ice packs intermittently to the perineal area for the first 24 hours for perineal trauma or edema.
2. Initiate the use of sitz baths tid for 15 to 20 minutes for perineal discomfort after the first 24 hours.
3. Instruct the woman to contract her buttocks before sitting and to use pillows to reduce perineal discomfort.
4. Teach the woman to use a peri-bottle and squirt warm water against her perineum while voiding.
5. Provide pads and witch hazel or topical anesthetic creams or ointments for perineum as indicated.
6. Administer pain medication as indicated.
7. If breasts are engorged and the woman is breast-feeding:

    a. Allow warm to hot shower water to flow over the breasts to improve comfort.

    b. Hot compresses on the breasts may improve comfort.

    c. Express some milk manually or by breast pump to improve comfort and make nipple more available for infant feeding.

    d. Nurse the infant.

8. If breasts are engorged and the mother is bottle-feeding:

    a. Wear a supportive bra night and day.

    b. Avoid handling the breasts because this stimulates more milk production.

    c. Suggest ice bags to the breasts to provide comfort.

Promoting Breast-Feeding

1. Have the mother wash her hands before feeding to help prevent infection.

2. Encourage the mother to assume a comfortable position, such as sitting upright, tailor sitting, or lying on her side.

3. Have the woman hold the baby so he or she is facing the mother. Common positions for holding the baby are the "cradle hold," with the baby's head and body supported against the mother's arm with buttocks resting in her hand; the "football hold" supports the baby's legs under the mother's arm while his or her head is at the breast resting in her hand; lying on the side with the baby lying on his or her side facing the mother.

4. Have the woman cup the breast in her hand in a "C" position with bottom of the breast in the palm of her hand and the thumb on top.

5. Have the woman place her nipple against the baby's mouth, and, when the mouth opens, guide the nipple and the areola into the mouth.

6. If the baby has "latched on" only to the nipple, have the mother take him or her off the breast by putting the tip of her finger in the corner of the baby's mouth to break the suction and then reposition on the breast to prevent nipple pain and trauma.

7. Encourage the woman to alternate the breast she begins feeding with at each feeding to ensure emptying of both breasts and stimulation for maintaining milk supply.
8. Advise the mother to use each breast at each feeding. Begin with about 5 minutes at each breast, then increase the time at each breast, allowing the infant to suck until he or she stops sucking actively.
9. Have the mother breast-feed frequently and on a demand schedule (every 2 to 4 hours) to help maintain the milk supply.
10. Have the mother air dry her nipples for approximately 15 to 20 minutes after feeding to help prevent nipple trauma.
11. Have the mother burp the infant at the end or midway through the feeding to help release air in the stomach.
12. Alert the mother that uterine cramping may occur, especially in multiparous women because of the release of oxytocin.
13. Teach the mother to provide for adequate rest and to avoid tension, fatigue, and a stressful environment, which can inhibit the letdown reflex and make breast milk less available at feeding.
14. Advise the woman to avoid taking medications and drugs because many substances pass into the breast milk and may affect milk production or the infant.

Promoting Postpartum Health Maintenance

1. Teach the woman to carry out perineal care: warm water over the perineum after each voiding, bowel movement, and routinely several times per day to promote comfort, cleanliness, and healing.
2. Teach the woman to apply perineal pads by touching the outside only, thus keeping clean the portion that will touch her perineum.
3. Advise the woman that healing occurs within 4 weeks; however, evaluation by the health care provider 4 to 6 weeks postpartum is necessary.

4. Inform the woman that intercourse may be resumed when perineal and uterine wounds have healed. Review methods of contraception.

5. Inform the woman that menstruation usually returns within approximately 3 months if bottle-feeding; if breast-feeding, menstruation usually returns within 4 to 8 months, but may return between 2 and 18 months postpartum. Nursing mothers may ovulate even if experiencing amenorrhea, so a form of contraception should be used if pregnancy is to be avoided.

6. Counsel the woman to rest for at least 30 minutes after she arrives home from the hospital and to rest several times during the day for the first few weeks.

7. Advise the woman to confine her activities to one floor if possible and avoid stair climbing as much as possible for the first several days at home.

8. Counsel the woman to provide quiet times for herself at home and help her establish realistic goals for resuming her own interests and activities.

9. Encourage the couple to provide times to reestablish their own relationship and to renew their social interests and relationships.

Teaching Postpartum Exercises

1. Instruct the woman in exercises for the immediate postpartum period (can be performed in bed).
   a. Toe stretch (tightens calf muscles): while lying on back, keep legs straight and point toes away from body, then pull legs toward body and point toes toward chest. Repeat 10 times.
   b. Pelvic floor exercise (tightens perineal muscles): contract buttocks for a count of 5 and relax. Contract buttocks, press thighs together for a count of 7, and relax. Contract buttocks, press thighs together, and draw in anus for a count of 10 and relax.

2. Teach exercises for the later postpartum period (after the first postpartum visit).
   a. Bicycle (tightens thighs, stomach, waist): lie on back on the floor, arms at sides, palms down. Begin rotating

legs as if riding a bicycle, bringing the knees all the way in toward the chest and stretching the legs out as long and straight as possible. Breathe deeply and evenly. Do the exercises at a moderate speed and do not tire yourself.

b. Buttocks exercise (tightens buttocks): lie on abdomen and keep legs straight. Raise left leg in the air, then repeat with right leg to feel the contraction in buttocks. Keep hips on the floor. Repeat 10 times.

c. Twist (tightens waist): stand with legs wide apart. Hold arms at sides, shoulder level, palms down. Twist body from side to front and back again to feel the twist in waist.

Assessment of the Neonate

The first 24 hours of life constitute a highly vulnerable time during which the infant must make major physiologic adjustments to extrauterine life.

General Physical Assessment

1. Assess posture: asymmetric posture may be caused by fractures of clavicle or humerus or by nerve injuries, commonly of the brachial plexus. Infants born in breech position may keep knees and legs straightened or in frog position, depending on the type of breech birth.
2. Assess length: ranges from 18 to 22 inches (46 to 56 cm).
3. Weigh neonate: average weight of male is $7\frac{1}{2}$ lb (3,400 g); female, 7 lb (3,200 g); 80% of full-term neonates will range from 6 lb 5 oz to 9 lb 2 oz (2,900 to 4,100 g).
4. Assess skin for hair distribution, turgor, and color.
   a. Term infant will have some lanugo over back; most of the lanugo will have disappeared on extremities and other areas of the body.
   b. *Acrocyanosis*, bluish color in hands and feet, is common because of immature peripheral circulation.
   c. Pallor: may indicate cold, stress, anemia, or cardiac failure.
   d. Plethora: reddish coloration may be caused by excessive red blood cells from intrauterine intravascular trans-

fusion (twins), cardiac disease, or diabetes in the mother.

e. Jaundice: physiologic jaundice caused by immaturity of liver is common beginning on day 2, peaking at 1 week, and disappearing by the second week.

f. Meconium staining: staining of skin, fingernails, and umbilical cord indicates compromise in utero unless infant was in breech position.

g. Harlequin color change: when lying on side, dependent half of body turns red, upper half pale; caused by gravity and vasomotor instability.

h. Dryness or peeling: marked scaliness and desquamation are signs of postmaturity.

i. Vernix: in full-term infants, most vernix is found in skin folds under the arms and in the groin.

5. Assess for skin lesions.

a. Ecchymoses: may appear over the presenting part in a difficult delivery; may also indicate infection or bleeding problem.

b. Petechiae: pinpoint hemorrhages on skin caused by increased intravascular pressure, infection, or thrombocytopenia; regresses within 24 to 48 hours.

c. Erythema toxicum ("newborn rash"): pink to red papular rash appearing on trunk and diaper areas; regresses within 24 to 48 hours.

d. Hemangiomas: vascular lesions present at birth; some may fade, but others may be permanent.

e. Telangiectatic nevi (stork bites): flat red or purple lesions most often found on back of neck, lower occiput, upper eyelid, and bridge of nose; regress by age 2.

f. Milia: enlarged sebaceous glands found on nose, chin, cheeks, and forehead; regress in several days to 1 or 2 weeks.

g. Mongolian spots: blue pigmentation on lower back, sacrum, and buttocks; common in African Americans, Asians, and infants of southern European heritage; regress by age 4.

h. Cafe-au-lait spots: brown macules, usually not significant; large numbers may indicate underlying neurofibromatosis.

i. Abrasions or lacerations can result from internal monitoring and instruments used at birth.

6. Examine head and face for symmetry, paralysis, shape, swelling, movement.

a. *Caput succedaneum*: swelling of soft tissues of the scalp because of pressure; swelling crosses suture lines. Associated with vacuum-assisted birth.

b. *Cephalohematoma:* subperiosteal hemorrhage with collection of blood between periosteum and bone that may result from vacuum-assisted birth; swelling does not cross suture lines.

c. *Molding:* overlapping of skull bones caused by compression during labor and delivery (disappears in a few days).

7. Measure head circumference: 13 to 14 inches (33 to 35 cm), approximately 1 inch (2.5 cm) larger than chest. Measure just above the eyebrows and over the occiput.

8. Palpate fontanelles: enlarged or bulging may indicate increased intracranial pressure; sunken often indicates dehydration; posterior fontanelle closes in 2 to 3 months; anterior closes in 12 to 18 months.

9. Palpate sutures (junctions of adjoining skull bones): may be overriding because of molding during labor and delivery; extensive separation may be found in malnourished infants and with increased intracranial pressure.

10. Examine eyes, ears, nose, and mouth for deformity, asymmetry, or any unusual discharge.

11. Examine neck for mobility, any abnormal positioning, and tone.

12. Assess chest circumference and symmetry: average circumference is 12 to 13 inches (30 to 33 cm), approximately 1 inch (2.5 cm) smaller than head circumference.

13. Observe breasts for engorgement: may occur at day 3 because of withdrawal of maternal hormones, especially estrogen; no treatment required; regresses in 2 weeks.

14. Assess respiratory rate, rhythm, and effort (diaphragmatic because of weak thoracic muscles), and auscultate breath sounds (mostly bronchial). Respiratory rate may be as high as 80 breaths/minute shortly after birth, then decrease to 35 to 50 breaths/minute. Apnea up to 15 seconds is not unusual in the neonatal period.

15. Assess heart rate and rhythm, and auscultate heart sounds for gallop (third and fourth sounds rarely heard) and murmurs (common, and most are transitory). Normal heart rate is 120 to 150 beats/minute, or greater when crying, lower while sleeping.

16. Palpate for presence of brachial, radial, pedal, and femoral pulses; lack of femoral pulses indicative of inadequate aortic blood flow.

17. Check blood pressure with the assistance of a Doppler for any signs of distress. Neonates weighing more than 6.6 lb (3 kg) have systolic blood pressure between 60 and 80 mm Hg; diastolic, between 35 and 55 mm Hg.

18. Assess for edema: some may be present over buttocks, back, and occiput if infant is supine; pitting edema may be due to erythroblastosis, heart failure, or electrolyte imbalance.

19. Examine abdomen for umbilical hernia or distention caused by bowel obstruction, organ enlargement, or infection. Bowel sounds are usually present 1 hour after delivery.

20. Examine umbilical cord: single artery associated with renal and other congenital abnormalities; redness and discharge indicate infection. By 24 hours becomes yellowish brown; dries and falls off in approximately 7 to 10 days.

21. Inspect genitalia for any abnormalities.
    a. White or pink vaginal discharge may be present because of the drop in maternal hormones; no treatment necessary.
    b. Edema may be present in scrotal sac if the infant was born in breech presentation; a frank collection of fluid in the scrotal sac is a *hydrocele*, which regresses in approximately 1 month.

22. Examine spinal column for normal curvature, closure, and presence of membranous sac, pilonidal dimple, or sinus.
23. Examine anal area for anal opening, response of anal sphincter, fissures.
24. Examine extremities for fractures, paralysis, range of motion, and irregular position; count fingers and toes.
25. Examine hips for dislocation: with the infant in supine position, flex knees and abduct hips to side and down to table surface; clicking sound indicates dislocation.

Neonatal Reflexes

Reflexes are important indices of infant neural development. Absence of neonatal reflexes or persistence of some reflexes beyond several months indicates neurologic immaturity or damage. Assess for:

1. Rooting: when corner of mouth is touched, turns mouth toward object and opens mouth.
2. Palmar grasp: pressure on palm elicits grasp (pressure on sole also elicits plantar flexion).
3. Tonic neck: when head is turned to one side with leg and arm on that side extended, the extremities on other side flex.
4. Neck righting: when head turned to one side, the shoulder, trunk, and then pelvis turn to that side.
5. Moro: sudden, loud noise causes body to stiffen and arms to go up, out, and then inward with thumbs and index fingers in "C" shape.
6. Babinski: scratching sole of foot causes great toe to flex and toes to fan.
7. Blink: eyes close and neck flexes when sudden light is shone (eyes also close when sudden, loud noise occurs).
8. Withdrawal: pricking sole of foot causes flexion at hip, knee, and ankle.
9. Parachute: if held prone and quickly lowered toward a surface, arms and legs will extend.

Neonatal Behavioral Assessment

1. Assess responses according to states of consciousness, which include quiet, deep sleep; light, active sleep; drowsy awake; quiet alert; active alert; and crying.
2. Assess sleeping patterns, which normally change with maturation of the central nervous system. Neonates usually sleep 20 hours per day.
3. Assess feeding pattern: Most neonates eat six to eight times per day, with 2 to 4 hours between feedings, and establish fairly regular feeding patterns in approximately 2 weeks.
4. Assess stools.
   a. Meconium (tarry, green-black stool) is usually passed in 24 hours and continues for 48 hours.
   b. Transitional stools (combination of meconium and yellow stools) are passed next.
   c. Milk stools (yellow) are passed by day 5.
   d. Neonate has up to six stools per day in the first weeks after birth.
5. Assess voiding: voids within first 24 hours; after first few days, voids 10 to 15 times per day.

Metabolic Screening Tests

Obtain blood sample as directed for the following tests:

1. *Phenylketonuria:* inability of the infant to metabolize phenylalanine; scheduled after 48 hours of protein feeding
2. *Galactosemia:* inborn error of carbohydrate metabolism, when galactose and lactose cannot be converted to glucose
3. *Hypothyroidism:* thyroid hormone deficiency
4. *Maple sugar urine disease:* inability to metabolize leucine, isoleucine, and valine
5. *Homocystinuria:* inborn error of sulfur amino acid metabolism
6. *Sickle cell anemia:* abnormally shaped red blood cells with lower oxygen solubility

Nursing Diagnoses

24, 48, 67, 135, 136

Neonatal Nursing Interventions
Bathing the Neonate
1. Make sure bath water is 98° to 100° F (37° to 38° C), and use neutral soap or plain water (if skin is dry).
2. Use cotton balls or soft disposable washcloths to wipe eyes (from inside corner outward), face, and outer ears.
3. Wash head using circular motions; tilt head back to expose skin folds to cleanse neck.
4. Bathe torso and extremities quickly to prevent unnecessary exposure and chilling.
5. Clean genital area of male. Retract foreskin gently to clean underneath, and replace quickly to prevent edema.
6. Clean genital area of female. Gently separate folds of the labia and remove secretions. Wipe vaginal area with cotton ball, using one stroke from front to back.
7. Bathe buttocks using a gentle, patting motion. Keep anal area clean and dry to prevent diaper rash. If rash does occur, apply protective ointment, such as zinc oxide or A&D, or expose buttocks to air or heat lamp.
8. Teach family the bathing procedure.

Providing Umbilical Care
1. Inspect the umbilical cord stump for bleeding or foul odor, which may indicate infection.
2. Apply a drying agent such as 70% alcohol or merthiolate to cord stump where it exits abdominal wall, using gauze or cotton swabs, three to four times per day.
3. Leave open to air; do not cover with diaper or use a dressing.
4. Teach care to family, and tell them to expect stump to dry up and fall off within 7 to 10 days.

Providing Circumcision Care
1. Place sterile petroleum gauze over area for 24 hours; change after voiding.
2. Observe hourly for bleeding for first 24 hours. If bleeds, apply gentle pressure or apply epinephrine solution as directed.

3. Position infant and diaper to prevent friction, which may cause bleeding and discomfort.
4. Teach circumcision care to family.

Feeding the Neonate

1. Give first feeding of sterile water to prevent injury to lungs if aspirated.
2. Initiate breast-feeding (see page 1015) or instruct family in bottle-feeding technique:
   a. Hold baby in semi-upright position.
   b. Position bottle so the neck of bottle is filled.
   c. Insert nipple into baby's mouth so baby's tongue is under nipple.
   d. Burp the baby during feeding while holding upright to expel air but not feeding.
3. Test blood for glucose, using Glucometer to identify hypoglycemia and need for frequent feedings.
4. Suggest feeding on demand schedule until more regular feeding schedule is established.

Ensuring Infant Safety

1. Instruct the family to contact the infant's health care provider for the following:
   a. Fever greater than 100° F (37.8° C)
   b. Loss of appetite for two consecutive feedings
   c. Inability to awaken baby to his or her usual activity state
   d. Vomiting all or part of two feedings
   e. Diarrhea: three watery stools
   f. Extreme irritability or inconsolable crying
2. Inform the family that, by law, infants and young children in cars are required to be in a car safety seat. Demonstrate and review the proper technique for use of the car seat.
3. Provide written instructions and educational material on infant care.
4. Provide reinforcement and reassurance to the family and ensure that they know whom to call with concerns.

COMPLICATIONS OF THE CHILDBEARING EXPERIENCE

ABORTION, SPONTANEOUS

Spontaneous abortion is the unintended termination of pregnancy at any time before the fetus has attained viability (20 weeks' gestation or fetal weight of 1.1 lb [500 g]). Spontaneous abortion may be classified as threatened, inevitable, habitual, incomplete, or missed. Cause is frequently unknown, but 50% are attributable to chromosomal anomalies. May also be related to exposure to or contact with teratogenic agents; poor maternal nutritional status; maternal viral or bacterial illness; chronic illness, such as diabetes and systemic lupus erythematosus; smoking or drug abuse; immunologic factors; postmature or imperfect sperm or ova; and structural defect in the maternal reproductive system. Complications include hemorrhage, uterine infection, septicemia, and disseminated intravascular coagulation (with missed abortion).

Assessment
1. Uterine cramping, lower back pain.
2. Vaginal bleeding usually begins as dark spotting, then progresses to frank bleeding as the embryo separates from the uterus.
3. Serum beta human chorionic gonadotropin levels may be elevated for as long as 2 weeks after loss of the embryo.

Diagnostic Evaluation
1. Ultrasonic evaluation of the gestational sac or embryo.
2. Visualization of the cervix shows dilation or tissue passing through cervical os.

Collaborative Management
Therapeutic Interventions
1. For threatened abortion, bed rest or limited activity may be advised and bleeding monitored.

Pharmacologic Interventions
1. For missed abortion (fetal death without passage of fetal tissue), oxytocin infusion to induce delivery.
2. RhoGAM injection may be necessary for maternal and paternal Rh incompatibility.

Surgical Interventions
1. For inevitable or incomplete abortion, dilatation and curettage with evacuation is performed.
2. For history of habitual abortions (spontaneous abortions with three or more consecutive pregnancies), workup to determine cause and possible suturing of cervix if incompetent cervix is a factor.

Nursing Diagnoses
5, 30, 123, 135

Nursing Interventions
Monitoring
1. Monitor amount and color of vaginal bleeding.
2. Monitor maternal vital signs for indications of complications, such as hemorrhage and infection.
3. Evaluate blood or clot tissue for the presence of fetal membranes, placenta, or fetus.

Supportive Care
1. Report tachycardia, hypotension, diaphoresis, or pallor, which indicates hemorrhage and shock.
2. Draw blood for type and screen for possible blood administration.
3. Establish and maintain an I.V. line with large-bore catheter for possible transfusion and large quantities of fluid replacement, if signs of shock are present.

4. Encourage the woman to discuss feelings about the loss of the baby; include effects on relationship with the father.
5. Do not minimize the loss by focusing on future child-bearing; rather acknowledge the loss and allow grieving.
6. Provide time alone for the couple to discuss their feelings.
7. Discuss the prognosis of future pregnancies with the couple.
8. If the fetus is aborted intact, provide an opportunity for viewing, if parents desire.

Education and Health Maintenance
1. Instruct the woman on perineal care to prevent infection.
2. Discuss with the couple the methods of contraception to be used.
3. Explain the need to wait at least 3 to 6 months before attempting another pregnancy.
4. Teach the woman to observe for signs of infection (fever, pelvic pain, change in character and amount of vaginal discharge), and advise her to report them to health care provider immediately.
5. Provide information about genetic testing of the products of conception if indicated; send the specimen according to facility policy.

ABRUPTIO PLACENTAE

An *abruptio placenta* is premature separation of the normally implanted placenta in the third trimester. There are two types of abruptio placentae: concealed hemorrhage and external hemorrhage. With a concealed hemorrhage, the placenta separates centrally, and a large amount of blood is accumulated under the placenta. When an external hemorrhage is present, the separation is along the placental margin, and blood flows under the membranes and through the cervix. Women at risk for developing abruptio placentae include those with history of hypertension or previous abruptio placenta, abdominal trauma during pregnancy, anomaly of the umbilical cord, uterine fibroids, advanced maternal age, cigarette smoking, and cocaine abuse. Complications include maternal shock, disseminated intravascular coagulation, anaphylactic syndrome of pregnancy, postpartum hemorrhage, prematurity, maternal or fetal death, adult respiratory distress syndrome, Sheehan's syndrome (postpartum pituitary necrosis), renal tubular necrosis, and rapid labor and delivery.

Assessment

1. Concealed hemorrhage: results in a change in maternal vital signs, but no visible bleeding is present.
2. External hemorrhage: vaginal bleeding is evident along with a change in maternal vital signs.
3. Fetal heart rate may change, depending on the degree of hemorrhage: tachycardia, late decelerations, and decreased variability.
4. Abdominal pain is usually present; nausea and vomiting.
5. Rapid progression of labor.

Diagnostic Evaluation

1. Diagnosis is usually made based on clinical signs and symptoms.
2. Ultrasound is done to exclude placenta previa, but it is not always sensitive enough to pick up abruptio placentae.
3. Laboratory screen for erythrocyte rosette test on mother's blood to check for fetal cells in maternal circulation.

Collaborative Management
Therapeutic Interventions

1. Hospitalization, bed rest, and continuous fetal monitoring.
2. Management of hemorrhagic shock with I.V. fluids and blood transfusions.
3. If the woman's status is stable, and there is no fetal distress, then a vaginal delivery may be considered.
4. Pediatric specialty team may be necessary at delivery because of prematurity and neonatal complications.

Surgical Interventions

1. Severe abruptions with fetal distress necessitate immediate delivery by cesarean birth.

Nursing Diagnoses

44, 88, 123

Nursing Interventions

Monitoring

1. Monitor amount of bleeding by weighing all pads and assess the presence or absence of pain.
2. Monitor maternal vital signs and fetal heart rate through continuous external fetal monitoring.
3. Monitor uterine contractions.
4. Measure and record fundal height, which may increase with concealed bleeding.
5. Monitor hemoglobin and hematocrit for blood loss.

Supportive Care

1. Position mother in the left lateral position, with the head elevated to enhance placental perfusion.
2. Administer oxygen through a face mask at 8 to 10 L/minute.
3. Establish and maintain large-bore I.V. line for fluids and blood products as directed.
4. Encourage relaxation techniques.
5. Inform the woman and her family about the status of both herself and the fetus.
6. Encourage the presence of a support person.

Education and Health Maintenance

1. Provide information to the woman and her family regarding cause of and treatment for abruptio placentae.
2. Encourage involvement from the neonatal team regarding education related to fetal or neonatal outcome.

ANAPHYLACTIC SYNDROME OF PREGNANCY

Anaphylactic syndrome of pregnancy, previously known as *amniotic fluid embolism*, is the escape of amniotic fluid containing debris, such as meconium, lanugo, and vernix caseosa into the maternal circulation, usually resulting in deposition of fluid or debris in the pulmonary arterioles, resulting rapidly in respiratory distress, shock, and the possible development of disseminated intravascular coagulation (DIC). The exact cause is unknown but predisposing conditions include abruptio placentae; uterine rupture; intrauterine fetal demise; advanced maternal age (older than age 35); polyhydramnios; short, tumultuous labor; oxytocin induction; and high parity. Anaphylactic syndrome of pregnancy is rare (1 in 8,000 births), unpreventable, and often fatal.

Assessment
1. Sudden dyspnea and chest pain
2. Cyanosis, tachycardia
3. Coughing with frothy, pink sputum
4. Seizures
5. Vomiting, shaking, chills; diaphoresis
6. Increasing restlessness and anxiety
7. Profound shock due to anaphylaxis, which causes vascular collapse and uterine bleeding with development of hypofibrinogenemia

Diagnostic Evaluation
1. Clinical picture of rapidly developing dyspnea, tachypnea, and cyanosis
2. DIC confirmed by coagulation studies (prolonged thrombin time, prothrombin time, and partial prothrombin time, decreased factor V, VIII, X; decreased platelets; increased fibrin split products)

Collaborative Management
Therapeutic and Pharmacologic Interventions
1. Transfer to tertiary care center for endotracheal intubation
2. Administration of I.V. crystalloid fluids, blood products, and heparin to combat DIC
3. Immediate delivery of the fetus

Nursing Diagnoses
6, 19, 23

Nursing Interventions
Also see *Disseminated Intravascular Coagulation*, page 301.

Monitoring and Supportive Care
1. Monitor maternal vital signs to assess for signs of shock.
2. Monitor for frank bleeding.
3. Monitor fetal heart rate for signs of distress (if situation happens before birth of infant).

> **EMERGENCY ALERT** Be alert for respiratory distress and alert medical staff immediately, and assist with emergency procedures such as delivery and with the cardiopulmonary resuscitation as needed.

4. Administer oxygen (8 to 12 L/minute) by way of snug face mask to assist respiratory status.
5. Provide information and comfort to the family or support persons. If unable to do this personally due to the emergent needs of the woman, delegate another member of the staff to stay with the family or support persons.

CESAREAN DELIVERY

Cesarean delivery is the surgical removal of the infant from the uterus through an incision made in the abdominal wall and the uterus. Size and location of incisions vary, but abdominal and uterine incisions of choice are low and horizontal. Vertical incisions may be necessary for quicker procedures, the presence of adhesions, and other complications. Indications for cesarean delivery include cephalopelvic disproportion; uterine dysfunction, inertia, and inability of cervix to dilate; neoplasm obstructing birth canal or pelvis; malposition and mal-

presentation; previous uterine surgery (cesarean delivery, myomectomy, hysterotomy) or cervical surgery — evaluated on
an individual basis; complete or partial placenta previa; premature separation of the placenta; prolapse of the umbilical
cord; fetal distress; active herpes outbreak; breech presentation; and need for cesarean hysterectomy. Indications for cesarean hysterectomy are ruptured uterus; intrauterine infection; hemorrhage due to uterine atony that does not respond
to oxytocin, prostaglandin, or massage; laceration of major
uterine vessel; severe dysplasia or carcinoma in situ of the
cervix; placenta accreta; and gross multiple fibromyomas.

Potential Complications

1. Increase in morbidity and mortality as compared with
   vaginal birth
2. Hemorrhage, endometritis
3. Paralytic ileus, intestinal obstruction
4. Pulmonary embolism, thrombophlebitis
5. Bowel or bladder injury
6. Respiratory depression of the infant from anesthetic drugs
7. Possible delay in maternal-infant bonding
8. Anesthesia complications

Nursing Diagnoses

3, 6, 132, 135

Collaborative Management and Interventions

Preoperative Care

1. Maintain NPO status (except possibly ice chips) and monitor maternal and fetal vital signs during labor.
2. Obtain blood sample for type and screen and possible
   crossmatch if needed; also obtain sample for baseline complete blood count.
3. Determine drug allergies and answer questions about anesthesia; option for regional or general, depends on the indication for surgery.
4. Establish a large-bore I.V. line and insert a Foley catheter.
5. Administer an antacid, as directed, to reduce gastric acidity and the risk of aspiration pneumonia.

6. Administer antibiotics prophylactically, as directed.
7. Assist with abdominal skin preparation and ensure that a grounding pad for electrocautery is applied to patient.
8. Encourage presence of support person throughout the delivery.
9. Explain that a sensation of pressure will be felt during the delivery, but that little pain will occur. Instruct that any pain should be reported.

Postoperative Care

1. Assess maternal vital signs and fundal firmness and position every 15 minutes the first hour, every 30 minutes the second hour, and hourly until she is transferred to the postpartum unit or per facility policy.
2. Assess type and amount of lochia and condition of the incision line or dressing.
3. Monitor urinary output and presence of bowel sounds.
4. Assess level and presence of anesthesia or pain, and medicate as indicated.
   a. Encourage use of relaxation techniques after medication has been given for pain.
   b. Monitor for respiratory depression up to 24 hours after epidural opioid administration.

⚡ **EMERGENCY ALERT** Do not administer parenteral opioids if receiving epidural opioids unless ordered by anesthetist.

5. Encourage support and splinting of the abdominal incision when moving or coughing and deep breathing.
6. Encourage frequent rest periods, and plan for them after activities.
7. Encourage ambulation to reduce pain caused by gas, and decrease chance of thrombophlebitis.
8. Provide aseptic dressing changes and encourage perineal care every 4 hours or as needed.
9. Encourage and assess infant bonding as soon as possible.

Education and Health Maintenance

1. Teach the woman the "football hold" for breast-feeding so the infant is not lying on mother's abdomen.

2. Teach the woman to observe for signs of infection (foul-smelling lochia, elevated temperature, increased pain, redness and edema at the incision site), and to report them immediately.
3. Assist family in planning for the assistance of friends, family, or hired help at home during the period immediately after discharge.

ECTOPIC PREGNANCY

Ectopic pregnancy is gestation located outside the uterine cavity. The fertilized ovum implants outside of the uterus, usually in the fallopian tube. Predisposing factors include adhesions of the tube, salpingitis, congenital and developmental anomalies of the fallopian tube, previous ectopic pregnancy, use of an intrauterine device for more than 2 years, multiple induced abortions, menstrual reflux, and decreased tubal motility.

Assessment

1. Abdominal or pelvic pain.
2. Amenorrhea in 75% of cases.
3. Vaginal bleeding, usually scanty and dark.
4. Uterine size is usually similar to what it would be in a normally implanted pregnancy.
5. Abdominal tenderness on palpation.
6. Nausea, vomiting, or faintness may be present.
7. Pelvic examination shows a pelvic mass, posterior or lateral to the uterus, and cervical pain on movement of the cervix.

EMERGENCY ALERT Pain may become severe if a tubal rupture occurs, and clinical presentation will be that of shock.

Diagnostic Evaluation

1. Serum progesterone level greater than 25 ng/mL indicates corpus luteum secretion of progesterone in a viable pregnancy; therefore rules out an ectopic pregnancy. Serum beta human chorionic gonadotropin (β-hCG), when done serially, will not show characteristic increase as in intrauterine pregnancy.

2. Transvaginal ultrasound may identify tubal mass, absence of gestational sac within the uterus.
3. Culdocentesis: bloody aspirate from the cul-de-sac of Douglas indicates intraperitoneal bleeding from tubal rupture.
4. Laparoscopy allows for visualization of tubal pregnancy.
5. Laparotomy may be done if there is any question about the diagnosis.

Collaborative Management
Therapeutic Interventions
1. Treatment of shock and hemorrhage, if necessary, with I.V. fluids and blood transfusions

Pharmacologic Interventions
1. In a hemodynamically stable woman, methotrexate therapy may be used, either single dose or every other day with leucovorin given on alternate days until adequate fall in b-hCG. Treatment with a single dose of methotrexate I.M. is increasingly being used as therapy.
   a. Goal is to preserve reproductive function.
   b. May be done as an outpatient procedure.

Surgical Interventions
1. Goal is preservation of maternal life, through removal of the pregnancy and reconstruction of the tube, if possible.
2. The surgical procedure depends on the extent of tubal involvement and if rupture has occurred. Procedures include removal of ectopic pregnancy with tubal resection, salpingostomy, salpingectomy, and possibly salpingo-oophorectomy.

Nursing Diagnoses
3, 5, 123

Nursing Interventions
Monitoring
1. Monitor maternal vital signs for hypotension and tachycardia caused by rupture or hemorrhage.

2. Monitor for presence and amount of vaginal bleeding, indicating hemorrhage.
3. Monitor for increase in pain and abdominal distention and rigidity, indicating rupture and possible intra-abdominal hemorrhage.
4. Monitor complete blood count (CBC) for amount of blood loss.

Supportive Care

1. Establish an I.V. line with a large-bore catheter and infuse fluids and blood products as prescribed.
2. Obtain blood samples for CBC and type, and screen for whole blood, as directed.
3. Administer analgesics as needed and directed.
4. Remain attentive and supportive to patient preoperatively, which may be a life-threatening period.
5. Provide emotional support after surgery, and help family explore and express their grief and sense of loss over the pregnancy.
6. Refer for counseling to local bereavement group, social worker, clergy, or psychologist.

Education and Health Maintenance

1. Teach patient the signs of postoperative infection, which include fever, abdominal pain, and increased or malodorous vaginal discharge.
2. Reinforce that chances of another ectopic pregnancy are increased and that subsequent conception potential may be decreased, based on health care provider's explanation.
3. Discuss contraception.
4. Teach patient the signs of recurrent ectopic pregnancy, which include abnormal vaginal bleeding, abdominal pain, and menstrual irregularity.

HYDRAMNIOS

Hydramnios (polyhydramnios) is caused by an excessive amount of amniotic fluid. Normal volume is 500 to 1,000 mL at term; in hydramnios, the amniotic fluid volume exceeds 2,000 mL between 32 and 36 weeks. Anomalies causing impaired fetal swallowing or excessive urination may contribute to the condition. It is associated with maternal diabetes, multiple gestation, and Rh isoimmunization. Other associated factors are anomalies of the central nervous system, including spina bifida and anencephaly, or anomalies of the GI tract, including tracheoesophageal fistula. In chronic hydramnios, the fluid volume gradually increases; in the acute type, the volume increases rapidly over a few days. Complications of hydramnios include preterm labor, dysfunctional labor with increased risk for cesarean delivery, and postpartum hemorrhage caused by uterine atony from gross distention of the uterus.

Assessment
1. Excessive weight gain, dyspnea.
2. Abdomen may be tense and shiny.
3. Edema of the vulva, legs, and lower extremities.
4. Increased uterine size for gestational age, usually accompanied by difficulty in palpating fetal parts and in auscultation of fetal heart.
5. Nonreassuring fetal heart rate tracing.

Diagnostic Evaluation
1. A diagnosis is made based on the presenting symptoms and ultrasound evaluation. The amniotic fluid index is greater than 10 inches (25 cm).
2. Ultrasound evaluation shows large pockets of fluid between the fetus and uterine wall or placenta.

Collaborative Management
Therapeutic Interventions
1. Depend on the severity of the condition and the cause; hospitalization is indicated for maternal distress.
2. If impairment of maternal respiratory status occurs, amniocentesis for removal of fluid may be performed.
   a. Amniocentesis is performed under ultrasound for location of the placenta and fetal parts.
   b. The fluid is then slowly removed.
   c. Rapid removal of the fluid can result in a premature separation of the placenta.

d. Usually 500 to 1,000 mL of fluid is removed.

Nursing Diagnoses
6, 62, 75, 88, 136

Nursing Interventions
Monitoring
1. Evaluate maternal respiratory status.
2. Inspect abdomen and evaluate uterine height and compare with previous findings.
3. Monitor fetal heart rate as indicated.

Supportive Care
1. Encourage positioning with head elevated to promote chest expansion, and on left side to promote placental perfusion. If unable to position on side, use a wedge to displace the uterus to the left.
2. Provide oxygen by face mask, if indicated.
3. Limit activities, and plan for frequent rest periods.
4. Maintain adequate intake and output through fluid intake.
5. Encourage passive or active assisted range of motion to the lower extremities.
6. Provide a diet adequate in protein, iron, and fluids.
7. Assist the woman with position changes and ambulation as needed.
8. Instruct the woman to wear loose-fitting clothing and low-heeled shoes with good support.
9. Prepare the woman for the type of delivery that is anticipated and for the expected finding at the time of delivery.

Education and Health Maintenance
1. Instruct the woman to notify her health care provider if experiencing respiratory distress.
2. Teach the woman signs of preterm labor and the need to report them to health care provider.

HYPEREMESIS GRAVIDARUM

Hyperemesis gravidarum is exaggerated nausea and vomiting during pregnancy persisting past the first trimester. Cause is unknown but may possibly result from high levels of human chorionic gonadotropin or estrogen. Psychological factors including neurosis or altered self-concept may be contributory. The persistent vomiting may result in fluid and electrolyte imbalances, dehydration, jaundice, and elevation of serum transaminase.

Assessment
1. Persistent vomiting; inability to tolerate anything by mouth
2. Dehydration: fever, dry skin, decreased urine output
3. Weight loss (up to 5% to 10% of body weight)

Diagnostic Evaluation
1. Tests may be done to rule out other conditions causing vomiting (cholecystitis, appendicitis).
2. Liver function studies: elevated aspartate aminotransferase and alanine aminotransferase up to four times normal in severe cases.
3. Blood urea nitrogen and creatinine may be slightly elevated.
4. Serum electrolytes may be hypokalemia, hyponatremia, or hypernatremia.
5. Urine for ketones is positive.

Collaborative Management
Therapeutic Interventions
1. Try withholding food and fluid for 24 hours, or until vomiting stops and appetite returns; then restart small feedings.
2. Control of dehydration through I.V. fluids — typically 1 to 3 L of dextrose solution.
3. Most women respond quickly to restricting oral intake and giving I.V. fluids, but repeated episodes may occur.
4. Rarely, total parenteral nutrition is needed.

Pharmacologic Interventions

1. Control of vomiting may require an antiemetic, such as prochlorperazine or promethazine in injectable or rectal suppository form; methyl prednisone, droperidol, and metoclopramide may also be used.
2. Potassium and vitamins may be added to I.V. fluids.
3. Bicarbonate may be given for acidosis.

Nursing Diagnoses
44, 51, 78, 123

Nursing Interventions
Monitoring

1. Evaluate weight gain or loss pattern.
2. Evaluate 24- or 48-hour dietary recall.
3. Monitor intake and output.
4. Monitor vital signs for tachycardia, hypotension, and fever caused by dehydration.
5. Assess skin turgor and mucous membranes for signs of dehydration.
6. Monitor serum electrolytes and report abnormalities.
7. Monitor fetal heart tones routinely.

Supportive Care

1. Maintain NPO status except for ice chips until vomiting has stopped.
2. Advise the woman that oral intake can be restarted when emesis has stopped and appetite returns.
3. Begin small feedings. Suggest or provide bland solid foods; serve hot foods hot and cold foods cold; do not serve lukewarm.
   a. Avoid greasy, gassy, and spicy foods.
   b. Provide liquids at times other than meal times.
4. Suggest or provide an environment conducive to eating.
   a. Keep room cool and quiet before and after meals.
   b. Keep emesis pan handy, yet out of sight.
5. Encourage patient to discuss any personal stress that may have a negative effect on this pregnancy.
6. Refer to social service and counseling services as needed.

Education and Health Maintenance

1. Educate the woman about proper diet and nutrition in pregnancy.
2. Educate the woman about healthy weight gain in pregnancy.
3. Ensure referral for prenatal care and social services as needed.

HYPERTENSIVE DISORDERS OF PREGNANCY

Hypertensive disorders of pregnancy are considered to be a disease of the placenta. The disorders are classified by onset and systemic effects (see *Maternity Box 3*). There are multiple theories about cause. Risk factors include chronic hypertension, hydatidiform mole, multiple gestation, polyhydramnios, and diabetes mellitus. These disorders are primarily seen in primigravidas and adolescents, and women older than age 35 are at higher risk. Complications include abruptio placentae, disseminated intravascular coagulation, prematurity, intrauterine growth retardation, and maternal or fetal death.

Assessment

1. Hypertension, which is defined as a blood pressure of 140/90 mm Hg or greater on two occasions at least 6 hours apart.
2. Proteinuria (300 to 500 mg/24 hours or 1+ to 2+ on urine dip test).
3. Oliguria ($\leq$ 400 to 500 mL/24 hours).
4. Nondependent edema, present after 8 to 12 hours of bed rest.
5. Frequently, a sudden weight gain will occur of 2 lb (1 kg) or more in 1 week, or 6 lb (2.7 kg) or more in 1 month. This often occurs before the edema is present.
6. Altered level of consciousness, visual changes, headache, blurred vision, scotoma.
7. Epigastric pain, right upper quadrant pain.
8. Hyperreflexia with or without clonus.
9. Seizures and possible coma in eclampsia.

Classification of Hypertensive Disorders of Pregnancy

Chronic Hypertension
Hypertension that is present and observable prior to pregnancy or that is diagnosed before the 20th week of gestation.

Preeclampsia
The diagnosis is determined by increased blood pressure (BP) accompanied by proteinuria. It is divided into mild and severe forms.
- Mild preeclampsia consists of systolic BP *greater than or equal to 140 mm Hg or diastolic BP greater than or equal to 90 mm Hg;* and urinary protein excretion of greater than or equal to 0.3 g in 24 hours.
- Severe preeclampsia consists of systolic BP of greater than or equal to 160 mm Hg or diastolic BP of greater than or equal to 110 mm Hg; and urinary protein excretion of greater than or equal to 2 g in 24 hours.
- Other features of severe preeclampsia are increased serum creatinine (greater than 1.2 mg/dL), persistent headache or cerebral or visual disturbances, persistent epigastric pain, platelet count less than 100,000/mm^3 and/or evidence of microangiopathic hemolytic anemia, and HELLP syndrome (See *Maternity Box 4,* page 1045.)

Eclampsia
Hypertension with convulsions (seizures) in a preeclamptic patient that cannot be contributed to an underlying neurologic condition. *Note:* Eclampsia was previously referred to as *toxemia* because it was thought to be caused by toxins. The term *eclampsia* is more commonly used.

Preeclampsia/Eclampsia Superimposed on Chronic Hypertension
Worsening of BP and new onset or worsening of proteinuria in women with previous hypertension.
- New-onset proteinuria, defined as the greater than or equal to 0.3 g protein in a 24-hour specimen, in women with hypertension but no proteinuria early in pregnancy (prior to 20 weeks' gestation)
- In women with hypertension and proteinuria prior to 20 weeks' gestation

(continued)

Classification of Hypertensive Disorders of Pregnancy *(continued)*

- Sudden increase in proteinuria — greater than or equal to 0.3 g protein in 24-hour specimen, or two dipstick tests of 2+ (100 g/dL), with values recorded at least 4 hours apart, with no evidence of urinary tract infection.
- Sudden increase in BP in a woman whose BP was previously well controlled.
- Thrombocytopenia (platelet count less than 100,000/mm^3)
- Increase in alanine aminotransferase and aspartate aminotransferase to abnormal levels.

Gestational Hypertension
BP elevation detected for first time in pregnancy, without proteinuria. If the woman does not develop preeclampsia and her BP has returned to normal by 12 weeks postpartum, the woman is given the diagnosis of *transient hypertension of pregnancy.*

Diagnostic Evaluation
1. 24-hour urine for protein greater than or equal to 300 mg.
2. Serum blood urea nitrogen and creatinine may be elevated.
3. Elevated liver enzymes and low platelet count in HELLP syndrome (see *Maternity Box 4*).
4. Sonogram or nonstress testing to evaluate placenta and fetus.

Collaborative Management
Therapeutic Interventions
1. Bed rest to help decrease blood pressure and maintain placental perfusion.
2. Increased dietary protein and possibly calories to ensure adequate nutrition.
3. Hospitalization for close monitoring and seizure prevention may be necessary.
4. If symptoms are uncontrollable, delivery is planned.

MATERNITY BOX 4 **HELLP Syndrome**

HELLP syndrome is a severe complication of gestational hypertension. It is comprised of Hemolysis, Elevated Liver enzymes, and Low Platelets.

- These findings are frequently associated with disseminated intravascular coagulation (DIC) and, in fact, may be diagnosed as DIC.
- The hemolysis of erythrocytes is seen in the abnormal morphology of the cells.
- The elevated liver enzyme measurement is associated with the decreased blood flow to the liver as a result of fibrin thrombi.
- The low platelet count is related to vasospasm and platelet adhesions.
- Treatment is similar to treatment for gestational hypertension with close monitoring of liver function and bleeding.
- These women are at increased risk for postpartum hemorrhage.

Pharmacologic Interventions

1. Magnesium sulfate ($MgSO_4$) may be given either I.V. or I.M. as loading dose, followed by maintenance dose to treat and prevent seizures.
2. Diazepam and amobarbital sodium may be used if convulsions occur that do not respond to $MgSO_4$.
3. Antihypertensive drug therapy may be used when the diastolic pressure is above 110 mm Hg or when stroke is impending.
   a. Hydralazine is the drug of choice; it relaxes the arterioles and stimulates cardiac output.
   b. Adverse effects include tachycardia, palpitations, dizziness, faintness, and headache.
4. Other drugs include:
   a. Labetalol may be used in place of hydralazine; contraindicated in women with asthma and second- or third-degree heart block.
   b. Methyldopa is relatively safe but has a delayed effect.

c. Nifedipine is a third-line agent; should not be given for hypertensive crisis—drops the blood pressure too quickly.

d. Sodium nitroprusside is used when all other agents have failed and the patient has life-threatening hypertension.

e. Nitroglycerin is indicated for hypertension refractory to conservative pharmacologic therapy.

Nursing Diagnoses
6, 19, 22, 42, 88, 136

Nursing Interventions
Monitoring

1. Monitor blood pressure in a sitting position and in the left lateral position to detect hypertension.
2. Monitor intake and output strictly and notify health care provider if output is less than 30 mL/hour.
3. Monitor vital signs every hour.
4. Auscultate breath sounds every 2 hours and report signs of pulmonary edema (wheezing, crackles, shortness of breath, increased pulse rate, increased respiratory rate).
5. Monitor protein level of spot urine specimens.
6. Evaluate edema, carefully noting the presence after 12 hours or more of bed rest.
7. Monitor daily weights for gain.
8. Evaluate deep tendon reflexes and clonus.
9. Monitor fetal activity and evaluate nonstress tests to determine fetal status.
10. Monitor for signs of $MgSO_4$ toxicity, including absent knee-jerk reflex, respiratory depression, and oliguria.

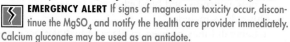 **EMERGENCY ALERT** If signs of magnesium toxicity occur, discontinue the $MgSO_4$ and notify the health care provider immediately. Calcium gluconate may be used as an antidote.

11. Monitor serum magnesium levels, as indicated by health care provider.

Supportive Care

1. Control I.V. fluid intake using a continuous-infusion pump.

2. Position the woman on left side to promote placental perfusion.
3. Encourage extra protein in diet to replace protein lost through kidneys.
4. Keep the environment quiet and as calm as possible.
5. If the woman is hospitalized, pad side rails and keep side rails up to prevent injury if seizure occurs.
6. If the woman is hospitalized, have oxygen and suction set up, along with a tongue blade and emergency medications immediately available for treatment of seizures.
7. Explain that pregnancy-induced hypertension does not lead to chronic hypertension and usually does not occur with subsequent pregnancies.

Education and Health Maintenance
1. Teach the woman the importance of bed rest in helping to control symptoms.
2. Encourage the support of family and friends while on bed rest.
3. Provide and suggest diversional activities while on bed rest.
4. Provide information on tests and procedures to evaluate maternal–fetal status, such as blood tests, sonogram, and nonstress testing.

INDUCTION OF LABOR

Induction of labor is the deliberate initiation of uterine contractions before their spontaneous onset. It is indicated when the woman's life or well-being is in danger or if the fetus may be compromised by remaining in the uterus any longer. *Augmentation of labor* refers to measures used to assist labor that has started spontaneously to be more effective. Contraindications include genital herpes outbreak, vaginal bleeding with known placenta previa, abnormal fetal presentation, previous uterine scar (controversial), known cephalopelvic disproportion, severe fetal distress, classic uterine incision, invasive cervical carcinoma, pelvic abnormalities, and fundal uterine scar. Complications include uterine hyperstimulation, fetal distress, and uterine rupture.

Collaborative Management
Therapeutic Interventions

1. Amniotomy (artificial rupture of membranes) — done to make contractions stronger
   a. Vulva is cleansed, amniohook is inserted through the cervix, and membranes are ruptured after evaluation of fetal presentation.
   b. Fetal heart tones are assessed continually for at least the next 20 minutes.
   c. Complications include umbilical cord prolapse or compression, maternal or fetal infection.
2. Stripping the membranes: separating the membranes from the lower uterine segment without rupturing the membranes
   a. Membranes and amniotic fluid then act as a wedge to dilate cervix.
   b. Maternal or fetal infection is a complication.

Pharmacologic Interventions

1. Oxytocin is given I.V. by infusion pump; 10 units of oxytocin are added to 1,000 mL I.V. solution such as 0.9% sodium chloride and piggybacked to primary I.V. infusion at the port of entry nearest the vein.
   a. Fetal monitoring is instituted. If membranes have ruptured, an intrauterine catheter and internal scalp electrode may be used.
   b. The dose is increased by institutional policy according to American College of Obstetrics and Gynecology guidelines.
   c. The goal is to establish a regular labor pattern — contractions occurring every 2 to 3 minutes, lasting 45 to 60 seconds, and having an intensity of 50 mm Hg (moderate) or Montevideo units greater than 180.
   d. Complications include uterine hyperstimulation, fetal distress, increased rate of cesarean delivery, maternal cardiac arrhythmias, severe water intoxication, and neonatal hyperbilirubinemia, possibly from red blood cell trauma from intense contractions or decreased maturity of the neonate.

2. Prostaglandin E_2 (PGE_2) — used before induction of labor for cervical ripening.
   a. If labor results from administration of PGE_2, it is similar to spontaneous labor.
   b. Prostaglandins are administered intracervically or vaginally as a solid, tablet, or gel form.
   c. Uterine hyperstimulation is a complication.

Nursing Diagnoses
3, 6, 88, 130

Nursing Interventions
Monitoring
Before Induction
1. Obtain a 20-minute strip for the fetal heart rate and uterine activity.
2. Evaluate maternal vital signs.
3. Evaluate the patency of the I.V. site.

After Administration of Oxytocin
1. Continuously monitor fetal heart rate and uterine activity, especially uterine resting tone.
2. Assess maternal vital signs in accordance with facility policy. Temperature is taken every 2 to 4 hours unless an amniotomy has been performed and then every 1 to 2 hours.
3. Monitor intake and output records, and watch for signs of water intoxication.

 EMERGENCY ALERT A major adverse reaction of oxytocin is water intoxication, which can lead to heart failure. Signs of water intoxication include headache, nausea and vomiting, mental confusion, decreased urine output, hypotension, tachycardia, and cardiac arrhythmia.

4. Evaluate I.V. site for patency and rate control for correct rate at least hourly.

Supportive Care and Education
1. Teach or review the use of relaxation and distraction techniques.

2. Before beginning any new procedure, explain the procedure to the woman and her support person.
3. Limit vaginal examinations, especially after membranes have ruptured.
4. Position mother on left side to enhance placental perfusion.
5. Have oxygen set up with a mask ready and administer as prescribed if fetal decelerations occur.
6. If hyperstimulation of the uterus or fetal distress occurs, discontinue the infusion, maintain the primary I.V., and notify the health care provider immediately.

PLACENTA PREVIA

Placenta previa is the development of the placenta in the lower uterine segment, partially or completely covering the internal cervical os (see *Maternity Box 5*). The cause is unknown, but a possible theory states that the embryo will implant in the lower uterine segment if the decidua in the uterine fundus is not favorable. Cause is unknown, but risk factors include abortion, cesarean delivery, and uterine scarring. Most occur in multiparas. Complications are immediate hemorrhage, shock, and maternal death; fetal mortality; and postpartum hemorrhage.

MATERNITY BOX 5	Classification of Placenta Previa

- Placenta previa — the placenta totally covers the cervical os.
- Partial placenta previa — the placenta partially covers the cervical os.
- Marginal placenta previa — the placenta lies within 0.75 to 1.2 inches (2 to 3 cm) of the internal os, but does not cover it.
- Low-lying placenta — the exact relationship of the placenta to the os has yet to be determined, or placenta previa is suspected prior to the third trimester.

Assessment

1. Characteristic sign is sudden onset of painless vaginal bleeding, which usually appears near the end of the second trimester or later.
2. Initial episode is rarely fatal and usually stops spontaneously, with subsequent bleeding episodes occurring spontaneously; each episode is more profuse than the previous one.
3. Bleeding from placenta previa may not occur until cervical dilation occurs and the placenta is loosened from the uterus.
4. With a complete placenta previa, the bleeding will occur earlier in the pregnancy and be more profuse.

EMERGENCY ALERT Never perform a vaginal examination on anyone who is bleeding until placenta previa has been ruled out. This may result in puncturing the placenta.

Diagnostic Evaluation

1. Transabdominal ultrasound is the method of choice, to show location of the placenta.
2. If findings are questionable, transvaginal ultrasound can improve the accuracy of diagnosis. Because of bleeding tendencies, however, this must be done by a highly skilled technician.

Collaborative Management
Therapeutic Interventions

1. Bed rest and hospitalization during any bleeding episode is usual.
2. If discharged, needs availability of immediate transport to the hospital for recurrent bleeding.
3. I.V. access and at least two units of blood available at all times.
4. Continuous maternal and fetal monitoring.
5. Amniocentesis may be done to determine fetal lung maturity for possible delivery.
6. Vaginal delivery may sometimes be attempted in a marginal or low-lying placenta previa without active bleeding.

7. A pediatric specialty team may be needed at delivery because of prematurity and other neonatal complications.

Surgical Interventions

1. Cesarean delivery is usually indicated and may be performed immediately on bleeding, depending on the degree of placenta previa.

Nursing Diagnoses
6, 88, 123, 135

Nursing Interventions
Monitoring

1. Monitor amount and type of bleeding.
2. Monitor and record maternal and fetal vital signs every 5 to 15 minutes while active bleeding is present.
3. Monitor for uterine contractions.
4. Monitor hemoglobin level and hematocrit for amount of blood loss.
5. Monitor temperature every 4 hours unless elevated; then evaluate every 2 hours.
6. Monitor white blood cell count for infection.

Supportive Care

1. Position mother on left side to promote placental perfusion and administer oxygen if there is evidence of fetal distress.
2. Establish and maintain a large-bore I.V. line, as directed, and draw blood for type and screen for blood replacement.
3. Position mother in a sitting position to allow the weight of fetus to compress the placenta and decrease blood loss during episode of bleeding.
4. Maintain strict bed rest during any bleeding episode.
5. If bleeding is profuse and delivery cannot be delayed, prepare the woman physically and emotionally for a cesarean delivery.

 EMERGENCY ALERT Women who have had a placenta previa are at risk for postpartum hemorrhage because of the decreased contractility of the lower uterine segment and the large space the placenta occupied.

6. Use aseptic technique when providing care, and teach perineal care and hand washing to prevent infection.
7. Provide emotional support and discuss the effects of long-term hospitalization or prolonged bed rest.

Education and Health Maintenance

1. Educate the woman and her family about the cause and treatment of placenta previa.
2. Advise the woman to inform medical personnel about her diagnosis and not to have vaginal examinations.
3. Educate the woman who is discharged from the hospital with a placenta previa about avoiding intercourse or anything per vagina; limiting physical activity; the need for an accessible person in the event of an emergency; and to go to the hospital immediately for repeat bleeding, or uterine contractions exceeding 6 per hour.

POSTPARTUM HEMORRHAGE

Postpartum hemorrhage involves a loss of 500 mL or more of blood; it occurs most frequently in the first hour after delivery. It may be caused by uterine atony (relaxation of the uterus) secondary to multiple pregnancy, hydramnios (excessive amniotic fluid), high parity, prolonged labor with maternal exhaustion, deep anesthesia, presence of fibromyoma, and retained placental fragments. Laceration of the vagina, cervix, or perineum secondary to forceps delivery, large infant, or multiple pregnancy may also cause postpartum hemorrhage.

Assessment

1. With uterine atony, uterus is soft or boggy, often difficult to palpate, and will not remain contracted; excessive vaginal bleeding occurs.
2. Hemorrhage usually occurs about the 10th postpartum day with retained placental fragments.
3. Lacerations of the vagina, cervix, or perineum cause bright red, continuous bleeding even when the fundus is firm.

Collaborative Management
Pharmacologic Interventions
1. For uterine atony, I.V. administration of oxytocin, I.M. administration of methylergonovine, or prostaglandins administered directly into the myometrium.
2. Pain medication may be needed to counter uterine contractions.

Surgical Interventions
1. If placental fragments have been retained, curettage of the uterus is indicated.
2. Lacerations may need to be repaired.

Nursing Diagnoses
23, 44, 135

Nursing Interventions
Monitoring
1. Monitor for hypotension, tachycardia, change in respiratory rate, decrease in urine output, and change in mental status; may indicate hypovolemic shock.
2. Monitor location and firmness of uterine fundus.
3. Percuss and palpate for bladder distention, which may interfere with contracting of the uterus.
4. Monitor amount and type of bleeding or lochia present and the presence of clots.
5. Inspect for intactness of any perineal repair.
6. Monitor complete blood count for anemia.

Supportive Care
1. Maintain a quiet and calm atmosphere.
2. Maintain or start a large-bore I.V. line if vaginal bleeding becomes heavy.
3. Ensure that crossmatched blood is available.
4. Infuse oxytocin, other contractile agents, I.V. fluids, and blood products at prescribed rate.
5. Provide information about the situation and explain everything as it is done; answer questions that the woman and her family ask.

6. Maintain aseptic technique and evaluate for infection. Report chilling, elevated temperature, changes in white blood cell count, uterine tenderness, and odor of lochia.
7. Administer antibiotics as directed.

Education and Health Maintenance
1. Educate the woman about the cause of the hemorrhage.
2. Teach the woman the importance of eating a balanced diet and taking vitamin supplements.
3. Advise the woman that she may feel tired and fatigued, and to schedule daily rest periods.
4. Advise the woman to notify her health care provider of increased bleeding or other changes in her status.

POSTPARTUM INFECTION

Postpartum (puerperal) infection is a postpartum infection of the genital tract, usually of the endometrium (endometritis), which may remain localized or may extend to various parts of the body, such as the connective tissue by way of lymphatic spread (parametritis). The main pathway for spread of the infection is the broad ligament. Risk factors include prolonged labor or preterm premature rupture of the membrane, vaginal examinations, infection elsewhere in the body, anemia, malnutrition, size and number of perineal lacerations, intrauterine manipulation, retained placental fragments, lapse in aseptic technique, poor perineal hygiene, Cesarean delivery, and instrumented delivery. Complications include thrombophlebitis, pulmonary embolus, and peritonitis.

Assessment
Diagnosis is made by sustained fever with oral temperature of 100.4° F (38° C) or higher occurring 6 hours apart on two occasions of the first 10 days postpartum, excluding the first 24 hours. Symptoms depend on site and extension of infection.

1. Postpartum endometritis — fever occurring around third day; uterus usually larger than expected for postdelivery day; uterus tender; lochia may be profuse, bloody, and foul smelling; chills; malaise; and fever occur if lochial discharge is obstructed by clots, white blood cell count greater

than 20,000/mm^3 with increased neutrophils, infection may spread to myometrium (endomyometritis), parametrium, uterine (fallopian) tubes, peritoneum, and blood.

2. Parametritis (Pelvic cellulites) — chills, fever (102° to 104° F [38.9° to 40° C]), tachycardia, severe unilateral or bilateral pain in lower abdomen, enlarged and tender uterus; uterine position may become fixed as it is displaced by the exudates along the broad ligament, often the result of an infected wound in the cervix, vagina, perineum, or lower uterine segment.

Collaborative Management
Therapeutic and Pharmacologic Interventions

1. Antibiotic therapy is instituted after cultures are obtained and causative agent is identified. Broad-spectrum antibiotics are the treatment of choice including penicillins, cephalosporins (cefoxitin, cefazolin), clindamycin (Cleocin), and aminoglycosides (gentamicin, tobramycin). Antibiotics are given until the woman is afebrile for 48 hours (maternal response is usually very quick, within 48 to 72 hours).

2. Encourage fluid intake of minimum of 6 to 8 glasses (1,500 to 2,000 mL) of water, milk, or juices (3,000 mL is preferred).

3. Encourage intake of 1,800 to 2,000 calories if lactating; 1,500 calories if not lactating. Diet should be a variety of foods, usually high in protein and vitamin C (promotes wound healing).

4. Supportive therapy is used to control pain and to maintain hydration and nutritional status.

5. Drainage is indicated for abscess development.

6. Administration of single-dose ampicillin or cephalosporins after umbilical cord clamping is considered effective prophylaxis for nonelective cesarean delivery.

DRUG ALERT Clindamycin/gentamicin treatment is successful in only 75% to 92% of cases and is associated with renal toxicity. It is not effective against enterococci — ampicillin is the drug of choice in this instance.

Nursing Diagnoses
3, 49, 123, 107

Nursing Interventions
Monitoring and Supportive Care

1. Perform postpartum assessment, noting uterine tenderness on palpation and the color, amount, and odor of lochia.
2. Monitor vital signs every 4 hours for signs of infection.
3. Assess knowledge and skill of perineal hygiene; teach proper technique and assist, if necessary.
4. Provide for adequate rest periods.
5. Increase fluid intake to meet recommendations.
6. Position the woman in high Fowler's position to promote drainage.
7. Administer antibiotics and analgesics, as directed.
8. Explain the benefit of perineal washing or sitz baths and demonstrate setup.
9. Explain the need for good hand-washing technique and how contamination of vagina from the rectum occurs.
10. Show how to place perineal pads and medications; encourage to change pads with each voiding, bowel movement, or every 4 hours while awake.
11. Encourage minimal separation from the infant and continuation of breast-feeding, as able.
12. Promote good hand-washing technique for the mother before contact with the infant.
13. Observe for signs of septic shock: tachycardia greater than 120 beats/minute, hypotension, tachypnea, changes in sensorium, and decreased urine output.
14. If pulmonary embolism in question, elevate the head of the bed and provide oxygen.

PRETERM LABOR

Preterm labor is defined as uterine contractions occurring after 20 weeks of gestation and before 37 completed weeks of gestation. Risk factors include multiple gestation; history of previous preterm labor or delivery; abdominal surgery during current pregnancy; uterine anomaly; history of cone biopsy;

multiple abortions; fetal or placental malformation; diethylstilbestrol (DES) exposure; bleeding after the first trimester;
maternal age younger than age 20 or older than age 35; poor
nutritional status; poor, irregular, or no prenatal care; emotional stress; smoking; and recreational drug use. Complications of preterm labor are prematurity and associated neonatal problems, such as lung immaturity.

Assessment

1. Abdominal cramps or contractions are less than 10 minutes apart.
2. Cervical changes result with cervical dilation of ¾ inch
   (2 cm) or effacement of 75%.

Collaborative Management

Therapeutic Interventions

1. Treatment is begun early with bed rest in a left lateral position.
2. Hydration with I.V. fluids and continuous monitoring of
   fetal status and uterine contractions.

Pharmacologic Interventions

1. If conservative therapy is not successful, tocolytic therapy is instituted. These drugs should be used only when
   the potential benefit to the fetus outweighs the potential
   risk.
2. Beta-mimetic agents, such as ritodrine and terbutaline.
   a. These drugs stimulate the beta$_2$-adrenergic receptors,
      which causes uterine relaxation.
   b. Ritodrine is administered I.V. or orally; terbutaline may
      be administered I.V., subcutaneously, or orally.
   c. Frequent monitoring is necessary to observe for adverse
      effects of increased pulse, shortness of breath, chest
      pain, decreased blood pressure, hypervolemia, decreased
      potassium concentration, hyperglycemia, and hyper-
      insulinemia.
   d. Baseline electrocardiogram and laboratory tests, in-
      cluding complete blood count with differential, elec-
      trolytes, glucose, blood urea nitrogen, creatinine, pro-

thrombin time, and partial thromboplastin time, are
obtained.

3. Magnesium sulfate: interferes with smooth muscle contractility.
   a. Administration is I.V. by infusion pump.
   b. Pulmonary edema, loss of deep tendon reflexes, decreased respirations, and hypotension are adverse reactions related to magnesium toxicity.
   c. Serum magnesium levels are monitored.
   d. Calcium gluconate is the antidote and should be at the
   bedside.
4. Indomethacin: prostaglandin inhibitor that inhibits contractions; given orally or rectally and usually well tolerated.
5. Nifedipine: calcium channel blocker that relaxes smooth
muscle; given orally, and adverse effects include headache,
nausea, and flushing from vasodilation.
6. Corticosteroid administration to accelerate fetal lung maturity for less than 32 weeks' gestation.
   a. Given before delivery to mother; try to postpone delivery for 48 hours.
   b. Usually I.M. administration of betamethasone with initial dose followed by second dose 24 hours later.
7. Artificial surfactant therapy.
   a. Decreases number of days of mechanical ventilation
   for infants with respiratory distress syndrome.
   b. Given after delivery to infant directly into lungs by way
   of endotracheal tube.

Nursing Diagnoses
6, 22, 78, 136

Nursing Interventions

DRUG ALERT Be alert for potential complications of tocolytic therapy. Beta-mimetic therapy may cause hyperglycemia, hypokalemia, hypotension, pulmonary edema, and myocardial ischemia.
$MgSO_4$ may cause respiratory depression, cardiac arrest, tetany, hypotension, and paralysis.

Monitoring

During tocolytic therapy, monitor the following:

1. Fetal status by electronic fetal monitoring
2. Uterine contraction pattern
3. Respiratory status for pulmonary edema
4. Muscular tremors
5. Symptoms of palpations and dizziness
6. Urinary output

Supportive Care

1. Provide accurate information on the status of the fetus and labor (contraction pattern).
2. Allow the woman and her support person to verbalize their feelings regarding the episode of preterm labor and the treatment.
3. If a private room is not used, do not place the woman in a room with an occupant who is in labor or who has lost an infant.
4. Encourage diversional activities while on bed rest and encourage visits from family.

Education and Health Maintenance

1. Educate the woman about the importance of continuing the pregnancy until term, or until there is evidence of fetal lung maturity.
2. Encourage the need for compliance with a decreased activity level or bed rest, as indicated.
3. Teach the woman the importance of proper nutrition and the need for adequate hydration, at least eight glasses of fluids per day.
4. Instruct the woman not to engage in sexual activity.
5. Advise the woman to report signs of infection.

PRETERM AND PRELABOR RUPTURE OF MEMBRANES

Preterm premature rupture of membranes (PPROM) is defined as rupture of the membranes before 37 completed weeks' gestation with or without the onset of spontaneous labor. *Premature rupture of membranes* (PROM) is also known as prelabor rupture of membranes and is defined as rupture of membranes before the onset of spontaneous labor. PROM at term may result from stretching of the membranes and fetal movements that cause the membranes to weaken. In PPROM, risk factors include infection, previous history of PPROM, hydramnios, incompetent cervix, multiple gestation, and abruptio placentae. Complications include preterm labor, prematurity and associated complications, maternal infection (chorioamnionitis), and fetal or neonatal infection.

Assessment

1. PROM is manifested by a large gush of amniotic fluid or leaking of fluid per vagina, which usually persists.

Diagnostic Evaluation

1. Sterile speculum examination for identification of "pooling" of fluid in the vagina.
2. Nitrazine test: positive test will change pH paper strip from yellow-green to blue in the presence of amniotic fluid taken from the vaginal canal.
3. Fern test: positive test will show ferning pattern of amniotic fluid on a slide viewed under a microscope.
4. Ultrasound assesses amniotic fluid volume.

Collaborative Management
Therapeutic Interventions

1. Once PROM is confirmed, the woman is admitted to the hospital and usually remains there until delivery.
2. The woman is evaluated to rule out labor, fetal distress, and infection, and to establish gestational age. If all factors are ruled out, the woman is managed expectantly.
3. Management of PROM at 36 weeks' gestation or greater focuses on delivery.
4. Vaginal examinations are kept to a minimum to prevent infection.

Pharmacologic Interventions

1. Tocolytics to prevent premature labor.

2. Corticosteroids to decrease the severity of respiratory distress syndrome in the premature infant are controversial.
3. Prophylactic antibiotics may be used.

Nursing Diagnoses
135

Nursing Interventions
Monitoring
1. Evaluate maternal blood pressure, respirations, and pulse every 2 to 4 hours, more frequently if elevated; monitor temperature every 1 to 2 hours.
2. Monitor the amount and type of amniotic fluid that is leaking, and observe for purulent, foul-smelling discharge.
3. Evaluate daily complete blood count (CBC) with differentials, noting any shift to the left (ie, increase of immature forms of neutrophils), indicating infection.
4. Evaluate fetal status every 4 hours or as indicated, noting fetal activity and heart rate; monitor for fetal tachycardia.
5. Determine if uterine tenderness occurs on abdominal palpation, indicating infection.
6. Minimize infection with decreased or no vaginal examinations, aseptic techniques, and appropriate perineal care.

Supportive Care
1. Place patient on disposable pads to collect leaking fluid and change pads every 2 hours or more frequently as needed.
2. Review the need for good hand-washing technique and hygiene after urination and defecation.
3. Report immediately any change in vital signs, uterine tenderness, CBC, or fluid leakage that may indicate infection.
4. Encourage diversional activities and involvement of support person.
5. Administer antibiotics as directed.

Education and Health Maintenance
1. Explain that the goal is to await the onset of natural labor while preventing infection.
2. Explain that, if signs of infection do develop, the baby will be delivered and infection will be treated.

PROLAPSED UMBILICAL CORD

A *prolapsed umbilical cord* slips in front or alongside the fetal presenting part. Types of cord prolapse include:

Complete — the cord can be felt on vaginal examination and be seen in the vaginal canal; membranes are ruptured. Changes in the fetal heart rate (FHR) are evident.

Occult — the cord cannot be felt on vaginal examination or be seen. The cord lies between the presenting part and the maternal pelvis; membranes can be intact or ruptured. Changes in the FHR are evident.

Forelying — the cord can be felt on vaginal examination but cannot be seen; usually contained within intact membranes. The cord lies in front of the presenting part. Predisposing factors include rupture of membranes before the presenting part is engaged in the pelvis, shoulder and foot presentations, prematurity, polyhydramnios, multifetal gestation, fetopelvic disproportion, abnormally long umbilical cord, and the result of interventions or maneuvers.

Assessment
1. Cord may be seen protruding from vagina or palpated in the vagina or cervix.
2. With compression, FHR pattern may show variable decelerations with contractions or between contractions; often fetal bradycardia is present.

 NURSING ALERT Prolapsed cord should be suspected with FHR deceleration after rupture of membranes.

Collaborative Management
Therapeutic Interventions
1. Delivery of the fetus as soon as possible.
2. Relief of pressure from the umbilical cord immediately.

3. Change maternal position — usually in knee-chest position to relieve pressure of presenting part.
4. Prepare for emergency delivery (vaginal or cesarean, whichever is deemed appropriate by situation).

Nursing Diagnoses
44, 88, 136

Nursing Interventions
Monitoring and Supportive Care

1. Observe for prolonged FHR deceleration.
2. Identify complete or forelying cord prolapse with a vaginal examination by a qualified nurse or health care provider. If the cord is exposed to cold room air, there may be a reflex constriction of the umbilical blood vessels that further restricts the oxygen flow to the fetus.
3. Do not pinch or squeeze the umbilical cord because it may cause the cord to spasm, which decreases umbilical blood flow and fetal oxygen leading to fetal hypoxia.
4. Explain procedures as much as possible to the woman during this emergent situation.
5. Administer oxygen by snug face mask at 8 to 12 L/minute.
6. Relieve pressure from the presenting part of the fetus off the umbilical cord by manually pushing the presenting part upward with a gloved hand. Pressure must be relieved until the fetus is delivered by way of cesarean or vaginally. Do not remove hand until delivery is imminent.
7. Provide constant reassurance to the woman and her support persons.
8. Encourage the woman to talk about her feelings regarding herself and the baby after delivery.

> **EMERGENCY ALERT** If prolapsed cord occurs at home with ROM, have the mother or partner look or feel in the vagina for the protruding cord. If the cord is visible or felt, push the fetal presenting part upward off the cord. Call 911. Have mother lie on floor or bed with hips and legs elevated above level of her head (Trendelenburg's position) until help arrives.

PROBLEMS OF INFANTS

PREMATURE INFANT

The *premature infant* is an infant born before the completion of 37 weeks' gestation.

A *low-birthweight* infant is one whose birthweight is less than 5 lb 8 oz (2,500 g) regardless of gestational age.

A *very-low-birthweight* infant is one whose birthweight is below 3 lb 5 oz (1,500 g) regardless of gestational age.

The premature infant has altered physiology due to immature and often poorly developed systems. The severity of any problem that occurs depends somewhat on the gestational age of the infant. Systems and situations that are most likely to cause problems in the premature infant include respiratory system, digestive system, thermoregulation, immune system, and neurologic system.

Assessment

1. Notice physical characteristics of the premature infant such as lanugo; poor ear cartilage; thin skin; lack of subcutaneous fat; smooth soles of feet; undescended testes; undeveloped labia majora; very fine rugae of scrotum; soft fingernails; relatively large abdomen; relatively small thorax; head appears disproportionately large; poor muscle tone; and poor, possibly weak reflexes.
2. Obtain accurate body measurements.
   a. Head circumference—frontal-occipital circumference one finger above eyebrows, using parallel lines of tape around head
   b. Abdominal girth—one finger above umbilicus, mark location
   c. Heel–crown
   d. Shoulder to umbilicus—used to calculate proper length of catheter for umbilical arterial catheter placement

    e. Weight in grams

3. Assess gestational age using a tool such as the Ballard scoring system (recommended by Committee of Fetus and Newborn of American Academy of Pediatrics).

4. Assist with laboratory testing as indicated for blood gases, blood glucose, complete blood count or hemoglobin and hematocrit, electrolytes, calcium, and bilirubin.

5. Monitor closely for respiratory or cardiac complications.

    a. Respirations above 60 per minute over a period of time may be indicative of respiratory difficulty.

    b. Expiratory grunting, retractions, chest lag, or nasal flaring should be reported immediately.

    c. Cyanosis (other than acrocyanosis — coldness and cyanosis of hands and feet) should be watched for along with other signs of respiratory distress.

    d. Increased (above 180 beats/minute) or irregular heart rate may indicate cardiac or circulatory difficulties.

    e. Muscle tone and activity should be evaluated.

    f. Hypotension, indicated by blood pressure measurement, may be due to hypovolemia.

    g. Hypoglycemia may result from inadequate glycogen stores, respiratory distress, and cold stress.

6. Institute cardiac monitoring and care for infant in isolette or radiant heater. Omit bath until infant's temperature has stabilized.

7. Observe for early signs of jaundice and check maternal history for any blood incompatibilities. Also, be aware of maternal factors that can lead to additional complications, such as drug use, diabetes, or infection.

8. Once the infant is admitted to the nursery, be aware that the first 24 to 48 hours after birth is a very critical time, often requiring constant observation and intensive care management. Make the following observations:

    a. Note bleeding from the umbilical cord — apply pressure, and notify the health care provider.

    b. Note first voiding — may occur up to 36 hours after birth; report any 4- to 6-hour period when voiding does not occur once the first voiding has occurred.

    c. Note stools—abdominal distention and lack of stool may indicate intestinal obstruction or other intestinal tract anomalies. Measure abdominal girth at regular intervals.

    d. Note activity and behavior—look for sucking movement, hand-to-mouth maneuver, which can help to determine oral feeding initiation.

    e. Observe for a tense and bulging fontanelle; feel suture lines noting separation or overriding—may indicate intracranial hemorrhage. Be alert to twitching and seizures.

    f. Note color of skin for cyanosis and jaundice, rashes, paleness, or ruddiness.

    g. Carefully monitor, record, and report vital signs.

Nursing Diagnoses
23, 75, 78, 134, 135, 136

Collaborative Management and Interventions

1. Have available resuscitative equipment, oxygen, and suction apparatus; a rubber ear bulb syringe is often all that is necessary.

2. Position infant to allow for easy ventilation, paying careful attention to maintaining body alignment and facilitating hand-to-mouth positioning.

    EMERGENCY ALERT Prone positioning offers some advantage for oxygenation in preterm infants with respiratory compromise. During the initial phase of illness, these infants are cared for with cardiorespiratory monitoring and may be placed prone according to facility policy. Before discharge, these infants should become accustomed to sleeping supine, and supine positioning should be reinforced with the infant's care providers.

3. Provide oxygen therapy with moisture in the percentage necessary to maintain appropriate blood gas values.

4. Monitor for apnea versus periodic breathing (regular repetition of breathing pauses of less than 15 seconds alternating with breaths of regularly increasing then decreasing amplitude for 10 to 15 seconds). Theophylline may be given to reduce apneic episodes.

5. Protect the infant from infection by following scrupulous hand-washing policy, minimizing infant's contact with unsterile equipment, and minimizing the number of people who come in contact with the infant.

6. Provide good skin care using water for bathing, an approved emollient for the skin, avoidance of adhesives, and providing adequate hydration.

7. Avoid cranial deformity by using gel head pillow, frequent turning, and upright position.

8. Protect the infant's eyes from bright lights.

9. Continue to provide I.V. and oral feedings according to infant's needs. Assist the mother with breast pumping as needed, and encourage both parents to hold and feed infant.

10. Continue to monitor for complications — hypoglycemia, hyperglycemia, respiratory distress syndrome (see page 795), apnea, infection, hypocalcemia, cardiac abnormalities, necrotizing enterocolitis, intracranial hemorrhage, and hyperbilirubinemia. Long-term complications may include retinopathy of prematurity, chronic lung disease, hearing loss, and learning disabilities.

11. Do not neglect the needs of the parents; instead, make every effort to include them in the infant's care and update them frequently on the infant's condition.

POSTMATURE INFANT

The *postmature infant* is one whose gestation is 42 weeks or longer and who may show signs of weight loss with placental insufficiency.

Assessment

1. Be alert for the physical appearance of a postmature infant. The following characteristics are most often seen in infant of 44 weeks' gestation or more: loose skin; long, curved fingernails and toenails; reduced amount of vernix caseosa; abundant scalp hair; wrinkled, macerated skin; possibly pale, cracked, parchmentlike skin; having the alert appearance of a 2- to 3-week-old infant after deliv-

ery; and greenish-yellow staining of skin, fingernails, or cord, indicating fetal distress.

2. Determine gestational age by physical examination. Measure weight, length, and head circumference, and plot on Colorado intrauterine growth chart. Compare percentiles.

3. Be alert for meconium aspiration; signs include thick meconium in amniotic fluid at time of delivery; tachypnea; increasing signs of cyanosis; difficulty breathing with need for ventilation; tachycardia; inspiratory nasal flaring and retraction of chest; expiratory grunting; increased anteroposterior diameter of the chest; palpable liver; crackles and rhonchi on chest auscultation; and concomitant cerebral irritation (jitteriness, hypotonia, seizures). Additional signs include metabolic acidosis, hypotension, hypoglycemia, and hypocalcemia.

Nursing Diagnoses
51, 75, 87, 119, 135

Collaborative Management and Interventions
1. Provide supportive treatment for meconium aspiration.
   a. Warmth — maintain thermally neutral environment so the infant uses fewer calories and less oxygen.
   b. Adequate oxygenation and humidification to maintain PaO_2 at 50 to 70 mm Hg.
   c. Respiratory support with ventilator; extracorporeal membrane oxygenation may be needed if persistent pulmonary hypertension of the neonate develops.
   d. Adequate administration of calories and fluid.
   e. Accurate monitoring of intake and output — assess possible alteration in kidney function due to hypoxia.
   f. Administration of antibiotics prophylactically.

   EMERGENCY ALERT Some cases of meconium aspiration can be prevented if meconium is removed from the mouth and trachea by proper suctioning before the infant takes first breath.

2. Provide oral feeding or I.V. glucose soon after birth to treat or prevent hypoglycemia. If oral feedings are not

contraindicated, they can begin 1 or 2 hours after birth. Monitor blood sugar every hour until condition stabilizes.

3. Be alert for persistent pulmonary hypertension of the neonate — physiologic disorder characterized by severe, labile cyanosis arising from persistent or return to suprasystemic pulmonary vascular resistance and pressure normally found in the fetus.
   a. Cyanosis, pronounced respiratory distress, presence of murmur or heart failure.
   b. Treatment is aggressive respiratory support in a tertiary care nursery.

4. Provide psychological support to the parents. Long-term sequelae common in the postmature infant are central nervous system problems.

INFANT OF A DIABETIC MOTHER

Infants born to mothers with overt or gestational diabetes are at risk for health problems. The severity of infant problems depends on the severity of the maternal diabetes. Hyperinsulinemia in utero secondary to elevated maternal glucose levels results in the following in the infant: macrosomia — increased amount of body fat, not edema; hypoglycemia; hypocalcemia; hyperbilirubinemia; prematurity; polycythemia; congenital anomalies, such as renal and central nervous system anomalies, caudal regression syndrome, facial clefts, patent ductus arteriosus, transposition of the great vessels, ventricular septal defect, and small colon syndrome; and infection.

Assessment

1. Be alert for typical appearance of an infant of a diabetic mother — macrosomia, cardiomegaly, hepatomegaly, large umbilical cord and placenta, plethora, full face, tendency to be large for gestational age (some may be normal weight or small for gestational age), abundant fat, abundant hair, extensive vernix caseosa, and hypertrichosis pinnae.

2. Assist with diagnostic tests — serum glucose, calcium, phosphorus, magnesium, electrolytes, bilirubin, arterial blood gas analysis, and blood hemoglobin and hematocrit.

Nursing Diagnoses
61, 131, 136

Collaborative Management and Interventions

1. Monitor for hypoglycemia.
   a. Monitor serum glucose levels every 30 to 60 minutes beginning immediately after birth for 24 hours every 4 to 8 hours until stabilized.
   b. May be asymptomatic or show signs of jitteriness, tremors, seizures, sweating, cyanosis, weak or high-pitched cry, refusal to eat, hypotonia, apnea, and temperature instability.
   c. Hypoglycemia may be prevented or treated by early feedings of 10% glucose or formula by nipple or gavage, if blood glucose is 20 to 40. If under 20, will require I.V. solution with appropriate glucose concentration.
2. Monitor infant closely for changes in acid-base status, respiratory distress, temperature instability, hypocalcemia, and sepsis.
3. Observe for hyperbilirubinemia. Levels will be elevated 48 to 72 hours after birth. The infant may need an exchange transfusion at relatively lower bilirubin levels (as in the premature infant) to prevent kernicterus. Phototherapy may need to be initiated early.
4. Monitor intake and output, ensure adequate fluid intake, and assess for dehydration.
5. Observe for possible cardiac anomalies and secondary heart failure.
6. Observe for other complications including respiratory distress syndrome, renal vein thrombosis, infection, hypermagnesemia or hypomagnesemia, birth injuries (cephalohematomas, facial nerve paralysis, fractured clavicles, brachial nerve plexus injuries), prematurity, asphyxia neonatorum, and organomegaly.
7. Support the family, especially the mother who may feel guilty about being responsible for the infant's problems.

JAUNDICE IN THE NEONATE (HYPERBILIRUBINEMIA)

Hyperbilirubinemia (jaundice) in the neonate is an accumulation of serum bilirubin above normal levels. Onset of clinical jaundice is seen when serum bilirubin levels are 5 to 7 mg/100 dL.

Kernicterus is a yellow discoloration of specific areas of brain tissue by unconjugated bilirubin; it can be confirmed only by death and autopsy. *Bilirubin encephalopathy* best describes the occurrence of the syndrome and the accompanying neurologic sequelae in neonates. *Physiologic jaundice* occurs 3 to 5 days after birth and is an increase in unconjugated bilirubin levels that do not exceed 5 mg/100 dL/day.

Assessment
1. Be alert for signs and symptoms of jaundice: sclerae appearing yellow before skin appears yellow; skin appearing light to bright yellow; lethargy; dark amber, concentrated urine; poor feeding; and dark stools.
2. Make observations in daylight, sunlight, or white fluorescent light.
   a. Blanch the skin during the observation to clear away capillary coloration. Forehead, cheeks, and clavicle sites allow for clear view.
   b. Be alert to the infant's age in connection with the appearance of jaundice.

Nursing Diagnoses
87, 136

Collaborative Management and Interventions
1. Assist with treatment.
   a. Fluids — to ensure adequate hydration
   b. Exchange transfusion — to mechanically remove bilirubin
   c. Phototherapy — to allow for utilization of alternate pathways for bilirubin excretion

d. Enzyme induction agent — to reduce bilirubin levels by inducing hepatic enzyme system involved in bilirubin clearance (ie, phenobarbital).

2. Provide nursing care related to phototherapy.

a. Photoisomerization of tissue bilirubin occurs when the baby is exposed to 420 to 460 nm of light.

b. Check light intensity for therapeutic range daily. Use commercial bili light.

c. Have the infant completely undressed so entire skin surface is exposed to light.

d. Keep the infant's eyes covered, unless using a biliblanket, to protect them from the constant exposure to high-intensity light, which may cause retinal injury.

e. Shield gonads.

f. Develop a systematic schedule of turning infant so all surfaces are exposed (ie, every 2 hours).

g. Maintain thermoneutrality — light affects the ambient temperature.

h. Shield the infant (by Plexiglas) from direct exposure of the lights.

i. Obtain bilirubin levels as directed. The diminishing icterus (ie, the lowering of unconjugated bilirubin from cutaneous tissue) does not reflect the serum bilirubin concentration. Lights should be turned off when blood is being collected to eliminate false-low bilirubin levels.

j. If possible, remove the infant from under the lights, remove eye covers, and encourage parents to hold the infant for feedings.

EMERGENCY ALERT If priapism occurs during phototherapy, turn the infant on his abdomen for short periods of time, and this will cease.

SEPTICEMIA NEONATORUM

Septicemia neonatorum (sepsis of the neonate) is a generalized infection that may occur in the neonate and is characterized by the proliferation of bacteria in the bloodstream and frequently involves the meninges (as distinguished from simple bacteremia, congenital infection, septicemia after major diseases or surgery, or major congenital anomalies). There is a high mortality rate.

The distribution of etiologic agents varies but may include gram-negative organisms such as *Escherichia coli*, *Klebsiella* (Enterobacteriaceae), *Pseudomonas*, *Proteus*, *Salmonella*, *Haemophilus influenzae*; gram-positive organisms including group B beta-hemolytic streptococcus, *Listeria monocytogenes*, *Staphylococcus aureus* (coagulase-negative and coagulase-positive), *Staphylococcus epidermidis*, *Streptococcus pneumoniae*, *Streptococcus faecalis*; and fungal infections.

Assessment

1. Be alert for early signs of sepsis, which are usually vague and subtle: poor feeding; gastric retention; weak sucking; lethargy, limpness; weak crying; temperature alteration—generally hypothermia, but infant may have hyperthermia; and hypo- or hyperglycemia.
2. Assist with diagnostic tests: cultures from the blood, urine, spinal fluid, skin lesions, nose, throat, rectum, gastric fluid; complete blood count and differential; blood chemistries—glucose, calcium, pH, electrolytes; C-reactive protein and erythrocyte sedimentation rate; bilirubin; TORCH screen (toxoplasmosis-rubella-cytomegalic inclusion virus-herpes-other) to detect antibodies against common intrauterine-infective agents; arterial blood gases; chest radiograph; and urinalysis.

Nursing Diagnoses
49, 123, 136

Collaborative Management and Interventions

1. Assist with treatment.
   a. Before the specific organism is identified, and after cultures have been obtained, the antibacterial therapy is based on the more common causative agents and their anticipated susceptibilities.
   b. Supportive therapy includes observation, isolation, hydration, nutrition, oxygen, regulation of thermal en-

vironment, blood transfusion to correct anemia and shock, and protection from further infection.

2. Observe for complications, such as meningitis (very common), shock, adrenal hemorrhage, disseminated intravascular coagulation, persistent pulmonary hypertension of the neonate, metabolic derangements, seizures, pneumonia, urinary tract infection, and heart failure.

INFANT OF SUBSTANCE-ABUSING MOTHER

Maternal abuse of substances, such as drugs, alcohol, and tobacco, may impact the growth, development, and well-being of her fetus or neonate.

Assessment

1. Obtain maternal history of drug, dosage, time of last dose. Be alert for onset of symptoms of opioid withdrawal.
   a. Heroin — several hours after birth to 3 to 4 days of life
   b. Methadone — 7 to 10 days after birth to several weeks of life
   c. Cardinal signs of neonatal opioid withdrawal include coarse, flapping tremors, irritability, hyperactivity, hypertonicity, persistent high-pitched cry, restlessness, and sleepiness

2. Be alert for fetal alcohol syndrome: difficulty establishing respirations; metabolic problems; irritability; increased muscle tone, tremulousness; lethargy; opisthotonus; poor sucking reflex; abdominal distention; seizure activity; and facial abnormalities.

3. Be alert for infant born to mother of cocaine abuse — does not appear to experience classic neonatal abstinence syndrome. Instead may exhibit mild tremulousness; increased irritability and startle response; muscular rigidity; difficult to console; pronounced state of lability; tachycardia and tachypnea; poor tolerance for oral feedings, diarrhea; and disturbed sleep pattern.

4. Collect urine for toxicology screen within 24 hours after birth. Obtain blood gases, blood glucose, and other lab-

oratory tests as indicated, including meconium stool sent for toxicology screen.

Nursing Diagnoses
51, 61, 75, 134, 136

Collaborative Management and Interventions

1. Administer opioid antagonist, such as naloxone (Narcan), for opioid-induced respiratory depression at birth.
2. Administer drugs for alleviation of opioid withdrawal symptoms. Duration of therapy using decreasing dosages may be from 4 to 40 days: paregoric (camphorated tincture of opium); phenobarbital; chlorpromazine; diazepam I.M.; methadone.
3. Provide nursing care to support infant and relieve symptoms.
   a. Irritability and restlessness, high-pitched crying: loosely swaddle; minimize handling; decrease environmental stimuli; organize care to allow for periods of uninterrupted sleep; prone positioning may help the infant organize movements; give medications with meals unless there is vomiting, then 30 minutes before.
   b. Floppy tremors — protect skin from irritation and abrasions: change position frequently; give good frequent skin care — keep the infant clean and dry.
   c. Frantic sucking — give pacifier between feedings; protect the infant's hands from excoriation.
   d. Poor feeding — give small, frequent feedings; maintain caloric and fluid intake requirement for the infant's desired weight.
   e. Vomiting or diarrhea — position the infant to prevent aspiration; provide good skin care to areas exposed to vomitus or stool.
   f. Muscle rigidity, hypertonicity: change position frequently to minimize development of pressure areas; use sheepskin and provide good skin care.
   g. Increased salivation and nasal stuffiness: aspirate nasopharynx; suction tracheal mucus; provide frequent

nose and mouth care; note respiration rate and characteristics and infant's color.

h. Tachypnea: note onset and severity of accompanying signs of respiratory distress; place the infant on respiratory monitor; position the infant for easier ventilation — semi Fowler's position; tilt head back slightly; minimize handling; have resuscitative equipment available.

i. Tachycardia and hypertension — monitor vital signs closely; cardiopulmonary monitor may be indicated.

4. Assist mother in learning to care for infant, efforts to promote bonding, and her own alcohol or drug rehabilitation efforts.

5. Obtain further information and resources from March of Dimes, *www.marchofdimes.com.*

NANDA International— Accepted Nursing Diagnoses

The numbered nursing diagnoses listed here correspond to the numbers listed under the *Nursing Diagnoses* headings in the text.

1.	Activity intolerance
2.	Acute confusion
3.	Acute pain
4.	Adult failure to thrive
5.	Anticipatory grieving
6.	Anxiety
7.	Autonomic dysreflexia
8.	Bathing or hygiene self-care deficit
9.	Bowel incontinence
10.	Caregiver role strain
11.	Chronic confusion
12.	Chronic low self-esteem
13.	Chronic pain
14.	Chronic sorrow
15.	Compromised family coping
16.	Constipation
17.	Death anxiety
18.	Decisional conflict (specify)
19.	Decreased cardiac output
20.	Decreased intracranial adaptive capacity
21.	Defensive coping
22.	Deficient diversional activity
23.	Deficient fluid volume
24.	Deficient knowledge (specify)
25.	Delayed growth and development
26.	Delayed surgical recovery
27.	Diarrhea

28.	Disabled family coping
29.	Disorganized infant behavior
30.	Disturbed body image
31.	Disturbed energy field
32.	Disturbed personal identity
33.	Disturbed sensory perception (specify: visual, auditory, kinesthetic, gustatory, tactile, olfactory)
34.	Disturbed sleep pattern
35.	Disturbed thought processes
36.	Dressing or grooming self-care deficit
37.	Dysfunctional family processes: Alcoholism
38.	Dysfunctional grieving
39.	Dysfunctional ventilatory weaning response
40.	Effective breast-feeding
41.	Effective therapeutic regimen management
42.	Excess fluid volume
43.	Fatigue
44.	Fear
45.	Feeding self-care deficit
46.	Functional urinary incontinence
47.	Health-seeking behaviors (specify)
48.	Hopelessness
49.	Hyperthermia
50.	Hypothermia
51.	Imbalanced nutrition: Less than body requirements
52.	Imbalanced nutrition: More than body requirements
53.	Impaired adjustment
54.	Impaired bed mobility
55.	Impaired dentition
56.	Impaired environmental interpretation syndrome
57.	Impaired gas exchange
58.	Impaired home maintenance
59.	Impaired memory
60.	Impaired oral mucous membrane
61.	Impaired parenting
62.	Impaired physical mobility
63.	Impaired skin integrity

64. Impaired social interaction
65. Impaired spontaneous ventilation
66. Impaired swallowing
67. Impaired tissue integrity
68. Impaired transfer ability
69. Impaired urinary elimination
70. Impaired verbal communication
71. Impaired walking
72. Impaired wheelchair mobility
73. Ineffective airway clearance
74. Ineffective breast-feeding
75. Ineffective breathing pattern
76. Ineffective community coping
77. Ineffective community therapeutic regimen management
78. Ineffective coping
79. Ineffective denial
80. Ineffective family therapeutic regimen management
81. Ineffective health maintenance
82. Ineffective infant feeding pattern
83. Ineffective protection
84. Ineffective role performance
85. Ineffective sexuality patterns
86. Ineffective therapeutic regimen management
87. Ineffective thermoregulation
88. Ineffective tissue perfusion (specify type: renal, cerebral, cardiopulmonary, gastrointestinal, peripheral)
89. Interrupted breast-feeding
90. Interrupted family processes
91. Latex allergy response
92. Nausea
93. Noncompliance (specify)
94. Parental role conflict
95. Perceived constipation
96. Posttrauma syndrome
97. Powerlessness
98. Rape-trauma syndrome
99. Rape-trauma syndrome: Compound reaction

100. Rape-trauma syndrome: Silent reaction
101. Readiness for enhanced communication
102. Readiness for enhanced community coping
103. Readiness for enhanced coping
104. Readiness for enhanced family coping
105. Readiness for enhanced family processes
106. Readiness for enhanced fluid balance
107. Readiness for enhanced knowledge (specify)
108. Readiness for enhanced management of therapeutic regimen
109. Readiness for enhanced nutrition
110. Readiness for enhanced organized infant behavior
111. Readiness for enhanced parenting
112. Readiness for enhanced self-concept
113. Readiness for enhanced sleep
114. Readiness for enhanced spiritual well-being
115. Readiness for enhanced urinary elimination
116. Reflex urinary incontinence
117. Relocation stress syndrome
118. Risk for activity intolerance
119. Risk for aspiration
120. Risk for autonomic dysreflexia
121. Risk for caregiver role strain
122. Risk for constipation
123. Risk for deficient fluid volume
124. Risk for delayed development
125. Risk for disorganized infant behavior
126. Risk for disproportionate growth
127. Risk for disuse syndrome
128. Risk for falls
129. Risk for imbalanced body temperature
130. Risk for imbalanced fluid volume
131. Risk for imbalanced nutrition: More than body requirements
132. Risk for impaired parent/infant/child attachment
133. Risk for impaired parenting
134. Risk for impaired skin integrity
135. Risk for infection
136. Risk for injury

137. Risk for latex allergy response
138. Risk for loneliness
139. Risk for other-directed violence
140. Risk for perioperative-positioning injury
141. Risk for peripheral neurovascular dysfunction
142. Risk for poisoning
143. Risk for posttrauma syndrome
144. Risk for powerlessness
145. Risk for relocation stress syndrome
146. Risk for self-directed violence
147. Risk for self-mutilation
148. Risk for situational low self-esteem
149. Risk for spiritual distress
150. Risk for sudden infant death syndrome
151. Risk for suffocation
152. Risk for suicide
153. Risk for trauma
154. Risk for urge urinary incontinence
155. Self-mutilation
156. Sexual dysfunction
157. Situational low self-esteem
158. Sleep deprivation
159. Social isolation
160. Spiritual distress
161. Stress urinary incontinence
162. Toileting self-care deficit
163. Total urinary incontinence
164. Unilateral neglect
165. Urge urinary incontinence
166. Urinary retention
167. Wandering

Newest NANDA-approved nursing diagnoses:

168. Impaired religiosity
169. Readiness for enhanced religiosity
170. Risk for dysfunctional grieving
171. Risk for impaired religiosity
172. Sedentary lifestyle

INDEX

i refers to an illustration; t refers to a table.

---

i refers to an illustration; t refers to a table.

i refers to an illustration; t refers to a table.

i refers to an illustration; t refers to a table.

i refers to an illustration; t refers to a table.

i refers to an illustration; t refers to a table.

i refers to an illustration; t refers to a table.

---

i refers to an illustration; t refers to a table.

i refers to an illustration; t refers to a table.

i refers to an illustration; t refers to a table.

i refers to an illustration; t refers to a table.

i refers to an illustration; t refers to a table.

i refers to an illustration; t refers to a table.

i refers to an illustration; t refers to a table.

---

i refers to an illustration; t refers to a table.

---

i refers to an illustration; t refers to a table.

---

i refers to an illustration; t refers to a table.

i refers to an illustration; t refers to a table.

i refers to an illustration; t refers to a table.

ers to an illustration; t refers to a table.